The Fenway Guide to Lesbian, Gay, Bisexual, and Transgender Health

D1231344

2nd edition

The Fenway Guide to Lesbian, Gay, Bisexual, and Transgender Health

2nd edition

Harvey J. Makadon, MD
Kenneth H. Mayer, MD
Jennifer Potter, MD
Hilary Goldhammer, MS

AMERICAN COLLEGE OF PHYSICIANS   PHILADELPHIA

Vice President, Publishing: Diane Scott-Lichter
Associate Publisher, Circulation, Licensing and Permissions: Aileen McHugh
Associate Publisher, New Product Development: Thomas McCabe
Books Associate: Charles Graver
Design: Michael Ripca
Composition: Aptara, Inc.

Printing/binding by Sheridan Books, Inc.
Printed in the United States of America

Library of Congress Cataloging-in-Publication Data

The Fenway guide to lesbian, gay, bisexual, and transgender health/[edited by]
Harvey J. Makadon, Kenneth H. Mayer, Jennifer Potter, Hilary Goldhammer. – 2nd edition.
    p. ; cm.
Includes bibliographical references and index.
ISBN 978-1-938921-00-1 (alk. paper)
    I. Makadon, Harvey J., editor. II. Mayer, Kenneth H., editor. III. Potter, Jennifer,
editor. IV. Goldhammer, Hilary, editor. V. American College of Physicians (2003-), issuing body.
    [DNLM: 1. Delivery of Health Care–United States. 2. Bisexuality–United States.
3. Transgender–United States.
4. Homosexuality–United States.   W 84 AA1]
    RA564.9.H65
    362.1086′6–dc23

                                                    2014024635

15 16 17 18 19 20 / 9 8 7 6 5 4 3 2 1

Contributors

Jonathan S. Appelbaum, MD, FACP, AAHIVS
Laurie L. Dozier Jr., MD, Education Director and Professor of Internal Medicine
Florida State University College of Medicine
Core Faculty
Florida State University–Tallahassee Memorial Healthcare Internal Medicine Residency Clinic
Tallahassee, FL

Stewart Adelson, MD
Assistant Clinical Professor, Divisions of Gender, Sexuality, and Health and Child and Adolescent Psychiatry
Columbia University College of Physicians & Surgeons
New York, NY

Kevin L. Ard, MD, MPH
Instructor of Medicine
Harvard Medical School
Assistant in Medicine
Division of Infectious Diseases
Massachusetts General Hospital
Boston, MA

Stefan Baral, MSc, MD, MPH, MBA, FRCPC, CCFP
Associate Professor, Department of Epidemiology
Director, Key Populations Program, Center for Public Health and Human Rights
Johns Hopkins Bloomberg School of Public Health
Baltimore, MD

Chris Beyrer, MD, MPH
Professor of Epidemiology, International Health, and Health, Behavior, and Society
Director, Center for Public Health and Human Rights
Johns Hopkins Bloomberg School of Public Health
Baltimore, MD

Bernadette V. Blanchfield, MA
Department of Psychology
University of Virginia
Charlottesville, VA

Melissa Boone Brown, PhD, MPhil
Postdoctoral Fellow
Pennsylvania State University
The Methodology Center/Prevention Research Center
State College, PA

Michael S. Boroughs, PhD, MA
Research and Clinical Fellow
Harvard Medical School
Massachusetts General Hospital
Boston, MA

Judith B. Bradford, PhD, MA
Director, Center for Population Research in LGBT Health
Co-Chair
The Fenway Institute, Fenway Health
Boston, MA

Sean Cahill, PhD
Director, Health Policy Research
The Fenway Institute, Fenway Health
Adjunct Assistant Professor, Public Administration
Robert Wagner School of Public Service, New York University
Boston, MA
New York, NY

Demetre C. Daskalakis, MD, MPH
Associate Professor of Medicine and
    Infectious Diseases
Icahn School of Medicine at Mount Sinai
New York, NY

John A. Davis, PhD, MD
Assistant Professor of Medicine
Associate Dean for Medical Education
Ohio State University College of
    Medicine
Columbus, OH

Madeline B. Deutsch, MD
Clinical Lead, Center of Excellence for
    Transgender Health
Assistant Clinical Professor
Department of Family & Community
    Medicine
University of California, San Francisco
San Francisco, CA

Manuel A. Eskildsen, MD, MPH, AGSF
Associate Chief of Geriatrics for
    Education
Director, Emory Geriatric Medicine
    Fellowship Program
Associate Professor of Medicine
Division of General Medicine and
    Geriatrics
Emory University School of Medicine
Atlanta, GA

Jamie Feldman, MD, PhD
Associate Professor, Program in Human
    Sexuality
Department of Family Medicine and
    Community Health
University of Minnesota
Minneapolis, MN

Robert Garofalo, MD, MPH
Professor of Pediatrics and Preventive
    Medicine
Feinberg School of Medicine,
    Northwestern University
Attending Physician, General Academic
    Pediatrics (Adolescent Medicine)
Medical Director, Adolescent HIV
    Services
Ann & Robert H. Lurie Children's
    Hospital of Chicago
Chicago, IL

Travis A. Gayles, MD, PhD
Instructor
Feinberg School of Medicine,
    Northwestern University
Fellow, General Academic Pediatrics and
    Adolescent Medicine
Ann & Robert H. Lurie Children's
    Hospital of Chicago
Chicago, IL

Marcy Gelman, RN, MSN, MPH
Director of Clinical Research
The Fenway Institute, Fenway Health
Boston, MA

Hilary Goldhammer, MS
Program Manager, National LGBT Health
    Education Center
The Fenway Institute, Fenway Health
Boston, MA

Joanne Greenfield, PhD
Licensed Psychologist, Private Clinical
    Practice
Cambridge and Lexington, MA

Luis Gutierrez-Mock, MPH, MA
TETAC Project Coordinator, Center of
    Excellence for Transgender Health
University of California, San Francisco
San Francisco, CA

Timothy M. Hall, MD, PhD, Dip ABPN, Dip ABAM
Clinical Instructor, Department of
Family Medicine
David Geffen School of Medicine,
University of California, Los Angeles
Los Angeles, CA

Kevin Kapila, MD
Medical Director of Behavioral Health
Fenway Health
Instructor in Medicine
Harvard Medical School
Boston, MA

Joanne G. Keatley, MSW
Director, Center of Excellence for
Transgender Health
University of California, San Francisco
San Francisco, CA

Scott Leibowitz, MD
Assistant Professor of Psychiatry and
Behavioral Sciences
Feinberg School of Medicine,
Northwestern University
Head Child and Adolescent Psychiatrist,
Gender and Sex Development
Program
Anne & Robert H. Lurie Children's
Hospital of Chicago
Chicago, IL

Kalvin Leveille, BS
Outreach Coordinator
Department of Sociomedical Sciences
Mailman School of Public Health,
Columbia University
New York, NY

Carmen Logie, MSW, PhD
Assistant Professor
Faculty of Social Work, University of
Toronto
Toronto, Ontario, Canada

Harvey J. Makadon, MD
Director, National LGBT Health
Education Center
The Fenway Institute, Fenway Health
Professor of Medicine
Harvard Medical School
Boston, MA

Gal Mayer, MD, MACP
Medical Director
Callen-Lorde Community Health Center
New York, NY

Kenneth H. Mayer, MD
Co-Chair and Medical Research Director
The Fenway Institute, Fenway Health
Professor of Medicine
Harvard Medical School
Infectious Disease Attending and
Director of HIV Prevention Research
Beth Israel Deaconess Medical Center
Professor in the Department of Global
Health and Population
Harvard School of Public Health
Boston, MA

Hilary Meyer, JD
Director, National Programs
SAGE
New York, NY

Matthew J. Mimiaga, ScD, MPH
Associate Professor of Psychiatry
Harvard Medical School
Associate Professor of Epidemiology
Harvard School of Public Health
Associate in Residence
Department of Psychiatry
Massachusetts General Hospital
Affiliated Senior Scientist
The Fenway Institute, Fenway Health
Boston, MA

Conall O'Cleirigh, PhD
Assistant Professor of Psychiatry
Harvard Medical School
Associate Director, Behavioral Medicine,
  Department of Psychiatry
Massachusetts General Hospital
Affiliated Scientist
The Fenway Institute, Fenway Health
Boston, MA

Jill Pace, MPH
Senior Program Coordinator
Department of Sociomedical Sciences
Mailman School of Public Health,
  Columbia University
New York, NY

Erin Papworth, MPH
Senior Technical Advisor, West and
  Central Africa
Key Populations Program, Center for
  Public Health and Human Rights
Department of Epidemiology, Johns
  Hopkins Bloomberg School of Public
  Health
Dakar, Senegal

Charlotte J. Patterson, PhD
Professor of Psychology, Department of
  Psychology
University of Virginia
Charlottesville, VA

Jennifer Potter, MD
Director, Women's Health Program
Fenway Health
Associate Professor
Harvard Medical School
Director, Women's Health Center
Beth Israel Deaconess Medical Center
Boston, MA

Anita Radix, MD, MPH, FACP
Director of Research and Education
Callen-Lorde Community Health Center
Clinical Assistant Professor of Medicine
New York University
New York, NY

Cathy J. Reback, PhD
Research Sociologist
David Geffen School of Medicine,
  Integrated Substance Abuse Programs
Semel Institute for Neuroscience and
  Human Behavior
University of California, Los Angeles
Senior Research Scientist
Friends Research Institute
Los Angeles, CA

Rachel G. Riskind, PhD
Assistant Professor of Psychology
Department of Psychology
Guilford College
Greensboro, NC

Steven A. Safren, PhD, ABPP
Professor in Psychology, Department of
  Psychiatry
Harvard Medical School
Director of Behavioral Medicine
Massachusetts General Hospital
Affiliated Scientist
The Fenway Institute, Fenway Health
Boston, MA

Jae M. Sevelius, PhD
Co-Principal Investigator, Center of
  Excellence for Transgender Health
Assistant Professor, Department of
  Medicine
University of California, San Francisco
San Francisco, CA

Steven Shoptaw, PhD
Professor and Vice Chair for Research
Director, Center for Behavioral and
  Addiction Medicine
Department of Family Medicine
David Geffen School of Medicine,
  University of California, Los Angeles
Los Angeles, CA

Mark J. Simone, MD
Instructor of Medicine
Harvard Medical School
Geriatrician and Associate Program
    Director-Primary Care, Mount
    Auburn Internal Medicine Residency
    Program
Mount Auburn Hospital
Boston and Cambridge, MA

Katherine Spencer, PhD
Assistant Professor
Coordinator, Transgender Health
    Services
University of Minnesota, Program in
    Human Sexuality
Department of Family Medicine and
    Community Health
Minneapolis, MN

Cynthia Telingator, MD
Assistant Professor of Psychiatry
Harvard Medical School
Senior Consultant
Cambridge Health Alliance
Boston and Cambridge, MA

Samantha Tornello, PhD
Assistant Professor of Psychology
Pennsylvania State University – Altoona
Altoona, PA

Aimee Van Wagenen, PhD
Director of Administration and
    Operations
The Fenway Institute, Fenway Health
Boston, MA

Hector L. Vargas Jr., JD
Executive Director
GLMA: Health Professionals Advancing
    LGBT Equality
Washington, DC

Jon Vincent, BA
Program Director, Prevention, Education
    and Screening
Fenway Health
Boston, MA

Patrick A. Wilson, PhD
Associate Professor, Department of
    Sociomedical Sciences
Mailman School of Public Health,
    Columbia University
New York, NY

Darrell P. Wheeler, PhD, MPH
Professor and Dean
Loyola University Chicago School of
    Social Work
Chicago, IL

Contents

Appendices

Visit www.lgbthealtheducation.org for
additional programs and materials on
LGBT health.

Preface

In recent years, lesbian, gay, bisexual, and transgender (LGBT) people have had a higher profile in public discourse across a wider range of issues than was true even a decade ago. The rationale for focusing on LGBT health as a distinct area of education for health professionals has long been discussed among a relatively small group of LGBT people and allies. However, publication of Healthy People 2020's goals for LGBT health and the Institute of Medicine's report on the "Health of Lesbian, Gay, Bisexual and Transgender People" has highlighted the existence of health disparities affecting LGBT communities and the need to urgently address these issues to ensure quality care and health equity for all. The recent implementation of the Affordable Care Act further underscores the importance of taking steps to facilitate affirmative and inclusive access to care for the many LGBT people who will be newly insured. This will mean ending LGBT invisibility in health care and training clinicians about the unique health needs of LGBT communities as well as about the diverse demographics of these communities in terms of race, ethnicity, and socioeconomic status. We will need to reassure the many people who have lacked access to or avoided care because of previous discriminatory experiences that clinicians are both interested and skilled in caring for LGBT people.

This second edition of the *Fenway Guide* is designed for health care providers, students, and trainees of all disciplines and specialties. Researchers, policymakers, and public health professionals will also find that many of the chapters are useful and relevant to their work. The book is meant to serve as a learning tool for individuals or as a teaching tool for use in a comprehensive LGBT health curriculum. However, each chapter is written so that it can stand alone and be incorporated into a variety of learning contexts. The sometimes differing terminology referencing LGBT people across chapters reflects a real-world diversity of language among people in the community. Ultimately, we seek to facilitate a dialogue with patients about their sexual orientation and gender identity, and offer LGBT patients high quality care in a welcoming and inclusive environment.

For this new edition, we did not include a chapter on Disorders in Sex Development (sometimes referred to as *intersex conditions*), believing this topic is unique and complex and deserves its own textbook. This new edition of the *Fenway Guide* builds on the first edition by including chapters that pay specific attention to emerging LGBT health issues, such as gender identity development in children and adolescents, global LGBT health and human rights, new standards for comprehensive care of transgender people, and advances in HIV/AIDS prevention, particularly for sexual and gender minorities who are at highest risk. This edition also embodies an enhanced appreciation of the social determinants of health as well as the intersectionality of diverse identities among LGBT people. We hope that this book will fill many gaps in health care education and facilitate the provision of equitable care for all.

Acknowledgments

We would like to thank the American College of Physicians for publishing a new edition of this ground-breaking text, and the individuals who have helped us along the way, including Adrianna Sicari, Jeffrey Walter, Scott Lundgren, Ida Bernstein, Ruben Hopwood, Raymond Powrie, Danya and Laura Potter, Joyce Collier, Marc Erickson, and the Shainker-Mayer family. We would also like to gratefully acknowledge Hilary Goldhammer for her work as both a coeditor and developmental editor.

In addition, we could not have done this without the support of the dedicated and inspiring team at The Fenway Institute and the whole Fenway Health family, who provide exceptional primary and behavioral healthcare and other clinical services, who work tirelessly to educate the community and advocate for change to enhance LGBT health care, and who are creating sustainable models of care for sexual and gender minorities and their families.

UNDERSTANDING LGBT POPULATIONS AND THEIR HEALTH CARE NEEDS

Chapter 1

Providing Optimal Health Care for LGBT People: Changing the Clinical Environment and Educating Professionals

HARVEY J. MAKADON, MD
HILARY GOLDHAMMER, MS
JOHN A. DAVIS, PhD, MD

Introduction

Perhaps no document has been more significant in focusing attention on health disparities affecting lesbian, gay, bisexual, and transgender (LGBT) people than the Institute of Medicine (IOM) report published in 2011, *The Health of Lesbian, Gay, Bisexual, and Transgender People: Building a Foundation for Better Understanding* (1). The report, which was written for the National Institutes of Health (NIH) to develop a research agenda for the future, begins with a clear statement that "lesbian, gay, bisexual, and transgender (LGBT) individuals experience unique health disparities." It goes on to explain that "although the acronym LGBT is used as an umbrella term, and the health needs of this community are often grouped together, each of these letters represents a distinct population with its own health concerns" (1).

In essence, the report establishes two critical points: 1) the evidence for LGBT health disparities and 2) the great diversity of the LGBT population. This report has become a keystone for advancing research, educational activities, and institutional change across many disciplines. Prior to this, other significant publications on LGBT health included the IOM's 1999 report *Lesbian Health: Current Assessment and Directions for the Future* (2); the LGBT companion document to Healthy People 2010 (3); the first edition of the *Fenway Guide to Lesbian, Gay, Bisexual, and Transgender Health* in 2008 (4); and the release of Healthy People 2020 (5), which for the first time set out strategies for overcoming health disparities specific to LGBT people.

Seen in this context, the publication of the 2011 IOM report represents the largest multidisciplinary effort of a national committee to date to summarize the evidence on LGBT health in order to learn more about the health needs of the LGBT community and what additional research is required for fully understanding those needs and addressing them. Over the years, teachers, clinicians, and students have looked to all of these documents as consolidated sources of information on a population that has been understudied and remains largely invisible to a health system despite the presence of disparities. It is our hope that with this new edition of the *Fenway Guide* we can provide clinicians and other LGBT health stakeholders with practical tools for addressing what has been learned about disparities thus far, and ultimately help bring an end to the invisibility of LGBT people in health care.

LGBT Terminology

As a start to ending LGBT invisibility, it is important to understand the terminology used to define sexual and gender minorities, keeping in mind that these terms are not static and can vary in different cultures. In general, *sexual orientation* describes a person's emotional and/or physical attraction to people of the same gender and/or a different gender. Most people identify themselves as *lesbian, gay, bisexual,* or *heterosexual,* but there are many other terms that people use to describe their sexual orientation. For example, a growing number of individuals, especially youth, identify with the term *queer,* which they see as more fluid and inclusive than the traditional sexual orientation categories.

Some individuals engage in sexual behaviors that do not fit with what is typically associated with their sexual identity. For example, studies have demonstrated that there are people who identify as heterosexual but who have intimate relations with members of the same gender (6–8); similarly, some people identify as gay or lesbian and have intimate relations with individuals of the opposite gender (9). Some individuals who engage in sexual activities with people from both genders identify as bisexual, but some do not (8,9). As later chapters in this book will demonstrate, it is important that we understand how people identify, how they behave, and what they desire so we can help them achieve healthy lives.

The *T* in LGBT stands for *transgender,* an umbrella term for people whose gender identity is not consistent with their assigned sex at birth. *Gender identity* refers to a person's internal sense of gender and is distinct from sexual orientation: All people have both a sexual orientation and a gender identity. Many gender minorities identify as transgender or use a related term, such as *transgender man* or *woman, trans man* or *woman,* or *MTF (male-to-female)* or *FTM (female-to-male).* Some transgender people just describe themselves as men or women. A transgender man would have been assigned the sex of a girl at birth, and a transgender woman would have been assigned the sex of a boy at birth. At some point in childhood, adolescence, or adulthood, transgender people recognize that their gender identity is different from their sex assigned at birth and will usually change their name, appearance, and other personal details in order to affirm their gender identity. Some reject the gender binary and prefer to use a term such as *genderqueer* to define their gender identity, and some may prefer no term. *Gender expression* differs from gender identity in that it refers to the spectrum of normative masculine or feminine characteristics, such as how people dress, how they cross their legs, and how they shake hands. The effect on health is not rooted in the individual's expression or identity but rather is based on the individual's and community's response to it. These concepts are explained in more detail in later chapters (see especially Chapters 16 and 17).

Understanding Disparities

LGBT people experience a higher prevalence of a range of medical and behavioral health issues. The research supporting the evidence on these issues is covered in detail in the 2011 IOM report mentioned earlier (1). Table 1-1 summarizes these disparities to the extent that they have been studied in any depth across the life course, from adolescence to late adulthood. As one can see from Table 1-1, these disparities include common clinical problems, such as smoking and obesity, which require appropriate inquiry but not always approaches that differ from those a clinician would use in the general population. These disparities also include more complex clinical issues, such as HIV infection, which may require clinicians to receive additional education and training, but can still be accomplished by a generalist in the primary care setting.

In summarizing a large body of knowledge, it is critical to recognize that LGBT health disparities largely track to a long history of societal

---

Table 1-1   Summary of LGBT Health Disparities

LGBT youth are more likely to attempt suicide and be homeless

LGBT populations have higher rates of tobacco, alcohol, and other drug use

LGBT populations have a higher prevalence of certain mental health issues

Transgender individuals have a high prevalence of attempted suicide and victimization

Gay, bisexual, and other men who have sex with men (MSM) are at higher risk for HIV and other sexually transmitted infections

Young MSM and transgender women, especially those who are black, are at especially high risk for HIV

Lesbians and bisexual women are more likely to be overweight or obese

Lesbians are less likely to get preventive services for cancer

Elderly LGBT individuals face additional barriers to optimal health because of isolation and a lack of culturally appropriate social services and providers

Data obtained from references 1 and 5.

stigma and discrimination directed at sexual and gender minorities (1). Herek has defined *sexual stigma* as that "attached to any non-heterosexual behavior, identity, relationship or community" (10). Lacking specific research, one might also talk about *transgender stigma* in a similar way (1). Stigma and discrimination can affect individuals directly (e.g., bias by health care professionals, violence fueled by hatred of LGBT people, and policies that deny health insurance coverage to same-sex partners) and indirectly, with discriminatory actions toward LGBT people around the world creating a negative environment for LGBT individuals wherever they may reside.

Despite growing cultural acceptance of LGBT people, a substantial portion of Americans still hold negative views of homosexuality. For example, a 2013 Pew Research Center study found that 33% of Americans believe society should not accept homosexuality (11). In a separate 2013 Pew Research study that surveyed a nationally representative sample of LGBT Americans, 53% of respondents said there is still a lot of discrimination against gays and lesbians, and an additional 39% said there is some discrimination. When asked if any of the following had ever happened to them as a result of being LGBT, 58% of respondents reported being subject to jokes or slurs, 26% reported being threatened or physically attacked, and 21% reported being treated unfairly by an employer (12).

Despite the existence of discrimination and disparities, it is important to keep in mind that a sizable majority of LGBT people live healthy, productive lives that are integrated into the activities and professions of general society. According to the 2013 Pew Research Center study of LGBT Americans, most respondents viewed their sexual orientation/gender identity as a positive aspect of their lives (34%) or as something that does not make much difference either way (58%) (12). An emerging theory suggests that LGBT people often become resilient in the face of marginalization and discrimination, but because of a lack of research, is it not yet possible to fully delineate predictors of resilience for specific LGBT populations (13–15).

Attitudes among Health Professionals

There is no question that the actions and inactions of health professionals have had a significant effect on the health of LGBT people. It was not until 1973 that the *Diagnostic and Statistical Manual of Mental Disorders* (DSM) removed homosexuality as a pathology (16), but even this did not mean that all health professionals immediately engaged in affirmative treatments for LGB people. Many health care professionals continued to offer reparative (or "conversion") therapies with the promise of "curing" homosexuality. Only starting in 2000 did the American Psychiatric Association officially oppose reparative therapy (17), and reparative therapies weren't banned by states across the country until 2013 (although some have brought lawsuits challenging these bans). It was also just in 2013 that the new fifth edition of the *DSM* (*DSM-5*) removed the diagnosis "gender identity disorder," which had the effect of pathologizing transgender people, and established the diagnosis "gender dysphoria" to describe those who experience clinically significant distress associated with feeling and seeing themselves as a gender that differs from the sex they were assigned at birth (18).

Studies show that physicians' attitudes toward LGBT people have changed markedly in recent years. For example, in a 1982 survey of physicians in San Diego, California, about 46% of respondents indicated that they would not refer a patient to an openly LGBT pediatrician, and 30% said they would not admit an openly LGBT person to medical school (19). When this survey was repeated in 1999, the percentages had decreased to 9% and 3%, respectively (20). Despite this positive shift in attitudes, there are still signs that full acceptance within the medical profession has not yet been achieved. A survey of medical students in 2005–2006 showed that 15% reported mistreatment of LGBT students at school and that 17% of LGBT students reported hostile working environments (21). The authors' experiences spending time with students at schools across the United States suggest this is a near-universal occurrence. Moreover, acceptance of transgender people in medical settings lags behind that of LGB people. In the 2011 National Transgender Discrimination Survey of more than 6400 transgender participants, 24% of respondents reported being denied equal treatment at a doctor's office or hospital (22).

Of note, some physicians still lack comfort and competency in caring for LGBT people. A 2002 Kaiser Family Foundation Survey reported that 6% of physicians nationally were uncomfortable treating gay or lesbian patients (23), and a 2003 survey of medical residents found that 71% did not ask sexually active adolescents about sexual orientation regularly; 93% of those reporting said this was because they were too uncomfortable to ask (24).

How Stigma and Discrimination Affect LGBT Health

And to the degree that the individual maintains a show before others that he himself does not believe, he can come to experience a special kind of alienation from self and a special kind of wariness of others.

—Erving Goffman, *The Presentation of Self in Everyday Life*, 1959 (25)

The stigmatized individual is asked to act so as to imply neither that his burden is heavy nor that bearing it has made him different from us; at the same time he must keep himself at that remove from us which assures our painlessly being able to confirm this belief about him. Put differently, he is advised to reciprocate naturally with an acceptance of himself and us, an acceptance of him that we have not quite extended to him in the first place. A PHANTOM ACCEPTANCE is thus allowed to provide the base for a PHANTOM NORMALCY."

—Erving Goffman, *Stigma: Notes on the Management of Spoiled Identity*, 1963 (26)

Erving Goffman's work on stigma dates back to the 1960s but is readily applicable to issues faced by LGBT people through the years up to the present time. Although many have developed resilience and remain unaffected, others live with a "phantom normalcy" or with strong feelings of "undesired differentness" (26). Many constructs have been applied to LGBT people to explain how stigma and discrimination affect them. Much of this work draws on the minority stress theory described by Meyer (27,28), who relates how stigmatized groups "experience excess stress and negative life events due to their minority status in addition to the general stressors experienced by all people" (28). Minority stress includes "internalized and external stress processes that can cause negative mental health outcomes" (1).

Stigma can act on multiple levels to create both personal and structural barriers to accessing care. These barriers may be reinforced for LGBT people who belong to more than one marginalized and stigmatized group related to their race, ethnicity, or socioeconomic status or who simply express themselves in ways that differ from accepted norms. This nexus, which results in accumulated stigma, leads to both medical and behavioral health disparities and reinforces barriers to care (29).

Social Determinants of LGBT Health

Social determinants of health refer to economic and social conditions that influence individual and group differences in health status. There are many constructs and many definitions, but taken together, social determinants tend to include social and economic resources, such as housing, education, employment, and health care, as well as government and institutional policies. Unequal access to these resources and policies across population groups contributes to disparities in morbidity and mortality (30,31). For LGBT people, social determinants of health are often linked to stigma and discrimination (5). For example, state legislation that denies marriage to same-sex couples can leave some families without adequate health insurance (32). Schools that do not include sexual orientation and gender identity/expression protections in their antibullying programs can leave LGBT youth vulnerable to verbal and physical harassment, which is associated with depression, suicidality, and risk for HIV and other sexually transmitted infections (33). Employment discrimination against transgender people can cause many to go without health care and can lead some to engage in the sex trade as a means of survival, putting them at risk for multiple health issues (34,35).

Unequal access to health care is of critical importance to all LGBT people, particularly those who are poor and/or living with HIV/AIDS. Even with the health care reforms under the Affordable Care Act, many who do not qualify for traditional Medicaid cannot access insurance in the states that have chosen not to expand their Medicaid programs; many of these same people will not be eligible for subsidies to purchase insurance in the health insurance marketplace (36). Beyond insurance issues, many LGBT people continue to lack access to providers who are knowledgeable about their unique health needs or who understand how to address them with cultural sensitivity (37). Although biases and lack of competency with LGBT people in health care have long been present, they are by no means inherent in our health care system.

Creating Affirmative and Inclusive Clinical Environments

While this book has been written to enhance clinical knowledge of LGBT health disparities and how to manage them in clinical settings, it is important to look at what needs to be done to create environments that will expand access to affirmative and inclusive care for LGBT people. This includes changes to the policies and practices of health care settings, as well as changes to how health professionals are trained.

Most of us can relate to the concept of how the environment of care can affect one's overall health care experience. It can begin well before a patient greets a clinician in the exam room. Imagine a gay man walking into a waiting room full of brochures that show images of heterosexual couples but none of same-sex couples. He then sits down to complete a registration form that has options only for single or married; he struggles to answer because he is in a long-term relationship in a state where he is legally unable to marry. How might this man feel about the environment of care at this office? It is unlikely that he feels included, affirmed, or even safe to disclose his sexual orientation to his provider. For transgender people, there are legions of embarrassing and hurtful stories reflecting lack of cultural competency in health care organizations. Common among these are being called by the wrong name and wrong pronoun in reception areas because of medical forms not matching current gender identity and preferred names.

The experience of many LGBT people as a population is that they are often invisible to the health care system in situations where knowledge of their identity may be critical to receiving appropriate preventive care or making appropriate diagnoses. For example, consider the case of a transgender woman who is hospitalized with pneumonia and develops a fever. The cause of the fever turns out to be acute prostatitis. Without knowing this patient was transgender and had a prostate, an appropriate diagnosis would be delayed at a minimum. These issues are discussed in more detail in other chapters but are highlighted here as they demonstrate the importance of an environment that is welcoming and encourages openness and frank discussion of sexual orientation and gender identity between patients and their providers.

In recent years, many resources have become available to help health care organizations consider ways to create more inclusive environments. There are also several incentives to do so, including provisions of the Affordable Care Act, which encourage management of the health of populations and looking at measurable change by tying goals to financial incentives. Perhaps the most exhaustive look at environmental change can be found in the Joint Commission's *Advancing Effective Communication, Cultural Competence, and Family- and Patient-Centered Care for the Lesbian, Gay, Bisexual and Transgender (LGBT) Community: A Field Guide* (38). The *Field Guide* is available online and highlights critical areas for organizational change, including chapters on leadership; provision of care; workforce; data collection and use; and patient, family, and community engagement. Also included are appendices with useful checklists for organizational assessment.

Two recommendations from the *Field Guide* specific to improving care environments for LGBT people have already been codified into Joint Commission requirements for hospital accreditation (39,40). These are RI.01.01.01: "The hospital respects, protects and promotes patient rights."

- EP 28: The hospital allows a family member, friend, or other individual to be present with the patient for emotional support during the course of the stay.
- EP 29: The hospital prohibits discrimination based on age, race, ethnicity, religion, culture, language, physical or mental disability, socioeconomic status, sex, sexual orientation, and gender identity or expression.

These 2 basic requirements can dramatically improve an LGBT person's experience of being in the hospital. First, allowing a patient to determine who can visit and who cannot, as opposed to using organizational rules that have historically limited visitation to members of immediate family, allows people with unmarried same-sex partners, or who rely primarily on friends because of intolerance from their biological families, to have the visitors that will support them the most. Second, requiring that nondiscrimination policies apply to sexual orientation and gender identity or expression gives LGBT people reassurance, as well as the basis for speaking up if they perceive that their care is not equitable. Beyond these critical requirements, organizations must take other steps toward achieving truly LGBT-inclusive and -affirming environments for care, as recommended by the Joint Commission and other organizations. Examples of these steps can be found in Appendix A; resources for improving the environment of care can be found in Appendix C.

Collecting Data on Sexual Orientation and Gender Identity

Both the *Field Guide* and the 2011 IOM report recommend that data on sexual orientation and gender identity be collected in electronic health records (EHRs) (1,38). However, the *Field Guide* goes further in explaining ways to accomplish this, and emphasizes the importance of allowing LGBT people to express their satisfaction with the care they receive (38). The central arguments for collecting data on sexual orientation and gender identity in EHRs are that 1) aggregated data will allow clinicians to recognize and respond to health disparities in their LGBT patient population and 2) asking these questions on forms is a sign to LGBT patients that the organization is interested in their health needs and that they will no longer be invisible to their providers. A 2013 study in 4 health centers that piloted sexual orientation and gender identity questions in registration forms found that patients both accepted and understood the questions (41). Data collection is not without controversy, however; there are important concerns that it not be implemented without expanded training of clinicians to provide culturally appropriate care (42). Nevertheless, change does not occur in a vacuum, and a case can be made that increased data collection will actually lead to greater educational efforts. Some of these concerns can also be alleviated by allowing patients to not answer these questions if they wish.

Data collection does not have to be the sole province of the primary clinician, nor should it always be delegated to a clerk. Perhaps the most efficient and confidential system for collecting these data is through electronic channels. Figure 1-1 is a schematic that highlights how data can be collected directly from patients electronically as part of the registration process, either in the privacy of their homes through a patient portal they can access on their computer or mobile device, or upon arrival at the site, ideally at a private kiosk with a computer or tablet. The primary clinician can then use this information for more nuanced discussion and clarification. If the patient does not complete a form with these questions, then the provider can be the one to ask and enter the information into the EHR. The fact that it will be available for other clinicians appropriately engaged in an individual's care will eliminate the need to repeat this discussion again and again. While some raise concerns about privacy and confidentiality with electronic data, these issues are in general more effectively managed than with use of traditional paper charts, where it is very difficult to track who looks at information concerning an individual patient.

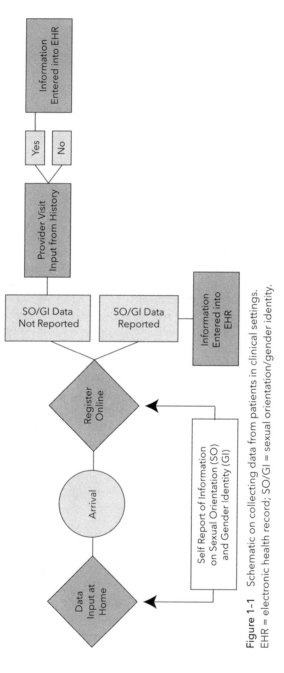

Figure 1-1   Schematic on collecting data from patients in clinical settings. EHR = electronic health record; SO/GI = sexual orientation/gender identity.

Regarding how to frame questions, different examples of questions on sexual orientation and gender identity have been developed. Appendix B provides an example of questions to use. More information can be found on the website of the Center of Excellence for Transgender Health at the University of California San Francisco (www.transhealth.ucsf.edu) and in the issue brief "Asking Patients About Sexual Orientation and Gender Identity in Clinical Settings: A Study in Four Health Centers" (41). These questions are discussed again in other chapters (see Chapters 8 and 17) but are presented here because they represent a critical first step in providing optimal care to LGBT people. Not only does this information help end LGBT invisibility in health care, but it can lead to provision of quality care responsive to their unique needs and experiences.

Standards-Based and Functional Assessments

Beyond the Joint Commission's *Field Guide*, other organizations have designed programs to help assess the degree to which a health care organization adopts leading practices designed to create an LGBT-inclusive environment. The Human Rights Campaign, a large LGBT civil rights organization based in Washington, DC, developed a resource tool for both health care and non-health care organizations to assess how well their policies and programs meet certain requirements for both quality care and a quality workplace for LGBT people. The Corporate Equality Index (CEI) was designed for non-health care organizations, and the Healthcare Equality Index (HEI) was developed for health care organizations. Through a survey process, the HEI identifies leading organizations that comply with criteria set out by the Human Rights Campaign and a group of advisors. Between 2012 and 2013, the number of organizations that completed the HEI increased from 122 to 309. The 309 respondents represented 718 health care facilities, as many of the respondents own more than one facility (43). Facilities that achieve HEI leadership status must demonstrate that they have achieved four core metrics, two of which are now Joint Commission requirements. The four metrics are as follows:

Patient Nondiscrimination Policies

- Patient nondiscrimination policy (or patients' bill of rights) includes the term *sexual orientation.*
- Patient nondiscrimination policy (or patients' bill of rights) includes the term *gender identity.*
- Patient nondiscrimination policy is communicated to patients in at least two readily accessible ways.

Equal Visitation Policies

- Visitation policy explicitly grants equal visitation to LGBT patients and their visitors.
- Equal visitation policy is communicated to patients and visitors in at least two readily accessible ways.

Employment Nondiscrimination Policies

- Employment nondiscrimination policy (or equal employment opportunity policy) includes the term *sexual orientation*.
- Employment nondiscrimination policy (or equal employment opportunity policy) includes the term *gender identity*.

Training in LGBT Patient-Centered Care

- To meet this criterion, facilities participating in the HEI for the first time in 2013 were required to document that they had enrolled at least one staff member in each of five designated work areas for at least 90 minutes of training.

In addition to the questions directed toward achieving leadership status, in 2013 the HEI asked 31 questions based on an "additional best practices checklist" (43).

The HEI has driven hospitals and health centers across the country to demonstrate their concern and make greater efforts to improve LGBT health equity at their institutions. The approach is broadly structural and therefore not tailored to specific organizational needs. On a smaller scale, other groups have focused on gaining a more functional understanding of how organizations approach issues of LGBT health equity in order to address specific needs identified through a participatory process. For example, the National LGBT Health Education Center has developed an online assessment for health care organizations that involves a survey for members of senior management and a survey for all staff (both clinical and nonclinical). Quantitative and qualitative responses are invited. The surveys are the first of a three-part process that involves administering the survey, analyzing the data and reporting back, and providing training and consultation that is tailored to an organization's identified challenges and needs. The results of the surveys might show, for example, that even though an organization has a nondiscrimination policy that includes sexual orientation and gender identity/expression, only 25% of the staff is actually aware of this policy. This suggests that compliance with a standard does not always translate to real-world practice and full achievement of health equity. Educating staff about the policies and helping staff develop protocols for reporting and resolving policy breaches could then become part of the suggested training program for that organization.

Achieving Life-Long Learning: Health Professional Education and LGBT Health Care

LGBT Issues in Health Care Education

Education is at the heart of the health care profession. As we know, when taught well, health care education affects the knowledge, attitudes, and skills of learners. Education, therefore, represents an opportunity to not only help the learner develop LGBT-care competence but also to help improve the care received by that learner's future patients, and, perhaps on a grander scale, to improve overall social equity for LGBT people.

Traditionally, medical, nursing, and other health professional school curricula have contained very little LGBT-specific content, in part at least because of pervasive homophobic attitudes among educators, the health care professions as a whole, and the population at large (as discussed earlier in this chapter). However, as cultural attitudes are shifting to regard LGBT people in the United States more positively, so have attitudes in health care and health care education. In addition to the national programs mentioned earlier that focus on improving LGBT health care, such as the HEI, the National LGBT Health Education Center, and the Joint Commission *Field Guide*, there has been an increased interest in adding LGBT-specific content to health professions curricula. Demonstrating this need is a recent study of medical school curricula reporting that more than 33% of medical schools reported 0 hours of LGBT-specific content delivered in the clinical years, and 6.8% of medical schools reported 0 hours of LGBT-specific content in the preclinical years (44). While the same study found that medical schools that responded had a median of 5 hours of LGBT-specific content in the course of the standard, 4-year curriculum, it is important to note that time devoted to subject-specific education does not necessarily equate to quality of education, nor does it necessarily lead to desirable learning outcomes (knowledge, skills, behaviors, attitudes).

Speaking more to such learning outcomes, another survey demonstrated that 10.5% of graduating U.S. medical school seniors did not agree with the statement that they could "provide safe sex counseling to a patient whose sexual orientation differs from mine," while only 4.5% of students did not agree with the statement that they could "care for patients from different backgrounds." The same survey places this in the broader context of relatively greater student dissatisfaction with education on topics of human sexuality (21.6% found content coverage inadequate) when compared to topics of culturally appropriate care (11.4% found content coverage inadequate) (45).

An increasing amount of curricular material is intended to help learners develop competency in LGBT care, and increasing numbers of resources are devoted to advancing LGBT health care (see Appendix C). Individual providers may find themselves with the opportunity to advance the LGBT-related knowledge/skills/attitudes of a learner or group of learners. With this in mind, the remainder of this chapter is devoted to the approaches a teacher in different educational settings can take to incorporate LGBT health into established curricula.

Learners in the Classroom Setting

In the classroom or other lecture-based setting, a large amount of teaching and learning deals with foundational science. Here, there are occasionally opportunities for dedicated time for LGBT-related content, particularly an introduction to definitions and concepts related to sexual orientation and gender identity. For those helping to design curricula with time allocated to LGBT-specific content, resources such as chapters of textbooks, or existing presentations (e.g., those available from the National LGBT Health Education Center website: www.lgbthealtheducation.org) are available to help as starting or focal points. However, it should be noted that culturally competent LGBT health care could be taught by introducing key principles in the context of other content. For instance, as a part of a cardiac pathophysiology activity, modifying a case meant to illustrate principles of congestive heart failure by using a patient who presents for care with her same-sex partner allows for exploration of the social determinants of health as they apply to LGBT populations. Likewise, other concepts can be introduced in the context of cases used throughout the preclinical curricula in most medical schools. The primary challenge in taking the latter approach is that it requires added diligence to ensure all key concepts are covered, and usually requires close work with faculty who are primarily responsible for other content areas to determine where concepts might be introduced.

Learners in the Clinical Setting

On occasion, teaching in the clinical setting may take the form of a didactic lecture or activity that is more similar in delivery to content encountered in the preclinical setting. In those instances, the suggestions offered in the preceding section apply. However, in contrast to the situation in the classroom setting, most teaching in the clinical setting centers on active participation by the learner in patient care, whether in a hospital or ambulatory site. The challenge in this setting is that it can be difficult to program in or engineer certain encounters. However, the benefit is that the setting is ideal for direct observation of skills that demonstrate competence in LGBT care. In the early stages, a learner may observe the instructor demonstrate these skills, such as taking a history that is inclusive of LGBT people; performing a physical examination in an appropriately sensitive and respectful way; or discussing care related to sex, sexual orientation, or gender identity. The clinical setting permits the instructor to then observe the more advanced learner put these skills into practice. It is not necessary for a patient to be LGBT in order for this demonstration of skills to happen; all patients can benefit from LGBT-competent care.

From a broader, curriculum-design standpoint, it is often desirable to measure or demonstrate mastery of LGBT-care skills. In these instances, incorporation of LGBT-related cases into the Objective Structured Clinical Exam setting permits demonstration of these skills along with many others. Examples of such cases are described, and some are available on the Association of American Medical Colleges' MedEdPortal (mededportal.org). The Objective Structured Clinical Exam and direct observation of competence together serve as complementary means of demonstration of skills mastery, and many educators prefer the combination as a means of competency assessment.

Learning in Graduate Professional Education

As learners advance, the service component of patient care can predominate, and learning often takes one of two forms: didactics offered by a graduate professional education program or self-directed (life-long) learning. From the didactic standpoint, while graduate learners may need some refinement of principles learned in the undergraduate professional education setting, most often reinforcement of principles is needed most; thus, lectures given in this setting will be quite similar to those given in the previous settings (see "Learners in the Classroom Setting" earlier in this section). Unfortunately, the demands placed on education program directors are many, and the time available for such didactics is little, so dedicated time for LGBT-specific (reinforcement of) education is rare. It is clear that attitudes of learners with respect to self-directed (life-long) learning are driven by the role modeling of teachers and mentors. Thus, it is helpful for those who are teaching in the clinical setting at the graduate professional level to point out instances when issues or topics relevant to the care of LGBT persons or populations are identified. Resources, such as this book, can provide some of the evidence base for what defines good clinical care and best practices for LGBT persons, and samples from that evidence base can serve as excellent launching points for discussion, reflection, and/or self-directed (life-long) learning.

Life-Long Learning and Continuing Professional Education

As part of a profession, and in keeping with the fundamental importance of practice-based and life-long learning as espoused by many professional societies (e.g., the American Medical Association, the American Nurses Association, the American Pharmacists Association), providers are expected to continually update knowledge, skill, and behavior domains of their practice. It is possible that some reading this book for the first time will be doing so in pursuit of that goal. Others, and even those just mentioned (after reading this book), may be in a position to offer education to their peers. Continuing professional education may take many forms, including didactics such as grand rounds (usually at medical centers), webinars or asynchronous learning (often offered by medical centers or societies), and conferences. For those looking to further their knowledge of LGBT care-related issues, it is important to take advantage of the many venues currently available for the delivery of such content, including journals and conferences (see Appendix C). Likewise, it is important to realize that the full potential of LGBT-related research is not achieved without appropriate dissemination and incorporation into practice, and thus it is critical that LGBT care-related research and issues be discussed in non–LGBT-specific journals/conferences. We must all continue to be producers and dissemi-nators of peer education content and provide these resources for those who identify, and would like to address, gaps in practice, skills, or knowledge.

Summary Points

- Lesbian, gay, bisexual, and transgender (LGBT) is an umbrella term for all sexual and gender minorities; however, LGBT people are very diverse, and many use different terminology to describe themselves.
- There has been growing awareness of LGBT health needs, culminating in the 2011 Institute of Medicine report on LGBT health disparities. This report has become a keystone for advancing LGBT health research, edu-cational activities, and institutional change across many disciplines.
- A long history of anti-LGBT stigma and discrimination has created both individual and structural barriers to accessing health care and achieving optimal health outcomes.
- Cultural attitudes are shifting more positively toward LGBT people in the United States, including attitudes in health care and health care education; nonetheless, many clinicians continue to experience dis-comfort, lack of knowledge, and/or lack of experience and training in caring for LGBT people.
- Establishing inclusive and welcoming health care environments for LGBT people can help eliminate disparities by 1) increasing access to and retention in care and 2) encouraging patients to be open about their sexual orientation and gender identity, thus enabling providers to offer more appropriate, targeted, and sensitive care.
- Examples of ways to create inclusive environments include nondis-crimination policies for LGBT patients and staff; hospital equal-visitation policies; training in LGBT patient-centered care for all staff members; health promotion and marketing materials that contain

LGBT visuals, such as images of same-sex couples and gender-noncon-forming people; engaging with LGBT community groups; and using inclusive language on registration and medical history forms.

- Collecting data on sexual orientation and gender identity in electronic health records allows clinicians to recognize and respond to health disparities in their LGBT patient population and signals to patients that the organization understands the importance of sexual and gender identity in providing optimal care.
- Organizations such as the Human Rights Commission and the National LGBT Health Education Center offer assessments and training for health care organizations interested in improving the quality of care for LGBT patients.
- A growing number of curricular materials and other resources can be used in educational settings to help learners develop competency in LGBT care.
- This material can be used for dedicated classroom time or can be incorporated into cases in the context of other topics. There are also opportunities for learning in the clinical setting through direct observation and practice.
- Learning about LGBT health care can be a life-long process; it is important to take advantage of the many venues currently offering continuing education on such content, including journals, webinars, grand rounds, and conferences.
- Despite the existence of discrimination and disparities, the sizable majority of LGBT people live healthy, productive lives.

References

1. **Institute of Medicine.** The Health of Lesbian, Gay, Bisexual, and Transgender People: Building a Foundation for Better Understanding. Washington, DC: National Academies Press; 2011.
2. **Institute of Medicine.** Lesbian Health: Current Assessment and Directions for the Future. Washington, DC: The National Academies Press; 1999.
3. **Gay and Lesbian Medical Association.** Healthy People 2010: A companion document for lesbian, gay, bisexual, and transgender (LGBT) health. April 2001. Available at www.glma.org/_data/n_0001/resources/live/HealthyCompanionDoc3.pdf.
4. **Makadon H, Mayer K, Potter J, Goldhammer H, eds.** The Fenway Guide to Lesbian, Gay, Bisexual, and Transgender Health. Philadelphia: American College of Physicians; 2008.
5. **U.S. Department of Health and Human Services, Office of Disease Prevention and Health Promotion.** Healthy People 2020. Lesbian, gay, bisexual, and transgender health. 2014. Available at: www.healthypeople.gov/2020/topicsobjectives2020/overview.aspx?topicid=25.
6. **Xu F, Sternberg MR, Markowitz LE.** Men who have sex with men in the United States: demographic and behavioral characteristics and prevalence of HIV and HSV-2 infection: results from National Health and Nutrition Examination Survey 2001-2006. Sex Transm Dis. 2010;37:399-405.
7. **Xu F, Sternberg MR, Markowitz LE.** Women who have sex with women in the United States: prevalence, sexual behavior and prevalence of herpes simplex virus type 2 infection—results

from National Health and Nutrition Examination Survey 2001-2006. Sex Transm Dis. 2010;37:407-13.

8. **Pathela P, Hajat A, Schillinger J, Blank S, Sell R, Mostashari F.** Discordance between sexual behavior and self-reported sexual identity: a population-based survey of New York City men. Ann Intern Med. 2006;145:416-25.

9. **Bailey JV, Farquhar C, Owen C, Whittaker D.** Sexual behaviour of lesbians and bisexual women. Sex Transm Infect. 2003;79:147-50.

10. **Herek GM.** Hate crimes and stigma-related experiences among sexual minority adults in the United States. Prevalence estimates from a national probability sample. J Interpersonal Violence. 2009;24:54-75.

11. **Pew Research Center.** Global divide on homosexuality: greater acceptance in more secular and affluent countries. June 4, 2013. Available at: www.pewglobal.org/2013/06/04/the-global-divide-on-homosexuality/.

12. **Pew Research Center.** A survey of LGBT Americans: attitudes, experiences and values in changing times. June 13, 2013. Available at: www.pewsocialtrends.org/2013/06/13/a-survey-of-lgbt-americans/3/.

13. **Herrick AL, Lim SH, Wei C, et al.** Resilience as an untapped resource in behavioral intervention design for gay men. AIDS Behav. 2011;15 Suppl 1:S25-9.

14. **Herrick AL, Stall R, Chmiel JS, et al.** It gets better: resolution of internalized homophobia over time and associations with positive health outcomes among MSM. AIDS Behav. 2013;17:1423-30.

15. **Herrick AL, Stall R, Goldhammer H, Egan JE, Mayer KH.** Resilience as a research framework and as a cornerstone of prevention research for gay and bisexual men: theory and evidence. AIDS Behav. 2014;18:1-9.

16. **American Psychiatric Association.** Homosexuality and sexual orientation disturbance. In: Diagnostic and Statistical Manual of Mental Disorders, 2nd ed. Arlington, VA: American Psychiatric Publishing; 1973:44.

17. **American Psychiatric Association.** Commission on Psychotherapy by Psychiatrists. Position statement on therapies focused on attempts to change sexual orientation (reparative or conversion therapies). Am J Psychiatry. 2000;157:1719-21.

18. **American Psychiatric Association.** Diagnostic and Statistical Manual of Mental Disorders. 5th ed. Arlington,VA: American Psychiatric Publishing; 2013.

19. **Mathews WC, Booth MW, Turner JD, Kessler L.** Physicians' attitudes toward homosexuality—survey of a California county medical society. West J Med. 1986;144:106-10.

20. **Smith DM, Mathews WC.** Physicians' attitudes toward homosexuality and HIV: survey of a California Medical Society-revisited (PATHH-II). J Homosex. 2007;52:1-9.

21. **Harris S.** Gay discrimination still exists in medical schools. AAMC Reporter. July 2007.

22. **Grant JM, Mottet LA, Tanis J, et al.** Injustice at every turn: a report of The National Transgender Discrimination Survey. National Center for Transgender Equality and National Gay and Lesbian Task Force. 2011. Available at: www.thetaskforce.org/reports_and_research/ntds.

23. **Kaiser Family Foundation.** National Survey of Physicians Part I: Doctors on disparities in medical care. Washington, DC: The Kaiser Family Foundation; 2002.

24. **Kitts RL.** Barriers to optimal care between physicians and lesbian, gay, bisexual, transgender, and questioning adolescent patients. J Homosexual. 2010;57:730-47.

25. **Goffman E.** The Presentation of Self in Everyday Life. Anchor Books; 1959.

26. **Goffman E.** Stigma: Notes on the Management of Spoiled Identity. New York: Simon and Schuster; 1963.

27. **Meyer IH.** Minority stress and mental health in gay men. J Health Soc Behav. 1995;36:38-56.

28. **Meyer IH.** Prejudice, social stress, and mental health in lesbian, gay, and bisexual populations: conceptual issues and research evidence. Psychol Bull. 2003;129:674-97.

29. **Krehely J.** How to close the LGBT health disparities gap: disparities by race and ethnicity. Center for American Progress. December 2009. Available at: www.americanprogress.org/press/release/2009/12/21/14895/how-to-close-the-lgbt-health-disparities-gap.

30. **Brennan Ramirez LK, Baker EA, Metzler M.** Promoting health equity: a resource to help communities address social determinants of health. U.S. Department of Health and Human Services, Centers for Disease Control and Prevention. 2008. Available at: www.cdc.gov/nccdphp/dch/programs/healthycommunitiesprogram/tools/pdf/SDOH-workbook.pdf.

31. **Commission on Social Determinants of Health.** Closing the gap in a generation: health equity through action on the social determinants of health. Final report of the Commission on Social Determinants of Health. World Health Organization. 2008. Available at http://whqlibdoc.who.int/publications/2008/9789241563703_eng.pdf.

32. **Badgett MVL.** The economic value of marriage for same-sex couples. Drake Law Review. 2010;58:1081-16.

33. **Russell ST, Ryan C, Toomey RB, Diaz RM, Sanchez J.** Lesbian, gay, bisexual, and transgender adolescent school victimization: implications for young adult health and adjustment. J Sch Health. 2011;81:223-30.

34. **Herman JL.** The cost of employment and housing discrimination against transgender residents of New York. The Williams Institute. April 2013. Available at: http://williamsinstitute.law.ucla.edu/research/transgender-issues/ny-cost-of-discrimination-april-2013/.

35. **Hoffman B.** An overview of depression among transgender women. Depression Res Treat. 2014:394283.

36. **Ranji U, Beamesderfer A, Kates J, Salganicoff A.** Health and access to care and coverage for lesbian, gay, bisexual, and transgender individuals in the U.S. The Kaiser Family Foundation. January 2014. Available at: http://kff.org/disparities-policy/issue-brief/health-and-access-to-care-and-coverage-for-lesbian-gay-bisexual-and-transgender-individuals-in-the-u-s.

37. **Lambda Legal.** When health care isn't caring: Lambda Legal's survey of discrimination against LGBT people and people with HIV. 2010. Available at: www.lambdalegal.org/health-care-report.

38. **The Joint Commission.** Advancing Effective Communication, Cultural Competence, and Family- and Patient-Centered Care for the Lesbian, Gay, Bisexual and Transgender (LGBT) Community: A Field Guide. Oak Brook, IL: The Joint Commission; October 2011.

39. **The Joint Commission.** Comprehensive Accreditation Manual for Hospitals, Update 1. January 2011.

40. **The Joint Commission.** Comprehensive Accreditation Manual for Critical Access Hospitals, Update 1. January 2011.

41. **Cahill S, Singal R, Grasso C, et al.** Asking patients about sexual orientation and gender identity in clinical settings: a study in four health centers. The Fenway Institute and the Center for American Progress. 2014. Available at: www.lgbthealtheducation.org/wp-content/uploads/COM228_SOGI_CHARN_WhitePaper.pdf.

42. **Institute of Medicine.** Collecting sexual orientation and gender identity data in electronic health records: workshop summary. Washington, DC: The National Academies Press; 2013.

43. **Human Rights Campaign.** Healthcare Equality Index. Available at: www.hrc.org/hei.

44. **Obedin-Maliver J, Goldsmith ES, et al.** Lesbian, gay, bisexual, and transgender-related content in undergraduate medical education. JAMA. 2011;306:971-7.

45. **American Association of Medial Colleges.** Medical Student Graduation Questionnaire. 2013 All Schools Summary Report. July 2013. Available at: https://www.aamc.org/download/350998/data/2013gqallschoolssummaryreport.pdf.

Chapter 2

What We Know and Don't Know About LGBT Demographics: Informing Clinical Practice

JUDITH B. BRADFORD, PhD, MA
KENNETH H. MAYER, MD

Introduction

Demography is the statistical study of human populations. Populations tend to be dynamic because of changes in fertility practices, migration, aging and death and may be significantly affected by geopolitical, social, and cultural changes; wars and famines; and societal evolution (e.g., contraception providing women with more autonomy in family planning). Understanding the demographic features of specific population groups enables governments and other administrative bodies to develop programs addressing the health care needs of population members. Lacking this information, appropriate services and associated resources cannot be successfully developed and implemented. The greatest challenge to accurately understanding specific health care needs of lesbian, gay, bisexual, and transgender (LGBT) patients has been the lack of sufficient demographic data about the many subgroups within this population. However, in recent years, the inclusion of sexual orientation and gender identity measures in a small, but growing, number of federally funded and state-level surveys has led to an increase in information about the characteristics and specific social and health-related needs of LGBT people and communities.

In this chapter, we describe the demographic characteristics of LGBT people across the United States so that clinicians and others involved in the health care of LGBT people can increase their understanding of this population as a whole. While other chapters in this book focus on health disparities and how to address them, this chapter will focus on the enumeration and geographic distribution of LGBT people, as well as look at racial/ethnic, socioeconomic, and other demographic characteristics. By offering this information, we hope to help diminish the "invisibility" of LGBT people in health care by highlighting these key points: 1) Millions of Americans identify as LGBT; 2) LGBT individuals and families live in all parts of the country; and

3) LGBT people are diverse in terms of race/ethnicity, socioeconomic status, and family structure. In addition, this chapter illuminates the current limitations of demographic data on LGBT people and argues for why the health and well-being of LGBT communities will benefit from some of the new efforts to include sexual orientation and gender identity measures on national government and privately funded surveys. Finally, we end the chapter with a discussion on how different conceptual frameworks on populations can inform clinical practice so that it is possible to provide enhanced care to LGBT patients.

The U.S. Census and the Enumeration of Same-Sex Households

The U.S. population is periodically counted in a variety of ways, but the official enumeration is conducted by the decennial U.S. census (1). Although the census forms do not ask about sexual orientation, male and female same-sex partners who live in the same household have been identifiable in the U.S. census since 1990. Gays and lesbians first became a subpopulation recognized by academics and government officials when social scientists published census data about same-sex partnered households from the 1990 Census (2).

Information about the distribution and characteristics of same-sex households was of tremendous value to organizations concerned about LGBT health across the country. Scientists, advocates, and providers formed the National Coalition for LGBT Health to raise awareness about the lack of LGBT inclusion in national health planning and service provision. Analysis of 2000 Census data by research and policy leaders led to the production and distribution of a "User's Guide" that Coalition members could take to congressional staff, containing specific numbers and locations of same-sex households throughout the country, for each state and each county (3). The robust discussions that took place with this information, made available in an easily accessible format, has facilitated enhanced collection of data regarding sexual and gender minority populations in other key demographic surveys in the United States and other countries.

In preparation for the 2010 Census, LGBT advocates and scientists worked with the Census Bureau to improve measurement of same-sex partnered households, contributing to more precise representation than in previous decades. When the count was completed and estimates adjusted for coding errors, it was concluded that there were approximately 646,450 same-sex couple households in the United States, representing an 80% increase from the 2000 census. In comparison, U.S. households overall increased by only 11% (4).

The 2010 census also identified same-sex couple households in 93% of all U.S. counties (5); however, their distribution varied substantially among geographic areas of the country. The preponderance of same-sex households was found along the coasts and in western and southern areas of the

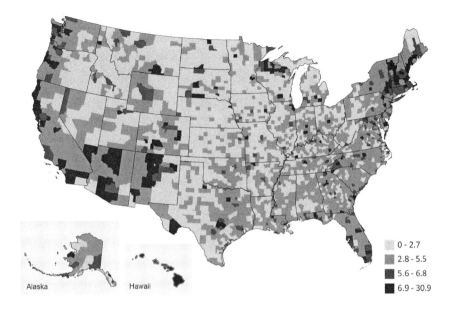

Figure 2-1 Same-sex couples per 1000 households by county (adjusted).

Figure used with permission from Gates GJ, Cooke AM. United States Census Snapshot: 2010. The Williams Institute, UCLA School of Law. September 2011. Available at http://williamsinstitute.law.ucla.edu/wp-content/uploads/Census2010Snapshot-US-v2.pdf?r.

country (Figure 2-1). Among the 10 jurisdictions with the highest density of same-sex households were the District of Columbia (18.08 per 1000 overall households) and the states of Vermont, Massachusetts, Maine, and Delaware on the East Coast; California, Oregon, and Hawaii in the West; and New Mexico in the Southwest (Table 2-1). The density of same-sex households in midsized cities, such as Fort Lauderdale, Florida, and Berkeley, California, approximated that in large cities, while the highest densities were reported in small cities and in primarily coastal communities (Table 2-2) (5).

Demographic Characteristics of Same-Sex Households

The ability to locate same-sex couple households within the census data has made it possible for researchers to explore the diversity within these households. More specific information about same-sex households and the nature of the householder/partner relationship has been derived by improved measurement techniques. Overall, the racial/ethnic makeup of 2010 householders did not differ substantially between same-sex and different-sex couples: Twenty-eight percent of householders in same-sex couples were nonwhite compared with 24% in different-sex married couples.

Table 2-1   Top 10 U.S. States/Jurisdictions Ranked by Number of Same-Sex Couples per
1000 Households

State	Same-Sex Couples per 1000 Households
District of Columbia	18.08
Vermont	8.36
Massachusetts	7.95
California	7.80
Oregon	7.75
Delaware	7.73
New Mexico	7.36
Washington	7.25
Hawaii	7.11
Maine	7.10

Data obtained from reference 5.

However, same-sex householders were more likely to be interracial or interethnic (20.6%) than were different-sex married couples (18.3%) and different-sex unmarried couples (9.5%) (4). Differences varied by geography: In Hawaii, more than half of same-sex couples were interracial or interethnic (53%); the percentages were 33% in California, 31% in New Mexico, and 30% in Nevada (4).

Seventeen percent of 2010 Census same-sex households reported raising their "own child" (defined as a biological child, adopted child, or stepchild younger than age 18 years) (5). Of these households, 73% reported having biological children only, 21% reported having adopted children or stepchildren only, and 6% reported a combination (6). Same-sex couples that included at least one person who was a racial or ethnic minority were more likely to be raising a child than same-sex couples in which both people in the couple were white (7).

An analysis of 2000 Census data showed that women in same-sex couples were 4 times more likely to be veterans than women in different-sex couples (about 13% of same-sex female couples include a veteran, compared with 3% of women in different-sex couples) (8).

In addition to the decennial census, the U.S. Census Bureau conducts the ongoing American Community Survey (ACS), which collects annual information about education, housing, jobs, and other characteristics of daily life in order to help determine the social and economic needs of communities throughout the country (9). The ACS randomly selects households from the U.S. Census survey; as such, it also provides valuable information on same-sex couples, helping us to understand variations in their characteristics and changes over time. A recent review of ACS data (as well as data from other national surveys) comparing demographic characteristics of same-sex

Table 2-2   U.S. Cities Ranked by Number of Same-Sex Couples per 1000 Households

City, State	Same-Sex Couples per 1000 Households
Large cities (population 250,000+)	
San Francisco, CA	30.25
Seattle, WA	23.06
Oakland, CA	21.84
Minneapolis, MN	21.74
Atlanta. GA	19.75
Portland, OR	19.25
Long Beach, CA	19.13
Washington, DC	18.08
Denver, CO	15.65
Boston, MA	14.70
Midsize cities (population 100,000–250,000)	
Fort Lauderdale, FL	31.08
Berkeley, CA	20.61
Salt Lake City, UT	15.36
Cambridge, MA	14.39
Orlando, FL	13.80
St. Petersburg, FL	13.78
Madison, WI	13.24
Alexandria, VA	11.39
Pasadena, CA	11.35
Jersey City, NJ	11.15
Small cities (population <100,000)	
Provincetown, MA	148.08
Wilton Manors, FL	125.33
Palm Springs, CA	107.28
Rehoboth Beach, DE	99.97
Guerneville, CA	80.36
West Hollywood, CA	62.05
Pleasant Ridge, MI	54.77
Rancho Mirage, CA	52.29
New Hope, PA	49.99
Oakland Park, FL	49.41

Data obtained from reference 5.

couples with those of different-sex couples found that individuals in same-sex couples have higher levels of labor force participation (82% compared with 69% of different-sex couples) and greater educational attainment—almost half of individuals in same-sex couples have a college degree (46%) compared with 32% in different-sex couples. Despite higher levels of education and employment, however, LGB Americans are more likely to be poor than heterosexuals. The analysis found that 7.6% of lesbian couple households reported living in poverty, compared with 5.7% of married different-sex couples and 4.3% of same-sex male couples. African-American same-sex couples have poverty rates more than twice those of their different-sex married counterparts (6,10).

Population-Based Surveys and the Enumeration of LGBT Individuals

Despite its power to map and describe certain characteristics of same-sex households, the decennial census and its companion ACS cannot provide sufficient data about LGBT individuals. This is because the Census is not able to identify LGBT people who are not living with a same-sex partner, nor can it provide information on same-sex couples at the individual level. A few government-funded recurring surveys include measures for sexual minorities and provide some specific demographic, attitudinal, and health-related information on LGB people (11–18). These "population-based" or "representative" surveys choose participants through a randomized method, such that each participant has a known likelihood of being selected. By randomized selection, results can be generalized to the overall population. Although these studies provide valuable information, variations in data collection methods and lack of consistent measures for sexual orientation result in different percentages of adults who identify as lesbian, gay, or bisexual. Moreover, as of 2013, no federal surveys have included a measure related to transgender identity. As a result of these limitations, no single survey offers a definitive estimate for the size of the U.S. LGBT community.

To arrive at a single estimate of the nation's LGB population, the Williams Institute of the UCLA School of Law conducted an analysis that averaged findings from 5 population-based surveys, as shown in Table 2-3. From this analysis, the authors estimated that LGB people make up about 3.5% of the adult population (1.8% bisexuals; 1.7% lesbian or gay). Among adult women, 1.1% were estimated to be lesbian/gay and 2.2% to be bisexual, for a total of 4,007,834 women. Among adult men, 2.2% were estimated as gay and 1.4% as bisexual, for a total of 4,030,946 men. Two of the studies also

Table 2-3   Survey Estimates of the Percentage of People Who are Lesbian, Gay, or Bisexual in the United States

Survey (Reference)	Lesbian/Gay (%)	Bisexual (%)	Total (%)
National Epidemiological Survey on Alcohol and Related Conditions, 2004–2005 (11)	1.0	0.7	1.7
National Survey of Family Growth, 2006–2008 (Age 18-44) (12)	1.4	2.3	3.7
General Social Survey, 2008 (13)	1.7	1.1	2.9
California Health Interview Survey, 2009 (14)	1.8	1.4	3.2
National Survey of Sexual Health and Behavior, 2009 (15)	2.5	3.1	5.6
Average of all surveys	1.7	1.8	3.5

asked about same-sex sexual attraction and behavior, finding that many more people report same-sex attractions and behaviors (7.5% to 8.8% of the U.S. population) than identify as LGB (19).

As discussed earlier, there is no national data set that includes transgender identity. To estimate the U.S. transgender population, the Williams Institute used data from 2 population-based state-run surveys (Massachusetts and California) that measured transgender identity. From these surveys, the authors estimated that approximately 0.3% (about 700,000) of U.S. adults identify as transgender (see also Chapter 17) (19).

Demographic Characteristics of LGBT Individuals

Important gaps in our knowledge of LGBT people have been addressed through privately funded probability studies, most of which are conducted at a single point in time, gathering a broad range of information designed to answer specific questions of interest to the funder. Two prominent examples are Gallup's inclusion of a new question for LGBT identification in its Daily Tracking survey (20) and the Pew Research Center's "A Survey of LGBT Americans: Attitudes, Experience and Values in Changing Times," conducted in 2013 (21).

In October 2012, Gallup released responses to the new LGBT identification question in a survey conducted from June 1 through September 20 (20). Among a random sample of 121,290 adults aged 18 years and older, living in all 50 U.S. states and the District of Columbia, 3.4% answered "yes" and 92.2% answered "no" (and 4.4% didn't know or chose not to answer) to the question: "Do you, personally, identify as lesbian, gay, bisexual, or transgender?" This finding was similar to that estimated by the Williams Institute (discussed in the previous section), further strengthening their estimation methods (19). In the Gallup survey, women were slightly more likely to identify as LGBT (3.6%) than men (3.3%). Young adults (age 18 to 29 years) were most likely to identify as LGBT (6.4%), whereas seniors age 65 years and older were least likely (1.9%) (20).

Specific information about demographic and lifestyle characteristics was also collected from Gallup survey respondents. Overall, a third of LGBT-identified respondents were nonwhite (33%), compared with 27% of non-LGBT individuals (20). Table 2-4 shows that greater percentages of Hispanic, black, and Asian respondents identified as LGBT compared with non-Hispanic white respondents. Contrary to other studies and to census data on same-sex households, LGBT Gallup respondents tended to have lower levels of education and income than non-LGBT respondents. Similar to other studies, the Gallup survey showed higher rates of poverty among LGBT people. LGBT adults living alone were more likely to live in poverty than non-LGBT adults living alone: 20.1% of LGBT men compared with 13.4% of heterosexual men and 21.5% of LGBT women compared with 19.1% of heterosexual women. Across the population, poverty rates were much

Table 2-4   Lesbian, Gay, Bisexual, Transgender Identity According
to Race/Ethnicity and Age

Variable	Do You, Personally, Identify as Lesbian, Gay, Bisexual, or Transgender?		
	Yes (%)	No (%)	Don't Know/Refused to Answer (%)
Race/ethnicity			
Non-Hispanic white	3.2	93.0	2.8
Black	4.6	90.1	5.3
Hispanic	4.0	90.2	5.8
Asian	4.3	92.0	3.7
Age range			
18–29 y	6.4	90.1	3.5
30–49 y	3.2	93.6	3.2
50–64 y	2.6	93.1	4.3
65+ y	1.9	91.5	6.5
Women age 18–29 y	8.3	88.0	3.8
Men age 18–29 y	4.6	92.1	3.3

Data obtained from reference 20.

higher in households with children and greater in same-sex couples than in different-sex households. For example, 2.7% of male same-sex couples in households without children lived in poverty; when children were present, 19.2% of same-sex male couples reported living in poverty (10).

With regard to relationships, 20% of LGBT respondents indicated that they were married and an additional 18% were in a domestic partnership or living with a partner; nearly half (48%) were single and never married. These percentages are different among non-LGBT respondents: Fifty-four percent were married, 4% were living with a partner, and 23% were single and had never been married. One third (32%) of non-LGBT and LGBT women alike have children under 18 years in the home; among men there are large differences. Sixteen percent of LGBT men are raising children compared with 31% of non-LGBT men. Ten percent of LGBT white men are raising children (29% of non-LGBTs), 39% of LGBT Hispanic men (44% of non-LGBTs), 14% of Asian men (34% of non-LGBTs), and 14% of African-American men (34% of non-LGBTs) (20).

A survey conducted in April 2013 by the Pew Research Center explored the attitudes, experiences, and "values in changing times" of LGBT Americans. A noteworthy nonpartisan fact tank that provides the U.S. public with information about demographic and social science research, Pew conducted a nationally representative survey of 1197 self-identified LGBT adults (398 gay men, 277 lesbians, 479 bisexuals, and 43 transgender participants) to gather information about key issues of concern to this population. Responses were statistically weighted to adjust for differences within each of these subgroups, with an acceptable margin of sampling error. Questions about social acceptance, coming out, marriage and parenting, identity and community, religion, and partisanship/policy views/values were explored. Survey results found that the LGBT population is distinctive in many ways beyond sexual orientation. Compared with the general population of Americans, LGBT respondents were more liberal, more Democratic, less religious, less happy with their lives, and more satisfied with the general direction of the country (21).

Few studies have collected robust data on bisexuals. In the Pew study, bisexuals were younger, had lower family incomes, and were less likely to be college graduates compared with lesbians and gay men. In addition, bisexuals were far more likely than gays and lesbians to keep their identity secret from all or most of the important people in their lives (sharing this information with 28%, compared with 77% of gay men and 71% of lesbians). Bisexual women were nearly 3 times more likely to share this information than bisexual men (33% versus 12%) (21).

Rationale for Increasing Demographic Data Collection of LGBT Populations

Changing policy and practice is to a large degree dependent on obtaining trustworthy data. Despite considerable progress in understanding the characteristics of sexual and gender minorities, the data are still limited not just by measurement challenges but by social stigma against LGBT people. Residual homophobia and stigma limit the willingness of many LGBT people to disclose their lives to strange interviewers, making the population very hidden in surveys and polls. Societal attitudes toward LGBT people have been changing, however, and in many important ways sexual and gender minorities are gaining civil rights equal to those of the general population. Improved access to the benefits of American society has been gained in large part by the acknowledgement that LGBT people are present throughout society. Increased knowledge about how LGBT people live and the challenges they face because of their differences has helped to moderate public attitudes and increase the engagement of sexual and gender minority individuals in civil society. Increased government inclusion of sexual minorities in demographic and health-related data collections has contributed to general knowledge of their prevalence in society and the health disparities they experience.

Only recently have federally supported data sets incorporated any measure of sexual orientation, and none yet consistently measures gender identity. At this time, standardized measures are being incorporated in an increasing number of government surveys, and ongoing cognitive testing provides a growing body of knowledge about the best ways to word sexual minority, gender identity, and behavioral questions for subpopulation cultural groups. In the future, clinicians will benefit from this improved information. In Table 2-5, sexual orientation measures, data collection methods,

Table 2-5   Recurring Federally Funded Surveys That Include Lesbian, Gay, and Bisexual Measures

Survey (Reference)	Topic Areas	Method of Data Collection	Sexual Orientation Measures
National Epidemiological Survey on Alcohol and Related Conditions (NESARC) (11) Wave 1: 2001–2002 Wave 2: 2004–2005 (longitudinal method)	Alcohol and drug use; alcohol and drug abuse and dependence; associated psychiatric and other medical comorbidities	CAPI: Computer-assisted personal interviews; flash card used to ask racial categories	Identity, behavior, attraction
National Survey of Family Growth (NSFG) (12) Annually since 1996	Family life, marriage and divorce, pregnancy, infertility, use of contraception, and men's and women's health	CAPI: Computer-assisted personal interviews (with assistance or on one's own)	Identity, behavior, attraction
General Social Survey (GSS) (13) Annually 1972–2012 Routinely asks the general population about attitudes toward LGBT-related concerns	A standard "core" of demographic, behavioral, and attitudinal questions, plus topics of special interest to describe the overall U.S. population	Multiple stage sample of geographic areas and corresponding frame of housing unit addresses	Identity, behavior, same-sex partner households
National Health and Nutrition Examination Survey (NHANES) (16)	A program of studies designed to assess the health and nutritional status of adults and children in the United States	Combined interviews and physical examinations	Identity, behavior
National Survey on Drug Use and Health (NHSDA) (17)	Alcohol, tobacco, and illicit drug use; measuring demographic correlates of drug use; providing information on related topics, including drug treatment	Self-completed questionnaire	Behavior: Sex or partners during last 12 mo Sexual orientation in 1996 only
National Health Interview Survey (NHIS) (18) Annually since 1957	Gathers a broad range of health topics from a representative sample of the U.S. civilian, noninstitutionalized population	Household interviews by study staff	Identity

and health-related topic areas are presented for 6 national, federally funded studies, notably including the National Health Interview Survey (NHIS), that began to include a measure of sexual orientation in 2012 (11–13,16–18). Because sexual minorities are a small subpopulation, only the NHIS collects sufficient sample sizes to generate annual comparisons of heterosexual and sexual minority men and women. Inclusion of a sexual orientation measure was added to the 2012 NHIS after discussion among scientists and the Office of the Secretary of Health and Human Services, responding to a recommendation from the Institute of Medicine's report (22). This action was a major step forward to increase inclusion of sexual and gender minority populations in prominent population-based surveys. Unfortunately, NHIS does not yet include a measure of gender identity and thus cannot track the health-related behavior and needs of transgender people. Inclusion of a standardized transgender measure in NHIS is currently targeted for 2015.

Despite these gains, significant gaps remain to be filled in order for LGBT people to attain full inclusion in U.S. society. In part, change will occur as heterosexual cisgender people have increased interaction with sexual and gender minorities who are open about their identities. Families, schools, religious communities, and other organizations will become more knowledgeable, resulting in greater acceptance and support. Important change in the national health care system under the Affordable Care Act presents additional, new challenges and opportunities. The growing use of electronic health records may allow for increased identification of LGBT patients if the appropriate questions are asked and if patients are comfortable with providing candid information (see Chapter 1). Electronic health technology can also benefit patient care by asking sensitive behavioral health questions that could be filled out online or in a waiting room before a clinical encounter. However, for all this information to benefit patient care, medical providers will need to be trained to provide culturally sensitive care to sexual and gender minority patients, and to understand the reasons for specific health disparities that are prevalent within different sexual and gender minority subpopulations.

The Relevance of a Population Approach for Clinicians

It is important for clinicians to be aware of demographic differences because of the effects that each factor may have on patient care. Moreover, understanding how demographic characteristics influence health outcomes is essential to understanding the challenges that LGBT people (and other minority groups) face in accessing care and modifying behaviors. The 2011 Institute of Medicine's report on the health of LGBT people (which reviewed the existing research evidence on LGBT health outcomes) (22) conceived of 4 conceptual frameworks through which to understand the health-related challenges of LGBT people. Each of these perspectives has been tested over time with populations that have greater than usual health disparities, focusing on the demographic characteristics and social conditions that define their daily lives and health. Each perspective provides a unique lens developed through research and practice experience that offers clinicians a way to see each patient as an individual and more clearly assess health-related stressors and needs. Each perspective also provides conceptual tools for better understanding health status, health needs, and health disparities in LGBT populations. The 4 frameworks are briefly described below.

Life Course: This perspective recognizes that people have different health care needs at different life stages. For example, LGBT youth may have concerns related to coming out to their families, while older LGBT adults may have concerns about loneliness and living without extended families. See Chapters 5 through 7 for an in-depth exploration of LGBT health needs throughout the life course.

Social Ecology: This framework emphasizes that characteristics of the social environment, including family, other relationships, the community, culture, and general society, can affect an individual's behavior and well-being. Recognizing how the social context of people's lives influences their health is therefore an important element of health care.

Minority Stress: This theory posits that sexual and gender minorities (like other minority groups) experience chronic stress arising from social stigmatization and manifested in both external and internal processes. Lack of social tolerance of homosexual behavior may result in stress-related disorders, such as depression, for LGBT people, especially in those who feel the need to be covert about their sexual orientation or gender identity.

Intersectionality: This perspective recognizes that social, racial/ethnic, religious, economic, cultural and other factors–in addition to sexual orientation and gender minority status–influence the identities, health, and lived experiences of LGBT people. In caring for patients, clinicians may need to explore and understand the role–and intersection–of different identities and other factors in their patient's lives. See Chapter 3 for more on intersectionality.

In summary, as clinicians become familiar with the increasing array of population-level data related to the social and cultural factors affecting their LGBT patients, their awareness of key components of care for sexual and gender minority patients should increase. This heightened awareness of the existence of health disparities may help to improve practice so that motivated clinicians can provide optimal and culturally appropriate care to all of their LGBT patients.

Summary Points

- It is important to be aware of demographic differences because of the effects that each factor may have on patient care, and because it leads to a better understanding of the challenges that LGBT people (and other minority groups) face in accessing care and modifying behaviors.
- The 2010 Census counted approximately 646,450 same-sex couple households in the United States.
- The 2010 Census also identified same-sex couple households in 93% of all U.S. counties.
- Based on limited data, an estimated 3.5% of the U.S. population identifies as lesbian, gay, or bisexual. Accurate estimates of the transgender population are difficult to make because of lack of data.
- A Gallup Daily tracking survey found that 33% of LGBT-identified respondents were a racial or ethnic minority.
- LGBT adults are more likely to be living in poverty compared with non-LGBT adults.
- Eighteen percent to 32% of LGBT people are raising children.
- Only recently have federally supported data sets incorporated any measure of sexual orientation, and none yet consistently measures gender identity.
- Improved understanding of the demographic features of the LGBT population will enable governments and other administrative bodies, as well as health care providers, to develop programs that address LGBT health care needs.

References

1. **United States Census Bureau.** Available at: www.census.gov.
2. **Black D, Gates G, Sanders S, et al.** Demographics of the gay and lesbian populations in the United States: evidence from available systematic data sources. Demography. 2000;37: 139-54.
3. **Bradford J, Barrett K, Honnold JA.** The 2000 Census and Same-Sex Households: A User's Guide. New York: The National Gay and Lesbian Task Force Policy Institute, the Survey and Evaluation Research Laboratory, and The Fenway Institute; 2002. Available at www.thetask-force.org/downloads/reports/reports/2000Census.pdf.
4. **Gates GJ.** Same-sex Couples in Census 2010: Race and Ethnicity. The Williams Institute, UCLA School of Law. April 2012. Available at http://williamsinstitute.law.ucla.edu/wp-content/uploads/Gates-CouplesRaceEthnicity-April-2012.pdf
5. **Gates GJ, Cooke AM.** United States Census Snapshot: 2010. The Williams Institute, UCLA School of Law. September 2011. Available at http://williamsinstitute.law.ucla.edu/wp-content/uploads/Census2010Snapshot-US-v2.pdf?r

6. **Lofquist D.** American Community Survey Briefs: same-sex couple households. U.S. Census Bureau. September 2011. Available at www.census.gov/prod/2011pubs/acsbr10-03.pdf.

7. **Gates GJ.** LGBT parenting in the United States. The Williams Institute, UCLA School of Law. February 2013. Available at http://williamsinstitute.law.ucla.edu/wp-content/uploads/LGBT-Parenting.pdf.

8. **Gates GJ.** Gay men and lesbians in the U.S. military: estimates from Census 2000. Urban Institute. September 2004. Available at www.urban.org/publications/411069.html.

9. **United States Census Bureau.** American Community Survey. https://www.census.gov/acs.

10. **Badgett MVL, Durso LE, Schneebaum A.** New patterns of poverty in the lesbian, gay, and bisexual community. Williams Institute, UCLA School of Law. September 2013. Available at http://williamsinstitute.law.ucla.edu/research/census-lgbt-demographics-studies/lgbt-poverty-update-june-2013/.

11. **U.S. Department of Health and Human Services.** Office of the Assistant Secretary for Planning and Evaluation. National Epidemiological Survey on Alcohol and Related Conditions (NESARC). Available at http://aspe.hhs.gov/hsp/06/catalog-ai-an-na/nesarc.htm.

12. **Centers for Disease Control and Prevention.** National Survey of Family Growth. Available at www.cdc.gov/nchs/nsfg.htm.

13. **General Social Survey.** Available at http://www3.norc.org/gss+website/.

14. **UCLA Center for Health Policy Research.** California Health Interview Survey. Available at http://healthpolicy.ucla.edu/chis/Pages/default.aspx.

15. **Center for Sexual Health and Promotion.** School of Health, Physical Health and Recreation, Indiana University. National Survey of Sexual Health and Behavior. Available at www.nationalsexstudy.indiana.edu/.

16. **Centers for Disease Control and Prevention.** National Health and Nutrition Examination Survey. Available at www.cdc.gov/nchs/nhanes.htm.

17. **LGBTData.com.** National Survey on Drug Use and Health. Available at www.lgbtdata.com/national-household-survey-on-drug-abuse-nhsda.html.

18. **Centers for Disease Control and Prevention.** National Health Interview Survey. Available at www.cdc.gov/nchs/nhis.htm.

19. **Gates GJ.** How many people are lesbian, gay, bisexual, and transgender? The Williams Institute, UCLA School of Law. April 2011. Available at http://williamsinstitute.law.ucla.edu/wp-content/uploads/Gates-How-Many-People-LGBT-Apr-2011.pdf.

20. **Gates GJ, Newport F.** Special report: 3.4% of U.S. adults identify as LGBT. Gallup. October 18, 2012. Available at www.gallup.com/poll/158066/special-report-adults-identify-lgbt-aspx?version=print.

21. A survey of LGBT Americans: attitudes, experiences and values in changing times. Pew Research Center. June 11, 2013. Available at www.pewsocialtrends.org/2013/06/13/a-survey-of-lgbt-americans/.

22. **Institute of Medicine.** The Health of Lesbian, Gay, Bisexual, and Transgender People: Building a Foundation for Better Understanding. Washington, DC: The National Academies Press, 2011.

Chapter 3

Intersectionality: Implications for Clinical Care of LGBTQ People

DARRELL P. WHEELER, PhD, MPH

Introduction

The goal of this chapter is to offer an approach to using key concepts of identity intersectionality for clinical care with lesbian, gay, bisexual, transgender, and queer/questioning (LGBTQ) persons. The focus is on developing an applied knowledge of the ways in which multiple facets of a person's identity converge or meld to create a unique and dynamic sense of self. When health care providers understand identity intersectionality, they are better able to optimize treatment outcomes with diverse LGBTQ individuals and groups. The intent of the chapter is not to provide an exhaustive theoretical discussion of intersectionality, nor to fully explicate each level or tier of identity; rather, the focus is to enhance the reader's awareness of how identity intersectionality can affect care.

A provider's ability to transform this awareness of identity intersectionality into effective practice is arguably a cornerstone to high-quality patient care. After all, patients come to the provider with a need, usually seeking help for a situation that is problematic, stressful, or harmful in some way. Ultimately, the provider's capacity to be open, knowledgeable, and receptive to the patient's needs is a crucial component in designing and delivering the best care possible. Content in this chapter, therefore, is intended to support the provider's critical thinking about the ways in which identities—both the patient's and the provider's—influence perceptions of problems, care options, and utilization of care.

Provoking critical thinking about these elements is a necessary step in awakening our own assumptions about the neutrality of our own roles as providers. As will be explored in this chapter, the provider's awareness of these issues may be as important as the provider's specific knowledge about any one fact about an LGBTQ person. After all, in the arena of health care delivery, the provider most often has a power advantage, with the ability to provide or deny access to care or treatment. Keeping this knowledge of the power dynamic in focus is important in understanding the relational aspects of care and treatment, which have been shown to be critical to optimal care outcomes (1).

Conceptualizing the Issues

One of the most obvious reasons for focusing on intersectionality is that, as providers, we want the best for our patients in terms of care, treatment, and outcomes. However, many of us, despite our best efforts, have seen repeatedly either in our own practices or through a fairly exhaustive literature that the inequalities and disparities for certain groups continue to grow (2,3). One prevailing perspective on such inequalities focuses on differences in health care outcomes—disparities—that are not attributable to other known factors (e.g., biomedical and physiologic differences). The disparities approach reinforces that there may be things about the person or group, such as race, class, gender, or sexual identities, that will consistently render that person or group at a "disadvantage" for achieving the best health outcomes.

Another perspective focuses on equity and equality in health care, wherein the most relevant theories, techniques, and technologies are appropriately applied to achieve the most desirable outcomes, for the intended group (4). In this perspective, knowledge, application, and outcomes are seen as mutable, and the problem is not seen as vested in the patient but in the ways in which practices are learned and applied. For the purposes of this chapter, we will focus on the latter perspective, as this is the one that is arguably more oriented to change and hope.

Applying this perspective to LGBTQ persons is certainly a matter of health equity. Understanding and deepening our understanding of the factors that contribute to health inequities and that can be overcome to achieve equitable care are important for us and the patients we serve. Furthermore, these are matters of ethical, professional, and organizational responsibility. There is increasing legal and regulatory emphasis on equity in care for all.

Health Inequalities: Theories and Perspectives

Estimates of the number of LGBTQ people vary, but as Chapter 2 explains, current estimates have found that approximately 3.5 % of the U.S. population identifies as LGBT (5) and that LGBT people live in nearly every U.S. county (6). Despite the uncertainty of the exact number, we can certainly assert that the health of 3.5% of our patients is well worth the effort of developing our knowledge and skills to bring about optimal health care outcomes for them. This is particularly important when we look at the body of available literature that suggests disproportionate negative health outcomes for LGBTQ persons, including depression, anxiety, tobacco use, substance use, HIV/AIDS, and lower use of preventive cancer screenings (3).

A variety of theories and perspectives have been posited as contributing to these disproportionate health outcomes (3). These include the following:

- LGBTQ patients' negative encounters with medical institutions
- Lack of attention on the part of health care providers and institutions to diversity in sexual expression, sexual health, and sexual well-being overall
- Interactions between sexual identity, social class, and race
- Roles of social networks that support and sustain apprehensions and fears about health care providers and systems of care
- Stigma and fear of being "outed" by health care providers
- Limited attention to the developmental needs of LGBTQ persons across the life span
- Religious and cultural norms.

In addition, the theory of minority stress suggests that members of stigmatized groups have chronically high levels of stress in response to stigma and prejudice, and that this stress causes responses such as high blood pressure and anxiety, which, in turn, increase the risk for negative health behaviors, such as substance use and high-risk sexual practices (7,8). Overall, it can be helpful to understand that biological, psychological, social, and spiritual factors can overlap and be experienced in ways that are greater than the effect of any single factor on its own.

Intersectionality: Many Identities, One Person

Intersectionality as a term is derived from feminist theoretical discourse and refers to the "intersection of multiple identities and experiences of exclusion and subordination" (9). In the application for health care, it speaks to the relationship of a person's many identities (e.g., sexual, racial, economic, geographic) that coexist and present in a way that is not singularly about any one identity, but about the "integrated" experience of all identities into a "new" whole. Bowleg's descriptive article title on male intersectionality captures this concept well: "Once You've Blended the Cake, You Can't Take the Parts Back to the Main Ingredients" (10). An integrated identity is influenced by internal perspectives; cultural views; and issues of social, economic, and political positioning with dominant groups (11,12). Intersectionality also recognizes that oppressive forces act overtly or covertly to disempower the manifestation of the intersected identity (13). Ultimately, it is about a person's understanding and lived experience of intersecting identities in a complex and dynamic context (14,15).

For the LGBTQ patient, intersecting identities are likely composed of gender and sexual expressions and identities, racial identities, ethnic identities, religious identities, geographic identities (including migration and immigration statuses), lifespan/age identities, and class (income, occupation, and education) identities. Clearly, the list of possible identities is not exhaustive but rather illustrates the range of forces that can affect patients' formulation of their understanding of themselves, and ultimately frame the ways in which they engage their world. Intersectionality also reminds us that LGBTQ people are not heterogeneous despite their shared status as sexual and gender minorities, and that they represent a diverse range of races, ethnicities, religions, and other identities.

The identities that people hold of themselves are not always the same as how others perceive them on the basis of outward physical appearances. Similarly, a person's sexual orientation or identity may not always be consistent with sexual behaviors or practices. It is important for providers to understand these issues in order to avoid assumptions when working with LGBTQ patients. See Chapter 1 for a discussion of different terms and definitions used to describe sexual and gender identities.

Four Perspectives on Awareness and Integration of Identities

Awareness (or lack of awareness) of identities can happen in many ways (16–18). Four of these perspectives are briefly presented here and are illustrated in Figure 3-1.

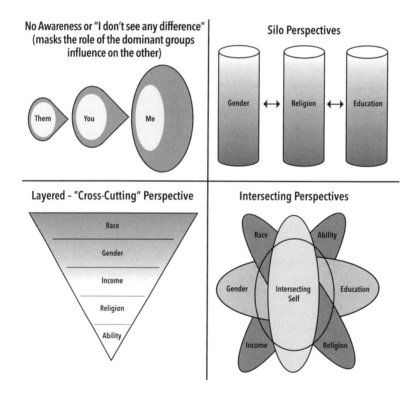

Figure 3-1 Four perspectives on awareness and integration of cultural identities.

One common perspective is nonawareness or a "universalist" approach. In this approach, a person might state, "I don't see race, or gender, or class . . . I just see a person." While this perspective appears neutral, it could potentially have a negative effect on the patient–provider relationship because suggesting that one does not see identity has the potential of shutting down a patient who wishes to open up. The implicit message is: "I do not want to see or know about your gender, class, race or sex."

A second perspective is the "silo perspective," in which one identity is selected or essentialized relative to another. This perspective acknowledges that multiple identities can exist but that only one defines the person. This perspective has the potential of negating the other identities, which may be of equal importance to the patient, and could lead to seeing an incomplete perspective on who the patient is.

A third perspective is the layered or cross-cutting perspective. In this perspective patients are seen as (and may see themselves as) composed of multiple coexisting but not integrated identities. The perspective may relate to patients' movement between identity statuses knowingly or unknowingly in order to "fit in" or because one or more of the identities is particularly more salient to how the patients view themselves at a moment in time.

A fourth perspective is an integration of the various identity statuses the patient holds. The intersected self may not look exactly like any one of the individual identity statuses but is affected by all identities and affects them in return. The patient's understanding of this may be influenced by social networks but equally may be the result of responses to exclusions and subordinations. The intersected identity of the patient becomes a construct that may or may not reflect an obvious association with the constituent identities if one attempted to understand them individually. Another way of saying this is that each of the constituent parts of the identity cannot be seen as additive to create a "known" whole, but may manifest as something other and understood uniquely from the perspective of the individual.

How Intersectionality Affects the Provision of Health Care

Identity formation and integration and ultimately intersected identities have implications for health care and health outcomes. Immediate implications would include assessing the extent to which any identity formation is creating emotional, physical, or social distress for the patient. A client/patient-centered approach to understanding what is being experienced provides a mechanism for doing this. Research (12) with LGB youth underscores that in addition to supporting LGB identity development, working on integrating of identities is essential to reducing psychological distress. See Chapter 4 for a discussion of supporting positive identity formation in LGBTQ clients.

As noted from the outset of this chapter, this work is equally about the providers' self-awareness as it is about knowing the many facets of the LGBTQ patient. This point should be critically clear here because any attempt to fully list all potential identities a person could hold would not be possible. Rather, the goal is that as providers we become aware of the potential range of identities and come to understand that these identities converge to create a unique experience for the patient. Knowledge alone about the various identities is insufficient in truly understanding how these identities are brought into a coherent whole for each unique patient. The coming together of the multiple components of LGBTQ persons' identities are not lived—and likely are not learned—in neat silos. They are contextual, derived, and melded over the life course and likely constructed, destructed, and reconstructed as well. In fact, there often is no readily accessible reference point to use in articulating who the patient is. It is therefore important to listen to and explore with the patient the meaning, perception, and impact of these identities.

An example could be gender-nonconforming patients who do not identify as male or female; as heterosexual, bisexual, or gay; or by a racial category. These individuals' understanding of themselves would have to be understood through their own lens and would require engagement by the provider to ascertain what this identity means for the individuals in their social milieu. Thus, the work for the provider is to be a partner in the process of exploring the meaning of identity for LGBTQ persons and helping patients recognize how to integrate different parts of their identity. Further, because we are humans ourselves, composed of many identities, the exchanges with our patients can be very overwhelming as we (knowingly or not) seek to differentiate our own expectations of who our patients are and should be from our patients' understanding of these.

Finally, providers should be aware that "provider positionality"—or the relationship of the provider's views interfacing at the clinical exchange with the patients' realities—is an important part of the health care experience (19,20–22). The point of interface between the patient and provider is an opportunity to facilitate or shut down productive health communications and ultimately outcomes (23,24). Understanding not just patients' physical but also their social, psychological, and identity issues provides a rich opportunity to support patient engagement and positive health and mental health outcomes (25,26).

Providing Care to LGBTQ Patients by Supporting Integrated Identities: Case Scenarios

This chapter concludes with three case scenarios to highlight and support the concepts explained throughout the chapter. These cases are meant to illustrate ways in which providers have attended to their patients' identity concerns while providing optimal care and treatment.

Case 1

A young black pre-med college student recovering from repair of a sports-related injury comes to his doctor to talk about switching pain medications. After some discussion, the patient reveals that he has been drinking alcohol more heavily to help with the pain "and some other stuff." When the doctor probes further, the patient confides that he has come to realize that he is attracted to both men and women and that while he has not yet been sexually active, the experience and process of coming to terms with his sexuality have caused him significant stress. The patient tells the doctor he felt he could express this to her because she does not "judge" others, and that her approach to him suggests that she is open to hearing his concerns. The patient is very worried that if he starts to date men, others will find out about his bisexuality, particularly his best friend and parents, and that they will tease and ostracize him. He also has developed some anxious feelings about becoming infected with HIV if he starts to have sex with men.

After hearing her patient's concerns, the doctor does not avoid discussions of sexuality as irrelevant to the presenting problem of pain medication, but rather takes the opportunity provided by the patient to more fully explore his many intersecting identities (athlete, son, friend, student, bisexual, black man). She does not focus on any one of these identities as defining him but builds on the patient's process of integrating these into a fuller understanding of his current situation. She affirms that bisexuality is a normal, healthy expression of sexuality, while also empathizing with the patient that societal and cultural acceptance of bisexuality is mixed. She encourages him to talk more about his fears of his friends and parents' reactions, and encourages him to seek additional support through a support group or counseling (she offers referrals). She also spends some time educating him about what is known about risk of HIV and how to use protection.

Case 2

A 75-year-old self-identified lesbian patient has undergone a major surgical procedure and will require in home and family assisted care. The nurse assigned to the case is aware that the patient has self-identified as lesbian but is unsure how this might affect the patient's home care. Instead of ignoring or making assumptions about the patient's lesbian identity, the nurse acknowledges his own limitations of understanding the patient's home situation and asks the patient to help identify the family and home-based supports she might have in place. The patient is pleased to share with the nurse about her long-term relationship with another woman who is currently healthy and able to provide support with meals and care. Together they identify action steps that are respectful and helpful to the patient. In this case, the nurse has assessed his own sensitivities about LGBTQ people and "joins" with the patient to gather and provide useful information that promotes positive outcomes.

Case 3

Malcolm is 29 years old and has a mixed ethnic background of white/Anglo, Caribbean and Spanish. He has lived in the United States for 14 years and works as a paralegal with a small firm in a non-urban Midwestern town. He is living with a woman but also engages in sex with other men and women regularly. He came to the clinic because he was feeling tired and has not been sleeping much during the past month or so. He reports limited "illegal" drug use but does use marijuana at least weekly and drinks 2 to 4 beers a day. He has 5 children: 3 with the woman he currently lives with and 2 others he rarely sees. In exploring his current situation the provider learns that Malcolm has a "steady" male sexual partner with whom he has a strong friendship and sexual relationship. He states that his "wife" is unaware of this and that he does not want anyone to know about this as both are married and have professional careers and children. His primary reason for coming in to the clinic is to get some help so he can get back to sleeping "normally" and feeling like his old self.

The provider assures Malcolm that she is there to work with him to understand the issues that have brought him to the clinic, and that she will be asking questions about his life and his physical health in order to get a better perspective on the ways she and the clinic team might help him. She also tells him that she will want to see him a few times to make certain that, whatever the course of action to which they both agree, it is working and that he is feeling like himself. The provider uses Malcolm's language of "feeling like himself" to ask questions that describe what this means and how this is different from the way he feels and acts now. She also informs him that some medical tests will be needed to make a comprehensive assessment. Malcolm is agreeable to the plan, participates with the assessment, and consents to the necessary medical and laboratory procedures. He follows up with the requested visits and is seen by the provider again appointments.

In this case the provider "suspends" her determination of who Malcolm is based on his ethnic and/or racial background (27–29), his economic status, and his sexual orientation and identity. The provider uses the skills of clinical engagement to allow Malcolm to guide her to a fuller and more nuanced understanding of his goals and how his current condition was perceived as different from his desired goal state (30). In addition, the provider understands that the perceptions she held about the potentially incongruent identities were actually part of an intersected identity for Malcolm that was not distressful to him (31).

Summary Points

- While the underlying biomedical parameters for LGBTQ persons may not be different from those for non-LGBTQ persons, many of the contributing and unaddressed social, contextual, psychological, developmental, interpersonal, and environmental factors can produce deleterious outcomes.

- Addressing issues arising from disparate care for LGBTQ patients can help improve health outcomes and eliminate inequities.
- Intersectionality speaks to the relationship of a person's many identities (e.g., sexual, racial, economic, geographic) that coexist and present in a way that is not singularly about any single identity but instead concerns the "integrated" experience of all identities into a "new" whole.
- Intersectionality is an important concept to incorporate when working with LGBTQ and other individuals facing multiple and complex identity integration.
- In constructing patient, family, provider and organizational responses to the needs of LGBTQ individuals, it is important to avoid essentializing, or reducing, the entire focus to sexual behaviors of the LGBTQ person.
- Understanding not just the physical but also the social, psychological, and identity issues of the patients provides a rich opportunity to support patient engagement and positive health and mental health outcomes.

References

1. **Lohr KN, Zebrack BJ.** Using patient-reported outcomes in clinical practice: challenges and opportunities. Qual Life Res. 2009;18:99-107.
2. **Williams DR, Mohammed SA, Leavell J, Collins C.** Race, socioeconomic status, and health: complexities, ongoing challenges, and research opportunities. Ann N Y Acad Sci. 2010;1186: 69-101.
3. **Institute of Medicine.** The Health of Lesbian, Gay, Bisexual, and Transgender People: Building a Foundation for Better Understanding. Washington, DC: The National Academies Press; 2011.
4. **Carter-Pokras O, Baquet C.** What is a "health disparity"? Public Health Rep. 2002;117: 426-34.
5. **Gates GJ.** How many people are lesbian, gay, bisexual, and transgender? The Williams Institute. April 2011. Available at: http://williamsinstitute.law.ucla.edu/wp-content/uploads/Gates-How-Many-People-LGBT-Apr-2011.pdf.
6. **Gates GJ, Cooke AM.** United States Census Snapshot: 2010. The Williams Institute. September 2011. Available at: http://williamsinstitute.law.ucla.edu/wp-content/uploads/Census2010Snapshot-US-v2.pdf?r.
7. **Meyer IH.** Prejudice, social stress, and mental health in lesbian, gay, and bisexual populations: conceptual issues and research evidence. Psychol Bull. 2003;129:674-97.
8. **Meyer IH.** Minority stress and mental health in gay men. J Health Soc Behav. 1995;36: 38-56.
9. **Davis K.** Intersectionality as buzzword: sociology of science perspective on what makes a feminist theory successful. Feminist Theory. 2008;9:67-85.
10. **Bowleg L.** Once you've blended the cake, you can't take the parts back to the main ingredients: black gay and bisexual men's descriptions and experiences of intersectionality. Sex Roles. 2013;68:754-67.

11. **Bowleg, L, Teti M, Malebranche DJ, Tschann JM.** "It's an uphill battle everyday": Intersectionality, low-income Black heterosexual men, and implications for HIV prevention research and interventions. Psychol Men Masculin. 2013;14:25-34.

12. **Rosario M, Schrimshaw EW, Hunter J.** Different patterns of sexual identity development over time: implications for the psychological adjustment of lesbian, gay, and bisexual youths. J Sex Res. 2011;48:3-15.

13. **Airhihenbuwa CO.** Health & Culture: Beyond the Western Paradigm. Thousand Oaks, CA: Sage; 1995.

14. **Rothblum ED.** From invert to intersectionality: understanding the past and future of sexuality. In: Das Nair R, Butler C, eds. Intersectionality, Sexuality, and Psychological Therapies: Working with Lesbian, Gay and Bisexual Diversity. Hoboken, NJ: Wiley; 2012:263-268.

15. **Crethar H, Rivera E, Nash S.** In search of common threads: linking multicultural, feminist, and social justice counseling paradigms. J Counsel Devel. 2008;86:269-78.

16. **Anderson RE, Carter I.** Human Behavior in the Social Environment, A Social Systems Approach. 3rd ed. New York: Aldine; 1984.

17. **Sue D.** Multidimensional facets of cultural competence. Counseling Psychologist. 2001; 29:790-821.

18. **Sue EE.** The model of cultural competence through an evolutionary concept analysis. J Transcultural Nurs. 2004;15:93-102.

19. **Niimura J.** A cross-cultural experience at midnight. Int J Nurs Pract. 2013;19 Suppl 2:59-60.

20. **Wheeler DP, Dodd S-J.** LGBTQ capacity building in health care systems: a social work imperative. Health Social Work. 2011;36:307-9.

21. **Kronenfeld JJ.** Social Sources of Disparities in Health and Health Care and Linkages to Policy, Population Concerns and Providers of Care. Bradford, United Kingdom: Emerald Group; 2009;27, V. v. 27.

22. **Van Den Bergh N, Crisp C.** Defining culturally competent practice with sexual minorities: Implications for social work education and practice. J Social Work Educ. 2004;40:221-238.

23. **Cooper LA, Ghods Dinoso BK, Ford DE, et al.** Comparative effectiveness of standard versus patient-centered collaborative care interventions for depression among African Americans in primary care settings: the BRIDGE Study. Health Serv Res. 2013;48:150-74.

24. **Gregory H Jr, Van Orden O, Jordan L, et al.** New directions in capacity building: incorporating cultural competence into the interactive systems framework. Am J Community Psychol. 2012; 50:321-33.

25. **Bidell MP.** The sexual orientation counselor competency scale: assessing attitudes, skills, and knowledge of counselors working with lesbian, gay, and bisexual clients. Counselor Educ Supervision. 2005;4:267-79.

26. **Brach C, Fraserirector I.** Can cultural competency reduce racial and ethnic health disparities? A review and conceptual model. Med Care Res Rev. 2000;57:181-217.

27. **Strunk JA, Townsend-Rocchiccioli J, Sanford JT.** The aging Hispanic in America: challenges for nurses in a stressed health care environment. Medsurg Nurs. 2013;22:45-50.

28. **Stepanikova I, Cook KS.** How do American black, white, Hispanic, and Asian health care users perceive their medical non-adherence? Social sciences of disparities in health and health care and linkages to policy. Sociol Health Care. 2009;27:47-66.

29. **Cheng TC, Robinson MA.** Factors leading African Americans and Black Caribbeans to use social work services for treating mental and substance use disorders. Health Social Work. 2013;38:99-109.

30. **Jani JS, Ortiz L, Pierce D, Sowbel L.** Access to intersectionality, content to competence: deconstructing social work education diversity standards. J Social Work Educ. 2011;47: 283-301.

31. **Ibrahim SA, Franklin PD.** Race and elective joint replacement: where a disparity meets patient preference. Am J Public Health. 2013;103:1077-e2.

CARING ACROSS THE LIFE CONTINUUM

Chapter 4

Coming Out: The Process of Forming a Positive Identity

JOANNE GREENFIELD, PhD

Introduction

In the most simple and common usage, *coming out* is the experience of becoming self-aware or the act of openly disclosing to others that one is lesbian, gay, bisexual, transgender, or queer/questioning (LBGTQ). The developmental process of clarifying and accepting one's LGBTQ identity (coming out to oneself) is inextricably linked to the process of readying oneself to reveal that identity publicly (coming out to others). Self-acceptance and whether, when, and how to come out to others are influenced by personal history and characteristics; ethnic, cultural, and religious background; experiences of victimization and prejudice; family and societal messages that often derail rather than facilitate adjustment; and the presence or absence of community supports. These factors, combined with the inherent complexity of gender identity and sexual orientation, make coming out a challenging, dynamic, and lifelong experience.

Health professionals can play a pivotal role in supporting patients who identify, or are beginning to identify as LGBTQ. Like everyone else, health professionals are subject to biased societal messages and often carry these prejudices into their work realms unwittingly (1–4). For LGBTQ patients, access to health care, quality of communication during a clinical encounter, and relevance of the care that is offered are compromised when health providers are homophobic, undereducated with regard to LGBTQ issues, or unaware of their patients' gender or sexuality (5–8). On the other hand, health providers who convey acceptance and affirmation can counteract the effect of confusing or negative messages LGBTQ patients receive elsewhere and can have an enormous influence on the development of positive self-esteem and a healthy life adjustment.

This chapter describes the nuances and complexity of the coming out process and suggests approaches clinicians can use to facilitate open and supportive communication with patients about gender identity and sexual orientation issues. The first section, "Identity Development," describes different models of gender identity and sexual orientation; addresses how language and stereotypes affect identity consolidation and development of self-esteem; and briefly reviews theories of identity development as they relate to LGBTQ populations. The second section, "Common Coming Out Patterns," reviews models of coming out that have been described in the literature and considers the consequences—both positive and negative—of various coping strategies used by LGBTQ individuals. The third section, "Barriers and Benefits to Coming Out," discusses the challenges and rewards of coming out with respect to self-esteem, relationships with family, ethnic and cultural diversity, interaction with the health care system, religion and spirituality, management of daily life dilemmas, and coming out as a health provider. The chapter closes with "What Providers Can Do to Help," a summary of ways in which clinicians can provide appropriate guidance and support for patients with regard to gender identity or sexual orientation issues.

Identity Development

The child development theorist Donald Winnicott describes how children develop a secure sense of self and positive self-esteem, in part through a process known as "mirroring," in which a child's feelings and behaviors are responded to empathically by parents and other critical role models. Through accurate mirroring, the child's experiences are validated and internalized, creating a "true self" (9). According to Winnicott, it is critical to develop a "true self" in order to achieve positive self-esteem and a sense of wholeness as a person. He states: "The true self feeling . . . requires a lived recognition of being the self one is, that this felt presence is one's true being" (10).

While development of a "true self" is complicated for anyone, it is particularly challenging for LGBTQ individuals. Culturally bound perceptions about gender and sexuality contradict the true identity of LGBTQ children and adolescents. Although some parents may deem heterosexuality and stereotypical gender presentations as "more appropriate," pressure in these directions does not alter a child's or later adult's identity; rather, it is confusing and destructive to the individual's positive self-development. Common language that is constrained by stereotypical conceptions frequently fails to accurately describe the internal experience of an LGBTQ person, which can make finding the right words to explain one's identity to others extremely challenging.

The next section examines the limitations of prevailing concepts of gender identity and sexual orientation, presents alternative models with expanded definitions, and considers possible solutions to the language problem.

Coming Out as What? Gender Identity, Sexual Orientation, and Language

Health professionals' understanding of patients' feelings, thoughts, and experiences surrounding gender and sexuality can have a large impact on patients' self-esteem and identity clarification. When clinicians confuse gender identity, gender role, and sexual orientation, patients who are in the midst of securing their identity become or remain confused, feel that aspects of their identity are blocked or degraded, and are hindered in the development of positive self-esteem. Such confusion by clinicians hinders the development of open and trusting therapeutic relations for both these patients and patients who are secure in their identity. The language we use, the questions we ask, and how we respond to patients' disclosures all determine whether we communicate bias or openness and whether we alienate patients or succeed in providing a warm welcome. Toward the goal of greater clarity, this chapter will now review and critique existing models of gender and sexuality.

According to psychobiologist J.D. Weinrich, overall gender identity consists of three main components: core gender identity, gender role, and sexual orientation (11). Core gender identity consists of biological factors (such as genetics and physical anatomy) as well as psychological factors related to a person's inner experience of gender. Gender role refers to social roles of males and females as defined by the society or culture at a particular time in history and can be observed in mode of dress, actions, or personal qualities. Gender role varies with historical and societal shifts and cultural differences. As with core gender identity, each person has a unique inner experience and behavioral style with regard to gender role. Sexual orientation refers to the propensity to be romantically and/or sexually attracted to and fall in love with people of a different gender, the same gender, or both. Specific terms associated with core gender identity, gender role, and sexual orientation are listed in Table 4-1. Chapters 1, 16, and 17 offer additional terms and definitions for these concepts.

Table 4-1   Common Terms Associated With Core Gender Identity, Gender Role, and Sexual Orientation

Concept	Terms
Core gender identity	man, woman, transgender, transsexual, intersex, queer,* questioning,[†] genderqueer[‡]
Gender role	masculine, feminine, effeminate
	Slang: butch (masculine-appearing or -acting lesbian woman or masculine person of any gender or sexual orientation), fem (feminine-appearing or -acting lesbian woman or feminine person of any gender or sexual orientation)
Sexual orientation	heterosexual, homosexual, bisexual, gay, lesbian, straight, queer, questioning
	Slang: used as prejudicial insults or with pride by LGBTQ people: dyke (lesbian), fag (gay man)

*Queer is a non-traditional gender identity *or* sexual orientation term preferred by some people who wish not to be more specifically categorized. Queer is sometimes used as an umbrella term for any LGBTQ person.

[†]A person who is in the process of actively exploring their sexual orientation and/or gender identity may use the term "questioning."

[‡]A genderqueer person is someone who blurs or bends the gender binary, identifies outside of the gender binary (i.e., neither male nor female, agender), and/or identifies as both male and female. Similar terms include gender variant and gender fluid.

Table 4–2   Binary/Unidimensional versus Complex/Multidimensional Gender and Sexuality Models

Concept	Binary and Unidimensional Models	Complex/Multidimensional Models	
Gender	Male | Female	Multiple and fluid gender constellations (e.g., male, female, transgender, intersex, transsexual, genderqueer, ambigender)	
Gender role	Masculine | Feminine Masculinity↔Femininity	High masculinity ↑ ↓ Low masculinity	High femininity ↑ ↓ Low femininity
		Multiple and fluid gender role qualities, each with its own continuum	
Sexual orientation	Heterosexual | Homosexual Hetero | Bisexual | Homo (Freud) Hetero 0 1 2 3 4 5 6 Homo (Kinsey)	High attraction to men ↑ ↓ Low attraction to men	High attraction to women ↑ ↓ Low attraction to women
		Multiple and diverse bases on which one may be attracted to others, each with its own continuum	

Over time, thinking of gender, gender role, and sexual orientation dichotomously or unidimensionally has shifted toward conceptualizing the components of gender and sexuality in more complex and multidimensional ways (see Table 4-2). Insisting that individuals conform to only a male or female category of gender means that people who wish to express their true selves in expanded ways—for example, as "genderqueer, radical transgenderists, ambigendered or a third gender"—find no vision or reinforcement of themselves in society (2). The perception of gender identity as nonbinary, with options that exist across a spectrum, acknowledges the existence of people with diverse and multifaceted gender identities. Similarly, with respect to gender role, use of a multidimensional model recognizes that people can have a variety of masculine and feminine qualities simultaneously.

Finally, sexual orientation has also been historically conceptualized according to dichotomous (heterosexual/homosexual) or unidimensional models. Examples of the latter include Freud's introduction of bisexuality in the early 1900s and Kinsey's 7-point scale with gradations from exclusively heterosexual to exclusively homosexual and degrees of bisexuality in between (12-14). More complex/multidimensional models of sexual orientation acknowledge that each individual can have different levels of attraction to men and/or women independently (11). For example, an exclusively gay man may be attracted only to men and not to women at all, while an exclusively lesbian woman may experience the reverse. Some individuals are attracted to both men and women to varying degrees along a continuum. While some of these people may embrace the concept of bisexuality as a description of their identity, others may use a label such as *gay* or *lesbian* rather than *bisexual* to describe their identity even though they have had fantasies, attractions, or experiences involving the other sex. Some people who have sex regularly or periodically with those of the same gender or both genders label themselves *heterosexual*. Finally, there are people who eschew labels as excessively constrictive or who consider sexual orientation to be fluid over time. Consider the following examples (all cases in this chapter are hypothetical):

> Mary, age 36, used to date men and was married for several years. After her divorce, she started dating women. Currently, she is single. When asked to describe her sexual orientation, she states: "When I dated men, I thought of myself as straight; when I dated women, I called myself lesbian. Some people would say I'm bisexual, but I've decided I don't really like labels."

> Noor, a 24-year-old woman, explains, "In high school, I dated boys, but was also attracted to girls and had some experiences with them. Now I notice I'm attracted to some guys and some women, but they all are pretty nontraditional in their gender identity or sexual orientation. I'm dating a person who has a trans identity now so it feels like *straight*, *lesbian*, or *bi* aren't really good descriptions for me. I like the term queer—it's open, inclusive, and more fluid. It doesn't pigeon hole me."

It is critical to find appropriate words to express oneself when trying to clarify feelings and sense of self in a confusing environment. This challenge is especially daunting in attempts to describe these aspects to another person. Clinicians who display awareness, openness, and flexibility about language options and alternative concepts of gender and sexual orientation are much more likely to be successful in establishing a productive therapeutic connection. Consider the following case:

> Lee is transgender (female-to-male) and is in the process of transitioning (altering female body and gender presentation to become male, through dress, behaviors, hormone treatments, and/or surgical interventions). Lee uses male self-references despite an androgynous appearance. He uses male gender words to refer to himself and does not like to refer to himself as queer or trans because he feels he is male. He presents saying "I used to be lesbian but now I don't know what to say about my sexual orientation."

In addition to dealing with gender identity terms, Lee is grappling with how to discuss his sexual orientation. Instead of using labels such as lesbian, gay, or straight, it is likely to be much more fruitful to help Lee think about sexual orientation by asking him if he knows to whom he's attracted (e.g., men, women, both, transgender men, transgender women). If he is clear about that, then it would be helpful to encourage him to first think and talk in terms of having attractions to one or more of these groups. From there, he can think about which, if any, labels fit his experience (e.g., *gay, straight, bi*) or whether he would like to just continue to express himself by saying "I am attracted to/interested in/like women/men, etc."

For some people, a term such as *queer* is more palatable due to its gender-neutral, inclusive, and more fluid nature. Listening to patients' language or asking them how they define or refer to themselves and using that same language not only allows for more openness about sexuality and gender between patient and health provider but also imbues more trust and safety in the relationship in general. For patients who are searching for or confused about their identity, using the models that allow for the most flexibility can be supportive and allow the patient to express or explore who they are from within rather than be constrained by external stereotypes or biases.

Our culture's tendency is to not only categorize dichotomously (male–female, feminine–masculine, heterosexual–homosexual) but also to link up these dichotomies in culturally traditional or stereotypical ways (see Table 4-3). For example, male is linked with masculine; female is linked with feminine. Messages that endorse the traditional view create additional identity development problems for people who do not fit these stereotypes. Consider the following example:

Sam, age 25, has been feeling panicky and is experiencing episodic chest pain and shortness of breath. He has been obsessing about his attractions to men, but says that it is impossible for him to be gay because he has always been very masculine, even playing football in college.

Similar worries might be seen in a "lipstick" or "fem" lesbian who presents as very feminine and is told she can't possibly be gay; a straight, artistic, nonathletic guy who is labeled, to his confusion, as gay; or a big, strong, straight girl on the high school hockey team who gets labeled as lesbian.

Table 4-3   Societal Stereotypes of Gender and Sexual Orientation

Traditional/Stereotypic	Nontraditional
Masculine–man–heterosexual	Masculine–man–homosexual
Feminine–man–homosexual	Feminine–man–heterosexual
Feminine–woman–heterosexual	Feminine–woman–homosexual
Masculine–woman–homosexual	Masculine–woman–heterosexual

More masculine, lesbian women report being mistaken for men or being accused of wanting to be men; similarly, feminine gay men or boys are often teased or bullied for being "too much like girls." Bisexual people may feel themselves pressured (within themselves and/or by others) toward a heterosexual or homosexual orientation based on their gender role characteristics, thereby invalidating their bisexuality.

Misperceptions encountered by transgender people abound. For example, assuming that a masculine-looking and masculine-acting biologic female is lesbian or that a feminine biologic male is gay rather than possibly transgender misses the true identity of the individual and confuses gender identity and sexual orientation. Repeated misreading of people who present themselves in nontraditional ways can be confusing and damaging to youth and adults who are exploring different presentations as part of the process of clarifying who they are. Informed and supportive health providers can help by pointing out to those coming out, parents and others who may be confounding these areas the difference among gender identity, gender role presentation, and sexual orientation and by affirming the existence of heterosexual, homosexual, bisexual, and transgender people who have both masculine and feminine attributes.

Identity Development Models and the LGBTQ Population

Research indicates that most LGB men and women realize their sexual orientation during their teens and early 20s, although some discover their orientation in early childhood or later in adulthood (15,16). Coming out to self (self-awareness/self-identification) evolves simultaneously with the emergence of other developmental capacities and in conjunction with other developmental milestones such as the emergence of puberty. Emerging awareness of oneself as a sexual being (sexual exploration with self and others) and a relational being (developing capacities and skills for emotional intimacy) interacts in complex ways with the development of one's emerging identity. Sometimes people become clearly aware of their sexual orientation prior to any sexual activity, while in other cases sexual exploration facilitates clarification of sexual orientation (16). While there is little research on identity development among transgender people, available data suggest an incremental process beginning in early childhood, when many children attempt to communicate their gender differences to parents and others; intensifying in puberty as physical changes that conflict with the developing sense of self take place; and culminating in adulthood, when many transgender people become more fully self-aware and reveal their gender identity to others (2,6). Transgender identity development is described in more detail in Chapter 17.

Exploration of same-sex experiences is common in adolescent development; this does not automatically imply a homosexual orientation but also does not mean that a youth is not gay, lesbian, or bisexual (15). Sexual experimentation can range from being wondrous and conflict-free to an experience riddled with shame, conflict, and confusion. Encountering heterosexist or homophobic attitudes and misconceptions during this developmental phase can inhibit and disrupt a young person's healthy exploration of sexual identity and budding sense of self. This can promote internalized homophobia, in which external negative messages and experiences become transformed into self-hatred, denial, and an impaired sense of self (17).

One problem for LGB adolescents is that many adults (e.g., parents and teachers) view homosexuality or bisexuality as a passing phase (15). A young LGB child, teen, or adult working to clarify sexual identity and develop a positive sense of self can become confused, depressed, and even suicidal when faced with erroneous and invalidating messages. The stressors that promote internalized homophobia can also result in additional problems, including substance abuse, smoking, eating disorders, poor academic performance, dropping out of school, delinquency, problems with intimacy, high-risk sexual behavior, prostitution, and running away (16,18,19). These stressors often lessen as people age but may still continue to varying extents throughout people's lives (20).

People who are bisexual face certain challenges that are unique. While gay and lesbian people who are coming out experience feelings of being different from heterosexual peers, they may be able to find community more easily than bisexual people. When bisexual men and women first become aware of their attraction to, or have actual sexual experiences with, same-gender partners, they may feel somewhat aligned with gay and lesbian peers. However, they are also acutely aware of being different from these men and women because of the presence of simultaneous other-gender attractions. To complicate matters, bisexual people who try to connect with gay and lesbian peers for support may find themselves accused of denying their "true homosexuality." This lack of validation, coupled with the oft-cited view that bisexuals are "confused" or "just going through a phase," can inhibit identity clarification and result in significant isolation. The following case illustrates the challenge bisexual people face in having to contend with both homophobia and biphobia simultaneously (21):

Bianca, age 17, dated girls for 2 years and is "out" as a lesbian to her friends and parents. Her parents told her she'll "grow out of it" and to "focus on boys." She just met a boy whom she feels attracted to and who feels the same way. Her lesbian and gay friends say she's in denial about being lesbian and just wants to conform. She knows she isn't straight because she still has attractions to girls. She doesn't want to identify as bisexual because she doesn't know which group of kids to hang out with. She doesn't want to tell her parents about the new boyfriend because they will be thrilled and think that dating girls was just a phase. On the other hand, she thinks that maybe her parents will be less angry with her if she pretends she is straight. It's all so weird. She doesn't know what to do, and she's starting to feel really depressed.

A health care appointment may be one of the few places where Bianca can discuss her concerns openly, without censorship or emotional repercussions. She needs to be told that her attractions are normal, that whoever she is in terms of sexual orientation is okay, and that she does not need to settle on a specific identity at this point in time. She also needs some guidance on how to talk with her parents without causing harm to herself or to her family relationships. It may be helpful to provide her with a list of local or web-based bisexual community resources and reading materials so she can discover other people like herself and feel less "weird" and alone.

Like bisexual people, transgender people also often feel isolated from lesbian and gay communities. While awareness about transgender issues is increasing in LGB communities, transgender people do not always feel supported by their LGB peers. Even supportive LGB peers may not understand or relate to the unique challenges transgender people encounter during their process of exploration and transition. To work through their own internal transphobia and arrive at a positive and solid sense of self, it is critical for transgender people to find and connect with transgender communities and other knowledgeable, supportive people.

Common Coming Out Patterns

To provide sensitive and appropriate assistance to patients who are grappling with gender or sexual orientation issues, health professionals must be able to identify where patients are in the process of self-awareness and how effectively they are coping with the challenges of coming out. While coming out is a complicated process that is unique for each individual, certain aspects are common to most people's experiences. This section presents coming out theories that describe the general progression of the coming out process; cases that illustrate both positive and maladaptive coping styles are presented. In addition to reading this section, it may also be useful for health professionals to read educational materials and coming out stories that demonstrate and normalize the range of possible experiences; when relevant, these readings may also be useful to patients.

Coming Out Theories

Early coming out theories developed in the 1970s and 1980s (see Table 4-4) (22–25) drew heavily from life crisis literature (26) and, in particular, from models of bereavement developed by Kubler-Ross and others (27). The LGB individual was seen as moving through specific stages—shock, denial, anger, sadness, negotiation, and acceptance—to eventually reach a healthy resolution of the life crisis. According to these early theories, coming out begins with a subconscious sense of being different, often without awareness of why. This is followed by more conscious questioning and exploration of

Table 4–4   Stage Theories of Coming Out

Theorist, Year (Reference)	Stages
Cass, 1979 (22)	Identity confusion, identity comparison, identity tolerance, identity acceptance, identity synthesis
Coleman, 1982 (23)	Pre-coming out, coming out, exploration, first relationships, integration
Sophie, 1984 (24)	Lesbian feelings, coming out to self, coming out to others
Devine, 1984 (25)	Subliminal awareness, impact, adjustment, resolution, integration

same-gender attractions and relationships without definitive belief that one is homosexual; the process eventually progresses to clarity and acceptance of gay or lesbian identity as a fact. Initially, this definitive belief does not translate into self-acceptance, pride, or readiness to be open with others: the gay or lesbian aspect of identity is not yet integrated into the rest of one's identity or life. Achieving an open, nondefensive, and positive sense of self as a gay or lesbian person (identity synthesis or integration) is considered the final step in the process. While early theorists focused on developing and integrating identity as gay or lesbian rather than as bisexual, the process is easily applicable to bisexual people with regard to their same-sex attractions. These early coming out theories did not address transgender individuals or coming out issues.

Later theorists criticized early coming out models as excessively linear and progressive and recognized that development is a process of adaptation where growth tasks, including coming out, are creatively worked and reworked throughout the life span as new life events trigger the re-emergence of old feelings (28,29). The following case provides a good example:

Jamal, age 47, has been happily out to everyone in his life as a gay man. Over the last 2 years, 2 of his friends developed HIV infection, and a third died of complications related to AIDS. Lately, he has been feeling anxious and worries constantly about his health even though he knows his HIV test result is negative. For the first time in his life, he is dreaming of having sex with women. He is starting to believe it is unhealthy or even wrong to be gay—thoughts he has never had in the past. He ignored these thoughts initially but is starting to think he should try being straight.

Jamal's dreams and the sudden emergence of internalized homophobia were triggered by recent traumatic events: He needs help processing his reactions to his friends' diagnoses and death. Referral to an informed and nonbiased therapist to work through his feelings is likely to be helpful. He might also benefit from a support group for gay men who are not HIV infected, if one is available in his area.

An LGBTQ person's identity is repeatedly challenged and consolidated at each instance of coming out to a new person or in a new environment. Because this identity is often invisible, LGBTQ people can often make a conscious choice about whether to come out at all, when to make the announcement, and with whom they wish to share this information. It is possible to be more or less "out" or "closeted" in different situations: Some LGBTQ people are out to everyone and everywhere, while others are selectively out to friends but not to family, at school or work, or elsewhere. In some cases, choosing not to come out to certain people or in certain situations is a healthy decision made for reasons related to opportunity and safety, rather than self-loathing or shame.

At times, people who believe they are free of internalized homophobia (or biphobia or transphobia) find that negative feelings re-emerge when they attempt to come out to a new person or in a new realm of their life:

Sara, age 38, identifies as lesbian, has been publicly involved in gay rights issues, and has been out to friends for years. She is involved with a woman with whom she wants to make a long-term commitment, and she wants to share her joy about the relationship with her devoutly Catholic parents. As she prepares to come out to them for the first time, she notices feelings of guilt and shame about herself and her partner. She is shocked by the re-emergence of feelings she thought she worked out years ago. She can't sleep and is having heart palpitations.

Sara could be referred to an affirming therapist (one who is supportive of patients finding their true identity without homophobic bias) to discuss her feelings about coming out to her parents and to work on her anxiety. She might benefit from reading books on coming out to parents and referral to her local PFLAG (Parents and Friends of Lesbians and Gays, discussed later in this chapter) organization to attend a support group and have an opportunity to talk to some parents who have already gone through this process with their sons and daughters. All of these interventions are also likely to be helpful for her parents; in addition, educational materials that address homosexuality and religion specifically may help her parents with any religious dilemmas.

For bisexual people, the coming out process often involves struggling with the question of which community they belong to and should spend time with (especially when interested in meeting eligible people with whom to develop intimate relationships). Some bisexual people initially feel that they straddle 2 worlds: the straight and the LGBTQ. While gay and lesbian people can be reasonably assured (even though it is still scary) that coming out to other gay and lesbian people will be a positive or neutral experience, bisexual people can experience negative reactions from straight, gay, and lesbian people alike. Bisexual people sometimes describe feeling incompletely seen or known by others when they are in a relationship because they are assumed to be straight when with a person of the same gender, and gay or lesbian when with a person of the opposite gender. To dispel these incorrect assumptions, bisexual persons may feel the need to come out repeatedly, even when in a stable relationship or being clear in their identity for a long time.

While coming out as lesbian, gay, or bisexual involves revealing a secret about oneself in terms of inner feelings and desires, coming out as transgender involves revealing one's inner sense of self as well as changes in gender, appearance, social role, and, for some, physical anatomy. Some transgender people are "forced" out of the closet by their nontraditional gender presentation or during the process of transitioning from one gender to another, while others have greater ability to choose the timing of their coming out to others (6). Many transgender people not only come out but "cross over" to the other gender (i.e., to male or female), while some transgender people come out without choosing a binary characterization of gender. Whether crossing over or not, transgender people grapple with the challenge of developing a physical (e.g., dress, manner, body) presentation of themselves that accurately expresses their inner experience of gender identity. Sometimes this involves experimenting with a spectrum of gender expressions before settling on one stable expression. As with LGB individuals, transgender people have to contend with shame both in the process of expressing their true selves and at times when they are hiding in order to protect themselves from attacks by others (2).

A person's stage of life, concurrent life events and experiences, motivations for coming out, and relationship to the persons to whom the person is coming out all create different contexts and result in a wide variety of experiences for both the person coming out and for those in whom the LGBTQ person confides (see Figure 4-1). Health providers who are attuned to these complexities can help patients understand their motivations for coming out, consider options for how they may wish to come out, and anticipate and ready themselves to handle people's reactions.

Common Coping Strategies

Youth and adults can use several strategies to cope with internal conflicts about coming out. Some people employ the strategy of "hiding" in which they try to act and appear more stereotypically heterosexual by altering their dress, speech, or mannerisms (15). This strategy can be exhausting for LGB teens and adults who, like their heterosexual peers, often just want to "fit in." Some people try or pretend to be straight, dating and sometimes becoming sexually involved with peers of another gender, while others avoid the dating scene altogether and gain approval and self-worth by immersing themselves in academic achievement, extracurricular activities, sports, religious or spiritual quests, and other pursuits. Still others may try to cope by suppressing their feelings and awareness of their true selves by engaging in

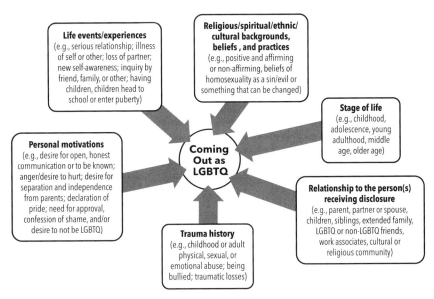

Figure 4-1 Influences on the coming out experience.

drug or alcohol abuse, sexual promiscuity, compulsive overeating, or other self-destructive behaviors that provide a diversion from unacceptable feelings and conflicts. People may also hide their secure or emerging gender status and sexual orientation from health providers. Creating an open and supportive atmosphere with affirmative literature in the office, clinic, or waiting area; asking questions and eliciting a history in open and nonbiased ways (orally and on forms); and being open-minded, flexible, and relaxed during discussions about gender and sexuality will encourage patients who hide elsewhere to consider being open in the health encounter.

Another common LGBTQ experience is one of social isolation, through either rejection by peers or dropping out of social interaction by choice. While some teens do come out, openly revealing their true selves, this can result in increased discrimination, taunting, violence, and other forms of victimization by peers, siblings, parents, and others. For LGBTQ youth who lack support, these negative messages can precipitate anxiety, depression, or suicidal behavior. Adults who are in certain geographic areas or who have not yet found or connected with local communities may also be isolated and experience similar outcomes.

Social support is a buffer that mediates the stresses related to growing up "different" (18,19). Support from family, LGBTQ community connections, and a positive intimate relationship can be especially helpful. Finding and interacting with LGB or LGBT communities and organizations can be instrumental in helping LGBTQ individuals develop more positive feelings about themselves and in combating feelings of isolation. LGBTQ support groups, gay/straight alliances that exist in some high schools, books, and web-based information can also be extremely helpful. Identifying bisexual and transgender resources can be more challenging because they are less numerous and more difficult to locate. Patients may need assistance with finding appropriate community organizations, online resources, and print materials.

While strategies such as hiding and isolation can be very prominent in adolescence, their impact is not exclusive to this age or period of development. Many adults who have not fully clarified or accepted their identity continue to use these coping strategies throughout life. Those who hid and isolated themselves as children and teens in order to cope and became more open as adults may later experience grief over having "lost time" during their younger years over being confused, closeted, self-hating, or isolated. Both teens and adults often need to work these issues out in therapy or through other forms of personal healing and development. Unfortunately, LGBTQ individuals who demonstrate gaps in development are sometimes diagnosed erroneously as having personality disturbances or other disorders. Health professionals should recognize that many LGBTQ patients require a "catch-up" period in which to experiment with what was missed earlier, including dating, exploring sexual likes and dislikes, and experiencing initial faltering attempts at developing intimate relationships. The following case describes a helpful intervention:

David (age 33) reflects on his teens and early 20s as a challenging time and recalls feeling very isolated. He found it difficult to trust others because he felt different and feared getting beaten up at school and being rejected by family and friends if he told them about his attractions to men. He avoided dating and other social activities with peers and threw himself into his schoolwork and music, excelling in those areas but missing out on some aspects of social development. Despite a successful early career life, he continued to be isolated as an adult and began to meet men at bars for anonymous sex. He started using designer drugs such as Ecstasy in the clubs, and when he got into crystal meth he spiraled downhill. His concerned health provider referred him to a gay-friendly rehab program. He is now doing 12-step work in Narcotics Anonymous and is in a gay men's support group. He feels he is gradually catching up on learning to trust other people, making friendships, and managing the dating scene. He is working avidly to overcome the shame and self-hatred he developed during years of hiding his identity. He is excited to be back at work and making new friends and feels his best years are ahead of him.

In a theory about lesbian identity "management," which also applies to GBT individuals, de Monteflores identified 4 types of adaptation approaches that are less than ideal: assimilation, confrontation, ghettoization, and

Table 4–5   Lesbian Identity Development Strategies

Defensive Strategies	Description
Assimilation	Passing as one of the mainstream group
Confrontation	Facing up to one's difference but coming out as a form of confrontation
Ghettoization	Living almost or totally exclusively within the subculture with energy put into avoiding intrusion by mainstream culture
Specialization	Seeing oneself and the subculture as possessing unique and superior qualities
Healthy integration	Recognition of sameness and difference, flexibility in boundaries between gay and straight world, inner sense of security about individual identity

Based on de Monteflores (31).

specialization (see Table 4-5) (30,31). All of these strategies are considered somewhat defensive, but de Monteflores goes on to describe a more integrated way of managing identity as follows: "The mature identity necessarily includes a recognition of sameness as well as difference. The articulation of these attributes requires a certain flexibility in boundaries, which comes out of an inner sense of security about individual identity" (31). While connection with the LGBTQ community is extremely important and supportive in healthy identity development, integration of a person's identity into non-LGBTQ venues and aspects of life is also critical for a full acceptance of self, which includes working through gender bias and internalized homophobia. In the case example above, as David becomes more secure, he comes out not only to gay friends but also to straight people. In his position as a high school music teacher, as he begins to feel more comfortable with himself over time, he comes out to colleagues and becomes the faculty advisor to the Gay-Straight Alliance in his school. Outside of school, he has started to play his trumpet in the orchestra for his town's community theater. He now feels comfortable moving between gay and straight communities.

Barriers and Benefits to Coming Out

As the coming out models describe, both self-awareness and disclosure to others are critical for development of positive self-esteem as well as for a sense of connection in relation to others. At the same time, it is important to recognize the real and formidable difficulties associated with coming out, such as stigmatization, discrimination, and even overt violence. LGBTQ individuals must negotiate numerous barriers in order to attain the benefits of coming out. This section looks more closely at some aspects of this journey.

Table 4-6   Theory of Stigmatization/Negative Attitudes toward Homosexuals

Experiential attitudes	Based on one's past interactions with homosexual people
Defensive attitudes	Reflected by people coping with their inner conflicts or anxieties about gender and sexuality by projecting them onto gay and lesbian people
Symbolic attitudes	Expressions of abstract ideologies that are close to one's notion of self and one's social network and reference group (e.g., teachings of one's religion or culture)

Based on Herek (33).

Stigmatization, Homophobia, Gender Prejudice, and Relationships With Others

Societal prejudice and stigmatization create many stresses that strongly influence LGBTQ people engaged in the developmental process of coming out (18). Collectively referred to as *minority stress*, contributing factors include subtle negative attitudes and messages; insults and discriminatory language; hate crimes (including violence assault); lack of acceptance by family members; and discrimination in many realms of daily life, such as employment, housing, child custody, adoption, tax code, and marriage (18). A parallel stigmatization occurs for people whose internal gender identity and/or external gender presentation is discordant with their biologic sex (6). If LGBTQ people recognize they will be in danger if they reveal themselves, secrecy becomes a survival strategy rather than an act of self-hatred or a sign of incomplete personal development (32). For example, silence may be the best option for a teen who lives with family and has reason to fear that she might be financially or physically abandoned or abused if she comes out, while an adult who would lose his job if he came out at work may choose to remain hidden.

According to Herek, heterosexual peoples' ambivalent or negative impressions of lesbians and gay men are shaped by experiential, defensive, and symbolically based attitudes (33) (see Table 4-6). Interestingly, experience is positively correlated with acceptance—that is, straight people with more gay or lesbian contact have less stereotyped and more positive attitudes toward gay and lesbian people. Defensiveness describes homophobic attitudes that some people project onto gay and lesbian (and bisexual) people in an attempt to cope with their own inner conflicts or anxieties about gender and sexuality. Symbolic attitudes refer to religious and/or cultural teachings that reject homosexuality. It is not hard to see how these concepts might also explain people's negative reactions to transgender people.

We are all subject to societal influences and are therefore vulnerable to making assumptions and judgments. As clinicians, we have an added duty to examine our conclusions to be sure they are soundly supported by existing data. We can check our attitudes and assumptions by asking ourselves questions such as "Do I feel negatively about this person and why?" or "Are my reactions due to ideologies I've been exposed to or a personal vulnerability or defensiveness?" or "How can I learn more about LGBTQ populations?"

Self-Esteem/Internal Issues

Herek's research explains not only the stigma and prejudice LGBTQ people experience from external sources but also illuminates how internalization of these same attitudes can lead to a deep sense of shame. The need to rid oneself of shame and to challenge stereotypes about sex and gender is clearly an issue not just for LGBTQ people but also for many straight and traditionally gendered people. However, the process of untangling feelings about issues such as body image; participation in various sexual activities; a history of childhood or adult emotional, physical, or sexual trauma; or expectations regarding sexual prowess is particularly complicated for a person who is simultaneously clarifying or coming out about their gender status or sexual orientation. The greater the level of internalized homophobia, biphobia, or transphobia, the more negative the impact on self-esteem.

As LGBTQ people encounter major life events, nontraditional gender identity and sexuality present challenges to coming out and self-esteem, which may evoke a variety of emotional reactions, such as a reawakening of shame or self-hatred, feelings of isolation, anger about societal prejudice, sadness or feelings of loss, and even rejecting or requestioning a previously solid identity. The list of potential triggering events is long and includes hormonal transitions (puberty, pregnancy, and menopause), social transitions (negotiating adolescence, changes in friendships, social communities, and intimate relationships; considering and becoming a parent; experiencing one's children's life stages or career milestones; illness and death of a parent), and experiencing illness and aging. The more unresolved childhood or adult trauma in a person's history, the greater the challenge: the more support available, the better for healing and positive development. Patients with more positive self-esteem will care for their health better than patients who are filled with shame and self-hatred. Psychotherapy with an LGBTQ-affirmative therapist can be a great resource in many situations. LGBTQ people who have strong supports and who have achieved a solid, positive gender and sexual identity frequently experience feelings of pride, strength, and accomplishment as life challenges are met successfully.

Coming Out Within the Family

Just as LGBTQ people's process of gaining self-acceptance and preparing for coming out to others takes months to years, it stands to reason that family members and others may require a parallel period in which to adjust to the news after a loved one has come out to them. While LGBTQ people may wish for rapid integration of the news and immediate acceptance, it is helpful to guide LGBTQ patients toward expectations of a process for others (parents, siblings, spouses, children, friends) that is parallel to their own process. Some of these people may then take on the additional challenge of coming out to others in their own lives about their loved one's identity. This secondary coming out involves a process that is very similar to the one the LGBTQ person experiences, sometimes requiring parents and others to grapple with insecurity, trepidation, and shame.

Families with good communication and processing skills have a far easier time with the tasks of assimilation, acceptance, and secondary coming out than families with conflict and difficult family system issues. However, all families can benefit from support: PFLAG is an excellent resource. A national organization of parents, families, and friends of LGBTQ people, PFLAG offers nonjudgmental support services in every state for parents, straight spouses, other family members, and friends, as well as LGBTQ people.

Ethnic and Cultural Diversity Issues and Coming Out

In recent years, more attention has been given to ethnic, cultural, and religious diversity issues with regard to sexual orientation, gender, and coming out. Each culture and ethnicity has its own unique nuances about gender and sexuality, the detailed examination of which is beyond the scope of this chapter. Even when speaking about what may seem to be one group, for example Latina/Latino people, there can be a multiplicity of ethnic/cultural, racial, and linguistic subgroups (34–36). Class and religious differences interact with culture and ethnicity, adding to the complexity of a person's experience of sexual and gender identity and how he or she chooses to communicate with others (37–40). This section highlights several well-documented, cross-cultural issues that affect the coming out process; however, readers should consult other resources for a greater understanding of concerns and needs of LGBTQ individuals in specific cultures, religions, and ethnicities.

In some Asian cultures, the taboo against public discussion of anything sexual creates a barrier for any discussion that might lead to coming out (41). Chan points out that in East Asian cultures, loyalty to the interests of family and community are dominant over the needs or wishes of the individual and that the concept of individual identity may not even exist (41).

Different cultures have varying norms with regard to same-gender relationships: These norms are reflected in the language that exists to describe these relationships. There are no words for *homosexuality* or *bisexuality* in some cultures (35,41). While a variety of sexual behaviors or even sustained relationships with same-gender partners may be seen as acceptable and not indicative of or described as homosexuality in some cultures, these behaviors may been seen as indicating a homosexual or bisexual identity in others (25,41,42).

Expectations of certain gender role behaviors (e.g., machismo in Latin cultures; female submissiveness in Asian cultures; and both, as in Greek culture) interact with expectations about heterosexuality, male dominance, and the family (34,41,43). Latino or African-American men may view sexual activity with other men as an acceptable part of their life while considering themselves straight, especially if they assume the "active" (dominant) rather than "passive" (receptive or submissive) position during sexual encounters, in keeping with the stereotypic masculine role. Emphasis on (heterosexual) family, child bearing and rearing, and creating future generations may also produce an intense pressure in some cultures (34,37,41).

Many models of identity development and theories about coming out consider coming out to others, for example family of origin, to be a critical and necessary step in fighting shame, denial, and self-hatred. However, accepting this concept as universal is culturally biased because independence and separation from family of origin are promoted as a sign of adult health and maturity in some cultures but not in others (32). Compromise in the service of preserving multiple aspects of one's identity is common. There are situations in which LGBTQ people can be strong and positive in their sense of self and make choices to remain closeted in some aspects of their life to preserve family connections and cultural identity. For example, in many Latin and African-American cultures, close connection to family of origin is of paramount importance, and individuals may therefore choose to conceal their LGBTQ identity in an effort to preserve their cultural identity (32,36).

Some families welcome, accept, and integrate significant others into the family without openly acknowledging the gay, lesbian, or bisexual family member's sexual orientation per se. In some cases, families can slowly be educated or conversations can be opened in incremental ways that do not destroy family cohesiveness or cultural ties. There are always costs involved in choosing incomplete disclosure, including lack of family support in understanding the burdens of living with oppression specific to life in a homophobic and gender-biased society. Clearly there are instances in which individuals choose to come out to the detriment of family relations and with loss of community connections. These losses must be grieved, and connection with other LGBTQ people from common cultural, ethnic, or religious backgrounds can be especially positive and healing in these circumstances.

Religion, Spirituality, and Coming Out

The task of reconciling one's sense of self with religious and spiritual beliefs that are frequently hostile to that identity can be extremely difficult. While some religious denominations have developed policies of being "welcoming communities" for LGBTQ people, many religious traditions continue to convey negative messages about homosexuality and gender nonconformity, including concepts of sin, eternal damnation, religious transgression, and ostracism from the spiritual community. This can lead LGBTQ people who were raised in such a tradition to a religious/spiritual crisis when coming out. Some people resolve this crisis by rejecting religion altogether, some shift to more accepting religious or spiritual traditions or form their own LGBTQ supportive religious communities, and some rework their relationship with their original spiritual or religious tradition in ways they can embrace. This can be a challenging, painful, confusing, and even frightening process. Consider the following example:

> William, age 49, is an evangelical Christian who has always believed homosexuality is sick and sinful. Although he has had close female friends for years, he reports little sexual attraction to women. He was engaged to a woman briefly but broke the engagement at the last minute. William has been aware of strong attractions to men since his early teens and has anonymous sex with men periodically, with each encounter followed by a period of severe guilt, shame, and suicidal thoughts. He sought religious counsel from his minister and was assured that he would find a spiritually healthy heterosexual life if his faith and prayer were strong enough. He has been working with a reparative therapist but continues to desire men. Feeling desperate, William presents to his doctor saying: "I can't keep living this way. Please tell me what I can do to stop thinking about men, and shift my attraction to women."

William is caught in a bind between his religious beliefs and what appears to be his natural sexuality. This is a serious situation: He needs to be carefully assessed for suicidality and should be referred to a mental health professional who has experience working in a nonjudgmental way with LGB people whose sexuality is in conflict with their religion. William needs to hear from his health provider that homosexuality is natural and healthy; that sexual orientation cannot be changed; and that many religious interpretations of the scriptures disagree with the concept of homosexuality as a sin. Referral to resources such as the website for Evangelicals Concerned (www. ecinc.org), an LGBTQ-affirming evangelical Christian community, and provision of written materials that address the intersection of homosexuality and spirituality may be very helpful. PFLAG has developed many informative pamphlets that can be ordered and displayed in waiting areas or handed out to patients.

Relationship With the Health Care System

Although the medical system considered homosexuality to be an illness for many years, this designation was dropped from the *Diagnostic and Statistical Manual of Mental Disorders* (*DSM*) in 1973 (44). "Gender identity disorder" was removed in May 2013 from the fifth edition of the *DSM* as a diagnostic category. It has been replaced by the diagnostic category "gender dysphoria," which describes people whose gender at birth is contrary to the one with which they identify. While this new categorization has been created in an attempt to be less stigmatizing than gender identity disorder, gender dysphoria is still categorized as a mental illness. The interpretation and classification of various types of transgenderism as mental illness, rather than simply as different expressions of gender or as physical variations, has a negative impact on self-esteem and efforts toward positive identity development of transgender people, much as the inclusion of homosexuality did for LGB people in the past (6).

Despite this progress, some clinicians continue to believe that homosexuality is a mental disorder and promote "conversion and reparative therapies"—"psychotherapeutic" interventions whose intent is the elimination of homosexual desire and behavior. These "treatments" directly oppose the research findings and policy statements of all the major relevant health and mental health professional associations, such as the American Psychiatric Association, American Psychological Association, National Association of Social Workers, American Academy of Pediatrics, American Counseling Association, and the American Medical Association. In 2001 the U.S. Surgeon General's "Call to Action to Promote Sexual Health and Responsible Sexual Behavior" asserted there is "no valid scientific evidence that sexual orientation can be changed" (45).

Each of the aforementioned organizations has strong policy statements opposing conversion or reparative therapies and any approach that portrays homosexuality as a disorder. The American Psychiatric Association's position statement states, in part, that "The potential risks of reparative therapy are great, including depression, anxiety and self-destructive behavior, since therapist alignment with societal prejudices against homosexuality may reinforce self-hatred already experienced by the patient" (46). The American Academy of Pediatrics statement (47) explains:

Confusion about sexual orientation is not unusual during adolescence. Counseling may be helpful for young people who are uncertain about their sexual orientation or for those who are uncertain about how to express their sexuality and might profit from an attempt at clarification through counseling or psychotherapeutic initiative. Therapy directed specifically at changing sexual orientation is contraindicated since it can provoke guilt and anxiety while having little or no potential for achieving changes in orientation.

It is not uncommon for LGBTQ people to experience periods in their coming out process when they wish they were not who they are. This phenomenon occurs both in people who are just beginning to explore their identity as well as in people who have been out for years and have had recent events or experiences that trigger old internal conflicts. It is critical that health professionals refrain from tacitly or openly suggesting that a patient's sexual orientation or gender status can or should be changed. All patients who are questioning should be directed to educational and therapeutic resources where internalized homophobia, biphobia, and/or transphobia can be addressed and feelings about possibly being gay, lesbian, bisexual, or transgender can be explored in a nonbiased and affirmative manner.

Daily Life Dilemmas and Coming Out

As discussed earlier, numerous daily life stresses are associated with being LGBTQ. Transgender people in particular face multiple unique stressors in their everyday life. For example, when transgender people are required to categorize themselves dichotomously by gender, such as on driver's license applications and other standard forms (insurance, doctor's office, hospital, marriage, and so on), they often find it necessary to come out in order to resolve the situation (2). Transgender people also face continual challenges to their identity in public venues, such as male/female restrooms, locker rooms, and dormitory sleeping arrangements (2). Whether they select the men's or women's facility, they often encounter hostility and even violence based on their choice. Transgender people encounter discrimination in every realm, including employment, housing, medical treatment, rape crisis centers, and homeless and battered women's shelters (6).

LGB people experience some of these problems as well. Discrimination, for example with regard to tax codes, insurance, and the completion of many forms, present LGB people with difficult choices that often do not reflect their identities. Many forms list a limited range of relationship options (single, married, widowed, divorced): This scheme offers no viable designations for the LGB person who is in a long-term relationship with a same-gender partner and unmarried (marriage only recently being an option in a very few places). When an LGB person lists his or her partner as next of kin or emergency contact, the door is opened to questions about the nature of that relationship and all of the risks of coming out (e.g., to a homophobic receptionist) ensue.

Health providers can help by creating intake forms that offer nonbiased options, signaling acceptance of LGBTQ people with a posted nondiscrimination policy and displays of inclusive educational materials in the waiting room, and offering sensitivity training to staff. In taking the medical history, inclusion of questions that elicit information about the entire range of gender and sexuality experiences will also promote a sense of safety and greater disclosure. Chapters 1 and 8 provide more information on these strategies.

Families with children encounter numerous dilemmas and frustrations in school systems where LGBTQ issues are not handled affirmatively. Despite the diversity of family structures across the United States, many teachers and school administrators continue to limit the notion of "family" to a mother, a father, and a child or children. They convey this bias to children and their families through insensitive comments, a lack of diversity of teaching materials in the classroom, exclusionary forms, and exercises such as Mother's or Father's Day card-making. Unfortunately, more extreme instances of outright homophobic, biphobic, or transphobic comments by teachers or by children that are tacitly condoned by teachers are still common. While these situations are clearly injurious to any child who does not fit the stereotype, they also pose stress for children of LGBTQ parents. Parents, both LGBTQ and straight, are affected by the stress being placed on their children, their family, and their own identities. While it is true that the judgment of peers can be brutal (as in the teasing or bullying of an LGBTQ youth because they are "different"), it is also true that peer voices have incredible power to effect change (witness the success of many gay/straight alliances in the schools). Health providers can serve as catalysts for change by referring families, school teachers, and administrators to programs such as PFLAG's Safe Schools Program, which provides resources to help schools become better educated and offer safer and healthier environments for children.

Coming Out as a Health Care Provider

Coming out as a health care provider can be a productive, educational, and rewarding experience for the clinician, patient, and colleagues (7) when the needs of the patient, the clinician's own motivations, and the costs and benefits of disclosure are all properly assessed. Reviewing all of the nuances of such an assessment is beyond the scope of this chapter; therefore, this section will highlight just a few major issues to be considered.

Clinicians may have a variety of motivations for coming out to a patient; similarly, patients may have many motivations for wanting (or not wanting) to know. Patients sometimes ask personal questions simply because it makes the clinician seem a little more real or human to know a little about their lives. LGBTQ patients may ask about a clinician's gender status or sexual orientation because they specifically want a provider who is LGBT; on the other hand, some patients may ask because they feel more comfortable with a provider who isn't. Reasons why clinicians may consider coming out include to reassure an LGBTQ patient that they can provide a sense of safety and support; to serve as a positive role model for both LGBTQ and heterosexual patients; and to maintain an atmosphere of openness rather than secrecy. Providers may also choose to come out to colleagues in order to relieve themselves of the burdens of hiding, to have more open collegial relationships, to be a resource or role model for other providers, or to dispel stereotypes and misperceptions about LGBTQ people.

When deciding whether to come out to a patient, clinicians should assess their own motivations carefully and consider both the potential positive and negative impact on the patient. Some patients (both heterosexual and LGBTQ) will welcome the news. On the other hand, this information might make LGBT patients feel pressured toward accepting a particular identity that may not be right or that they are not yet prepared to accept; a biased, heterosexual patient might feel frightened or alienated. When a patient asks about a clinician's identity, providers can better assess their patient's motivations and the pros and cons of coming out if they ask the patient about why she is inquiring, what she expects the answer to be, and what she would hope for and why. The provider must take the lead in helping patients to process their feelings about these issues because patients are often inhibited in this area. While choosing not to share information is a reasonable option, lying to a patient is fraught with risks to the therapeutic relationship. If tacitly or intentionally misleading information is discovered, it can cause breach of trust in or fracture of the entire alliance. It is important that providers, whether they come out or not, make it clear that they will accept the patient with whatever sexual orientation or gender identity the patient decides is right. Timing of any decision to come out is critical, especially when patients are unclear about their identity.

If for any reason a clinician feels confused or conflicted about how to approach these issues with a patient, the clinician should seek consultation from a qualified, nonjudgmental colleague.

What Providers Can Do to Help

Health professionals can play a pivotal role in the lives of LGBTQ patients who are securely established or struggling with gender identity or sexual orientation identity by providing appropriate guidance and support. The clinician–patient relationship itself can facilitate healing in that it provides a venue in which to normalize a developing LGBTQ person's questioning and an opportunity to "mirror" their emerging sense of self. This experience can be extraordinarily rewarding. Below are suggestions for how clinicians can create practices that are supportive of LGBTQ patients, particularly patients who are in the process of forming an LGBTQ identity.

Attitudes and Awareness

- Remain open to flexible, nonbinary models of gender and sexuality with all patients (not everyone initially shares their gender or sexual identity).
- Avoid assumptions based on conventional stereotypes of how LGBTQ people look and behave.
- Understand the coming out process; consider where in the coming out and life development process a person might be; what factors (internal and external) might be affecting their sense of self; and how that might be affecting their life choices, self-care, and other decisions.

- Develop awareness of how race, ethnicity, class, and religion can affect a patient's circumstances and perspective of their gender and sexuality and the process of coming out.
- Become aware of and sensitive to the bigotry and stigmatization that LGBTQ patients and their families experience in daily life and the stress it places upon them.

Skills and Practices

- Listen to how patients describe themselves and mirror their language; use nonbiased language to describe and discuss issues related to gender, sexuality, and relationships.
- Communicate that homosexuality, bisexuality, and nontraditional gender are healthy, normal, and positive expressions of gender and sexuality.
- Assess a patient's level of self-esteem and how it might be related to internalized homophobia.
- Assess a patient's connection to or isolation from LGBTQ resources and communities.
- Remain positive and affirming when talking to patients about their sexuality and gender identity.
- Include specific nonbinary questions about gender and sexuality on intake forms and in history-taking exams and discussions.
- Affirm the patient's true sense of self and/or their desire to find their true self-identity.
- Have available: (1) referrals to LGBTQ affirmative support groups, community organizations, and specialized professional mental health and health providers; (2) information on relevant LGBTQ community organizations and resources; (3) reading materials and/or lists of readings and web-based materials on LGBTQ health issues and supportive resources; and (4) resources for friends and family members of LGBTQ patients. Some family members will already be very supportive and knowledgeable while others will be uninformed and/or in crisis.
- Coming out as a health provider can be a productive, educational, and rewarding experience. The needs of the patient, the clinician's own motivations, and the costs and benefits of a disclosure must be properly assessed.

Conclusion

Coming out is a gradual and lifelong process. Healthy adjustment requires both achieving a positive sense of self and learning how to negotiate successful relationships in a world that is filled with intolerance. Clinicians can have positive, sometimes even life-altering, effects on their patients by educating themselves about and being sensitive to the needs of LGBTQ patients and family members. Understanding the nuances and complexities of "coming out" as LGBTQ will lead to more open, productive, and communicative relationships with LGBTQ patients.

Summary Points

- Coming out is the process of clarifying and accepting one's identity as LGBTQ and, when ready, revealing that identity to others. Self-acceptance of an LGBTQ identity typically evolves gradually over a period of many years.
- Gender and sexual orientation are complex and multidimensional rather than binary or unidimensional.
- Personal history and characteristics as well as the presence or absence of family and community supports all influence the experience and process of coming out. The diversity of beliefs and norms about gender and sexuality among different ethnicities, cultures, and religions also make the coming out process unique for each individual.
- Most LGB people realize their sexual orientation during their teens and early 20s, although some discover their orientation in early childhood or later in adulthood. Sometimes people become clearly aware of their sexual orientation prior to any sexual activity, while in other cases sexual exploration facilitates clarification of sexual orientation.
- Coming out as transgender involves revealing one's inner sense of self as well as changes in gender, appearance, social role, and, for some, physical anatomy. Some transgender people are "forced" out of the closet by their nontraditional gender presentation or in the process of transitioning from one gender to another, while others have greater ability to choose the timing of their coming out to others.
- Coming out to others is a dynamic and lifelong challenge. Every time LGBTQ people encounter a new person or environment they make a conscious choice about whether, when, and to whom they wish to share their identity.
- LGBTQ people may internalize societal prejudice and stigmatization and consequently develop a sense of shame, isolation, and loneliness affecting their coming out process. Social support from family, LGBTQ community connections, or a positive intimate relationship can help reduce the stresses related to feeling "different" and can promote formation of a positive identity.
- People who have difficulty with the process of self-acceptance and coming out cope with the challenges in a variety of ways. Some try to appear more stereotypically heterosexual; some become sexually and

romantically involved with other gender peers; some avoid dating altogether and immerse themselves in academic achievement and other activities that validate their self-worth; still others engage in drug and/or alcohol abuse, sexual promiscuity or other self-destructive behaviors that provide a diversion from unacceptable feelings.

- To best assist a patient who is grappling with gender or sexual orientation issues, health professionals must also be able to identify where the patient is in the process of self-awareness and how effectively they are coping with the challenges of coming out.
- Health professionals can play a pivotal role in the lives of patients who are struggling with gender or sexual identity by communicating that the patient's questioning about gender and sexuality is normal and that being LGBTQ is healthy and positive; by providing appropriate referrals; and by connecting patients to LGBT communities, organizations, publications, and support groups.

References

1. **Smith EM, Johnson SR, Guenther SM.** Health care attitudes and experiences during gynecologic care among lesbians and bisexuals. Am J Public Health. 1985;75:1085-7.
2. **Gagne P, Tewksbury R, McGaughey D.** Coming out and crossing over: identity formation and proclamation in a transgender community. Gender Society. 1997;11:478-508.
3. **Beehler GP.** Confronting the culture of medicine: gay men's experiences with primary care physicians. J Gay Lesbian Med Assoc. 2001;5:135.
4. **Rondahl G, Innala S, Carlsson M.** Nursing staff and nursing students' emotions towards homosexual patients and their wish to refrain from nursing, if the option existed. Scand J Caring Sci. 2004;18:19-26.
5. **Cole SW, Kemeny ME, Taylor SE, Visscher BR.** Elevated physical health risk among gay men who conceal their homosexual identity. Health Psychol. 1996;15:243-51.
6. **Gainor KA.** Including transgender issues in lesbian, gay and bisexual psychology: implications for clinical practice and training. In: Greene B, Croom GL, eds. Education, Research and Practice in Lesbian, Gay, Bisexual and Transgendered Psychology: A Resource Manual. Thousand Oaks, CA: Sage Publications; 2000:131-60.
7. **Potter JE.** Do ask, do tell. Ann Intern Med. 2002;137:341-3.
8. **Bonvicini KA, Perlin MJ.** The same but different: clinician-patient communication with gay and lesbian patients. Patient Educ Counsel. 2003;51:115-22.
9. **Winnecott DW.** Mirror-role of mother and family in child development. In: Playing and Reality. New York: Basic Books; 1967:111-18.
10. **Winnecott DW.** Ego distortion in terms of true and false self. In: Winnecott DW, ed. The Maturation Processes and the Facilitating Environment. New York: Int Univ Pr; 1965.
11. **Weinrich JD.** Sexual Landscapes. New York: Charles Scribner's Sons; 1987.
12. **Freud S.** Three Essays on the Theory of Sexuality. New York: Basic Books; 1962.
13. **Kinsey AC, Pomeroy WB, Martin CE.** Sexual Behavior in the Human Male. Philadelphia: WB Saunders; 1948.
14. **Kinsey AC, Pomeroy WB, Martin CE, et al.** Sexual Behavior in the Human Female. Philadelphia: WB Saunders; 1953.

15. **Hunter J, Mallon GP.** Lesbian, gay and bisexual adolescent development: dancing with your feet tied together. In: Greene B, Croom GL, eds. Education, Research, and Practice in Lesbian, Gay, Bisexual, and Transgendered Psychology: A Resource Manual. Thousand Oaks, CA: Sage Publications; 2000:226-43.

16. **D'Augelli AR.** Lesbian, gay, and bisexual development during adolescence and young adulthood. In: Cabaj RP, Stein TS, eds. Textbook of Homosexuality and Mental Health. Washington, DC: American Psychiatric Pr; 1996:267-88.

17. **Malyon AK.** The homosexual adolescent: developmental issues and social bias. Child Welfare. 1981;60:321-30.

18. **DiPlacido J.** Minority stress among lesbians, gay men and bisexuals; a consequence of heterosexism, homophobia, and stigmatization. In: Herek GM, ed. Stigma and Sexual Orientation: Understanding Prejudice Against Lesbians, Gay Men and Bisexuals. Thousand Oaks, CA: Sage Publications; 1998:138-59.

19. **Meyer IH, Dean L.** Internalized homophobia, intimacy and sexual behavior among gay and bisexual men. In: Herek GM, ed. Stigma and Sexual Orientation: Understanding Prejudice Against Lesbians, Gay Men and Bisexuals. Thousand Oaks, CA: Sage Publications; 1998: 160-86.

20. **The Medical Foundation.** Health Concerns of the Gay, Lesbian, Bisexual and Transgender Community. 2nd ed. Boston: Massachusetts Department of Public Health; June 1997.

21. **Fox RC.** Bisexuality in perspective: a review of theory and research. In: Greene B, Croom GL, eds. Education, Research, and Practice in Lesbian, Gay, Bisexual, and Transgendered Psychology: A Resource Manual. Thousand Oaks, CA: Sage Publications; 2000:161-206.

22. **Cass VC.** Homosexual identity formation: a theoretical model. J Homosex. 1979;4:219-35.

23. **Coleman E.** Developmental stages of coming out. J Homosex. 1982;7:31-43.

24. **Sophie J.** A critical examination of stage theories of lesbian identity development. J Homosex. 1984;12:39-51.

25. **Devine JL.** A systemic inspection of affectional preference orientation and the family of origin. J Social Work Human Sexual. 1984;2:9-17.

26. **Lazarus RS, Folkman S, eds.** Stress, Appraisal, and Coping. New York: Springer; 1984.

27. **Kubler-Ross E.** On Death and Dying. New York: MacMillan; 1969.

28. **Weick A.** A growth-task model of human development. Social Casework. 1983;64:131-7.

29. **Raphael B.** The Anatomy of Bereavement. New York: Basic Books; 1983.

30. **Falco KL.** Psychotherapy With Lesbian Clients: Theory Into Practice. New York: Brunner/ Mazel; 1991.

31. **de Monteflores C.** Notes on the management of difference. In: Stein TS, Cohen CJ, eds. Contemporary Perspectives on Psychotherapy with Lesbians and Gay Men. New York: Plenum; 1986:73-101.

32. **Smith A.** Cultural diversity and the coming out process: implications for clinical practice. In: Greene B, ed. Ethnic and Cultural Diversity Among Lesbians and Gay Men. Thousand Oaks, CA: Sage Publications; 1997:279-300.

33. **Herek GM.** Beyond homophobia: a social psychological perspective on attitudes towards lesbians and gay men. J Homosex. 1984;10:1-21.

34. **Gonzalez FJ, Espin OM.** Latino men, Latina women and homosexuality. In: Cabaj RP, Stein TS, eds. Textbook of Homosexuality and Mental Health. Washington, DC: American Psychiatric Pr; 1996:583-602.

35. **Nakajima GA, Chan YH, Lee K.** Mental health issues for gay and lesbian Asian Americans. In: Cabaj RP, Stein TS, eds. Textbook of Homosexuality and Mental Health. Washington, DC: American Psychiatric Pr; 1996:563-82.

36. **Greene B.** Ethnic minority lesbians and gay men: mental health and treatment issues. In: Greene B, ed. Ethnic and Cultural Diversity Among Lesbians and Gay Men. Thousand Oaks, CA: Sage Publications; 1997:240-8.

37. **Dworkin SH.** Female, lesbian and Jewish: complex and invisible. In: Greene B, ed. Ethnic and Cultural Diversity Among Lesbians and Gay Men. Thousand Oaks, CA: Sage Publications; 1997:63-87.

38. **Haldeman D.** Spirituality and religion in the lives of gay and lesbian Americans. In: Cabaj RP, Stein TS, eds. Textbook of Homosexuality and Mental Health. Washington, DC: American Psychiatric Pr; 1996:881-96.

39. **Cerbone AR.** Symbol of privilege, object of derision: dissonance and contradictions. In: Greene B, ed. Ethnic and Cultural Diversity Among Lesbians and Gay Men. Thousand Oaks, CA: Sage Publications; 1997:117-31.

40. **Tafoya T.** Native gay and lesbian issues: two spirited people. In: Greene B, ed. Ethnic and Cultural Diversity Among Lesbians and Gay Men. Thousand Oaks, CA: Sage Publications; 1997:1-10.

41. **Chan CS.** Don't ask, don't tell, don't know: the formation of a homosexual identity and sexual expression among Asian American lesbians. In: Greene B, ed. Ethnic and Cultural Diversity Among Lesbians and Gay Men. Thousand Oaks, CA: Sage Publications; 1997:240-8.

42. **Kite ME.** When perceptions meet reality: individual differences in reactions to lesbians and gay men. In: Greene B, Herek GM, eds. Lesbian and Gay Psychology: Theory, Research and Clinical Applications. Thousand Oaks, CA: Sage Publications; 1994:25-53.

43. **Fygetakis LM.** Greek American lesbians: identity odysseys of honorable good girls. In: Greene B, ed. Ethnic and Cultural Diversity Among Lesbians and Gay Men. Thousand Oaks, CA: Sage Publications; 1997:152-90.

44. **Greene B.** Lesbian and gay sexual orientations: implications for clinical training, practice and research. In: Greene B, Herek GM, eds. Lesbian and Gay Psychology: Theory, Research and Clinical Applications. Thousand Oaks, CA: Sage Publications; 1994:1-24.

45. U.S. Surgeon General's Call to Action to Promote Sexual Health and Responsible Sexual Behavior. Washington, DC: U.S. Department of Health and Human Services; July 9, 2001.

46. **American Psychiatric Association.** Position statement (1998): psychiatric treatment and sexual orientation. In: Just the Facts About Sexual Orientation and Youth: A Primer for Principals, Educators, and School Personnel. Washington, DC: American Psychological Association; 2008. Available at: www.apa.org/pi/lgbc/publications/justthefacts.html.

47. **American Academy of Pediatrics.** Policy statement (1993): homosexuality and adolescence. Just the Facts About Sexual Orientation and Youth: A Primer for Principals, Educators, and School Personnel. Washington, DC: American Psychological Association; 2008. Available at: www.apa.org/pi/lgbc/publications/justthefacts.html.

Chapter 5

Caring for LGBTQ Youth

TRAVIS A. GAYLES, MD, PhD
ROBERT GAROFALO, MD, MPH

Introduction

Adolescence and young adulthood (ages 12 to 24 years) is a time when most people begin to explore and construct their own identities, sometimes clashing with parental and community norms. Youth who come to recognize they are lesbian, gay, bisexual, transgender, and/or queer/questioning (LGBTQ) must not only navigate traditional developmental milestones but often do so within the context of stigma, discrimination, and societal and familial disapproval of their sexual and/or gender identity. To put this in some perspective, an online survey of over 10,000 adolescents found that while non-LGBTQ youth listed grades, college, and career as their top three concerns, LGBTQ youth listed nonaccepting families, school/bullying problems, and fear of being out as their chief concerns (1).

Economically and socially, adolescents are largely dependent on family and peers for guidance. When these networks do not permit adequate room for communication and connection with individuals who have similar experiences, LGBTQ youth may find themselves with insufficient support (2–4). As a result, some LGBTQ adolescents may feel isolated and marginalized; they may internalize feelings of shame and hatred. Such psychological and social stressors can have significant, negative effects on health and well-being: For example, LGBTQ youth are at higher risk than the general youth population for suicide attempts, bullying victimization, substance abuse, homelessness (due to family rejection), and sexual risk behaviors (2,5–9). However, despite this grim picture, most LGBTQ youth manage to overcome these challenges successfully and go on to lead healthy, well-adjusted lives, largely without additional stressors.

Health care providers are well positioned to assist LGBTQ-identified youth, as well as youth who are struggling with emerging sexual or gender identity issues, in making this developmental stage a time of healthy discovery, self-acceptance, and increasing autonomy. This requires creating a welcoming clinical environment and learning how to ask nonjudgmental questions about sexuality, sexual orientation, and gender identity, as not all adolescents will describe themselves as openly LGBT or Q at the time of their initial presentation. Primary care providers must also learn to address concerns about sexual and gender identity, as well as social and psychological stressors that may accompany sexual or gender minority status, with the same vigor as they would with any physical ailment. The clinical setting may be the only environment in which a youth feels safe enough to seek assistance and guidance.

Goals When Treating the Adolescent Patient

For adolescents, access to health services is influenced by the balance between their status as minors, their budding sexuality, and their need for confidential, culturally competent care. Traditionally, reproductive rights, access to contraception, and sexual health topped the list of topics related to adolescent medicine. In the 1960s, the women's rights movement forced society to deal with young people's ability to consent to medical treatment and thereby increased their access to informed, confidential health care. For LGBTQ youth, the HIV epidemic further highlighted the importance of access to culturally competent sexual health care for minors and adolescents. Today, adolescent patients often present for medical care with concerns about sexuality or sexual risk behaviors. As a result, adult and pediatric providers need to overcome any feelings of discomfort with these issues and prepare themselves to address sexuality and sexual activity as part of routine care for their adolescent patients.

Overall, the goals for LGBTQ health care are identical to those of any adolescent population: 1) to promote healthy development, 2) to promote social and emotional well-being, and 3) to promote and ensure physical health (10). Thus, health care providers should view LGBTQ adolescents within the context of general adolescent development while maintaining a firm understanding of specific issues this population may face as a result of their emerging sexual and/or gender identity.

The Clinical Environment

Patient-Provider Relationship

The quality of the patient–provider relationship is of key importance in facilitating adherence of LGBTQ youth to recommended screenings and easing the transition to healthy adulthood. A first medical visit often sets the tone for future access to care, risk reduction, help-seeking behavior, and adult physical and social health. While communication can be challenging, creating a safe, open, and honest dialogue should be the provider's primary objective with all adolescent patients, including those who may be LGBTQ.

Obtaining a truthful history and making an adolescent feel comfortable within the clinical encounter are critical first steps in addressing a youth's comprehensive health care needs.

When dealing with adolescents, the patient–provider relationship is a balancing act for both parties. The patient, caught between being a child and adulthood, is often uncomfortable discussing sensitive topics with parents or guardians in exam rooms or, conversely, accessing health care alone for the very first time. Adolescents seeing a clinician with their parents present may have reasonable fears about disclosure of their sexual orientation or gender identity, causing some to withhold information. For youth experiencing difficulties at home, this can result in missed opportunities to obtain needed support and guidance and can be particularly distressing. These issues highlight the need for providers to interview adolescents without parents or others in the examination room. A provider might introduce this process by saying something like: *"Today we're going to spend some time talking together about Robin's health. I'll address any questions you or she have, and then I'll also spend some time alone with Robin. At the end of the visit we'll come back together and talk again."* If the parent or patient shows reluctance, the provider could try framing the process in the context of adolescent self-responsibility and self-reliance.

When accessing health care alone, however, LGBTQ youth may struggle with language and with initiating discussion about potentially embarrassing topics such as sexual activity. They may be evasive when asked about their lives, health, or reason for the medical visit. Without the traditional buffer of having a parent or caregiver present, office procedures and exams may be uncomfortable or unfamiliar.

Ultimately, it is the provider who bears responsibility for carefully navigating the adolescent visit and for firmly establishing a level of trust and privacy. It is important to remember that even at a very young age, some LGBTQ adolescents engage in risky behaviors that can negatively affect their health (11). The provider serving the LGBTQ adolescent patient will need to deftly elicit a medical history while allowing the patient to feel both autonomous and safe during the visit. Safety starts with making the office space welcoming with posters or flyers that are not exclusively heterosexual in nature (see Appendix A for other suggestions). In addition, support staff require training about issues of importance to adolescent patients such as privacy and autonomy. Once engaged in the clinical encounter, it is the provider, rather than the patient, who must conduct a complete psychosocial and physical assessment and develop a health care plan that addresses each patient's unique needs.

Confidentiality

As previously mentioned, confidentiality is a major concern for LGBTQ adolescents (3). Many adolescents report forgoing health care that they believed was necessary, in part because of the fear that their parents will discover they attempted to access care (12,13). For LGBTQ adolescents, concerns regarding confidentiality may be complicated by additional fears concerning the advertent or inadvertent disclosure of their sexual orientation or gender identity (3). For example, even when the medical provider prioritizes patient confidentiality, other members of the health care team, such as medical assistants, receptionists, or nursing staff, can accidentally or purposefully disclose a youth's LGBTQ identity. Therefore, it is critically important that confidentiality be safeguarded by everyone in the medical environment.

Providers need to familiarize themselves with individual state laws and the statutes that govern adolescents' right to access confidential health care services. In every state, statutes differ regarding consent and parental notification (see www.guttmacher.org/graphics/gr030406_f1.html for a summary by state); however, each state allows minors to consent to treatment without parental consent under certain circumstances, such as seeking family planning services, treatment for sexually transmitted infections or HIV, and emergency care.

Parameters surrounding the confidentiality of health care services, including circumstances in which confidentiality may be broken (e.g., when an adolescent is acutely suicidal) should be reviewed on the first visit and then regularly thereafter. It is important to also inform parents or guardians about the parameters and importance of confidential care. Finally, providers should always clarify with patients what information is okay to share with parents.

Access to Care

Behavioral and physical health care tailored to the unique developmental needs of adolescents is often difficult to find and navigate, especially for those who are LGBTQ. Financing a health care visit can also be particularly challenging for many LGBTQ adolescents, who may fear an inadvertent disclosure of their sexual and/or gender identity should their parents' health insurance be used to cover a visit. Providers should be aware that the "Explanation of Benefits" form that parents may receive from a medical insurance company following a visit may pose a risk to an adolescent's desire to remain anonymous. Youth older than age 18 years may face additional challenges because they may be too old for state or federally funded health insurance programs but are not yet qualified for employer-based coverage. Fortunately, new provisions of the Affordable Care Act offer dependent coverage under a parent's insurance plan until a youth reaches the age of 26, which will help to address coverage lapses.

However, despite improved insurance coverage, the availability of truly culturally competent care for LGBTQ adolescents continues to be elusive. Barriers created by pervasive societal stigma, secrecy surrounding sexual orientation or gender identity, and a lack of knowledge about where to find

LGBTQ-friendly providers make access to care especially challenging for this population (2,3). In order to offer comprehensive care to LGBTQ youth, resources must be established that are readily available and barrier-free. For example, "closeted" LGBTQ youth may be able to seek health care services only in public health clinics, facilities catering to the uninsured, or other medical settings where they may more easily maintain their anonymity (5). Disproportionate socioeconomic factors, such as unemployment, homelessness, and lack of transportation, pose additional challenges for some young LGBTQ patients. For these youth, social and financial support, such as case management, bus tokens, and support groups, may help promote and facilitate access to care.

Conducting the Patient Interview

The chief medical complaint is frequently not the primary cause for an adolescent visit. Healthy adolescents seldom have reason for a "physical," but they trust that the questioning of an astute clinician may ultimately lead to a discussion of their true concern. Sometimes, however, the medical visit is prompted by symptoms the patient considers related to a sexually transmitted infection (STI) or to anxiety following an anonymous or otherwise high-risk sexual encounter. These visits represent opportunities for both medical care and significant education regarding sexual risk behaviors and family planning. In the adolescent population, even the most benign chief complaints can sometimes evolve into more complicated discussions offering the provider an opportunity for further investigation into potential areas of concern. Therefore, whether the presenting complaint is acne or cold symptoms, the primary care provider should always ask: "Do you have any other problems, have any questions, or want anything else checked out while you're here?"

With an adolescent, the patient interview is the most vital element of the office visit. As noted above, a thorough, guided history provides more information than a youth will generally volunteer. With adolescents, a thorough history is a dialogue that not only elicits information but also helps establish rapport. During the taking of a history, LGBTQ youth begin to understand what topics are relevant and important for present and future visits. Sensitive topics need to be addressed carefully and unapologetically with language that is easy to understand.

Discussing Sexual Orientation and Gender Identity

The goal of the medical history is not to identify all youth who identify as gay, lesbian, or transgender but rather to create an environment in which all adolescents, including those with emerging LGBTQ identities, feel comfortable asking questions, can seek help and support, and can obtain appropriate medical services. In general, providers should avoid making assumptions about a patient's self-identification or the extent to which LGBTQ youth have already shared their sexual orientation or gender identity with friends or family members. Providers need to give youth space in which to self-define and should rely on those definitions when they address clinical issues. It can be helpful to ask, "Do you consider yourself gay, lesbian, bisexual, hetero-sexual (straight), or some other term, or are you not sure?" Terms used in self-identification may vary considerably across racial or ethnic, gender, and socioeconomic groups. For example, many youth prefer to self-identify as *queer*, which they may see as a more empowering, gender neutral, and inclusive term than *gay* or *lesbian*. Some young men, particularly those from rural areas or communities of color, may identify as publicly hetero-sexual but engage in same-sex behavior with other men (5). Youth from these communities may not feel comfortable disclosing their sexual and/or gender identity to health care providers until they have fully integrated and accepted it themselves. Chapter 4 discusses the use of self-identification terms in more detail.

Taking the Social History

Although adolescents tend to be physically healthy, risk reduction in the realms of social and behavioral health is a cornerstone of the adolescent visit. The first step toward addressing risk is to thoughtfully and caringly assess and screen for leading health risks. This is done primarily through the social history. As with all adolescents, social history-taking from LGBTQ youth can be guided by the acronym HEADS: *H*—home; *E*—education; *A*—activities; *D*—depression/drugs/diet; *S*—safety/sexuality. Providers not only should recognize social issues that arise in general adolescent popula-tions but must also become adept at addressing issues and health threats unique to the LGBTQ experience (Table 5-1). A thorough social history also includes an assessment of the amount of exposure to and effect of social

Table 5–1   Top Health Risks of Lesbian, Gay, Bisexual, Transgender, Queer/Questioning Adolescents

HIV/AIDS

Smoking and other substance use

Depression and suicide

Sexually transmitted infections

Abuse and victimization

Stigma and heterosexism

Homelessness

Access to care

Isolation, marginalization, and lack of social support

media (e.g., Facebook, Twitter, text messaging) and other Internet-based media. On the plus side, the Internet can serve as a powerful social networking tool among youth, especially those who have little familial and environmental support. It allows access to online LGBTQ communities that have been traditionally difficult to find and can provide LGBTQ youth with health-related information (14). On the negative side, the Internet provides ready access to anonymous and high-risk sexual encounters, with attendant risks of intimidation and victimization, which will be discussed later in this chapter.

The following section considers "can't miss" clinical issues and key aspects of the social history that should be covered during the LGBTQ patient interview. Many of these issues are dealt with in greater detail elsewhere in this book; therefore, our discussion will focus on issues specific to the LGBTQ adolescent experience. Table 5-2 provides examples of adolescent-friendly questions that may facilitate the interview.

Table 5-2   Adolescent Patient Interview: Sample Questions

Sexual activity history

Do you have sex with men (boys), women (girls), or both?

Some of my patients your age begin to find themselves attracted to other people. Have you ever been romantically or sexually attracted to men (boys), women (girls), or both?

Have you ever dated or gone out with someone? Are you currently dating or in a relationship with a boy or a girl?

There are many ways of being sexual or intimate with another person: kissing, hugging, touching, having oral sex, anal sex, or vaginal sex. Have you ever had any of these experiences? Which ones? Were they with boys, girls, or both?

How do you protect yourself against sexually transmitted infections and pregnancy?

When you use condoms for anal (or vaginal) sex do you use them 5%, 50%, 75%, or 100% of the time? Are there times that you don't use condoms when you are having sex?

Do you have sex (oral, anal, or vaginal) with anyone other than your boyfriend or girlfriend? If so, how often do you use condoms in these situations?

Has anyone ever pressure you or forced you into doing something sexually that you didn't want to do?

Disclosure of sexual and gender identity

What term (if any) do you prefer that I use to best describe your sexual orientation? For example, do you consider yourself gay, lesbian, bisexual, heterosexual (straight), another term, or are you not sure?

Have you ever talked to your parents, brothers or sisters, or any other adult besides me about this? Any of your friends? What did they say?

Have you thought about disclosing your sexuality to your parents or friends? Are you concerned at all about their response or your safety?

Was coming out stressful? Or, do you get stressed out thinking about coming out?

It is normal for young people to sometimes be confused about their feelings and experiences. Do you have any questions you'd like to ask me or things you would like to talk about?

(continued)

Table 5–2   Adolescent Patient Interview: Sample Questions (*Continued*)

Mental health and depression

Over the past few weeks, have you ever felt down or depressed? Have you had less interest in doing things that you normally enjoy?

Have you ever thought about hurting yourself? Have you ever actually tried to hurt yourself? What did you do and tell me what happened?

Have you ever been treated for depression or other psychological issues? Have you ever been in the hospital for these issues or for trying to hurt yourself?

Who do you turn to when you are down or lonely or need someone to talk to?

Do you have a close friend or family member that is a good source of support?

Have you ever thought about seeing a counselor or therapist? Do you think that might be helpful?

Tobacco, alcohol, and other substance use

Do you currently smoke cigarettes? How much and for how long? Have you ever tried quitting? Do you need or want help quitting?

Do you drink alcohol? How often? Where do you get it, and who do you drink with? How many drinks do you typically have? Do you ever get drunk?

Have you ever used any other drugs such as marijuana, cocaine, Ecstasy, GHB, crystal meth? Which drugs do you currently use? How often?

Do you think your alcohol or drug use is a problem? Would you like help in trying to quit?

Do you have any questions about any drugs or drug use that I might be able to answer?

Do you ever have sex while drunk or high? Have you ever done something sexually while high or drunk that you regretted or didn't really want to do?

Have you ever driven a car or motor vehicle while high or drunk? Have you ever taken a ride from someone else who was high or drunk?

Safety and violence

How are things going at home or at school? Do you feel safe when you are at home? Do you feel safe in your neighborhood and at school?

How would you describe your school, home, neighborhood in terms of support for LGBTQ people?

Has anyone ever picked on you? Can you tell me about it? Was this because you are LGBTQ?

Have you ever missed school because of feeling unsafe?

Have you ever been in a fight at school with someone who was picking on you?

Have you ever brought a weapon to school because of feeling unsafe?

Have you stopped participating in any activities due to being picked on?

Who can you turn to for advice, support or protection?

Have you ever picked on anyone? Can you tell me about it? What was your reasoning for doing so?

Are you in a relationship? If so, do you feel safe with your partner?

Social media

Do you use social media, such as Facebook or Twitter? If so, tell me about it (How often? What do you use if for? Are your parents aware?)

How do you find out information about health related issues?

Do you have a cell phone? If so, what do you use if for? How often? Are your parents aware?

Do you use the Internet? If so, what do you use it for?

GHB = gamma-hydroxybutyrate.

Sexual History and Sexual Health

Questions and concerns regarding sex, dating, and sexuality are often foremost in the minds of adolescents during a nonurgent primary care visit. Nonetheless, LGBTQ adolescents may hide their concerns because of fear, shame, or embarassment, particularly if it requires them to disclose same-sex sexual activity or attraction. When approaching the sexual history with LGBTQ adolescents, it is helpful to normalize this part of the interview by using the same relaxed and open tone of voice as when discussing the rest of the social history. If patients seem hesitant, reminding them that the discussion is confidential may help. Providers should be prepared to hear about a variety of sexual behaviors and sexual partners, all of which can be an integral part of healthy identity formation (3).

Asking straightforward questions, such as, "Have you ever dated or gone out with someone?"

"Are you currently dating or in a relationship with a boy or a girl?" "Are you having sex?" is an excellent way to initiate the discussion. Following up with "Do you have sex with men (boys), women (girls), or both?" allows patients to know that it is okay to disclose same-sex activities. Note that the commonly used question "Are you sexually active?" can be misinterpreted in terms of meaning as well as timeframe and should be used with caution. For youth who have not yet initiated sexual activity, providers may wish to ask, "Are you romantically or sexually attracted to men (boys), women (girls), or both?" This allows LGBTQ youth to discuss their emerging feelings and understand it is safe to come out in this setting. Ask these questions of all patients: Avoid making assumptions about who is and who is not sexually active. For example, do not assume a younger adolescent or an "honors student" has not had sex. Similarly, do not assume that an LGBTQ adolescent has had sex. Many are aware of their sexuality before they have engaged in any sexual activity. To assume otherwise can be very damaging to the patient–provider relationship.

After the opening questions, it is important to follow-up with more detailed questions about types of sexual activity as well as use of protection, not only for risk assessment purposes but also because "sex" can be interpreted in multiple ways. Masturbation, petting, and oral sex are associated with vastly different risks for the acquisition of STIs, but to many youth, each may fall under the category of "not really" sex at all. Even anal sex, particularly for some young women, may not be considered "being sexually active" since it does not carry the risk of pregnancy, and for some, allows them to preserve their virginity. Providers should therefore ask specific questions, without judgment, about the types of sex patients are having to get an accurate picture of the sexual risk behavior profile of each LGBTQ adolescent patient. This includes asking about anal and oral sex, regardless of the patient's gender or gender identity. Providers should use anatomically specific terminology, avoid medical jargon, and ask questions and deliver information in language easily understood by the adolescent. By asking these questions, providers avoid making assumptions about which patients are at risk for pregnancy, HIV, and other STIs. This is beneficial not only for appropriate screening, care, and education but also for patient rapport.

Health protective behaviors (e.g., consistency of condom use), age of sexual debut, and history of sexual trauma (at any age) are also important lines of questioning. When asking about condom use, providers should avoid yes/no questions such as, "Do you use condoms for sexual activity?" and use open-ended questions instead, such as, "What do you use for protection when you have sex?" and "When you use condoms for anal (or vaginal) intercourse do you use them 5%, 50%, 75%, or 100% of the time?" When an adolescent reports less than 100% condom use, the provider has an opportunity to explore the social context of inconsistent condom use. This information is likely to be invaluable in designing a targeted prevention strategy that is relevant and meaningful for the adolescent.

Regarding sexual trauma, the tragic reality is that sexual abuse, incest, and rape may expose adolescents to STIs and HIV, without consent, at an early (or any) age. A history of sexual trauma is seldom identified without specific questions in this area. Adolescents with a sexual trauma history may not report these experiences during the routine sexual history because the abuse was neither consensual nor initiated by the patient, and therefore they do not perceive themselves as having been "sexually active." Unfortunately, however, the risk for infection or pregnancy may still be present, highlighting the need for specific questioning. Youth experiencing sexual trauma may present with other confounding symptoms (e.g., depression, cutting behavior) and need additional support. Some research suggests that rates of childhood sexual abuse may be higher among LGBTQ youth and that these experiences are associated with future negative health outcomes, such as high-risk sexual behaviors, substance use, and psychological distress (15,16).

Asking about partnerships and same-sex loving relationships can also help to establish an open line of communication between the LGBTQ adolescent and the medical provider. When asking about dating, romantic, or sexual partners, providers should use gender neutral language (e.g., avoid using terms such as *boyfriend* or *girlfriend*) unless instructed otherwise. This sends a subtle but important message to the LGBTQ adolescent that the provider is open to discussing same-sex relationships or concerns and may facilitate disclosure of same-sex feelings or behaviors when the adolescent is comfortable doing so. Whenever a same-sex relationship is disclosed, acknowledgment and acceptance are critical, as is routine inquiry into the overall quality and safety of the relationship (just like with any patient).

The fluidity of sexual expression in the young LGBTQ population can present a challenge to sexual history-taking and discussions regarding sexual activity, as many youth today may not identify with a binary or finite model of sexual and/or gender identity. Reclaiming of the term *queer* as an affirmative and often preferred term of self-identification is a perfect example of the fluidity of sexual expression and demonstrates how this generation of youth is to a large extent dissatisfied with traditional labels of sexual orientation and sexual expression. This may make providers uncomfortable, particularly those accustomed to thinking of "queer" as a pejorative term. Whether self-identified as gay, lesbian, or queer, it is not uncommon for a young person to have concerns about their "girlfriend" on one visit but then change this to "boyfriend" on a subsequent visit. Young patients may have started dating a partner of a different gender or may simply have become more comfortable now disclosing the true gender of their partner to a trusted provider over time. Or, as in the case of some transgender youth, where gender differs from anatomically defined sex, they or their partner may have changed their own gender identity. Overall, with the adolescent patient, nonbinary models of sexual orientation and gender identity are common and labels are often difficult to characterize. Whether or not youth classify themselves as LGBTQ, careful and thorough history-taking—particularly with regard to the sex and gender of partners, types of sexual activity, and consistency of safe sexual activity—will give providers the information needed to provide accurate and helpful preventive health education and medical advice.

Although discussions of sexual activity among LGBTQ youth are often directed toward young gay and bisexual men or transgender youth because of their disproportionate risk for acquiring HIV or other STIs, specific mention should be made regarding how to address sexual health issues with young lesbian and bisexual women. When young women have sex with women or self-identify as lesbian, gay, or bisexual, their sexual behavior and identity, like other developmental constructs in adolescence, may be permanent, nonexclusive, or fluid. In all cases, in obtaining a thorough risk assessment it is best to ask, "Some lesbians have also had sex with men. Have you ever had sex with men? If so, when was the last time?" While lesbian and bisexual young women are often perceived as a "low-risk" group, in reality women who have sex with women can be at risk for many STIs and may engage in risky sex with male partners.

For example, in a Chicago-based study of women who have sex with women aged 16 to 24 years, 58% reported a history of oral sex with a male partner (41% in the past year), 20% reported a history of pregnancy, and 26% reported a history of receptive anal intercourse with a male partner (17). Young lesbian and bisexual women, like other adolescents, are more likely to engage in high-risk sexual behaviors under the influence of drugs or alcohol (17). When caring for a young lesbian or bisexual woman, it is therefore important to take a comprehensive substance use history alongside the sexual history and to provide counseling about health risks, including the need for safer-sex precautions, contraception, and routine gynecological care, as appropriate. It is also important to ask about sexual or romantic desire or attraction and to keep in mind that definitions of sexual activity may vary.

Psychological History and Mental Health

LGBTQ youth experience the same range of mental health concerns as all adolescents, with additional distress at times created by the need to manage stigma associated with their sexual minority identity (3,18). Adolescence is a time when mental heath issues, including depression, anxiety, psychosis, and bipolar symptoms, may first emerge. Mental health needs identified in adolescence may present in atypical ways, such as missed school or withdrawal from previously enjoyed activities and hobbies. As in adults, adolescent mental health needs can be chronic or episodic. In the case of depression, vulnerabilities and external stressors unique to adolescence or the LGBTQ adolescent experience may trigger a major or episodic depressive episode. For example, "coming out" or beginning to experiment with same-sex sexual partners can be distressing to LGBTQ youth and may cause internal psychological conflict or perceived or actual conflict with family and peers (7). In addition, life changes and transitions that by and large define adolescence are often major psychological stressors, such as adjusting to a new school or peer group, entering college, transition to independent living, and/or finding employment. Compounding the problem, these life challenges often occur simultaneously or in quick succession, which may further accentuate the stress experienced by some LGBTQ youth. In general, life problems that may seem minor to some adults, such as breaking up with a boyfriend or girlfriend or unhappiness with physical appearance caused by acne or obesity, can be major triggers in youth.

Suicide is a leading cause of death among U.S. adolescents overall and has been postulated as the leading cause of death among LGBTQ youth. Much has been written about suicide risk in LGBTQ youth, and although available data consistently support the notion of "increased suicide risk" in this population, this interpretation requires caution (19–23). In a Massachusetts study, lesbian, gay, and bisexual youth were more than 3 times more likely to self-report "a suicide attempt in the past 12 months" compared with their heterosexual peers (19). However, the precise clinical meaning of the self-reported term "suicide attempt" is unclear when considered in the context of a broad continuum that extends from suicidal thoughts and feelings on the one hand to behaviors including actual attempts and completed suicides on the other hand. In reality, little is known about the actual number of suicides among LGBTQ youth or related to distress over sexual orientation or gender identity specifically, as data collected from death certificates and psychological autopsies cannot accurately ascertain sexual orientation or gender identity status. Moreover, many LGBTQ youth who attempt or commit suicide may never have discussed their sexual orientation or identity with anyone because of fear and anxiety surrounding disclosure.

While it may be tempting to discount alarming statistics about LGBTQ suicide that seem inconsistent with clinical experience, it is important for providers to remain mindful of this possibility (10,21). Suicide risk in all adolescents is associated with a common set of predisposing influences, including family dysfunction, depression, isolation, loss of family or friends, and alcohol and other substance use—issues that may be exacerbated in LGBTQ youth, particularly those youth who lack appropriate social support (3,19,24,25). Research shows that distressed patients frequently visit their primary care providers in the days, weeks, or months preceding a successful suicide, highlighting the importance of conducting a thorough psychological assessment in the primary care setting (26). Prompt identification of distress provides an opportunity for early intervention, when needed.

The psychological health and well-being of LGBTQ youth can be assessed by asking specific questions about behavioral health history, including hospitalization for issues such as clinical depression or suicidal ideation and/or use of psychoactive medications. This history should be obtained in person, although some clinicians may opt to include questionnaires or patient-administered self-assessment tools as adjuncts to the provider interview. It is also important to ascertain a family history of mental illness because depression, bipolar disease, and psychosis can all have a hereditary component. Inquiry regarding a family history of mental illness may need to be done initially with a parent or guardian present, as many adolescents may not be aware of these issues. Providers caring for LGBTQ youth may also wish to use general screening questions for depression, such as, "Over the past 2 weeks have you felt down, depressed, hopeless?" or "Over the past 2 weeks, have you felt little interest or pleasure in doing things?" Affirmative responses to either or both questions may warrant further assessment or intervention. Asking about available sources of support with questions such as, "Who do you turn to when you feel sad or need someone to talk to?" may help identify LGBTQ youth who are marginalized from family or peers and who feel particularly isolated or alone. In addition, specific questions regarding comfort level with their sexual minority identity or inquiries into how things are going at school, home, or with peers may help further identify adolescents who may benefit from referral to community-based support groups for LGBTQ youth (if and when available) or those in need of additional mental health support services.

Tobacco, Alcohol, and Other Substance Use

Alcohol and tobacco companies aggressively market products to the LGBTQ community; youth are highly vulnerable to these efforts (27). For example, a 2001 literature review found that smoking among LGB youth ranged from 38% to 59%, compared with 28% to 35% for adolescents in the general population (28). More recent studies confirm that smoking rates are disproportionately high among LGBTQ adolescents (29). Therefore, providers who care for LGBTQ youth need to inquire about current and past smoking behavior and should be prepared to offer adolescents assistance in quitting when desired. This may include providing access to nicotine replacement medications or assisting youth in finding culturally appropriate behavioral options, such as LGBTQ youth-focused smoking cessation support groups, when available.

Experimentation with tobacco, alcohol, or drugs can often be part of normal adolescent development. However, some adolescents use drugs or alcohol to self-medicate underlying depression or to relieve the pain associated with loneliness, rejection, and isolation (30). LGBTQ adolescents are no exception; in fact, for some LGBTQ youth, underlying depression or anxiety is often compounded by a paucity of venues in which safe social interaction with peers can occur (5). Consequently, LGBTQ youth may frequent bars, clubs, or other social settings that normalize the use of illicit substances or where alcohol use is ever-present. A meta-analysis of 18 published studies found that LGB youth were 190% more likely to use tobacco, alcohol, or an illicit substance compared with their heterosexual peers. Youth who identified as bisexual and/or who were female had remarkably higher rates of substance use (340% and 400%, respectively) compared with heterosexual peers (31). Alcohol and illicit drug use among all adolescents, including those who may be LGBTQ, are linked to other destructive behaviors and negative outcomes including high-risk sexual behaviors, suicide attempts, and motor vehicle accidents (32,33).

Although marijuana is the most commonly used illicit drug in adolescence, "club drugs" are taking hold in the LGBTQ youth community, particularly among young gay and bisexual men. Club drugs such as Ecstasy, methamphetamine, gamma-hydroxybutyrate (GHB), and ketamine are used by adolescents to create a sense of euphoria, social disinhibition, and heightened sexuality. There is often a perceived link between club drugs, social desirability, and popularity, resulting in limited stigma surrounding their use in some LGBTQ youth circles. Most club drugs such as Ecstasy and GHB are used episodically, either alone or in combination, within specific social environments (e.g., clubs, dances, or circuit parties). Others, however, such as methamphetamine, can be extremely physically addictive and lead to frequent if not daily use. Methamphetamine in particular has been strongly linked to high-risk sex in young gay and bisexual men, and the substance has emerged as a major risk factor for the acquisition of HIV infection and other STIs (34–36).

When assessing use of alcohol and illicit drugs, providers should ask LGBTQ youth direct questions in a nonjudgmental and unbiased manner. As much as possible, health care providers need to familiarize themselves with commonly used "street terms" for various drugs but should never be afraid to ask an adolescent patient for clarification if an unknown term or substance is mentioned during the interview. For many LGBTQ youth who use drugs or abuse alcohol, the private and confidential confines of the clinical exam room may be the only setting in which they feel able to disclose their behavior or express concerns about dependence or abuse. LGBTQ youth may ask questions regarding potential deleterious effects of alcohol, marijuana, and/or club drugs, such as hallucinations, seizures, hyperthermia, depression, erectile dysfunction, and irritability (37). Information regarding deleterious effects of alcohol and drug use and prevention education should be delivered in a firm, knowledgeable, but nonalarmist manner, affording the opportunity to continue the dialogue with the provider in future clinical encounters. Education should be broad-based, promoting both abstinence and harm reduction. Harm reduction strategies acknowledge that for many LGBTQ youth, drug and/or alcohol use is not likely to stop at the present time. Harm reduction emphasizes personal safety (e.g., consistent condom use, not driving under the influence) as well as avoidance of peer pressure that may contribute to substance use during adolescence.

Safety, Violence, and Victimization

Violence is a leading cause of morbidity and mortality among U.S. adolescents, and personal safety is often a primary concern of LGBTQ youth (1,38–41). An alarming number of sexual and gender minority youth experience violence directly related to their sexual orientation and gender identity. Safety threats can range from verbal taunts to physical or sexual harassment to dating violence.

Bullying and interpersonal violence against LGBT adolescents is not a new phenomenon but has received significantly more attention over the past several years because of many high-profile suicides and violent episodes. Evidence of bullying directed at gay and lesbian adolescents was first reported in 1995 (38), and even today, LGBTQ youth continue to experience high rates of verbal abuse, threats of physical violence, and overt physical assault (1,41). A 2013 study suggests that LGBTQ youth may also experience higher rates of dating violence, including physical, psychological, and cyber abuse (42). Research confirms that persistent exposure to bullying and victimization can lead to manynegative health outcomes, including anxiety, depression, underage alcohol and drug use, and unprotected sex (43).

Emerging data indicate that schools are frequent sites at which bullying and victimization of LGBTQ youth take place. According to the 2011 National School Climate Survey conducted by the Gay, Lesbian & Straight Education Network, of more than 8500 teens surveyed, 8 of 10 LGBT students experienced harassment, 63.5% felt unsafe at school because of their sexual orientation, and 44% felt unsafe because of their gender expression (41). As a result of this harassment, 32% of LGBT youth reported missing at least 1 day of school because they felt unsafe. Students who experienced higher levels of victimization based on their sexual orientation or gender expression had lower grade point averages and higher rates of depression than students with lower levels of victimization (41).

Experiencing antigay violence at home or at school is profoundly traumatic for LGBTQ youth since these environments are precisely the ones that should be the most predictable, reliable, safe, and nurturing. Family and/or school violence may leave LGBTQ youth feeling unsure of whom to turn to for advice, guidance, support, and protection. Under these circumstances, an astute provider can be of invaluable assistance. When asking adolescents about their experience with violence, it is best to start the inquiry using open-ended rather than yes/no questions, such as: "How are things going at home or at school?" Providers may then follow up by asking specifically about "being picked on by siblings, parents, relationship partners, or peers" or "feeling safe" within settings such as home, neighborhoods, relationships or school. Important clues to the presence of underlying distress include unspoken body language and unexplained changes in scholastic performance or participation in previously pleasurable hobbies or sports. When bullying or interpersonal violence are identified, providers can be integral in identifying community resources that provide support.

It is important that LGBTQ adolescents understand the precise legal limits of the confidentiality of the clinical encounter before beginning to answer questions regarding safety, as this allows them to be in control of the information they choose to disclose. Inadvertent disclosure of abuse or violence may trigger mandatory reporting obligations on the part of the health care provider that the LGBTQ adolescent may not perceive to be in their best interest. LGBTQ youth may use the clinical setting to discuss fears or safety concerns regarding self-disclosure of their sexual orientation or gender identity to parents or family members. They may realistically fear expulsion from their homes if their parents or guardians become aware of their sexual orientation or gender identity and may lack appropriate social support to deal with these stressors (3). As such, LGBTQ youth are the best to judge how their parents or families may react. Providers need to use extreme caution in offering specific advice, instructions, and guidance that might be construed as encouraging coming out. Deciding to come out is a highly personal and often frightening decision for LGBTQ youth (3). It is not the role of the health care provider to give specific advice or instructions regarding timing of the coming out process. Rather, providers should offer general support, suggest referrals to community resources when needed, and make it clear that they will be available to the adolescent as needed for future advice or assistance. Table 5-3 lists some examples of national resources for LGBTQ youth and

---

Table 5-3   Resources for Youth and Their Families

The Trevor Project: www.thetrevorproject.org

Gay, Lesbian & Straight Education Network (GLSEN): www.glsen.org

Safe Schools Coalition: www.safeschoolscoalition.org

Hetrick-Martin Institute: www.hmi.org

Centers for Disease Control and Prevention Lesbian, Gay, Bisexual and Transgender Health (Youth): www.cdc.gov/lgbthealth/youth.htm

Advocates for Youth: www.advocatesforyouth.org

National Youth Advocacy Coalition: www.nyacyouth.org

National Center for Transgender Equality: www.transequality.org

Parents, Families, Friends, and Allies United with LGBT People to Move Equality Forward: www.pflag.org

Family Acceptance Project: familyproject.sfsu.edu

their families, many of which offer community-level support groups and other programs.

Conducting a Physical Examination and Providing Appropriate Screening Recommendations

Primary health care recommendations for LGBTQ adolescents should generally follow the American Medical Association Guidelines for Adolescent Preventive Services (GAPS), including annual visits and health care screenings (44). Annual visits should include a comprehensive physical exam and appropriate screening for a variety of previously described health issues, including STIs, substance abuse, and mental health concerns. Additionally, given that some research suggests a higher prevalence of obesity in adolescent sexual minority females (45) and of eating disorders in adolescent bisexual and gay males (46), clinicians should pay careful attention to eating habits and levels of physical activity.

Immunizations

According to the Advisory Committee on Immunization Practices, all youth should receive age-appropriate vaccines, including hepatitis A and B and meningococcal vaccines. In addition, beginning at ages 11 to 12 years, all adolescent females should be offered the human papillomavirus (HPV) vaccine for cervical cancer prophylaxis even if they only report being sexually active with other females. To provide prophylaxis against the development of genital and anal warts and anal cancer, HPV vaccine may also be given to adolescent males (47).

Exams With Transgender Patients

For transgender individuals, the physical examination can be an unsettling experience. Transgender youth may be extremely uncomfortable exposing their genitalia as part of the routine clinical encounter; this discomfort is most pronounced with the gynecologic examination in female-to-male transgender youth. Providers should therefore proceed slowly and use caution when doing an external or internal genitourinary examination, as described in detail in Chapter 8. In the absence of symptoms or other clinical indications that make a genitourinary examination important, providers may wish to defer this aspect of the physical exam to a future visit to allow for a stronger clinical relationship to be established.

Screening for STIs and HIV

Sexually transmitted infections remain a concern for all adolescents, as young people are at increased risk of acquiring STIs, such as chlamydia, gonorrhea, and HIV infection (48). Young men who have sex with men (MSM [used to describe all men who have sex with men, including those who may not identify as gay]) are at particularly high risk for STIs (48,49). Screening for HIV and other STIs needs to be guided by the adolescent's sexual behavior, not orientation (as described in the section on taking a sexual history) and should be done whenever appropriate or indicated. For sexually active adolescents, particularly gay/bisexual youth, and transgender youth who have sex with males, HIV and STI screening should occur at least once per year (50).

Cervical cytology or Papanicolaou tests should be performed in young lesbian and bisexual women at the same intervals as for other young women, starting at age 21; similarly, these tests are indicated for transgender men (female-to-male) who have a cervix. Providers need to be aware that sexual minority youth often delay seeking care in this area, making patient education regarding the need for routine gynecologic exams of the utmost importance (2).

With regard to HIV, young MSM, especially those of color, are at a disproportionately higher risk. In 2010, young MSM (age 13 to 24 years) made up 30% of all new HIV infections among MSM and accounted for 72% of new HIV infections among all people in the same age range. Black MSM accounted for 36% of new HIV infections among MSM. From 2008 to 2010, new HIV infections increased by 20% among young black MSM (51). Young transgender women are also thought to be at greatly increased risk for HIV, although not many studies have been conducted with this population (52,53).

These disparities persist despite aggressive outreach efforts to increase testing in high-risk populations. Public health campaigns promoting safer sex were successful in achieving behavior change decades ago, but this success now appears to be waning (5). Young MSM in particular continue to engage in high-risk sexual behaviors, particularly when under the influence of alcohol or other drugs, such as methamphetamine. Reasons for this may include "prevention fatigue" related to exposure to continual reminders about the risk for HIV, lack of perceived risk due to adolescent beliefs of invulnerability, and reduced fear created by the success of new and improved HIV treatments. Use of the Internet for seeking and meeting romantic and sexual partners, socialization in adult environments such as bars and clubs, and/or sexual activity with older partners further accentuate the increased HIV risk for young MSM (54). Targeted, broad-based HIV prevention efforts tailored to the unique mechanisms of HIV risk need to be implemented in this population, particularly in communities of color.

Management of adolescents who are HIV infected highlights the need for health care delivery that is sensitive to the needs of young people. Providers caring for HIV-infected youth often need to be extremely flexible with their schedules, in terms of open office hours and late arrival policies; this is an often difficult task in more traditional adult-oriented health care environments. Confidentiality, lack of insurance, secrecy, shame, and stigma may pose particular roadblocks for HIV-infected youth and compromise clinical care, as illustrated in the following clinical case vignette:

> L.M. is an 18-year-old newly diagnosed HIV-infected male who was lost to care for approximately a year after his initial diagnosis because of feelings of shame about his HIV status. When he did seek care a year later, he disclosed that, in addition to not being out to his family about his sexual identity, he had not revealed and did not wish to reveal his HIV status to his family. As a result, he often had to lie to his mother about his whereabouts when he had medical appointments and hide his medications at home in a vitamin container.

HIV education is often a time-consuming process for these patients, but it is an element of primary care that is crucial in order to maintain optimum future health because there are frequently many barriers to adherence. While a medical provider may wish to discuss T cells, viral load, or other HIV-specific medical issues, many HIV-infected adolescents prefer to focus on bread-and-butter adolescent primary care issues, such as acne, family conflict, dating concerns, or counseling on high-risk sexual activity. Many face challenges in disclosing their diagnosis to others, particularly parents, family members, and romantic or sexual partners. For youth who have not disclosed their HIV-infected status or their sexual or gender identities, these issues seem inextricably linked. For youth who are financially dependent and reliant on parents or family for support, the possibility of a negative reaction can be an overwhelming concern. As a result, some HIV-infected youth forgo recommended medical treatment (e.g., highly active antiretroviral therapy) for fear that medications will be discovered at home or at school. Others, such as youth who are homeless, may not have a safe or reliable place to store their medications. Some HIV-infected youth may simply decide to abandon medical care completely. Adolescent HIV providers must not only be astute in the management of HIV-related disease but also be adept at managing the entire range of adolescent health care and social concerns.

Other Important and Emerging Issues

Homelessness

LGBTQ youth experience homelessness frequently; most commonly, this occurs because of conflict with parents over the adolescent's sexual orientation or gender identity (3,55,56). Some LGBTQ youth are asked or forced to leave their homes when parents or guardians discover or suspect a sexual or gender minority identity (2). Disclosure can occur directly (e.g., coming out) or inadvertently when parents discover gay or lesbian erotica, overhear phone conversations, or witness same-sex physical contact or cross-dressing. For other LGBTQ youth, leaving home is a voluntary decision or means of escaping a home situation that is rendered unsafe because of verbal or physical antigay harassment or parental attempts to convince adolescents to undergo psychological counseling or reparative therapy to "become heterosexual."

Once on the streets, LGBTQ youth typically find that employment, housing, and support are temporary, precarious, or both. Lacking a means of financial independence and stability leaves them vulnerable to numerous health risks. Unable to obtain legitimate or stable employment, some homeless LGBTQ youth trade sexual activity for food, money, drugs, or shelter (57–60), putting them at increased risk for HIV infection and other STIs. Substance use and exposure to violence or victimization may further complicate their lives.

Homeless LGBTQ youth are often forced to present to the emergency department for primary medical care, where they may be further marginalized and their primary health care issues ignored because of a focus on evaluating their acute physical symptoms. Access to care can be further complicated by legal constraints associated with young age and lack of proper identification. The bureaucracy of medicine can be difficult to navigate even for high-functioning adolescents; for homeless youth, culturally competent, comprehensive care is frequently an elusive goal.

Emerging Transgender Population

In recent years, increasing numbers of children are beginning to express transgender identity and at earlier ages. Despite this growing population, few medical centers specialize in addressing the needs of transgender and other gender-nonconforming children, and no formal, research-tested protocols have evaluated the use of clinical therapies, such as pubertal blockers and cross-sex hormones, in transgender youth. As a result, families who have questions and anxiety about their children's gender identity and expression may initially present to their primary care provider with questions and concerns. The primary care clinician can provide invaluable assistance by offering validation and support, directing them to resources that provide evidenced-based information, and making referrals to subspecialists, where available. Because providers are often the first point of contact for these families, the initial interaction has enormous power in shaping downstream experiences and expectations. It is therefore crucial for providers to create an environment that is comfortable and culturally competent, which includes maintaining an atmosphere of respect at all times, training all personnel to use preferred pronouns, and documenting alternate names in the medical record. Providers also have a professional duty to acquire and maintain a basic knowledge of issues pertinent to transgender children. Chapter 16 provides detailed information on offering care to transgender children and their families.

While there are currently no universal, evidenced-based protocols for prescribing hormone therapies in this population, several research centers, including the Children's Hospital of Los Angeles, Boston Children's Hospital, and the Ann & Robert H. Lurie Children's Hospital of Chicago, are developing multidisciplinary approaches to treating transgender children. These programs use teams of physicians from specialties of adolescent medicine, endocrinology, general surgery, and urology, as well as behavioral health specialists, to provide support for families and refine clinical techniques to improve patient outcomes. The primary care provider may play additional roles that include coordinating care and/or administering treatment (e.g., hormone shots) themselves, particularly in geographic areas that lack proximity to specialists. Consider the following case:

> P.J. is a 16-year-old transgender (male-to-female) patient who presented to a Midwestern regional center for gender dysphoria, where she and her mother received education on cross-sex hormone therapy and were instructed in self-injection techniques. Since P.J.'s family lived approximately 6 hours away, the center staff worked closely with her local pediatrician to design a lab follow-up schedule and address any acute concerns that might arise in between specialty visits, such as medication side effects. This collaboration facilitated a team approach to care and avoided unnecessary and costly trips into the city.

Conclusion

While most of this chapter has focused on how to meet the unique health needs of LGBTQ adolescents, in many ways these youth are similar to their heterosexual peers and should be viewed broadly within the context of general adolescent health and development. Adolescence is a challenging developmental phase in which youth must confront a variety of emotional, physical, and sexual changes. For LGBTQ youth, this developmental phase may be complicated by pervasive disapproval they perceive from society, family, and friends. As a result, although the vast majority of LGBTQ youth demonstrate remarkable strength and resilience and grow up to lead healthy lives as adults, there are still too many who are victims of violence; too many who are infected with HIV; and too many who contemplate suicide. To be able to provide optimal care, providers need to become aware and remain mindful of the unique issues and health risks that frequently affect LGBTQ adolescents, while remembering to address each patient as an individual.

Summary Points

- The goal of the clinical encounter is to promote social, emotional, and physical well-being. This includes creating a safe environment in which LGBTQ youth feel comfortable asking questions and seeking advice and support.

- Explicit discussion of confidentiality is critical. For LGBTQ adolescents, concerns about confidentiality may be complicated by realistic fears concerning the intentional or inadvertent disclosure of their sexual orientation or gender identity.
- Leading health risks for LGBTQ youth include HIV/AIDS, smoking, substance abuse, depression and suicide, STIs, abuse and victimization, external and internalized stigma, homelessness, and access to care.
- Risk reduction regarding social and behavioral health issues is the cornerstone of the adolescent visit. Screening for leading health risks is done primarily through the social history, guided by asking questions according to the following acronym: HEADS: *H*—home; *E*—education; *A*—activities; *D*—drugs/depression/diet; *S*—safety/sexuality.
- Primary care providers need to develop comfort discussing sexual activity with LGBTQ adolescents, which includes learning how to ask specific, nonjudgmental questions about types of sexual activity with various sexual partners and consistency of condom use for protection against pregnancy and HIV infection/STIs. Fluidity of sexual expression among adolescents can complicate sexual history-taking, as some may not identify with a binary model of sexual and/or gender identity.
- LGBTQ youth experience the same range of mental health concerns as all adolescents. However, stigma associated with sexual minority status may cause additional stress. Clinicians should be on the lookout for distress among youth who are beginning to experiment with same-sex partners or youth who are coming out, as these youth may experience internal psychological conflict and/or direct conflict with family and peers, requiring assistance or support.
- Although experimentation with alcohol, tobacco, and drugs may be a part of normal adolescence, LGBTQ youth in general smoke, drink, and use drugs more frequently than their heterosexual peers. In addition to remaining focused on primary prevention, primary care providers should educate LGBTQ youth about harm reduction strategies, including refraining from driving while under the influence and avoiding risky sex while high or drunk.
- Personal safety is often a primary concern of LGBTQ youth who may experience verbal taunts or physical or sexual harassment. Asking about "feeling safe" at home, school, within romantic relationships, and other settings is a critical aspect of the LGBTQ youth's social history, as these youth may be reticent to initiate discussion of these issues if a strong clinical relationship has not yet been established.
- Social media, including use of tools such as Facebook, Twitter, and text messaging, are playing an ever-increasing role in adolescents' lives in terms of how they access information and communicate with their peers. While these communication modalities present new opportunities to form connections, they may also be used to intimidate and

to facilitate high risk behaviors. Providers should therefore inquire routinely about the use and extent of use of social media.

- LGBTQ youth are the best to judge how parents or friends will react to their coming out. It is not the role of the provider to give specific advice regarding the timing of coming out. Rather, providers should offer general support and assure youth that they are available to offer assistance if needed.

- Physical examination maneuvers, screening tests, and preventive health interventions for LGBTQ adolescents should follow the American Medical Association Guidelines for Adolescent Preventive Services (GAPS). Screening for HIV and other STIs should be guided by the adolescent's sexual behavior, not orientation.

- HIV remains an area of special concern. Young gay and bisexual men and male-to-female transgender youth are the highest behavioral risk groups for adolescent or young adult HIV. These youth, particularly from communities of color, require targeted screening and HIV.

- The number of transgender adolescents is increasing, and research on this population is emerging. However, little information is available to guide evidence-based practice, and few clinical specialists have expertise in this area. It is therefore crucial for primary care clinicians to acquire a basic knowledge of relevant issues, as these providers are frequently the first points of contact for transgender children and their families.

References

1. **Human Rights Campaign**. Growing up LGBT in America: HRC Youth Survey Report Key Findings. Available at: www.hrc.org/youth.
2. **Remafedi G**. Fundamental issues in the care of homosexual youth. Med Clin North Am. 1990;74:1169-79.
3. **Ryan C, Futterman D**. Lesbian and gay youth: care and counseling. Adolesc Med. 1997;8: 207-374.
4. **Harper GW, Schneider M**. Oppression and discrimination among lesbian, gay, bisexual, and transgendered people and communities: a challenge for community psychology. Am J Community Psychol. 2003;31:243-52.
5. **Garofalo R, Harper GW**. Not all adolescents are the same: addressing the unique needs of gay and bisexual male youth. Adolesc Med. 2003;14:595-611, vi.
6. **Savin-Williams RC**. Verbal and physical abuse stressors in the lives of lesbian, gay male, and bisexual youths: associations with school problems, running away, substance use, prostitution, and suicide. J Consult Clin Psychol. 1994;62:261-69.
7. **Rosario M, Hunter J, Maguen S, et al**. The coming-out process and its adaptational and health-related associations among gay, lesbian, and bisexual youths: stipulation and exploration of a model. Am J Community Psychol. 2001;29:133-60.
8. **Coker T, Austin SB, Schuster MA**. The health and health care of lesbian, gay, and bisexual adolescents. Annu Rev Public Health. 2010;31:457-77.
9. **Needham BL, Austin EL**. Sexual orientation, parental support, and health during the transition to young adulthood. J Youth Adolesc. 2010;39:1189-98.

10. **Garofalo R, Katz E.** Health care issues of gay and lesbian youth. Curr Opin Pediatr. 2001;13:298-302.

11. **Garofalo R, Wolf CR, Kessel S, et al.** The association between health risk behaviors and sexual orientation among a school-based sample of adolescents. Pediatrics. 1998;101: 895-902.

12. **Klein J, McNulty M, Flatau CN.** Adolescents' access to care: teenagers' self-reported use of services and perceived access to confidential care. Arch Pediatr Adolesc Med. 1998;152: 676-82.

13. **Samargia L, Saewyc EM, Elliott BA.** Foregone mental health care and self-reported access barriers among adolescents. J School Nurs. 2006;22:17-24.

14. **Garofalo R, Bush S.** Addressing LGBT youth in the clinical setting. In: Makadon HJ, Mayer KH, Potter J, Goldhammer H, eds. Fenway Guide to Lesbian, Gay, Bisexual, and Transgender Health. Philadelphia: American College of Physicians; 2008:75-99.

15. **Saewyc EM, Bearinger LH, Blum RW, et al.** Sexual intercourse, abuse and pregnancy among adolescent women: does sexual orientation make a difference? Fam Plan Perspect. 1999; 31:127-32.

16. **Saewyc E, Skay C, Richens K, et al.** Sexual orientation, sexual abuse, and HIV-risk behaviors among adolescents in the Pacific Northwest. Am J Public Health. 2006;96:1104-10.

17. **Herrick A, Matthews AK, Garofalo R.** Health risk behaviors in an urban sample of young women who have sex with women. J Lesbian Stud. 2010;14:80-92.

18. **Perrin E, Cohen KM, Gold M, et al.** Gay and lesbian issues in pediatric health care. Curr Prob Pediatr Adolesc Health Care. 2004;34:355-98.

19. **Garofalo R, Wolf RC, Wissow LS, et al.** Sexual orientation and risk of suicide attempts among a representative sample of youth. Arch Pediatr Adolesc Med. 1999;153:487-93.

20. **Remafedi G.** Suicide and sexual orientation: nearing the end of controversy? Arch Gen Psychiatry. 1999;56:885-6.

21. **Savin-Williams RC.** A critique of research on sexual-minority youths. J Adolesc. 2001;24: 5-13.

22. **Almeida J, Johnson RM, Corliss HL, Molnar BE, Azrael D.** Emotional distress among LGBT youth: the influence of perceived discrimination based on sexual orientation. J Youth Adolesc. 2009;38:1001-14.

23. **Jiang Y, Perry DK, Hesser JE.** Suicide patterns and association with predictors among Rhode Island public high school students: a latent class analysis. Am J Public Health. 2010;100: 1701-7.

24. **Rosewater K, Burr BH.** Epidemiology, risk factors, interventions, and prevention of adolescent suicide. Curr Opin Pediatr. 1998;10:338-43.

25. **Low B, Andrews SF.** Adolescent suicide. Med Clin North Am. 1990;74:1251-64.

26. **Schulberg H, Bruce ML, Lee PW, et al.** Preventing suicide in primary care patients: the primary care physician's role. Gen Hosp Psychiatry. 2004;26:337-45.

27. **Washington HA.** Burning love: Big tobacco takes aim at LGBT Youths. Am J Public Health. 2002;92:1086-95.

28. **Ryan H, Pascale M, Eaton A.** Smoking among lesbian, gay, and bisexuals: a review of the literature. Am J Prev Med. 2001;21:142-9.

29. **Easton A, Jackson, K, Mowery P, Comeau D, Sell R.** Adolescent same-sex and both-sex romantic attractions and relationships, implications for smoking. Am J Public Health. 2008;98:462-97.

30. **Rosario M, Schrimshaw EW, Hunter J.** Disclosure of sexual orientation and subsequent substance use and abuse among lesbian, gay, and bisexual youths: critical role of disclosure reactions. Psychol Addict Behav. 2009;23:175-84.

31. **Marshal MP, Friedman MS, Stall R, King KM, Miles J, et al.** Sexual orientation and adolescent substance use: a meta-analysis and methodological review. Addiction. 2008;103:546-56.

32. **Crumley F.** Substance abuse and adolescent suicidal behavior. JAMA. 1990;263:3051-7.

33. **Remafedi G.** Predictors of unprotected intercourse among gay and bisexual youth: knowledge, beliefs, and behavior. Pediatrics. 1994;94(2 pt 1):163-8.

34. **Mansergh G, Shouse RL, Marks G, et al.** Methamphetamine and sildenafil (Viagra) use are linked to unprotected receptive and insertive anal sex, respectively, in a sample of men who have sex with men. Sex Transm Infect. 2006;82:131-4.

35. **Colfax G, Coates TJ, Husnik MJ, et al.** Longitudinal patterns of methamphetamine, popper (amyl nitrite), and cocaine use and high-risk sexual behavior among a cohort of San Francisco men who have sex with men. J Urban Health. 2005;82(1 suppl 1):i62-70.

36. **Forrest DW, Metsch LR, LaLota M, Cardenas G, Beck DW, Jeanty Y.** Crystal methamphetamine use and sexual risk behaviors among HIV-positive and HIV-negative men who have sex with men in South Florida. J Urban Health. 2010;87:480-5.

37. **Tellier P.** Club drugs: is it all ecstasy? Pediatr Ann. 2002;31:550-5.

38. **Pilkington N, D'Augelli AR.** Victimization of lesbian, gay, and bisexual youth in community settings. J Community Psychol. 1995;23:34-56.

39. **Waldo CR, Hesson-McInnis MS, D'Augelli AR.** Antecedents and consequences of victimization of lesbian, gay, and bisexual young people: a structural model comparing rural university and urban samples. Am J Community Psychol. 1998;26:307-34.

40. **D'Augelli AR, Grossman AH, Starks MT.** Childhood gender atypicality, victimization, and PTSD among lesbian, gay and bisexual youth. J Interpers Violence 2006;21:1462-82.

41. **Kosciw JG, Greytak EA, Bartkiewicz MJ, Boesen MJ, Palmer NA.** The 2011 National School Climate Survey: The experiences of lesbian, gay, bisexual and transgender youth in our nation's schools. New York: GLSEN. Gay, Lesbian, and Straight Education Network (GLSEN), 2012. Available at glsen.org/nscs.

42. **Dank M, Lachman P, Yahner J, Zweig JM.** Dating violence experiences of lesbian, gay, bisexual, and transgender youth. Washington, DC: Urban Institute, 2013. Available at www.urban.org/publications/412892.html.

43. **Smokowski PR, Kopasz KH.** Bullying in school: an overview of types, effects, family characteristics, and intervention strategies. Children Schools. 2005;27:101-9.

44. **Elster A, Kuznets NJ, eds.** AMA Guidelines for Adolescent Preventive Services (GAPS): Recommendations and Rationale. Chicago, IL: American Medical Association; 1994.

45. **Austin SB, Ziyadeh NJ, Corliss HL, et al.** Sexual orientation disparities in weight status in adolescence: findings from a prospective study. Obesity (Silver Spring). 2009;17:1776-82.

46. **Austin SB, Ziyadeh NJ, Corliss HL, et al.** Sexual orientation disparities in purging and binge eating from early to late adolescence. J Adolesc Health. 2009;45:238-45.

47. **Advisory Committee for Immunization Practices.** ACIP vaccine recommendations. Available at: www.cdc.gov/vaccines/hcp/acip-recs/index.html.

48. **Centers for Disease Control and Prevention.** Sexually Transmitted Disease Surveillance 2012. Atlanta, GA: U.S. Department of Health and Human Services; 2013.

49. **Mayer KH.** Sexually transmitted diseases in men who have sex with men. Clin Infect Dis. 2011;53(suppl 3):S79-S83.

50. **Workowski, KA, Berman S.** Sexually transmitted diseases guidelines, 2010. MMWR Recommend Rep. 2010;59:1-110.

51. **Centers for Disease Control and Prevention.** HIV among gay and bisexual men. March 2013. Available at: www.cdc.gov/hiv/pdf/risk_gender_238900B_HIV_Gay_Bisexual_MSM_FS_final.pdf

52. **Garofalo R, Deleon J, Osmer E, Doll M, Harper GW.** Overlooked, misunderstood and at-risk: exploring the lives and HIV risk of ethnic minority male-to-female transgender youth. J Adolesc Health. 2006;38:230-36.

53. **Wilson EC, Garofalo R, Harris RD, et al.** Transgender female youth and sex work: HIV risk and a comparison of life factors related to engagement in sex work. AIDS Behav. 2009;13:902-13.

54. **Garofalo R, Herrick A, Mustanski B, Donenberg GR.** Tip of the iceberg: young men who have sex with men, the internet, and HIV risk. Am J Public Health. 2007;97:1113-7.

55. **Kruks G.** Gay and lesbian homeless street youth: special issues and concerns. J Adolesc Health. 1991;12:515-8.

56. **Rew L, Whittaker TA, Taylor-Seehafer MA, et al.** Sexual health risks and protective resources in gay, lesbian, bisexual, and heterosexual homeless youth. J Special Pediatr Nurs. 2005;10: 11-9.

57. **Cochran BN, Stewart AJ, Ginzler JA, et al.** Challenges faced by homeless sexual minorities: comparison of gay, lesbian, bisexual, and transgender homeless adolescents with their heterosexual counterparts. Am J Public Health. 2002;92:773-7.

58. **Rew L, Fouladi RT, Yockey RD.** Sexual health practices of homeless youth. J Nurs Scholarship. 2002;34:139-45.

59. **Kipke MD, O'Connor S, Palmer R, MacKenzie RG.** Street youth in Los Angeles: profiles of a group at high risk for human immunodeficiency virus infection. Arch Pediatr Adolesc Med. 1995;149:513-9.

60. **Rice E, Barman-Adhikari A, Rhoades H, et al.** Homelessness experiences, sexual orientation, and sexual risk taking among high school students in Los Angeles. J Adolesc Health. 2013;52:773-8.

Chapter 6

LGBT Relationships and Family Lives

CHARLOTTE J. PATTERSON, PhD
BERNADETTE V. BLANCHFIELD, MA
SAMANTHA L. TORNELLO, PhD
RACHEL G. RISKIND, PhD

Introduction

Lesbian, gay, bisexual, and transgender (LGBT) relationships and people have lately been in the public eye more than ever. Despite greater public attention, however, many aspects of LGBT relationships and family lives are still not well known. How do LGBT people experience intimate relationships? How do LGBT people form families? How do the families of LGBT people function, and how do children of LGBT parents develop? What do answers to these questions mean for health care providers? In this chapter, we provide an overview of research on intimate relationships and parenting among LGBT people and on children with LGBT parents, and we consider implications of the research findings in the health care setting.

The research literature that we draw on is much stronger in its exploration of some topics than others. Considerable research has focused on couple relationships and parenting among lesbian and gay people, but much less has explored these topics among bisexual or transgender individuals. More information is available about white couples and families than about people of color, and more research has been conducted with relatively affluent than with economically challenged families. Little research has investigated the intersections of such issues. Within the constraints of the available work, we seek to provide a broad overview of the research on couples and families as well as its applications to health care. We begin with research on LGBT couples and other intimate relationships, then we turn to LGBT parenting and to children of LGBT parents. We conclude with implications of these research findings for development of competence among health care providers.

Couple and Other Intimate Relationships

The following section provides an overview of the expansive body of research on LGBT individuals' intimate relationships. Frequently investigated aspects of these relationships include love and commitment, power and division of labor, sexual behavior, relationship satisfaction, and relationship problems and conflict. For another recent review, see Fingerhut and Peplau (1).

Love and Commitment

As they look ahead to the future, many lesbian and gay youth hope to be involved in coupled relationships. For example, when D'Augelli and his colleagues interviewed lesbian- and gay-identified adolescents and young adults about their plans for the future, the youth described relationships as extremely important (2). Fully 82% of young men and 92% of young women expressed a desire to be a member of a couple at some point; most of them also hoped that they would someday marry a same-sex partner. Thus, involvement in an intimate relationship with a partner was an important part of these youths' visions of their future lives.

Survey data suggest that many LGBT individuals are indeed involved in same-sex relationships. Results vary from one survey to another, but anywhere from 45% to 80% of lesbian women and 40% to 60% of gay men have reported that they are currently in same-sex partnerships (3–5). In a probability sample of adult lesbian and gay individuals living in California (6), 51% to 62% of lesbian women and 37% to 46% of gay men reported current involvement in couple relationships.

How do the partners in same-sex couples meet? In the past, prospective partners often met at work, at school, or through their families. In recent years, the rise of the Internet has increasingly allowed LGBT people to make contact with potential partners online. Perhaps because there have been relatively few safe venues in which LGBT people could meet prospective partners, this has been especially important for those seeking same-sex partners. Meeting online was, in fact, recently reported to be more common among LGBT couples than among than heterosexual couples (7). Meeting online brings opportunities but also carries health-related risks, such as a possibly heightened risk for exposure to sexually transmitted infections.

Recent years have also seen growing legal recognition of same-sex couple relationships in the United States. As this volume goes to press, marriages of same-sex couples are legally recognized in 32 states and the District of Columbia, and cases are pending in other states. The 2010 U.S. Census allowed same-sex couples to report being married (as distinct from cohabitating) for the first time. In that Census, 25.7% of all same-sex couple households reported that they were spouses (8). Whether or not the law recognized these spousal relationships cannot be determined from the Census data. In a Pew Research Center survey of more than 1000 LGBT people in the

United States, for which data were collected in April 2013, 16% of respondents reported being legally married and another 21% reported living with a same-sex partner to whom they were not legally married. Those who reported being legally married also reported better mental health (9) than did those whose relationships were not legally recognized. Many same-sex couples have responded to recent legal changes by choosing to marry.

Same-sex couples responding to surveys have reported being as satisfied with their relationships as have their heterosexual counterparts (10–12). One recent study found that lesbian and gay individuals in dating, engaged, and married relationships were indistinguishable in attachment security and relationship quality from their heterosexual counterparts (10). A longitudinal study yielded similar results, finding that sexual minority and heterosexual individuals reported being equally satisfied with their couple relationships (12). Further, although relationship satisfaction tended to decline over the years for all couples in this study, there were no significant differences in the amount of change in relationship satisfaction as a function of sexual orientation over the 5 years of the study.

Research has identified several correlates of relationship satisfaction for lesbian and gay individuals that are similar to those for heterosexual individuals (13). For example, lesbian and gay respondents report greater satisfaction in their relationships when partners are similar to one another, when they perceive strong social support, and when they avoid "ineffectual arguing" (14,15). Other individual differences account for perceptions of relationship quality, including values, perceptions of autonomy and equality within the relationship, desires for strong attachment between partners (16), and, in some cases, extent of sexual identity disclosure (17,18). The relevance of differences between partners in disclosure or coming out in same-sex couple relationships is one of the few issues that is unique to same-sex relationships, and this points to the role that stigma may play in the experiences of LGBT individuals (1).

Power and Division of Labor

Power, as described by social exchange theory, is afforded to the partner in a relationship who has access to more resources, such as higher income or education (19). Among gay male couples, older and wealthier partners have been reported to have greater power (20,21). Results for lesbian women have been less clear. In one study, wealth and education were positively correlated with partner power (22), but in another study, wealth was not associated with power among lesbian women (23). Further research is needed to understand power dynamics in same-sex relationships (1).

While many people endorse the notion of equality within relationships, almost all lesbian and gay couples describe the ideal balance of power in their relationships as exactly equal (19). Reports on the actual balance of power within relationships, however, have been less clear. In one study,

48% of heterosexual men and women reported an equal balance of power in their relationships, as compared with 59% of lesbians and 38% of gay men (1). Other studies have reported higher rates of equal power among sexual minorities, with up to 60% of gay men (21) and 59% of lesbian women (24) reporting equal power within couples.

Much less is known about how bisexual and transgender people navigate these issues. Whereas many lesbian and gay couples seem to reject traditional gender norms, these roles may be more salient to transgender individuals, for whom gender affirmation may be especially important (25,26). Moreover, the adoption of traditional gender roles may place transgender women at high risk for victimization (26,27). Further research in this area could clarify ways in which bisexual and transgender people are similar to or different from others.

Self-reports about division of childcare among same-sex couples with children reveal a more egalitarian division of labor than is customary among heterosexual couples with children (28–33). Except for de facto stepfamily situations, in which one partner brings children to a new relationship from a former one (34,35), an egalitarian pattern of dividing childcare labor seems to predominate among same-sex couples. Questions have been raised about self-report methods used in much of this research (36), but a recent study found that these self-reports were consistent with observational findings (37).

Sexual Behavior

Sexuality is an important element of intimate relationships. A common assessment of sexual behavior among couples tallies their frequency of sexual relations. On average, gay male couples report greater frequency of sexual relations than do heterosexual couples, and heterosexual couples report greater frequency of sexual relations than do lesbian couples (32,38,39). Frequency of reported sexual relations decreases over time for all couple types, but the decline is greatest among lesbian couples and smallest among gay couples (38). Many interpretations and explanations have been offered for these findings, but none has been entirely supported by data (40–42).

Another dimension of sexual behavior is that of sexual exclusivity. Researchers have repeatedly reported that gay couples are less likely than other couple types to espouse monogamy (23,43). In the 1980s, Blumstein and Schwartz (23) found that 82% of gay couples reported nonmonogamy, but only 28% of lesbian couples and only 23% of heterosexual couples reported that they were not monogamous. More recent studies have also reported relatively high rates of agreement about nonmonogamy among gay men, relative to other couple types (44,45). Overall, lesbian and heterosexual couples seem more likely than gay couples to value and practice monogamy.

A recent large survey explored these questions among transgender individuals (46). Majorities of both transgender men and transgender women reported that they were engaged in sexually monogamous relationships, with only 21% of trans men and 26% of trans women describing themselves as being involved in nonmonogamous relationships. Thus, most transgender individuals endorsed monogamy as a value in their relationships.

Conflict

In general, lesbian and gay couples have been found to experience conflict over much the same issues as do heterosexual couples. In one study, Kurdek (13) asked couples to tell him what topics they fought over and found that most items on lesbian and gay couples' lists were similar to those of heterosexual couples. For instance, couples were likely to say that they fought over finances, driving style, intimacy, and division of labor (13). One type of disagreement that was relatively specific to same-sex couples, however, was the degree to which partners were comfortable disclosing their relationships in public (13,47). The ability to resolve such disagreements in ways that were acceptable to both partners was associated with relationship longevity and durability (13,48).

Conflict may erupt into actual violence between partners, and intimate partner violence does occur among same-sex couples (49). Recent surveys that have included heterosexual comparison groups have found that those in same-sex couples report similar or even higher rates of intimate partner violence than do those in mixed-sex couples. In two recent survey studies, bisexual respondents reported higher rates of intimate partner violence than did lesbian or gay respondents. Because of uncertainty about how much authorities can or will help, much intimate partner violence may go unreported (49) (see Chapter 11 for more on intimate partner violence).

Not every relationship can survive conflict. Kurdek and Schmidt (14) studied attractions as well as barriers to leaving relationships among lesbian, gay, and heterosexual couples. All couple types reported similar attractions in their relationships, but married heterosexual couples reported the greatest barriers to exit. Lesbian and gay couples, whose relationships were not recognized by law at the time, described the fewest barriers to leaving their relationships. Consistent with these findings, Blumstein and Schwartz (23) reported that 18-month breakup rates among couples who had been together 2 years or more before the study began were higher among lesbian, gay, and heterosexual unmarried couples and lowest among married heterosexual couples. Thus, legal marriage was associated with relationship stability. This finding raises questions about whether marriage equality may increase relationship stability among same-sex couples.

Less is known about the relationships of bisexual and transgender individuals than about those of lesbian and gay people. In particular, little research has focused on the special issues that transgender and bisexual individuals may bring to their couple relationships. It is important to recall that sexual identity labels can change over time, especially during transitions from one gender to another. More research on these topics would certainly be valuable.

Alternative Relationships

While most LGBT people report that they want to participate in couple relationships, others prefer alternatives. Some LGBT individuals—especially gay men—participate in consensually nonmonogamous relationships (50,51). Some of these involve a primary dyad, with one or another partner's additional sexual relationships taking place outside the dyad; others may involve both members of a primary dyad engaging in sexual encounters with a third person together. Still others may involve three or more partners of one or multiple genders becoming involved with one another in polyamorous relationships (52,53). Such alternative relationship patterns may or may not involve written agreements and may be especially common among bisexual individuals (52). Those who participate in alternative relationship patterns describe themselves as being as satisfied with their relationships as do those in monogamous couple relationships (12,53,54). Some recent studies have reported lower levels of sexual jealousy but similar overall relationship satisfaction among consensually nonmonogamous gay men than among their monogamous peers (44,45,53). Much remains to be learned about the dynamics of alternative relationship patterns.

Relationship Stigma

Many sexual minority individuals establish and maintain healthy couple relationships, but negative social climates can nevertheless create problems. Discriminatory laws and policies play an important role here, but qualities of interpersonal interactions may also be significant. For example, Walters and Curran (55) found that when same-sex couples went shopping, they received lower-quality service and more negative attention from shop clerks than did heterosexual couples. Similarly, in another study (56), hotel employees were less likely to provide room reservations to lesbian or gay couples than to heterosexual couples. Common discourse depicts bisexual relationships as promiscuous, shallow, and short-lived—stereotypes that have proven especially damaging to the health of bisexual women (52,57,58) and have contributed to instances of rejection from lesbian and gay communities (59).

Although intimate relationships of LGBT people are still stigmatized in many ways, attitudes have shifted in a positive direction in recent years. In a 2011 U.S. Gallup poll, a majority (53%) of Americans reported that they supported marriage equality for same-sex couples (60). This favorable majority opinion was maintained through 2012, as was the belief reported by 64% that consensual same-sex sexual behavior should not lead to legal repercussions (61). In a Pew Research Center report (62), for which data were collected in May 2013, 51% of people in the United States reported that they favored marriage equality. Results of these polls indicate growing support for sexual minority relationships, and this in turn may create more positive social climates for same-sex couples over time.

Summary and Thoughts for Health Care Providers

Overall, the relationship experiences of LGBT individuals are highly varied but do show some clear trends. Many sexual minority individuals express a desire to form couple relationships, and many succeed in forming happy and committed partnerships that endure over time. Despite stigma, LGBT individuals who are in relationships report being highly satisfied with their love lives and sexual relationships. Same-sex couples often report more egalitarian relationships than do heterosexual couples. Relationships of sexual minority individuals share many issues with those of heterosexual individuals, but same-sex couple relationships also involve some special concerns, such as disclosure. More research is needed, especially to learn more about the relationship experiences of bisexual and transgender individuals.

Health care providers should bear in mind that LGBT individuals may have very diverse sexual and romantic histories. Sexual attractions, sexual behaviors, and sexual identities may or may not be consistent at any given time in a person's life, and may also shift over time. Thus, health care providers should be open to the variety of personal histories and current relationships in which LGBT people may be involved. LGBT individuals may use any of a variety of terms to refer to their family members (e.g., *partner, spouse, girl/boyfriend, husband, wife*), and these may not always be reflected in the forms used in any particular health care setting. Health care providers who understand these issues and can use a patient's preferred terms stand a better chance of creating positive working relationships with LGBT patients. In addition, health care providers should become aware of variations in legal recognition for LGBT relationships across jurisdictions because these may have many implications for health care.

LGBT Parents and Parenting

In a 2013 poll, 51% of LGBT adults in the U.S. reported that they are either already parents or would like to have children someday (62). Indeed, LGBT people become parents in many ways (63–65). In some families, children were born or adopted in the context of heterosexual relationships that later dissolved when one or both parents came out as LGBT. In other families, children were born or adopted after parents had affirmed LGBT identities. Most families of the first type have experienced the challenges that accompany parental separation and divorce. Families of the second type, however, have not necessarily experienced parental separation or divorce. Therefore, the experiences of family members are likely to be quite different. For this reason, we present recent research on each in separate sections below. Patterson (66) has reviewed this material at greater length.

Lesbian Mothers Who Had Children in the Context of Heterosexual Marriages

Many parents who had children in the context of heterosexual marriages and later came out as LGBT—often in the context of a divorce—have faced legal challenges in the U.S. courts (67). Lawyers, judges, and others have sometimes voiced derogatory stereotypes and negative assumptions about LGBT people (68). For instance, disputes about child custody and visitation rights have included questions about the mental health and parenting abilities of LGBT parents (69). Negative stereotypes have sometimes been used to justify removal of children from the custody of LGBT parents (70).

Much early research compared mental health and parenting ability of divorced lesbian mothers and divorced heterosexual mothers. Such studies consistently reported that lesbian mothers were at least as likely as heterosexual mothers to enjoy good mental health and to exhibit good parenting abilities (64). Early research did, however, find that divorced lesbian mothers reported more fears about loss of child custody than did divorced heterosexual mothers (71,72). Thus, although lesbian and heterosexual mothers did not differ in their overall mental health or parenting abilities, lesbian mothers nevertheless had some special concerns.

Some might be tempted to dismiss these findings as outdated, but recent evidence suggests that many divorced lesbian mothers remain concerned about their legal rights. Shapiro and colleagues (73) studied mental health among lesbian and heterosexual mothers living in Canada or in the United States, most of whom were divorced. The international contrast was of interest because, despite many similarities between the two countries, Canada provides a more supportive legal climate for lesbian mothers and their children. For example, marriage rights are available to all lesbian mothers in Canada, but these rights are not available to lesbian mothers in many parts of the United States. In addition, several U.S. states do not allow joint or second-parent adoption. Shapiro and colleagues (73) found that lesbian mothers in the United States reported more concern about legal problems and about discrimination based on sexual orientation—but not more general family worries—than did lesbian mothers in Canada. Among heterosexual mothers whose family relationships enjoyed protection of the law in both countries, there were no differences across national boundaries. Thus, contextual factors may be important influences on mental health among lesbian mothers.

Gay Fathers Who Had Children in the Context of Heterosexual Marriages

Probably because most divorced gay fathers have lived apart from their children after divorce (74), little research has evaluated the mental health and parenting abilities of gay fathers. Available evidence suggests that gay fathers who were once married to women describe similar reasons for becoming parents and show parenting abilities that are at least as well developed as those of divorced heterosexual fathers (74,75). In this way, findings from research on divorced gay fathers have paralleled, to some degree, those from research on divorced lesbian mothers.

Research has addressed changes over time in gay father identity among those who were once married to women. Early work by Miller (76,78) and Bozett (78–80) attempted to conceptualize the processes through which men who considered themselves heterosexual fathers came to view themselves as gay fathers. Both authors emphasized the pivotal nature of identity disclosure and also of others' reactions to this disclosure. Emerging relationships in the gay community were seen as crucial to men's integration of their parental and sexual identities. As men came out, fell in love, and disclosed gay relationships to others, while remaining connected to their children, they came to integrate their parental and sexual identities (74).

Heterosexual relationships were once the main pathway through which gay men became fathers. Today, as gay men come out earlier and consider other pathways, heterosexual marriages may be less common, but divorced gay men still constitute an important group of nonheterosexual parents. In a recent web-based study of gay fathers from Australia, Canada, New Zealand, and the United Kingdom, more than half of the participants under 50 years of age reported that they had become parents through a previous heterosexual relationship; this was also the case for more than a third of gay fathers under 50 who lived in the United States (81). Thus, even though some gay men are now becoming parents after coming out, there are still many divorced gay fathers (74).

Planned LGB-Parent Families

Coming out as a lesbian woman or as a gay man once carried with it the assumption that one would never have children. Today, this is less and less the case. Increasingly, LGB adults are choosing to become parents after coming out (63,82–84), forming what may be called planned LGB-parent families. As LGB people increasingly choose to become parents, questions about desire for children, pathways to parenthood, transition to parenthood, and related issues become increasingly important (85).

Parenting Intentions and Desires

What proportion of lesbian and gay people want to have children? To become parents, both lesbians and gay men must first overcome popular stereotypes that parenting is an exclusively heterosexual prerogative (83,86,87). Results of recent research suggest that they are doing so with increasing frequency. Gates and his colleagues (88) analyzed data from the 2002 U.S. National Survey of Family Growth, a nationally representative sample of Americans in childbearing years. They found that 41% of childless lesbians and 52% of childless gay men expressed a desire to have children; these numbers were somewhat lower than those for heterosexual adults. In further analyses of this dataset, gay men who expressed a *desire* to become parents were found to be less likely than their heterosexual peers to express the *intention* to become parents (89). In other words, there was a bigger gap between desire and intention for gay than for heterosexual men. This was not true for women; lesbian women who desired parenthood were just as likely as other women to intend to become parents (89). Similarly, in a recent study of Israeli gay men, many men expressed the desire to become parents but reported that they did not expect this to happen; these men reported more depressive symptoms than did men who expected to fulfill their dreams of parenthood (90). A recent Pew Research Center (62) poll of LGBT people in the United States reported that 28% of those who were childless said that they would like to become parents, and 34% said that they were not sure. Overall, it appears that many lesbians and gay men do wish to become parents but that some may be uncertain about how or if they could do so. Those who do not believe that they can fulfill parenting desires may be at risk for internalizing problems, such as depression.

Barriers to and Supports for Parenthood Outside of Heterosexual Relationships

After deciding to pursue parenthood, same-sex couples and LGBT individuals (65,91,92) are likely to encounter many issues. Some of these issues are interpersonal in nature. For example, family members may express disapproval of parenthood outside of a heterosexual relationship (91), even in cases when they had accepted their loved one's LGBT identity. Similarly, it may be difficult for LGBT individuals to find accurate information about routes to parenthood.

Medical, legal, and financial issues may also influence LGBT adults' experiences as they consider parenthood (93). Many adoption agencies across the United States work with LGB prospective adoptive parents (94), but it may be difficult for some individuals to identify these agencies. Reproductive health services that welcome LGBT adults can be found, but some individual health care providers may refuse to provide services on the basis of client sexual orientation or marital status (95). It may be challenging in some geographic areas to locate agencies and clinics that are open to all, let alone to find agencies and clinics that can address the unique needs of LGBT individuals and same-sex couples in a competent manner. Even after appropriate services are located, the financial costs associated with adoption or reproductive health services may be important barriers. These and related issues are likely to emerge for LGBT individuals as they begin to pursue parenthood (92).

Many lesbian and gay adults in the United States feel confident about overcoming such barriers, but some do not. Barriers to the pursuit of parenthood loom particularly large for lesbian and gay adults who are older, who believe that children with lesbian and gay parents are more likely to experience psychological difficulties as a result of parental sexual orientation, and who live in social climates that are unfavorable to them (93). Little is yet known about attitudes or beliefs of bisexual adults, transgender adults, and lesbian and gay adults outside the United States in this regard.

Pathways to Parenthood

LGBT people can become parents through many different pathways (66,96). As discussed above, many become parents in the context of heterosexual marriages before coming out, and the great majority of these conceive children via heterosexual intercourse. For those who seek parenthood after coming out, pathways are more varied (85). Women may conceive via donor insemination, and men may become fathers via surrogacy. LGBT individuals and same-sex couples may become foster or adoptive parents.

For many lesbian and bisexual women, use of donor insemination is a preferred pathway to parenthood. Whether using sperm from a known donor (e.g., a male friend or relative) or from an unknown donor (e.g., via the resources of a sperm bank), women who conceive via donor insemination will be genetically linked with their offspring. For some female couples, one partner might serve as the genetic and one as the gestational parent, using in vitro fertilization to fertilize one woman's egg and then insert it into her partner's body. Known as partner-assisted reproduction (97), this procedure is still unusual, even among affluent groups in the United States. Many lesbian and bisexual women do, however, use some form of donor insemination to have children. For gay and bisexual men, surrogacy is an increasingly common pathway to parenthood (81,98). In this case, a woman serving as a surrogate carries a baby conceived either with her own egg or with a donor egg. The intended father, whose sperm were used to fertilize the egg, will be genetically linked with the child. Surrogacy is, however, costly, and the law in some jurisdictions prohibits its use. Thus, surrogacy may be a viable pathway to parenthood for some gay and bisexual men, but not for others.

Transgender men and women who wish to have biological children face specific challenges because cross-sex hormone therapies and gender affirmation surgeries can reduce or eliminate fertility. Nonetheless, transgender people have become parents through various means, including donor insemination, surrogacy, and egg or embryo freezing and sperm banking before initiating hormone treatment. Chapter 17 offers more detailed information about fertility options for transgender people.

LGBT individuals and same-sex couples may also become parents via foster care or adoption (37,99). Some LGBT adults agree to become foster parents for children in hopes of ultimately adopting the children; others foster children whom they do not intend to adopt. Adoptions may be arranged via public or private agencies, and they may involve children born in the United States or in another country (99). They may involve children to whom the adoptive parent is genetically related (e.g., nieces and nephews), but they more commonly involve genetically unrelated children. Adoptions may also vary in the extent to which there is contact among birth parents, adoptive parents, and adoptive children (i.e., in their extent of openness) (37). Finally, some LGBT individuals and couples undertake informal parenting arrangements that remain undocumented.

Thus, many options are now available to LGBT people who want to become parents. Choices among the options may be affected by financial matters, medical issues, and legal concerns, as well as by individual preferences and characteristics of social networks. Whatever pathway is selected, many LGBT people are becoming parents in the United States today.

Transition to Parenthood

Becoming a parent is a major life transition, and it can be both exciting and stressful (100). As happy as new parents may be, they must also master new tasks, cope with new demands on their time, and grow accustomed to new roles. These realities characterize the transition to parenthood for LGBT parents, just as they do for heterosexual parents (83,87,98,101). Satisfaction with couple relationships often declines during this transition, and this seems to be as true of same-sex couples as it is of others (101,102). Qualitative research suggests that time and energy for relationship maintenance and sexual activity may decrease over same-sex couples' transitions to parenthood (103).

Although there are many similarities, the transition to parenthood also varies as a function of sexual orientation and gender identity (91,104,105). Prospective parents who identify as lesbian or gay are less likely than heterosexual couples to feel supported by their friends and by members of their families of origin. For instance, Gartrell and her colleagues (106) reported that, at the time of a child's birth, most lesbian mothers in their sample expected to receive at least some support from relatives. There were, however, some—about 15%—who did not expect any of their family members to recognize the baby as a relative. In a more recent study, some pregnant lesbian women, interviewed in their third trimester, reported a lack of support from their families of origin (107). Three months after the baby's birth, however, these women reported that their families had become more supportive (107). In one of the only studies to examine the experiences of bisexual people across the transition to parenthood, pregnant bisexual women reported more depressive symptoms than did their lesbian and heterosexual peers (104). In a study of same-sex couples in the United States, those who had high levels of internalized stigma and who lived in states with laws that were unfavorable to lesbian and gay parents reported the greatest increases in depressive and anxious symptoms over the first year of parenthood (108). Much remains to be learned about the ways in which transitions to parenthood are experienced by LGBT individuals. Certainly, one might expect variation in such experiences as a function of social context (85).

Family Processes

What are the characteristics of families headed by LGBT parents? How are they similar to or different from families headed by heterosexual parents? Research in this area has focused mainly on describing families headed by lesbian mothers. However, research is increasingly focusing on the experiences of people in families headed by gay fathers, as well. Very little research has focused on the characteristics and experiences of families headed by bisexual or transgender parents.

Research on family relationships within lesbian-mother families suggests that they are generally positive (109). In study after study, both children and adolescents have been found to enjoy warm and supportive relationships with their lesbian mothers (37,110–113). As mentioned above, observations of family interactions have led to the same conclusion.

Research on lesbian mothers has highlighted that social (i.e., nonbiological) mothers report being more involved in childcare than do fathers or stepfathers in heterosexual-parent families (114). This pattern has been reported both in families formed using donor insemination and in families formed via adoption (39). In many studies, lesbian couples have reported sharing childcare more evenly, on average, than do heterosexual couples (66).

Fewer data are available on families headed by gay fathers, but existing findings suggest that relationships are also generally warm and positive in these families (39,115). In an early study, divorced gay fathers described themselves as more responsive to their children, more likely to use reasoning during disciplinary encounters, and somewhat more strict in setting standards than did divorced heterosexual fathers (116–118). In other work, gay fathers who had partners were more likely to express satisfaction with their lives and described themselves as being more successful at meeting common challenges involved in parenting than did those who were single (35,115).

More recent work has focused on family relationships among gay adoptive fathers. In a sample of adoptive families headed by lesbian, gay, or heterosexual couples, parents in all family types reported long-term, relatively harmonious relationships as well as high relationship satisfaction (39). There were no differences in these variables as a function of family type. Evidence from this sample also suggested that male and female couples who have adopted children together divide childcare tasks in a relatively egalitarian fashion (37). In another recent study, gay fathers who reported more positive gay identities reported less parenting stress than did those with more negative gay identities (119).

Contextual Influences

In what kinds of social contexts do LGBT parents rear their children? How might these social contexts be similar to or different from the contexts in which heterosexual parents live? Little research has explored these issues among children with bisexual, transgender, or gay parents; therefore, we describe research on lesbian mothers and their families.

Research has focused on children's contacts with members of their extended family, especially contact with grandparents (120,121). Patterson and her colleagues found that most lesbian mothers in their sample (121) reported that their children enjoyed regular contact with grandparents. In a study that included children of lesbian and heterosexual parents, there were no differences in frequency of contact with grandparents as a function of parental sexual orientation (120). Additional research has also suggested that a majority of grandparents acknowledged the children of lesbian daughters as grandchildren (122). Thus, findings suggest that intergenerational relationships in lesbian-parented families are generally satisfactory.

Researchers have also assessed children's contacts with adult friends of their lesbian mothers (111,120,121). All of the children in these studies were described as having contact with adult friends of their mothers, and most lesbian mothers reported that their friends were diverse in sexual orientation; they included lesbian, gay, and heterosexual individuals. Children of lesbian mothers were no less likely than those of heterosexual mothers to have social contact with adult men who were friends of their mothers (120). Thus, findings to date suggest that children of lesbian mothers have positive contacts with many adults in the context of their family lives.

Issues may emerge for some lesbian and gay parents as they decide how open to be about their nonheterosexual identities. For instance, some lesbian mothers have reported withholding information about their sexual identities in health care settings, particularly in situations they perceived to be unsafe (123,124). Some lesbian and gay parents also report selective disclosure at their children's schools, based on their evaluations of individual attitudes as well as overall school climate (123,125). Most lesbian and gay parents express desire for as much openness as possible in the context of maintaining a safe and welcoming environment for themselves and their children (126).

Summary and Thoughts for Health Care Providers

Families with LGBT parents are diverse. Some were formed in the context of heterosexual marriages that have since broken up, and others were formed in the context of LGBT identities. When LGBT individuals and couples decide to have children, they may do so via one of many pathways, such as donor insemination, adoption, and surrogacy. Experiences of parents and children may reflect differences in family formation. Because family relationships may be recognized under law in some jurisdictions but not in others, contextual factors loom especially large in the lives of LGBT parents. Becoming aware of the diversity among LGBT parents and their families assists health care providers in their efforts to provide quality care.

Because decision-making for LGBT prospective parents can be complex, planning may often involve legal and financial as well as medical decision-making, and health care providers should be prepared to offer salient referrals. As LGBT individuals and couples pursue pathways to parenthood, health care providers should be aware that stressors may include encounters with various forms of stigma, lack of support from family members, friends, and health care personnel, and/or problems with additional barriers that may be legal, financial, or medical in nature. After a child is born, LGBT couples in some jurisdictions must struggle to establish the legitimacy of the parent who is not legally or biologically linked with the child; in other jurisdictions, both parents are recognized in law and this issue does not loom as large. Health care providers who are aware of contextual factors such as the legal status of LGBT-parent families in their area are better equipped to advise prospective and current LGBT parents about how to ensure the best care for themselves and for their family members.

Children of LGBT Parents

Considerable research over the past decades has focused on development of children reared by LGBT parents. Most of this research has focused on children with lesbian mothers. Only a handful of studies have examined the development of children with gay fathers (38) or transgender parents (127,128); no comparable studies have focused on the experiences of bisexual parents. While research surrounding lesbian and gay parenting has found no negative associations between parental sexual orientation and developmental outcomes, some interesting variations have been observed (66,74,96,109,129).

Gender and Sexual Identity

Considerable research has focused on gender development among children of lesbian and gay parents. For example, this work has focused on questions about gender role behavior, gender, and sexual identities among children who grow up with same-sex parents. In general, researchers have found that children of lesbian and gay parents show gender and sexual development that is similar to that evinced by their peers with heterosexual parents (39,110,111,113,130,131).

Three different aspects of gender and sexual development have been considered. *Gender identity* is usually defined as an individual's self-identification as male, female, or otherwise. *Gender-role behaviors* are the behaviors seen as relevant to gender that determine how closely an individual exemplifies cultural norms about masculine and feminine behavior—for example, in play behavior or occupational aspirations. *Sexual identity* and *sexual orientation* refer to an individual's feelings of being attracted to sexual partners of same and/or different sexes. We review the findings relevant to each of these three areas below.

The gender identity of children with LGBT parents has been examined with a variety of methods, including projective tests (132), interviews with parents (111), and self-report questionnaires completed by children (129). None of these approaches has revealed differences in gender identity among children with lesbian mothers as compared to those with heterosexual parents. For instance, Bos and Sandfort (129) compared gender identity among children (8 to 12 years of age) who were being reared by lesbian mothers and same-aged children being reared by heterosexual parents in the Netherlands. A questionnaire was used to measure different aspects of gender identity, such as feelings about gender typicality and happiness with gender assignment. Results showed that children of lesbian mothers reported gender identities much like those of heterosexual parents (130).

In related research, Brewaeys and colleagues (110) compared gender role development of 4- to 8-year-old children of lesbian mothers conceived through donor insemination with that among same-aged children of heterosexual parents who conceived using donor insemination and with that among same-aged children of heterosexual parents who conceived via sexual intercourse. Using a standardized parent-report instrument called the Preschool Activities Inventory (PSAI), Brewaeys and colleagues found no differences in children's reported gender-role behavior across the three family types. In another study using the PSAI, Farr and her colleagues (39) reported no differences in gender development among preschool-aged children with lesbian, gay, or heterosexual adoptive parents. In both studies, gender role behavior of children with lesbian or gay parents was similar to that of other children.

In contrast, Goldberg and colleagues (133) also used the PSAI to assess play behavior of young adopted children (2 to 4 years of age) with heterosexual, gay, and lesbian parents. These researchers found that children of lesbian or gay parents were described as engaging in less gender-typed play than were children of heterosexual parents (133). Descriptions of behavior among children of lesbian and gay parents did not, however, differ from those given in a standardization sample of families with heterosexual parents.

In a related study, Bos and Sandfort (130) explored the gender-relevant beliefs and psychological development of children, 8 to 12 years of age, who had lesbian or heterosexual parents. Children of lesbian mothers reported less parental pressure to conform to gender stereotypes, were less likely to report their own gender as superior, and were more likely to question whether or not they would have future heterosexual relationships. Similarly, MacCallum and Golombok (134) reported that sons of lesbian mothers and single heterosexual mothers had higher femininity scores than their peers with two heterosexual parents; however, they found no differences in boys' masculinity scores across groups and no differences on either scale for girls.

With some variations, children with lesbian and gay parents have thus been found to show typical gender role development. Research examining variations in gender role behaviors and activities of children has found that these differences are linked to parental attitudes regarding gender roles, rather than to parental sexual orientation. All researchers have reported that gender role behavior of children with lesbian and gay parents follows culturally expected patterns.

Research on sexual orientation and sexual behavior among offspring of lesbian and gay parents has likewise found few differences in sexual development of adolescents and adults. In a study of adult children of gay fathers, Bailey and colleagues (135) found that the vast majority identified as heterosexual. Huggins (136) compared the sexual orientation of adolescents, half with divorced lesbian mothers and the other half with divorced heterosexual mothers. In this study, all of the children of lesbian mothers identified themselves as heterosexual, and all but one of the children of heterosexual mothers identified as heterosexual (136). These are two examples drawn from a larger research literature (113,127,131,137).

Some research has also explored dating and sexual behavior of children of same-sex parents. Wainright and colleagues (113) used data from a national dataset to examine the romantic relationships and sexual behavior of adolescents with same-sex parents, compared with those of a matched group of youth with different-sex parents. There were no differences in the rates of same-sex attraction, numbers of romantic relationships, or frequency of engaging in heterosexual sexual intercourse. Similarly, Gartrell and colleagues (137) explored sexual orientation, sexual behavior, and sexual risk among adolescents with lesbian mothers versus a representative U.S. sample of adolescents; they found that family type was unrelated to adolescent sexual identity. Female adolescents with lesbian mothers were, however, more likely than those in the national sample to report engaging in same-sex sexual behavior (137).

Very little research has been reported on children with transgender parents. In one study, Green (127) found that all who were old enough to interview reported heterosexual sexual behaviors and thoughts. More research on transgender parents and their children is needed.

Social Development

Research has also examined social development among children of lesbian or gay parents. This work has explored children's friendships and social networks, as well as their experiences of bullying and victimization. Some children have reported negative experiences, but most have shown normal growth on important dimensions of social development.

Overall, children with lesbian and gay parents establish and maintain social relationships with peers in much the same ways as do children with heterosexual parents (111,138,139). Golombok and colleagues (111) found no difference in number of friends or in quality of peer relationships among children being raised by divorced lesbian mothers versus divorced heterosexual parents. Wainright and Patterson (138) explored peer relationships of adolescents with same-sex parents and of adolescents with different-sex parents from a nationally representative U.S. dataset. On measures that included number of friends, presence of a best friend, and amount of support from closest friends, they reported no differences in peer relationships as a function of family type (138).

Gartrell and colleagues (122) reported that among their sample of 10-year-old children of lesbian mothers, 43% of the children reported having experienced homophobic comments. Most of those who heard such comments reported being upset or bothered by them (122). In a study of Australian youth with lesbian and gay parents, almost half of the children from grades 3 through 10 reported being bullied or teased because of their parents' sexual orientation (139). In the United States, most (89%) LGBT-parented adolescents in a large survey reported hearing negative comments about LGBT people (140). One question raised by these findings is whether children of lesbian or gay parents are at elevated risk for difficulties as a result of exposure to homophobic comments, teasing, and victimization.

Research on the incidence of peer victimization has found similar rates of bullying and victimization among heterosexual-parented and LGBT-parented children (137,141). Two studies—one of U.S. adolescents (141) and one of adolescents in the United Kingdom (142)—compared adolescents of same-sex parents with those of heterosexual parents and found that both groups had similar rates of reported victimization. Thus, although homophobic bullying does occur, the likelihood of victimization does not appear to be elevated among the offspring of lesbian and gay parents.

Other Aspects of Development

Many other aspects of development have also been studied among the offspring of lesbian and gay parents. Research findings suggest that children with lesbian and gay parents develop cognitively (132,143,144) and behaviorally (28,39,10,145,146) in similar ways to children with heterosexual parents. Research has also revealed that development of self-concepts is similar, regardless of parental sexual orientation (113,130,146). Overall, research results have supported the conclusion that important variations in children's development are not associated with parental sexual orientation.

Summary and Thoughts for Health Care Providers

Research on children of LGBT parents has generally found them to be developing in ways that are similar to development among children with heterosexual parents. Across a wide range of samples, research methods,

Table 6–1   Resources for LGBT Individuals and Their Families

AdoptUSKids www.adoptuskids.org
This website, which is operated by the Adoption Exchange Association, offers resources and assistance to LGBT parents interested in fostering or adopting.

American Fertility Association www.theafa.org/family-building/lgbt-family-building
The American Fertility Association offers comprehensive resources such as articles, fact sheets, handbooks, and videos on LGBT family building. Among their website resources is information about medical and legal issues facing LGBT parents and a directory of LGBT-friendly doctors, lawyers, sperm banks, adoption agencies, and egg donor/surrogacy agencies.

Children of Lesbians and Gays Everywhere (COLAGE) www.colage.org
COLAGE is a national support and empowerment network for people with LGBT parents and offers resources for both LGBT parents and children of LGBT parents. COLAGE includes many community-based groups across the United States.

Family Equality Council (FEC) www.familyequality.org
Family Equality Council connects, supports, and represents parents who are LGBT in the United States, as well as their children. FEC is changing attitudes and policies to ensure that all families are respected, loved, and celebrated—especially families with parents who are lesbian, gay, bisexual, or transgender. Their website includes many resources for parents, including maps that outline legal rights in different states, and sample forms for protecting families

Gay, Lesbian & Straight Education Network (GLSEN) www.glsen.org
GLSEN is an organization that focuses on providing LGBT-safe and friendly schools. The group empowers students, parents, and teachers with knowledge of LGBT issues through local community chapters, educator resources, and student support.

Human Rights Campaign (HRC) www.hrc.org
The HRC is the largest LGBT civil rights organization in the United States and provides resources for LGBT individuals on a diverse array of family and relationship issues, including marriage, adoption, assisted reproduction, and schooling.

Lambda Legal www.lambdalegal.org
Lambda Legal is a national organization working to achieve civil rights equality for LGBT individuals through impact litigation, education, and public policy work. It provides information on varied legal and policy issues affecting LGBT individuals, couples, and families across the United States.

Parents, Families, and Friends of LGBT People (PFLAG) www.pflag.org
PFLAG is a nonprofit organization composed of parents, families, friends, and straight allies of LGBT individuals, offering community help lines, support group meetings, and resources to the LGBT community. PLFAG also provides education for communities and families on gender, sexuality, and LGBT issues.

World Professional Association for Transgender Health (WPATH) www.wpath.org
This organization is dedicated to promoting evidence based care, education, advocacy, public policy, and respect in transgender health.

and family types, children of LGBT parents have been found, on average, to be flourishing. Many children of LGBT parents encounter negative attitudes toward their families, or even outright victimization. Children describe these as negative experiences but do not generally seem to be marked by them in any permanent way.

Health care providers should be aware of diversity in family configu-
rations among children who have LGBT parents, and of the variation in
terms that children use to refer to their parents and other family members. For example, a child with two fathers may call one "Papa" and the
other "Dad," may call both "Dad," or may use different names. Awareness
that children of LGBT parents may encounter stigma may also be valuable. As in other areas, readiness to refer a young patient to supportive
providers of health care can be invaluable (see Table 6-1 for a list of
resources).

Conclusions

There has been a substantial amount of research on couple relationships,
parenting, and family issues among LGBT people. Findings reveal that many
aspects of couple relationships are similar to those among heterosexual couples. There are, however, also some issues (such as the extent of legal recognition for family relationships) that are specific to LGBT people. It is clear
that many LGBT adults are or want to become parents, and research findings
suggest that lesbian women and gay men are at least as competent as their
heterosexual counterparts in parental roles. It is also clear that LGBT people
are achieving parenthood via many pathways, including prior heterosexual
marriages, donor insemination, surrogacy, and adoption. Finally, a substantial body of research indicates that, even though some encounter prejudice
against their families, the offspring of lesbian and gay parents generally
develop in positive ways.

The research literature in this area has many strengths but also some
limitations. Notable among the limitations is that relatively little is yet
known about intersectionality and its role in structuring couple and family
relationships. In other words, much of the research has focused on middle-
and upper-middle class Euro-American participants, and with few exceptions (147), little is known about racial, ethnic, and other forms of diversity.
Another important limitation is in the study of bisexual and transgender
issues. Much more of the research has focused on relationships of lesbian
and gay individuals than on relationships of bisexual and transgender people. Thus, much remains for future research to learn about LGBT relationships and family lives. At the same time, however, much that can be of value
to health care providers has been learned, and some of the clearest lessons
are outlined below.

First, health care providers should be aware of the great diversity of intimate relationships, sexual practices, and family ties among LGBT people. As
an example, the fact that gay men are involved in longstanding couple relationships does not mean that they are monogamous; they may be, or they
may have agreed upon other arrangements. Some men and women in LGBT
communities are involved in polyamorous rather than coupled relationships.

In addition, LGBT parents may or may not be genetically linked with their children. Many such variations can have important implications for the providers of health care (148).

Second, health care providers should be aware that many LGBT people who are not parents may nevertheless hope to have children in the future. It is clear that LGBT people are pursuing various pathways to parenthood today, including donor insemination, surrogacy, and adoption. Choices among pathways to parenthood may vary as a function of a person's sex, gender identity, sexual orientation, and financial circumstances, as well as local law and policy. LGBT prospective parents may call upon health care providers to provide information and education along with medical services (85).

Another issue is that legal recognition for LGBT couple relationships varies widely across jurisdictions, both in the United States and abroad. For instance, a same-sex couple may be legally married in one jurisdiction, but their marriage may not be recognized in another jurisdiction. Thus, a same-sex spouse may be eligible for health insurance coverage through the spouse's job in one jurisdiction, but she may be regarded as a legal stranger and hence be ineligible for health insurance coverage in another area. Moreover, in at least some jurisdictions, the law is changing rapidly, creating additional challenges and opportunities for LGBT parents and their children. When important family relationships are not recognized, this may pose problems in health care settings. For example, in some jurisdictions, LGBT spouses and parents may not be empowered to make medical decisions for one another or for some or all of their children (148).

Health care providers should also bear in mind that biological links between parents and children that are often taken for granted between heterosexual parents and their children may or may not exist among LGBT parents and their children. When lesbian couples have children via donor insemination or when gay male couples have children via surrogacy, only one of the two same-sex parents is usually biologically linked with their children. In health care settings, the lack of a biological link with one parent may affect the amount of information available about genetic risks and other medical issues.

Finally, the family lives of LGBT people are deeply affected by the legal and policy environments in which they live (see Chapter 19 for more on policies and laws that affect LGBT people). Research is beginning to reveal some of the ways in which discriminatory laws and policies, as well as the debates surrounding them, have a negative impact on the health of LGBT people (149). As family relationships of LGBT people are increasingly recognized in law and policy, this situation is changing. In the meantime, however, health care providers should be aware of the many ways in which the family lives of LGBT people are affected by living in social and legal environments that discriminate against them.

Summary Points

- Like other people, LGBT individuals form couple relationships that may last for many years; for LGBT people, these relationships are recognized by law in some but not other jurisdictions in the United States and around the world.
- Same-sex and opposite-sex couple relationships are similar in some respects but differ in others. As examples of difference, consider that same-sex couples may be more egalitarian than opposite-sex couples in division of household labor and that gay male couples may be less committed to monogamy than other couples.
- There is great diversity in the intimate relationships of LGBT people, and some pursue intimate relationships that may involve three or more people.
- Many LGBT people are parents and many more hope to become parents.
- At one time, LGBT people had children mainly in the context of heterosexual marriages, but now many LGBT individuals become parents after coming out, via adoption, foster care, donor insemination, and surrogacy.
- Biological linkages between parents and children should not be taken for granted in LGBT populations; children of LGBT parents may or may not be biologically linked with parents or with one another.
- Children of LGBT parents have been found to be developing in generally healthy ways; these children seem to show the range of common behaviors and problems that any ordinary sample of children would show—no more, and no less than typical.
- Legal and policy environments are highly variable in the United States and abroad, and this is a fact with great significance for LGBT couples and parents, and also for their children.

References

1. **Fingerhut AW, Peplau LA.** Same-sex romantic relationships. In: Patterson CJ, D'Augelli AR, eds. Handbook of Psychology and Sexual Orientation. New York: Oxford University Press; 2013:165-78.
2. **D'Augelli AR, Rendina HJ, Sinclair KO, Grossman AH.** Lesbian and gay youth's aspirations for marriage and raising children. J LGBT Issues Couns. 2006/07;1:77-98.
3. **Peplau LA, Cochran SD.** A relationship perspective on homosexuality. In: McWhirter DP, Sanders SA, Reinisch JM, eds. Homosexuality/Heterosexuality: Concepts of Sexual Orientation. New York: Oxford University Press; 1990:321-49.
4. **Peplau LA, Veniegas RC, Campbell SM.** Gay and lesbian relationships. In: Savin-Williams RC, Cohen KM, eds. The Lives of Lesbians, Gays, and Bisexuals: Children to Adults. New York: Harcourt Brace; 1996:250-73.
5. **Morris JF, Balsam KF, Rothblum ED.** Lesbian and bisexual mothers and nonmothers: demographics and the coming-out process. J Fam Psychol. 2002;16:144-56.

6. **Carpenter C, Gates GJ.** Gay and lesbian partnership: evidence from California. Demography. 2008;45:573-90.

7. **Rosenfeld MJ, Thomas RJ.** Searching for a mate: the rise of the internet as a social intermediary. Am Sociol Rev. 2012;77:523-47.

8. **Lofquist D.** American Community Survey Briefs: same-sex couple households. 2011; ACSBR/10-03.

9. **Wight RG, LeBlanc AJ, Badgett MVL.** Stress and mental health among midlife and older gay-identified men. Am J Public Health. 2012;102:503-10.

10. **Roisman GI, Clausell E, Holland A, Fortuna K, Elieff C.** Adult romantic relationships as contexts of human development: a multimethod comparison of same-sex couples with opposite-sex dating, engaged, and married dyads. Develop Psychol. 2008;44:91-101.

11. **Peplau LA, Padesky C, Hamilton M.** Satisfaction in lesbian relationships. J Homosex. 1982; 8:23-35.

12. **Kurdek LA.** Relationships outcomes and their predictors: longitudinal evidence from heterosexual married, gay cohabiting, and lesbian cohabiting couples. J Marriage Fam. 1998;60: 553-68.

13. **Kurdek LA.** What do we know about gay and lesbian couples? Curr Dir Psychol Sci. 2005;14:251-54,309.

14. **Kurdek LA, Schmitt JP.** Relationship quality of partners in heterosexual married, heterosexual cohabiting, and gay and lesbian relationships. J Pers Soc Psychol. 1986;51:711-20.

15. **Kurdek LA.** Are gay and lesbian cohabiting couples really different from heterosexual married couples? J Marriage Fam. 2004;66:880-900.

16. **Eldridge NS, Gilbert LA.** Correlates of relationship satisfaction in lesbian couples. Psychol Women Q. 1990;14:43-62.

17. **Berger RM.** Passing: impact of the quality of same-sex couple relationships. Soc Work. 1990;35:328-32.

18. **Caron SL, Ulin M.** Closeting and the quality of lesbian relationships. Fam Soc. 1997;78: 413-9.

19. **Peplau LA.** Human sexuality: how do men and women differ? Curr Dir Psychol Sci. 2003;12:37-40.

20. **Harry J.** Gay Couples. New York: Praeger; 1984.

21. **Harry J, DeVall W.** Age and sexual culture among homosexually oriented males. Arch Sex Behav. 1978;7:199-209.

22. **Caldwell MA, Peplau LA.** The balance of power in lesbian relationships. Sex Roles. 1984; 10:587-99.

23. **Blumstein P, Schwartz P.** American Couples: Money, Work, Sex. New York: William Morrow and Company, Inc.; 1983.

24. **Reilly ME, Lynch JM.** Power-sharing in lesbian partnerships. J Homosex. 1990;19:1-30.

25. **Melendez RM, Pinto R.** 'It's really a hard life': love, gender and HIV risk among male-to-female transgender persons. Cult Health Sex. 2007;9:233-45.

26. **Schilt K, Westbrook L.** Doing gender, doing heteronormativity: 'gender normals', transgender people and the social maintenance of heterosexuality. Gend Soc. 2009;23:440-64.

27. **Bockting WO, Robinson E, Rosser BRS.** Transgender HIV prevention: a qualitative needs assessment. AIDS Care. 1998;10:505-26.

28. **Chan RW, Brooks RC, Raboy B, Patterson CJ.** Division of labor among lesbian and heterosexual parents: associations with children's adjustment. J Fam Psychol. 1998;12: 402-19.

29. **Gartrell N, Banks A, Hamilton J, et al.** The national lesbian family study: 2. interviews with mothers of toddlers. Am J Orthopsychiatry. 1999;69:362-9.

30. **Kurdek LA.** The allocation of household labor by partners in gay and lesbian couples. J Fam Issues. 2007;28:132-48.

31. **Patterson CJ, Sutfin EL, Fulcher M.** Division of labor among lesbian and heterosexual parenting couples: correlates of specialized versus shared patterns. J Adult Dev. 2004;11: 179-89.

32. **Solomon SE, Rothblum ED, Balsam KF.** Pioneers in partnership: lesbians and gay men couples in civil unions compared with those not in civil unions, and married heterosexual couples. J Fam Psychol. 2004;18:275-86.

33. **Sullivan M.** Rozzie and Harriet? Gender and family patterns of lesbian coparents. Gend Soc. 1996;10:747-67.

34. **Moore M.** Gendered power relations among women: a study of household decision making in Black lesbian stepfamilies. Am Sociol Rev. 2008;73:335-56.

35. **Crosbie-Burnett M, Helmbrecht L.** A descriptive empirical study of gay male stepfamilies. Family Relations. 1993;42:256-62.

36. **Carrington C.** No Place Like Home: Relationships and Family Life Among Lesbians and Gay Men. Chicago: University of Chicago; 1999.

37. **Farr RH, Patterson CJ.** Lesbian and gay adoptive parents and their children. In: Goldberg AE, Allen KR, ed. LGBT-Parent Families: Innovations in Research and Implications for Practice New York: Springer; 2013:39-55.

38. **Kurdek LA.** Lesbian and gay couples. In: D'Augelli AR, Patterson CJ, eds. Lesbian, Gay and Bisexual Identities Over the Lifespan: Psychological Perspectives. New York: Oxford University Press; 1995:243-61.

39. **Farr RH, Forssell SL, Patterson CJ.** Parenting and child development in adoptive families: does parental sexual orientation matter? Appl Dev Sci. 2010;14;164-78.

40. **Peplau LA, Cochran SD, Mays VM.** A national survey of the intimate relationships of African American lesbians and gay men: a look at commitment, satisfaction, sexual behavior, and HIV disease. In: Thousand Oaks, CA: Sage Publications; 1997:11-38.

41. **Peplau LA, Fingerhut A, Beals KP.** Sexuality in the relationships of lesbians and gay men. In: Harvey J, Wenzel A, Sprecher S, eds. Handbook of Sexuality in Close Relationships. Mahwah, NJ: Lawrence Erlbaum Associates; 2004:349-70.

42. **Rothblum ED.** An overview of same-sex couples in relationships: a research area still at sea. In: Hope DA, ed. Contemporary Perspectives on Lesbian, Gay, and Bisexual Identities—Nebraska Symposium on Motivation. New York: Springer; 2009;54:113-39.

43. **Bryant AS, Demian.** Relationship characteristics of American gay and lesbian couples: findings from a national survey. J Gay Lesbian Soc Serv. 1994;1:101-17.

44. **Parsons JT, Starks TJ, Gamarel KE, Grov C.** Non-monogamy and sexual relationship quality among same-sex male couples. J Fam Psychol. 2012;26:669-77.

45. **Hoff CC, Beougher SC.** Sexual agreements among gay male couples. Arch Sex Behav. 2010; 39:774-87.

46. **Iantaffi A, Bockting WO.** Views from both sides of the bridge? Gender, sexual legitimacy and transgender peoples' experiences of relationships. Cult Health Sex. 2011;13:355-70.

47. **James SE, Murphy BC.** Gay and lesbian relationships in a changing social context. In: Patterson CJ, D'Augelli AR, eds. Lesbian, Gay and Bisexual Identities in Families: Psychological Perspectives. New York: Oxford University Press; 1998:99-121.

48. **Peplau LA, Fingerhut AW.** The close relationships of lesbians and gay men. Annu Rev Psychol. 2007;58:405-24.

49. **Balsam L, Hughes T.** Sexual orientation, victimization, and hate crimes. In: Patterson CJ, D'Augelli AR, eds. Handbook of Psychology and Sexual Orientation. New York: Oxford University Press; 2013:267-80.

50. **Barker M.** This is my partner, and this is my . . . partner's partner: constructing a polyamorous identity in a monogamous world. J Constr Psychol. 2005;18:75-88.

51. **Barker M, Langdridge D.** Whatever happened to non-monogamies? Critical reflections on recent research and theory. Sexualities. 2010;13:748-72.

52. **Rust P.** Monogamy and polyamory: relationship issues for bisexuals. In: Garnets LD, Kimmel DC, eds. Psychological Perspectives of Lesbian, Gay, and Bisexual Experiences. New York: Columbia University Press; 2003:475-96.

53. **Bricker ME, Horne SE.** The impact of monogamy and non-monogamy on relational health. J Couple Relatsh Ther. 2007;6:27-47.

54. **LaSala MC.** Comparing monogamous and nonmonogamous relationships. Fam Soc. 2004; 85:405-12.
55. **Walters AS, Curran M.** "Excuse me, sir? May I help you and your boyfriend?": Salespersons' differential treatment of homosexual and straight customers. J Homosex. 1996;31:135-52.
56. **Jones DA.** Discrimination against same-sex couples in hotel reservation policies. J Homosex. 1996;57:153-9.
57. **Herek GM.** Heterosexuals' attitudes toward bisexual men and women in the United States. J Sex Res. 2002;39:264-74.
58. **Klesse C.** Bisexual women, non-monogamy and differentialist anti-promiscuity discourses. Sexualities. 2005;8:445-64.
59. **Israel T, Mohr JJ.** Attitudes toward bisexual women and men: current research, future directions. J Bisex. 2004;4:117-34.
60. **Gallup Politics.** For first time, majority of Americans favor legal gay marriage. May 20, 2011. Accessed at: www.gallup.com/poll/File/147671/Gay_rights_110520.pdf.
61. **Gallup Politics.** Half of Americans support legal gay marriage. May 8, 2012. Available at: www.gallup.com/file/poll/154538/Gay_Marriage_120508.pdf.
62. **Pew Research Center.** A survey of LGBT Americans: attitudes, experiences and values in changing times. June 13, 2013. Available at: www.pewsocialtrends.org/files/2013/06/SDT_LGBT-Americans_06-2013.pdf.
63. **Johnson SM, O'Connor E.** The Gay Baby Boom: The Psychology of Gay Parenthood. New York: New York University Press; 2002:1-193.
64. **Patterson CJ.** Children of lesbian and gay parents. Child Dev. 1992;63:1025-42.
65. **Patterson CJ.** Sexual orientation and family life: a decade review. J Marriage Fam. 2000; 62:1052-69.
66. **Patterson CJ, D'Augelli AR, eds.** Handbook of Psychology and sexual Orientation. New York: Oxford University Press; 2013.
67. **Joslin CG, Minter SP.** Lesbian, Gay, Bisexual, and Transgender Family Law. Eagan, MN: West Publishing; 2009.
68. **Patterson CJ, Redding RE.** Lesbian and gay families with children: implications of social science research for policy. J Soc Iss. 1996;52:29-50.
69. **Falk PJ.** The gap between psychosocial assumptions and empirical research in lesbian-mother child custody cases. In: Gottfried AE, Gottfried AW, eds. Redefining Families. New York: Plenum Press; 1994:131-56.
70. **Richman KD.** Courting change: Queer Parents, Judges, and the Transformation of American Family Law. New York: New York University Press; 2009.
71. **Lyons TA.** Lesbian mothers' custody fears. Women Ther. 1983;2:231-40.
72. **Pagelow MD.** Heterosexual and lesbian single mothers: a comparison of problems, coping, and solutions. J Homosex. 1980;5:189-204.
73. **Shapiro DN, Peterson C, Stewart AJ.** Legal and social contexts and mental health among lesbian and heterosexual mothers. J Fam Psychol. 2009;23:255-62.
74. **Golombok S, Tasker F.** Gay fathers. In: Lamb ME, ed. The Role of the Father in Child Development. 5th ed. New York: Wiley; 2010:319-40.
75. **Patterson CJ.** Families headed by lesbian and gay parents. In Lamb ME, ed. Nontraditional Families: Parenting and Child Development. 2nd ed. Hillsdale, NJ: Lawrence Erlbaum Associates; 1998:397-416.
76. **Miller B.** Adult sexual resocialization: adjustments toward a stigmatized identity. Altern Lifestyles. 1978;1:207-34.
77. **Miller B.** Gay fathers and their children. Fam Coord. 1979;28:544-52.
78. **Bozett FW.** Gay fathers: how and why they disclose their homosexuality to their children. Fam Relations. 1980;29:173-9.
79. **Bozett FW.** Gay fathers: evolution of the gay father identity. Am J Orthopsychiatry. 1981; 51:552-9.
80. **Bozett FW.** Children of gay fathers. In: Bozett FW, ed. Gay and Lesbian Parents. New York: Praeger; 1987:39-57.

81. **Patterson CJ, Tornello SL.** Gay fathers' pathways to parenthood: international perspectives. Zeitschrift fur Familienforschung, Sonderheft. 2010;5: 103-11.

82. **Hermann-Green LK, Gehring TM.** The German lesbian family study: planning for parenthood via donor insemination. J GLBT Fam Stud. 2007;3:351-96.

83. **Mallon GP.** Gay Men Choosing Parenthood. New York: Columbia University Press; 2004.

84. **Rabun C, Oswald RF.** Upholding and expanding the normal family: future fatherhood through the eyes of gay male emerging adults. Fathering. 2009;7:269-85.

85. **Patterson CJ, Riskind RG.** To be a parent: issues in family formation among gay and lesbian adults. J GLBT Fam Stud. 2010;6:326-40.

86. **Berkowitz D, Marsiglio W.** Gay men: negotiating procreative, father, and family identities. J Marriage Fam. 2007;69:366-81.

87. **Gianino M.** Adaptation and transformation: the transition to adoptive parenthood for gay male couples. J GLBT Fam Stud. 2008;4:205-43.

88. **Gates G, Badgett LMV, Macomber JE, Chambers K.** Adoption and foster care by gay and lesbian parents in the United States. Los Angeles, CA: UCLA School of Law Williams Institute; 2007.

89. **Riskind RG, Patterson CJ.** Parenting intentions and desires among childless lesbian, gay, and heterosexual individuals. J Fam Psychol. 2010;24:78-81.

90. **Shenkman G.** The gap between fatherhood and couplehood desires among Israeli gay men and estimations of their likelihood. J Fam Psychol. 2012;26:828-32.

91. **Goldberg AE.** Lesbian, gay, and bisexual family psychology: a systemic, life-cycle perspective. In: Bray JH, Stanton M, eds. The Wiley-Blackwell Handbook of Family Psychology. West Sussex, UK: Wiley-Blackwell; 2009:576-87.

92. **Patterson CJ.** Lesbian and gay couples considering parenthood: an agenda for research, service, and advocacy. J Gay Lesbian Soc Serv. 1994;1:33-55.

93. **Riskind, RG, Patterson CJ, Nosek BA.** Childless lesbian and gay adults' self-efficacy about achieving parenthood. Couple Family Psychol. 2013;2:222-35.

94. **Brodzinsky DM, the Staff of the Evan B.** Donaldson Adoption Institute. Adoption by Lesbians and Gays: A National Survey of Adoption Agency Policies, Practices, and Attitudes. New York: Evan B. Donaldson Adoption Institute; 2003.

95. **Gurmankin AD, Caplan AL, Braverman AM.** Screening practices and beliefs of assisted reproductive technology programs. Fertil Steril. 2005;88:61-7.

96. **Goldberg AE.** Studying complex families in context. J Marriage Fam. 2010;72:29-34.

97. **Riskind RG.** Sexual orientation and use of assisted reproductive technology: social and psychological issues. In Schenker J, ed. Ethical and Legal Aspects of ART. Berlin: Walter de Gruyter; 2011:233-44.

98. **Bergman K, Rubio RJ, Green R, Padrón E.** Gay men who become fathers via surrogacy: the transition to parenthood. J GLBT Fam Stud. 2010;6:111-41.

99. **Brodzinsky DM, Pertman A, eds.** Adoption by Lesbians and Gay Men: A New Dimension in Family Diversity. New York: Oxford University Press; 2012.

100. **Cowan CP, Cowan PA.** Who does what when partners become parents: implications for men, women, and marriage. Marriage Fam Rev. 1988;12:105-31.

101. **Goldberg AE, Sayer A.** Lesbian couples' relationship quality across the transition to parenthood. J Marriage Fam. 2006;68:87-100.

102. **Goldberg AE, Smith JZ, Kashy DA.** Pre-adoptive factors predicting lesbian, gay, and heterosexual couples' relationship quality across the transition to adoptive parenthood. J Fam Psychol. 2010;24:221-32.

103. **Huebner DM, Mandic CG, Mackaronis JE, et al.** The impact of parenting on gay male couples' relationships, sexuality, and HIV risk. Couple Fam Psychol. 2012;1:106-19.

104. **Ross LE, Steele L, Goldfinger C, Strike C.** Perinatal depressive symptomatology among lesbian and bisexual women. Arch Womens Ment Health. 2007;10:53-9.

105. **Pfeffer CA.** Normative resistance and inventive pragmatism: negotiating structure and agency in transgender families. Gender Soc. 2012;26:574-602.

106. **Gartrell N, Hamilton J, Banks A, et al.** The national lesbian family study: 1. interviews with prospective mothers. Am J Orthopsychiatry. 1996;66:272-81.

107. **Goldberg AE.** The transition to parenthood for lesbian couples. J GLBT Fam Stud. 2006;2: 13-42.

108. **Goldberg AE, Smith JZ.** Stigma, social context, and mental health: lesbian and gay couples across the transition to adoptive parenthood. J Couns Psychol. 2011;58:139-50.

109. **Biblarz TJ, Stacey J.** How does the gender of parents matter? J Marriage Fam. 2010;72:3-22.

110. **Brewaeys A, Ponjaert I, Van Hall EV, Golombok S.** Donor insemination: child development and family functioning in lesbian mother families. Human Reproduct. 1997;12:1349-59.

111. **Golombok S, Spencer A, Rutter M.** Children in lesbian and single-parent households: psychosexual and psychiatric appraisal. J Child Psychol Psychiatry. 1983;24:551-72.

112. **Kirkpatrick M, Smith C, Roy R.** Lesbian mothers and their children: a comparative survey. Am J Orthopsychiatry. 1981;51:545-51.

113. **Wainright JL, Russell ST, Patterson CJ.** Psychosocial adjustment, school outcomes, and romantic relationships of adolescents with same-sex parents. Child Dev. 2004;75:1886-98.

114. **Tasker FL, Golombok S. Growing Up in a Lesbian Family: Effects on Child Development.** New York: Guilford Press; 1997:i1-194.

115. **Barrett H, Tasker F.** Growing up with a gay parent: views of 101 gay fathers on their sons' and daughters' experiences. Educat Child Psychol. 2001;18:62-77.

116. **Bigner JJ, Jacobsen RB.** The value of children to gay and heterosexual fathers. J Homosex. 1989;18:163-72.

117. **Bigner JJ, Jacobsen RB.** Parenting behaviors of homosexual and heterosexual fathers. J Homosex. 1989;18:173-86.

118. **Bigner JJ, Jacobsen RB.** Adult responses to child behavior and attitudes toward fathering: gay and nongay fathers. J Homosex. 1992;23:99-112.

119. **Tornello SL, Farr RH, Patterson CJ.** Predictors of parenting stress among gay adoptive fathers in the united states. J Fam Psychol. 2011;25:591-600.

120. **Fulcher M, Chan RW, Raboy B, Patterson CJ.** Contact with grandparents among children conceived via donor insemination by lesbian and heterosexual mothers. Parenting Sci Pract. 2002;2:61-76.

121. **Patterson CJ, Hurt S, Mason CD.** Families of the lesbian baby boom: children's contact with grandparents and other adults. Am J Orthopsychiatry. 1998;68:390-9.

122. **Gartrell N, Deck A, Rodas C, et al.** The National Lesbian Family Study: 4. Interviews with the 10-year-old children. Am J Orthopsychiatry. 2005;75:518-24.

123. **Perlesz A, Brown R, Lindsay J, et al.** Family in transition: parents, children and grandparents in lesbian families give meaning to 'doing family.' J Fam Ther. 2006;28:175-99.

124. **Weeks J, Heaphy B, Donovan C.** Same-sex Intimacies: Families of Choice and Other Life Experiments. London: Routledge; 2001.

125. **Casper V, Schultz SB.** Gay Parents/Straight Schools. New York: Teachers College Press; 1999.

126. **Tasker F, Patterson CJ.** Research on lesbian and gay parenting: retrospect and prospect. J GLBT Fam Stud. 2007;3:9-34.

127. **Green R.** Sexual identity of 37 children raised by homosexual or transsexual parents. Am J Psychiatry. 1978;135:692-7.

128. **White T, Ettner R.** Adaptation and adjustment in children of transsexual parents. Eur Child Adolesc Psychiatry. 2007;16:215-21.

129. **Bos HMW, van Balen F, van den Boom DC.** Lesbian families and family functioning: an overview. Patient Educ Couns. 2005;59:263-75.

130. **Bos HMW, Sandfort TGM.** Children's gender identity in lesbian and heterosexual two-parent families. Sex Roles. 2010;62:114-26.

131. **Golombok S, Tasker F.** Do parents influence the sexual orientation of their children? Findings from a longitudinal study of lesbian families. Dev Psychol. 1996;32:3-11.

132. **Green R, Mandel JB, Hotvedt ME, et al.** Lesbian mothers and their children: a comparison with solo parent heterosexual mothers and their children. Arch Sex Behav. 1986;15:167-84.

133. **Goldberg AE, Kashy DA, Smith JZ.** Gender-typed play behavior in early childhood: adopted children with lesbian, gay, and heterosexual parents. Sex Roles. 2012;67:503-15.

134. **MacCallum F, Golombok S.** Children raised in fatherless families from infancy: a follow-up of children of lesbian and single heterosexual mothers at early adolescence. J Child Psychol Psychiatry. 2004;45:1407-19.

135. **Bailey JM, Bobrow D, Wolfe M, Mikach S.** Sexual orientation of adult sons of gay fathers. Dev Psychol. 1995;31:124-9.

136. **Huggins SL.** A comparative study of self-esteem of adolescent children of divorced lesbian mothers and divorced heterosexual mothers. J Homosex. 1989;18:123-35.

137. **Gartrell N, Bos H.** US National Longitudinal Lesbian Family Study: Psychological adjustment of 17-year-old adolescents. Pediatrics. 2010;126:28-36.

138. **Wainright JL, Patterson CJ.** Peer relations among adolescents with female same-sex parents. Dev Psychol. 2008:44;117-26.

139. **Ray V, Gregory R.** School experiences of the children of lesbian and gay parents. Fam Matters. 2001;59:28-35.

140. **Kosciw JG, Diaz EM.** Involved, Invisible, and Ignored: The Experiences of Lesbian, Gay, Bisexual, and Transgender Parents and Their Children in Our Nation's K-12 Schools. New York: GLSEN; 2008.

141. **Wainright JL, Patterson CJ.** Delinquency, victimization, and substance use among adolescents with female same-sex parents. J Fam Psychol. 2006;20:526-30.

142. **Rivers I, Poteat VP, Noret N.** Victimization, social support, and psychosocial functioning among children of same-sex and opposite-sex couples in the United Kingdom. Dev Psychol. 2008;44:127-34.

143. **Flaks DK, Ficher I, Masterpasqua F, Joseph G.** Lesbians choosing motherhood: a comparative study of lesbian and heterosexual parents and their children. Dev Psychol. 1995;31:105-14.

144. **Lavner JA, Waterman J, Peplau LA.** Can gay and lesbian parents promote healthy development in high-risk children adopted from foster care? Am J Orthopsychiatry. 2012;82:465-72.

145. **Bos HMW, van Balen F, van den Boom DC.** Child adjustment and parenting in planned lesbian-parent families. Am J Orthopsychiatry. 2007;77:38-48.

146. **Shechner T, Slone M, Lobel TE, Shechter R.** Children's adjustment in non-traditional families in Israel: the effect of parental sexual orientation and the number of parents on children's development. Child Care Health Dev. 2011;39:178-84.

147. **Moore M.** Invisible Families: Gay Identities, Relationships, and Motherhood Among Black Women. Berkeley, CA: University of California Press; 2011.

148. **Institute of Medicine.** The health of Lesbian, Gay, Bisexual, and Transgender People: Building a Foundation for Better Understanding. Washington, DC: The National Academies Press; 2011.

149. **Hatzenbuehler M.** Social factors as determinants of mental health disparities in LGB populations: implications for public policy. Soc Issues Policy Rev. 2011;4:31-62.

Chapter 7

Caring for LGBT Older Adults

MARK J. SIMONE, MD
HILARY MEYER, JD
MANUEL A. ESKILDSEN, MD, MPH
JONATHAN S. APPELBAUM, MD

Introduction

Like lesbian, gay, bisexual, and transgender (LGBT) people of all ages, LGBT older adults may experience disparities in physical and mental health and often lack access to clinicians trained in LGBT health needs and sensitivity (1–4). For example, a study that analyzed 7 years worth of data from Washington State found that LGB older adults reported higher rates of disability, poor mental health, smoking, and excessive drinking compared with older heterosexuals (1). Lesbian and bisexual women reported higher rates of cardiovascular disease and obesity and were less likely to have screening mammography than heterosexual women; gay and bisexual men reported higher rates of poor physical health and living alone compared with heterosexual men (1). To understand the unique health challenges faced by LGBT older adults, it is important to recognize that most have experienced a lifetime of widespread discrimination, forcing them to hide their sexual orientation or transgender identity from their health care providers, their families, their employers, and sometimes even from themselves. Although social acceptance of LGBT people has grown considerably in recent years, older LGBT adults continue to be affected by past and ongoing social stigma, which can have an important effect on their health.

This chapter focuses on the unique medical, mental health, and end-of-life needs of older LGBT adults based on evidence of disparities in the general LGBT population, as well as on the growing body of literature specific to older LGBT adults (1–4). We generally use age 65 years and older throughout this chapter as the definition of older adults, although some cited references use age older than 50. The chapter also explores challenges that are more prevalent among older LGBT adults, including feelings of invisibility and isolation, lack of social supports and community engagement, high levels of discrimination in long-term care facilities, and policies that affect the financial security and medical decision-making of same-sex couples. Finally, the chapter concludes with a discussion of ways that providers can support their patients by connecting them to community-based resources that are available to meet the needs of this underserved group.

Background

Demographic Characteristics

Currently, an estimated 1 to 2 million older LGBT adults are living in the United States (5–7). By 2030, these numbers are expected to rise considerably, along with the overall aging U.S. population (5,6). The exact number of LGBT people is unknown and probably under-represented because of a lack of data, differing estimates by experts in related fields, and stigma that prevents LGBT people from identifying as such on surveys. However, although the data are limited, evidence suggests that older LGBT people are as racially and economically diverse as the general U.S. population (5–7). See Chapter 2 for more on the demographic characteristics of LGBT populations.

History of Stigma and Prejudice and Their Effect on LGBT Older Adults

Older LGBT adults came of age during a time in the United States when being a sexual or gender minority was viewed in an especially negative light. The experiences of older LGBT adults are influenced in part by whether they are part of the baby boomer generation (born between 1946 and 1964) or whether they were born before 1946. Those born before 1946 lived much of their lives in a society where the expression of their sexual orientation was criminalized by the government and pathologized by the medical community. For instance, it was not until 1962 that the first state decriminalized private, consensual homosexual acts, and it wasn't until 2003 that the last antisodomy laws were struck down (6). Being gay was considered not only a crime, but also a mental illness until 1973, when the American Psychiatric Association stopped designating homosexuality as a disorder that could be treated and cured (6). As a result, LGBT persons could have been involuntarily hospitalized or treated against their will, with understandable long-term consequences on this older generation's ability to trust the medical profession and seek psychiatric care.

A survey from 1967 by the Opinions Research Corporation, as commissioned by CBS News and reported by Mike Wallace, illustrates the historic prejudice and stigma experienced by this generation. In a televised report (8), Mike Wallace stated that "Americans consider homosexuality more harmful to society than adultery, abortion, or prostitution. Most Americans are repelled by the mere notion of homosexuality . . . 2 out of 3 Americans look upon homosexuals with disgust, discomfort, or fear; 1 out of 10 says hatred; the vast majority say it is an illness . . . [and] the majority of Americans favor legal punishment, even for homosexual acts performed in private between consenting adults." Given this widespread discrimination, it is no surprise that older LGBT adults are likely to have kept, and continue to keep, their sexual orientation and/or transgender identity hidden.

Society's views of homosexuality did not begin to change until the late 1960s and 1970s, and then only slowly. The Stonewall Riots of 1969, a series of violent demonstrations by LGBT people in New York City opposing ongoing police harassment, is considered to be the beginning of the modern gay civil rights movement in the United States. Baby boomers came of age during this social unrest of the 1960s, and as such have reaped the benefits of the gay civil rights movement that previous generations could not. To varying degrees, they have been more likely to come out of the closet. For example, a marketing survey of about 1000 LGBT people in the baby boomer generation conducted by the American Society on Aging and MetLife Mature Market Institute in 2009 indicated that 74% to 76% of lesbian and gay respondents were "completely or mostly out," while 16% of bisexual and 39% of transgender respondents were "completely or mostly out" (9). Although many baby boomers have lived openly and achieved a great deal, many have still experienced their share of homophobia and transphobia. Sadly, the baby boomer generation may again have to decide whether to be out of the closet if they need long-term care in an assisted-living facility or nursing home, out of fear of mistreatment by staff or isolation by other residents.

What does this mean for the health and health care of aging and older LGBT adults? For one, older LGBT people may be more susceptible to poor health because of the stresses associated with long-term concealment of sexual identity and many years of exposure to discrimination (10). Older adults are more likely to have experienced homophobia in health care situations and are understandably much less likely to be open about their sexuality or gender identity when seeking health care (11,12), hindering a trusting provider–patient relationship (6). Unfortunately, studies suggest that nondisclosure of sexual orientation can be associated with lower life satisfaction, lower self-esteem, depression and suicide, substance abuse, delay in seeking medical treatment, and increase in risk for illness (13,14). Medical mistrust is cited as a major reason why gay people, especially lesbians, do not always receive appropriate preventive care (15). Fear of culturally incompetent or discriminatory health care providers can result in LGBT people avoiding care until they have reached a crisis level, such as needing to go to an emergency department for treatment rather than using routine checkups for preventive care (16).

Asking About Sexual Orientation and Gender Identity

To provide optimal care of older LGBT adults, it is important to create an environment that allows this population to feel welcome, respected, and safe to disclose their identity as LGBT. Chapters 1 and 8, and Appendix A offer guidelines on how to create such an environment. An important part of offering appropriate, targeted health care requires providers to ask their older patients about their sexual orientation and gender identity. However, as discussed above, older LGBT adults may be unwilling to risk disclosing their sexual orientation or transgender identity to their health care providers, even if asked directly. It is therefore important for providers to be sensitive when asking about the sexual and gender identity of older adults and to offer a safe and confidential environment for disclosure, without forcing labels or outing someone if he or she is not ready to disclose. This same sensitivity should be used when asking about all aspects of the social history and sexual history because these are areas where patients may feel the need to hide details of their lives (see Table 7-1 for communication strategies to use when taking a sexual history with older adults). For more on asking

---

Table 7–1   Communication Strategies for Taking a Sexual History With Older LGBT Adults

Ensure confidentiality

Explain why you are asking the questions

Acknowledge when it can be uncomfortable information to share

Ask about social ties and support
    "Who do you live with?"
    "Who are the important people in your life?"
    "Who do you turn to for support?"

Do not make assumptions about the gender of the patient's significant other (i.e., do not assume that your patient is heterosexual)
    "What's the name of your spouse/partner?"

Be sensitive to the fact that many older LGBT adults never had the opportunity to get married
    Ask "Are you in a relationship?" instead of "Are you married?"

Ask about sexual activity and don't make assumptions about lack of risk or lack of sexual activity
    "Are you sexually active?" "With whom?"
    "Do you have any worries or concerns related to sex?"
    "Do you use condoms?"
    "Have you been tested for HIV?"

Ask about sexual orientation and gender identity, but be sensitive to the possibility that a patient may not be ready to disclose
    "Are you comfortable with your sexuality?"
    "Are you comfortable with me documenting this information in the chart?"

Do not force labels or out a patient if he or she is not ready to disclose

Have referrals on hand for LGBT-friendly community and mental health supports

Have signs, fliers, or symbols visible in your practice setting to signal an LGBT-friendly environment

Use inclusive forms and encourage all office staff to use inclusive language

about sexual orientation and gender identity of older adults, see *Inclusive Questions for Older Adults: A Practical Guide to Collecting Data on Sexual Orientation and Gender Identity*, which can be found at www.lgbtagingcenter. org/resources/resource.cfm?r=601.

Medical Issues in Older LGBT Adults

While LGBT older adults can experience the same geriatric syndromes as their heterosexual counterparts, and as a result need much the same health promotion and maintenance, certain issues require particular attention in LGBT older adults because of differential risk factors in these communities (1–4). These issues are explained in more detail below.

Cardiovascular Health

Cardiovascular disease (CVD) is the leading cause of death for all populations. Although no evidence suggests that LGBT people experience CVD at higher rates than the general population, research studies have consistently found higher rates of certain CVD risk factors in LGBT populations (described below). As with all patients, providers may be able to help modify risk factors through education, counseling, and referrals to individual and group interventions and programs.

Cardiovascular Risk in Older Gay and Bisexual Men

Cardiovascular disease, despite a decline in incidence, still kills more men than cancer does. Mitigating or removing traditional cardiac risk factors is the key to prevention. Because gay men have an increased rate of recreational drug use and smoking (17,18), attention to the traditional cardiovascular risk factors is important (19,20). The combination of smoking and HIV infection is particularly deadly (21); in a cohort of mostly men, the all-cause mortality was 4 times higher in HIV-infected smokers than never smokers. More than 12 life-years were lost from smoking compared with 5.1 life-years lost from HIV infection alone (22). Obtaining age-appropriate targets for blood pressure, cholesterol, and diabetes is also important in managing CVD risk.

Cardiovascular Risk in Older Lesbians

Cardiovascular disease is the number 1 killer of women in the United States and therefore is likely a primary health threat for older lesbians. Although CVD used to be considered a man's disease, 25% of women older than age 65 have CVD, and women older than 60 years of age develop CVD at the same rate as men. In the course of a lifetime, a woman is 10 times more likely to get CVD than breast cancer. Therefore, prevention of CVD in women should be as important as getting regular mammograms (23).

Traditional modifiable CVD risk factors are identifiable in the lesbian and bisexual female population, including higher rates of smoking and obesity (24). The National Lesbian Health Care Survey found that about 30% of lesbians smoke compared with about 23% of all women in the United States (25). In the Women's Health Initiative, a study of women age 50 to 79 years, twice as many lesbians reported themselves to be heavy smokers compared with heterosexual women (18,24).

Obesity is an independent CVD risk factor for women. Lesbians and bisexual women, on average, have a higher body mass index (BMI) than heterosexual women (26). In the Nurses' Health Study, risk for CVD was more than 3 times higher among women with a BMI greater than 29 kg/m², and even a moderate increase in BMI (25 to 28.9 kg/m²) was associated with a doubling of CVD risk (27).

Cardiovascular Risk in Older Transgender Adults

Transgender patients also face CVD risk factors. There is evidence of increased cigarette smoking in the transgender population (28). In addition, the pharmacologic use of sex hormones is known to increase the risk for CVD (29). For instance, estrogen has the potential to increase the risk for venous thromboembolism, blood pressure, and blood glucose and to cause water retention. Some studies suggest a possible increase in cardiovascular risk over time for transgender women taking feminizing hormones (see Chapter 18), but transgender men taking testosterone do not appear to have an increased risk for CVD (29,30).

Cancer Risk in Older LGBT Adults

Older LGBT adults may also have higher risk factors for certain cancers. As with all older patients, the risks and benefits of screening should be discussed and individualized to the patient, keeping in mind the patient's wishes as well as his or her life expectancy.

Anal Cancer

Anal cancer, like cervical cancer, is caused by infection with human papillomavirus (HPV). Anal HPV infection disproportionately affects men who have sex with men (MSM) compared with the general population of men (31). The prevalence of anal HPV infection in HIV-positive MSM is extremely high, ranging between 72% and 90%; in HIV-negative MSM, the prevalence is 57% to 61% (31). Evidence suggests that the incidence of anal cancer in HIV-negative MSM approaches the historic levels of cervical cancer in women before the widespread use of the Papanicolaou (Pap) smear (31). Risk factors for anal cancer include receptive anal intercourse and degree of immunosuppression, such as nadir CD4 count and higher HIV viral load (32). While there are no recognized guidelines for routine anal cancer screening, some organizations have proposed annual anal cytology for HIV-infected MSM, and screening every 2 years for HIV-uninfected MSM (31).

Prostate Cancer

Although there are no data on the incidence of prostate cancer in gay and bisexual men, prostate cancer is the second leading cause of cancer deaths among men in the general population. Among gay couples, there is a 28% chance that prostate cancer will be diagnosed in 1 partner and a 3% chance that both partners will get the disease (33). Risk factors include African-American race, high-fat diet, and family history of prostate cancer. While there is no evidence that gay and bisexual men are more likely than heterosexuals to develop prostate cancer, prostate cancer can affect the sexual health of gay and bisexual men in ways that are different from those in heterosexual men. The prostate gland is involved in the sexual response to receptive anal intercourse, and the effect on sexual health should be discussed with gay and bisexual men when treatment options for prostate cancer are considered (33).

Cervical Cancer

Cervical and breast cancer screening rates have historically been lower among lesbians than heterosexual women. For instance, a survey of 225 lesbians found that 29% did not have routine Pap smears (34). Fear of discrimination and not disclosing sexual orientation were associated with decreased likelihood to have Pap screening (34). Findings from the Boston Lesbian Health Project II suggest that lesbians have increased their use of Pap smear screening and mammography but still have not yet reached the same rate of screening as heterosexual women (35). Lesbians and bisexual women remain at risk for cervical cancer, partly because many have had intercourse with a man at some point in their lives and therefore need to be screened according to guidelines for all women. Surveys from self-identified lesbians show that 70% have had penile-vaginal intercourse (6% within the past year), 17% have had an abnormal Pap smear, and 17% have had anal intercourse (36).

The U.S. Preventive Services Task Force (USPSTF) updated their cervical cancer screening recommendations in 2012 to advise that all women age 21 to 65 years be screened every 3 years by using cytology; for women between 30 and 65 years, the screening interval can be lengthened to every 5 years if the screening combines cytology and HPV testing. Most women can discontinue screening after age 65 if they have had 3 consecutive negative Pap smears (37).

Breast Cancer

The primary risk factor for breast cancer is age; other risk factors include family history, obesity, smoking, alcohol use, and nulliparity. While some studies report that lesbians may have greater risk factors for breast cancer

(38,39), no prospective study has definitively shown an increased risk. However, older lesbians may receive fewer mammograms than heterosexual women (24), and studies suggest higher rates of obesity and alcohol use among lesbians (1,24). Current recommendations from the U.S. Preventive Services Task Force suggest that women age 50 to 74 undergo biannual screening mammography (40).

Additional Cancers

Older LGBT adults also have a higher prevalence of certain risk factors for the following cancers, although there is no evidence of a higher incidence of these cancers in LGBT populations.

- Lung cancer: Evidence suggests that lesbians and gay men have a higher lifetime prevalence of smoking (18), and because smoking is still the major risk factor for lung cancer, both medical and behavioral methods for smoking cessation can greatly benefit patients.
- Ovarian cancer: Nulliparity is a risk factor for ovarian cancer, although it is important to remember that many lesbians have given birth. Family history of ovarian cancer or breast cancer and genetic markers such as *BRCA1* and *BRCA2* are important indicators for high-risk patients. Unfortunately, no recommended screening test is available for ovarian cancer (41).
- HIV-related cancers: Kaposi sarcoma, lymphoma, and other cancers may be higher among older adults with HIV infection and may appear relatively early in the course of the illness. In fact, many malignancies not usually associated with immune compromise have been seen in older patients infected with HIV and are now one of the leading causes of death in these patients (42).
- Liver cancer: Gay and bisexual men have a higher risk for hepatitis B and C (43,44), thus potentially putting them at greater risk for liver cancer.

Cancer Screening in Transgender Older Adults

As transgender patients age, they may encounter health issues that correspond to their biological sex. Therefore, the major concern relates to appropriate health screening for biological sex, such as prostate examinations in transgender women (male-to-female) and pelvic examinations in transgender men (female-to-male). For instance, a person whose assigned sex at birth is male and who has transitioned to a woman may develop prostate cancer if the prostate was not removed. Similarly, a person born female who transitioned to a man may develop uterine cancer if the female sexual organs were not removed. These patients understandably may feel additional stress in coping with a disease or condition associated with the gender they have left behind (45). Hormone-related cancer in transgender persons is very rare (there are, however, case reports of breast cancer in male-to-female transgender patients). See Chapter 18 for more on cancer screening in transgender adults.

Sexual Health of Older LGBT Adults

It is important to address sexual function and sexual health in all older LGBT patients. Providers sometimes feel uncomfortable discussing sexual issues with their patients, particularly those who are old enough to be their parents or even grandparents. However, most older LGBT patients can benefit greatly from routine sexual history taking and risk-reduction counseling. Chapters 8 and 12 provide suggestions on how to talk with patients about their sexual health and provide effective risk reduction counseling.

Prevention of HIV and Sexually Transmitted Infection in Older LGBT Adults

More than half of seniors age 65 to 75 report being sexually active, and one quarter of those age 75 to 85 are sexually active (46). Sexually active older adults, however, are much less likely to use condoms than younger adults; a national survey of sexual practices found that older adults at risk for HIV infection were one sixth as likely as younger adults to use condoms during sex and one fifth as likely to have been tested for HIV infection (47,48). Older patients also report receiving little information about sexual health, HIV infection, and other sexually transmitted infections (STIs) from their physicians (46,49), and there are reports of increasing rates of syphilis and chlamydia in older adults and in counties with a high number of retirees (50).

For all of these reasons, providers need to take routine and thorough sexual and substance use histories from all of their older patients, regardless of sexual orientation or gender identity. Prevention of HIV and STI transmission also requires that clinicians provide counseling on safer sex practices and offer, when appropriate, information on the use of HIV postexposure prophylaxis and pre-exposure prophylaxis. More on the prevention of HIV and STIs can be found in Chapters 12 and 13.

Unfortunately, there are several barriers to optimal prevention and detection of HIV and other STIs in older adults, which providers should attempt to address. These include the following:

- Lack of knowledge about HIV/AIDS by older adults: A study of older women showed poor knowledge about HIV risk factors (51). Unfortunately, older adults are also often ignored or forgotten in typical prevention campaigns that generally target youth (52). Many older people do not consider themselves at risk for contracting HIV and therefore do not get tested (53).
- Underestimation of risk by health care providers: Health care providers may not consider discussing HIV/AIDS with older patients and may also lack the correct knowledge about risk factors in older patients (54). They may incorrectly assume that older patients are not sexually active or do not use drugs, or they may be uncomfortable raising these issues with older patients (53).

- Misdiagnosis: Diagnosing HIV/AIDS in older adults can be challenging because the symptoms can mimic normal aging or other medical conditions common in the elderly, such as fatigue, weight loss, and mental confusion (55).
- Stigma: Older adults with HIV infection may be more likely to experience greater stigma from their peers because of the association of HIV with homosexuality and substance abuse, leading them to hide their diagnosis or risk factors from providers or family (53).
- Finally, as discussed earlier, older LGBT adults often hide their sexual behavior and orientation from health care providers, which can further impair effective communication and reduction of sexual risk factors (56).

Sexual Risk in Older Gay and Bisexual Men

Gay, bisexual, and other MSM remain the group at greatest risk for acquisition of HIV, with MSM older than age 50 accounting for more than 25% of all new HIV infections (57). Older adults who are racial/ethnic minorities appear to be at increased risk for death from HIV/AIDS (57).

Sexually active men MSM who engage in high-risk sexual behavior need to be routinely assessed for gonorrhea, chlamydia, syphilis, herpes simplex virus, and human papillomavirus (HPV) risk per Centers for Disease Control and Prevention (CDC) guidelines (58). HIV risk assessment should be done at the same time as assessment for other STIs; the CDC has recommended that HIV testing be a regular part of primary care (59). Although the CDC's universal screening recommendations only go up to 64 years of age, providers should also screen MSM over 65 years of age based on individual risk behaviors (59,60).

Erectile dysfunction is more common as men age. With direct-to-consumer advertising of phosphodiesterase type 5 (PDE-5) inhibitors, such as sildenafil (Viagra), more men are willing to bring up this issue. Of note, all PDE-5 inhibitors interact with HIV protease inhibitors and can also cause hypotension if used along with nitrates (nitroglycerin, isosorbide, and "poppers") or α-blockers. There is also suggestion that the abuse of PDE-5 inhibitors is more prevalent in MSM and is associated with increased rates of high-risk sexual behavior and HIV transmission (61).

Sexual Risk in Older Lesbian and Bisexual Women

Many lesbians and bisexual women have been sexually active with both women and men. Therefore, taking a complete sexual history and providing sensitive risk reduction counseling is recommended. Lesbian and bisexual women can develop the same STIs as heterosexual women. In addition, lesbians have a higher incidence of bacterial vaginosis, and women can transmit candidiasis and *Trichomonas vaginalis* to their female partners. The use of barriers ("dental dams") is recommended for oral-vaginal and oral-anal contact.

Women who are exclusively sexually active with other women have a low risk for acquiring HIV infection, but because many lesbians and bisexual women have had heterosexual experiences, following the current HIV screening recommendations is important. Older women who have sex with men may be at increased risk for HIV because of age-related vaginal thinning and dryness (62). In addition, older women starting a new sexual relationship after many years of being in a monogamous relationship may find it difficult to initiate discussions about risks and the use of condoms (53).

Sexual Risk in Transgender People

HIV risk is high among transgender women, and frequent screening is important. Transgender women who engage in sex work and injection drug use are at extremely high risk for STIs and HIV infection. A study in San Francisco, California, found that 35% of transgender women respondents were HIV positive, with African Americans having an even higher rate of HIV infection (63). The African-American transgender community has one of the highest prevalence rates of HIV infection in the United States (64).

HIV/AIDS Treatment and Care

Among older patients, AIDS tends to be diagnosed much later in the course of the infection, primarily because the diagnosis is not considered and because older people are less likely to get tested (53). HIV/AIDS-related symptoms and associated diseases can be easily mistaken for other problems typically seen in older persons. In addition, because aging naturally weakens the immune system and comorbid conditions are more likely to exist, AIDS may progress more rapidly in older persons. In the D:A:D (Data Collection on Adverse Events of Anti-HIV drugs) study, older patients presenting with advanced HIV infection were 14 times more likely to die within a year of diagnosis compared with older adults in whom infection was not diagnosed late (65).

At the same time, patients older than age 50 who take antiretroviral medications seem to respond virologically as well as younger patients do, but they do not have as robust a return of their immune system. Treating older patients with HIV/AIDS adds a layer of complexity to care because many of these patients have other underlying illnesses; take several medications; and may additionally be dealing with some of the issues of aging, such as sensory loss, frailty, and dementia (66). Recently, the American Academy of HIV Medicine, the American Geriatrics Society, and the AIDS Community Research Initiative of America published a compendium of recommended treatment approaches to caring for this population (67). The latest set of HIV treatment guidelines suggests 2 important approaches for the older patient with HIV: early treatment is advised, regardless of baseline CD4 count, and treatment protects against the spread of this disease (68).

Mental Health, Social, and Economic Issues Affecting Older LGBT Adults

Mental Health

The link between mental health disorders and discrimination in LGBT populations has been well documented (3). Discrimination is present not only in health care but also in employment, housing, civil rights, federal laws, and organizational policies, all of which must be accounted for in addressing the psychosocial needs of older LGBT adults. The coming-out process for an older LGBT person, who has lived most of his or her life in a hostile or intolerant environment, can induce significant stress and contribute to lower life satisfaction and self-esteem (13). For older adults, managing social stressors such as prejudice, stigmatization, violence, and internalized homophobia over long periods of time can result in higher risks for depression, suicide, risky behavior, and substance abuse (13). However, while little is known about the actual prevalence of mental health disorders in LGBT adults, even less is known about the prevalence of mental health disorders in older LGBT adults. The studies that do exist have found elevated levels of current or lifetime depression among older LGBT adults, with rates possibly being the highest among transgender people (69–71). Among MSM, depression and emotional distress were associated with being single, experiencing antigay harassment or violence, feeling alienated from the gay community, or not identifying as gay (69).

Suicide rates are alarmingly high in young LGBT persons, and suicidality may persist throughout adulthood into old age. A 2001, self-administered survey of 416 LBG adults age 60 to 91 years found that 29% of participants rarely considered suicide, 8% sometimes considered suicide, and 2% often considered suicide, while 12% had suicidal thoughts in the past year (72). Most, however, did not relate their suicidal thoughts to their sexual orientation. Notably, better mental health was predicted in part by a higher percentage of people who knew about the participants' sexual orientation, including their health care provider (72).

Transgender persons may experience mental health problems, such as adjustment disorders, anxiety disorders, post-traumatic stress disorder, depression, and substance abuse, that are similar to those experienced by other persons who endure major life changes and discrimination (73,74). A survey of transgender adults found that 13% reported abusing alcohol or drugs as a means to cope with mistreatment, and 16% had attempted suicide at least once in their lifetimes (75).

Substance Use

Although LGBT youth have higher rates of alcohol and tobacco use compared with heterosexual peers, some of those behaviors differ on the basis of sexual orientation and do not appear to persist in older age. For instance, older lesbians and bisexual men are more likely to be current smokers than heterosexuals of the same gender after age 50, while older gay men and bisexual women have no difference compared with heterosexuals (18,24). Alcohol use in older LGB adults is similar to that in heterosexuals, with the caveat that binge drinking behavior is more common in older lesbian women and less likely in gay men compared with heterosexuals (18). However, a more recent survey of LGB older adults in Washington State found that all LGB older adults, regardless of gender, were more likely to smoke and drink excessively compared with older heterosexuals (1).

Concerns About Aging

LGBT adults may approach the aging process differently from their peers, and this approach may also differ by gender. Although some theories state that homosexuals are better able to cope with aging than heterosexuals because of the development of adaptive skills and the reconstruction of their identities during the coming-out process (76,77), a study published in 2005 found that 88% of younger gay men and 73% of older gay men felt that gay society viewed aging as a negative process (78). Lesbians, however, felt that lesbian society viewed aging in a positive manner (78). This difference may be due to the influence of youth and physical attraction in gay male subculture, thus subjecting older gay men to ageism from within their own community.

Older lesbian and gay adults generally have the same concerns about aging (such as loneliness, health, and income) as do their heterosexual counterparts, with the additional fears of rejection by their children and grandchildren, uncertain support, and concerns of discrimination in health care, employment, housing, and long-term care (76). About one third of gay men and one quarter of lesbians identified discrimination due to their sexual orientation as their greatest concern about aging (77,79).

Isolation and Social Support

LGBT older adults often find themselves without traditional familial and social supports to help them with age-related needs (80–83). A lack of spousal or familial support can be especially problematic as older LGBT adults find they must rely on the support of others as they age. Studies show that compared with heterosexual older adults, gay or bisexual men are twice as likely to be living alone and lesbian or bisexual women are one third more likely to be living alone (9,80). Moreover, studies show that older LGB adults are half as likely to have a significant other, half as likely to have close relatives to call for help, and three to four times more likely to not have children (6,9). Older LGBT adults may also have strained relationships with their extended family or children as a result of lack of acceptance of their sexuality or as a result of attempting to remain deeply closeted.

Given these diminished social connections, it is not surprising that isolation and loneliness are higher among LGB older adults than among their non-LGB peers (84). Research also shows that diminished social supports have been correlated with a wide range of health problems that can have serious consequences for older people, including premature institutionalization and early death (85).

Despite these grave statistics, however, many LGBT older adults do have various forms of support and are not entirely isolated. One study commissioned by the National Institutes of Health and the National Institute on Aging, in which 2560 LGBT people age 50 to 95 years participated, found that the picture of LGBT older adults' social support can be complex. For instance, while two thirds of LGBT older adult participants (67%) reported that they have someone to help with daily chores if they are sick, 1 in 3 (33%) reported that they do not (16). This study also showed that LGBT older adults have positive feelings of belonging to the LGBT community (16), which can lead to feelings of inclusion.

In addition, LGBT adults are sometimes able to rely on "nontraditional" family structures (6). For example, some form "families of choice" (86), a term used to describe diverse family structures that include close friends, partners, or significant others who are not biologically or legally related but nonetheless are the source of social and caregiving support (87). Reliance on families of choice poses some difficulties, however, because they are not recognized by law. For example, a chosen family member cannot make care decisions for a patient unless he or she has been named in an advance directive (see below for more on this topic).

Given all of these issues, it is vital for providers to recognize families of choice, be aware of the possibility of isolation and severe loneliness, and have referral points set up to assist LGBT older adults with services targeted especially for LGBT older adults or culturally competent care in traditional service settings.

Challenges With Financial Security

Older LGBT adults are more likely to live in poverty than their heterosexual counterparts. The rate of poverty is 4.6% among senior heterosexual couples, compared with 4.9% for senior gay male couples and 9.1% for senior lesbian couples (88). Older lesbian couples are likely poorer than senior gay couples, in part because of gender wage disparities in the general population.

The financial security of older LGBT persons can be severely affected by unequal access to benefits programs. While many large private companies provide benefits to unmarried same-sex couples, this is not required. Same-sex couples whose marriages are not recognized by their state are unable to access certain state and federal benefits that protect married spouses from financial hardship that are more likely to occur at an older age (e.g., Social Security survivorship benefits and eligibility under Medicare for joint placement in nursing homes across the country) (89). Up until the Supreme Court ruling against the Defense of Marriage Act (DOMA) in June 2013, federal benefits for spouses were denied to same-sex couples even if their marriage was recognized by their state. At the time of this publication, legal recognition of same-sex marriage is rapidly evolving, with rulings across the United States expanding equal marriage to an ever-increasing number of states.

End-of-Life Issues for Older LGBT Adults

Palliative Care Needs

Older adults who are LGBT may have unique palliative and end-of-life care needs. Minority stress, internalized homophobia, stigma, and misconceptions can all affect the mental health needs of older LGBT adults at the end of life. These issues may be magnified if the LGBT older adult is struggling with issues of disclosure of sexual orientation, fear of discrimination, and estrangement from family when approaching death. A 2012 systematic review of studies on the palliative care needs of LGBT people found that health care professionals 1) need training in the needs of LGBT older adults, 2) should explore the sexual orientation of their patients, 3) should avoid heterosexist assumptions, and 4) should recognize the importance of partners in decision making (90). Disenfranchised grief is another important topic to note, which refers to the ignored and unrecognized needs of a surviving same-sex spouse if that relationship is not recognized and validated by family, health care providers, or the legal system. For instance, a surviving same-sex partner may be intentionally or unintentionally excluded from making funeral arrangements if not legally married. They may also not feel welcome in support groups or community agencies, and as a result, may experience additional grief.

Elder Housing and Long-term Care

Studies show that LGBT older adults fear rejection and discrimination by both the staff and other seniors in long-term care facilities. For example, a survey reported that 578 of 649 respondents (89%) predicted that LGBT people would be discriminated against by staff at a long-term care facility (91). In that same study, 328 respondents (43%) reported 853 mistreatment incidents, including verbal or physical harassment from other residents and/or staff, refused admission or attempted discharge from facilities, denial of medical treatment, restriction of visitors, refusal by staff to accept medical power of attorney, and/or staff refusal to refer to transgender residents by preferred name or pronoun. In an attempt to address such concerns, there have been some legislative moves to mandate training; for example, California passed a law that requires health care staff in senior care settings to be trained in LGBT culturally competent care (92). Despite some advances, most states require no such training.

A 2009–2010 survey found that many LGBT older adults would prefer to age alongside other LGBT older adults if they are unable to, or choose, to age outside of their homes, citing safety as the main reason (93). At the time of this writing, no skilled nursing facilities are targeted to LGBT communities, although some may be opening in future years. Beyond skilled nursing, however, the idea of LGBT-targeted housing for older adults has resonated conceptually, although there are very few such places across the country. Examples are Rainbow Vision in New Mexico, which was built to offer LGBTQI (lesbian, gay, bisexual, transgender, queer, and intersexed) people an opportunity to live in a community, along with straight allies, in what is now called a Community of Living Diversity (94), and GLEH (Gay and Lesbian Elder Housing) in Los Angeles, California, which offers affordable housing for those who are low-income or living at or near the poverty line, including LGBT people and people living with HIV/AIDS and/or homelessness (95). However, not all older LGBT adults wish to live in an LGBT-targeted facility, and some older adult residential settings have begun to be trained in providing LGBT culturally competent care so that LGBT older adults' real and perceived fears of mistreatment may be alleviated (96).

Overcoming Barriers Through Outreach, Training, and Advance Care Planning

Community-Based Outreach

LGBT older adults access essential services, such as visiting nurses, food stamps, senior centers, and group meals, less frequently than the general aging population (5,13,77). Community resources for the general aging population are not guaranteed to understand or be inclusive of the needs of LGBT older adults. In addition, many of the social and support outlets for LGBT people are youth-oriented, making it difficult for older adults to feel comfortable accessing these organizations. For these reasons and others, government and foundation funding has been increasing for initiatives that support targeted LGBT older adult programs addressing health and wellness, some of which are described below. Two examples of community-based organizations that offer programming and supports for LGBT older adults are the LGBT Aging Project, based in Boston, Massachusetts, and Services & Advocacy for Gay, Lesbian, Bisexual, and Transgender Elders (SAGE), based in New York City, both of which integrate congregate and social services to support the healthy aging of the local LGBT population. For example, the LGBT Aging Project (www.lgbtagingproject.org) offers caregiver support groups, healthy aging education and services, and bereavement counseling, among other services. SAGE also offers health and wellness programming, such as in-house nursing, testing, and vaccination services; information exchanges with geriatric specialists; exercise classes; and access to local YMCA facilities. All of these not only help LGBT older adults learn about and navigate the health care system but also help reduce isolation and stigma that can result in poor fol-low-up and adherence to health regimens. SAGE has many affiliates across the country that provide similar programs targeted to LGBT older adults to enhance health outcomes. These programs are expanding rapidly and can be found by contacting the national SAGE office (www.sageusa.org).

Both SAGE and the LGBT Aging Project, along with several other organi-zations in different states, including Illinois (Center on Halsted) and Missouri (SAGE Metro St. Louis), also offer congregate meal programs to LGBT older adults. These programs are designed to give people age 60 and older a free, hot meal in a social setting. The congregate meal program increases seniors' access to nutritional meals, as well as reducing social iso-lation by having a centralized setting where LGBT and LGBT-friendly seniors can eat together without concern for harassment and discrimination.

Training and Resources

Health care and service providers seeking in-person training to better equip staff to provide culturally competent services to LGBT older adults can con-tact the National Resource Center on LGBT Aging (NRC), led by SAGE, which provides training as well as information dissemination through a website (www.lgbtagingcenter.org) (Table 7-2). The NRC not only educates aging ser-vices organizations about the existence and special needs of LGBT elders but also sensitizes LGBT organizations about the existence and special needs of older adults. They also bring information to LGBT older adults about a vari-ety of topics of importance to healthy aging. The NRC also serves as a resource to the medical community as well as other providers, and as a point of entry for information related to health, wellness, and many other topics for LGBT

Table 7–2   Resources on LGBT Aging for Providers and Patients

Services & Advocacy for Gay, Lesbian, Bisexual, & Transgender Elders (SAGE): www.sageusa.org

National Resource Center on LGBT Aging: www.lgbtagingcenter.org

LGBT Aging Project: www.lgbtagingproject.org

American Society on Aging: www.asaging.org

Transgender Aging Network: www.forge-forward.org/aging

Prime Timers World Wide: www.primetimersww.com

Old Lesbians Organizing for Change: www.oloc.org

Human Rights Campaign. Advance directives and visitation resources: www.hrc.org/resources/entry/protecting-your-visitation-decision-making-rights

older adults. Health professional training can also be accessed through the LGBT Aging Project and its partner at The Fenway Institute, the National LGBT Health Education Center (www.lgbthealtheducation.org).

Advance Care Planning

Health care providers have an important role in helping adults plan for the end of their lives and for eventualities in which they may not be able to make their own health decisions. This is why the discussion of advance directives plays an important role in the primary care of older adults. Advance directives, which are defined as a written statement of a person's wishes regarding medical treatment, can include living wills, do-not-resuscitate orders, and health care power of attorney.

A living will is defined as a document that outlines patients' preferences in case they become incapable of making their own decisions. These preferences relate to whether a person would want medical interventions, such as artificial feeding if it were necessary to sustain nourishment or the insertion of breathing tubes in case of respiratory failure. A health care power of attorney, on the other hand, does not state these preferences but designates an individual who would be legally empowered to make decisions for the patient in case of incapacity.

Older LGBT persons who live in states where their unions are not legally recognized have a particular need for advance directives. If they become severely ill and incapacitated, for example, they may be subject to state laws that give priority to blood relatives over their same-sex partner in medical decision-making and visitation rights. This could result in health decisions that run counter to the patient's desires and best interests. The LGBT Movement Advancement Project categorizes states by how they designate default decision makers as follows (6):

- "Gay-inclusive" states: These are states where same-sex couples can legally wed or that offer other forms of legal recognition, such as civil unions or domestic partnerships.
- "Close friend" states: These states include a "close friend" option among the list of relationships that are recognized as potential surrogates. However, blood relatives are usually given priority over close friends.
- "Legal stranger" states: They offer no "close friend" option, so same-sex partners are unlikely to be given a choice to be decision makers unless it was explicitly stated in a valid health care power of attorney document.

A signed health care power of attorney would help overcome these state laws and ensure that a same-sex partner or other "close friend" is the designated decision maker. On occasion, unfortunately, health providers decide not to recognize legally drafted advance directives. This was laid bare in the case of Lisa Pond, a woman who was about to go on a cruise from Florida and collapsed from an intracranial hemorrhage before departing (97). In a

Miami hospital, her partner and children were not allowed by hospital staff to be at her bedside even as she was dying. The case was the subject of a federal lawsuit, which the partner, Janice Langbehn, ultimately lost. Partly as a result of this case, President Barack Obama issued an executive order in 2010 that directed all facilities that accept Medicare and Medicaid patients to honor advance directives, including those from LGBT patients (98). In response, the Department of Health and Human Services in 2011 implemented regulation that all Medicare/Medicaid facilities must allow patients to decide who has visitation rights and who can make medical decisions for them, regardless of sexual orientation, gender identity or family makeup.

Conclusion

Many older LGBT adults have faced a lifetime of discrimination and health disparities. Health care providers must be sensitive to the specific challenges faced by this group, and provide the compassionate care, appropriate support, and resources that address their needs. As with all cross-cultural topics, however, one should not assume that the negative experiences and health disparities described in this chapter are automatically true for every individual LGBT older adult, as there are many examples of happy, healthy, and successful individuals who are all the more remarkable for having overcome significant obstacles to live enriched and inspiring lives. Yet many older LGBT adults continue to be invisible and ignored by today's society and health care system, and it is the responsibility of the health care profession, and society in general, to ensure that we provide the culturally sensitive care and services that all older LGBT adults deserve.

Summary Points

- Older LGBT people face the same health challenges as other American elders but also have specific medical, psychological, and social needs.
- Older LGBT adults are often invisible to the health care system and may have difficulty disclosing their sexual orientation and transgender status because of past negative experiences and from enduring a lifetime of discrimination. They came of age in an era of greater intolerance, and for this reason, many do not come out to others, including health care providers.
- As transgender patients age, they may be more likely to encounter health issues that correspond to their biological sex; these patients may need help in coping with a disease or condition associated with the gender they have left behind.
- LGBT older adults are more likely to live alone, be single, and not have children. They may rely more on extensive networks of friends rather

than family. Therefore, as they age, they may be at greater risk of isolation and need greater supports.

• Not all LGBT older adults are isolated and lonely; in fact, many LGBT older adults have partners, rich social lives, and extended families (including children and grandchildren).

• Many LGBT social and support outlets are youth-oriented, and LGBT older adults may not feel comfortable accessing these organizations. Mainstream community resources vary in terms of their understanding of the needs of LGBT older adults, and training opportunities exist to better inform the staff of outreach organizations.

• Health care providers must provide the appropriate support and resources that address and are sensitive to the needs of LGBT older adults.

• Clinicians should seek training and familiarize themselves with later-life and end-of-life issues faced by LGBT older adults and be prepared to make referrals to lawyers, elder housing, and assisted care facilities that are welcoming to LGBT people and that understand how legal policies affect older LGBT.

References

1. **Fredriksen-Goldsen KI, Kim H, Barkan SE, Muraco A, Hoy-Ellis CP.** Health disparities among lesbian, gay, and bisexual older adults: results from a population-based study. Am J Public Health 2013;103:1802-9.

2. **Healthy People 2020.** Lesbian, gay, bisexual, and transgender health. Available at: www. healthypeople.gov/2020/topicsobjectives2020/overview.aspx?topicid=25.

3. **Institute of Medicine.** The Health of Lesbian, Gay, Bisexual, and Transgender People: Building a Foundation for Better Understanding. Washington, DC: The National Academies Press; 2011. Available at: www.iom.edu/Reports/2011/The-Health-of-Lesbian-Gay-Bisexual-and-Transgender-People.aspx.

4. **Wallace SP, Cochran SD, Durazo EM, Ford CL.** The Health of Aging Lesbian, Gay and Bisexual Adults in California. Los Angeles: University of California, Los Angeles Center for Health Policy Research; 2011.

5. **Grant JM.** Outing Age 2010: Public Policy Issues Affecting Lesbian, Gay, Bisexual and Transgender Elders. Washington, DC: The National Gay and Lesbian Task Force Policy Institute; 2009. Available at: www.thetaskforce.org/reports_and_research/outing_age_2010.

6. **LGBT Movement Advancement Project and SAGE (Services and Advocacy for Gay, Lesbian, Bisexual and Transgender Elders).** Improving the lives of LGBT older adults. March 2010. Available at: www.lgbtagingcenter.org/resources/resource.cfm?r=16.

7. **Gates GJ, Newport F.** Special Report: 3.4% of u.s. adults identify as LGBT. Gallup. October 18, 2012. Available at: www.gallup.com/poll/158066/special-report-adults-identify-lgbt.aspx.

8. **Wallace M.** The homosexuals: a CBS Reports rrogram. CBS. 1967. Available at www.youtube.com/watch?v=-AXAOT_swIE.

9. **American Society on Aging and MetLife Mature Market Institute.** Still Out, Still Aging: The MetLife Study of Lesbian, Gay, Bisexual, and Transgender Baby Boomers. 2010. Available at: https://www.metlife.com/assets/cao/mmi/publications/studies/2010/mmi-still-out-still-aging.pdf.

10. **Pérez Benítez CI, O'Brien WH, Carels RA, Gordon AK.** Cardiovascular correlates of disclosing homosexual orientation. Stress Health. 2007;23:141-52.

11. **Eliason MJ, Dibble SL, Robertson PA.** Lesbian, gay, bisexual, and transgender (LGBT) physicians' experiences in the workplace. J Homosex. 2011;58:1355-71.

12. **Lambda Legal.** When Health Care Isn't Caring: Lambda Legal's Survey of Discrimination Against LGBT People and People with HIV. New York: Lambda Legal; 2010. Available at: www.lambdalegal.org/health-care-report.

13. **Brotman S, Ryan B, Cormier R.** The health and social service needs of gay and lesbian elders and their families in Canada. Gerontologist. 2003;43:192-202.

14. **Cole SW, Kemeny ME, Taylor SE, Visscher BR.** Elevated physical health risk among gay men who conceal their homosexual identity. Health Psychol. 1996;15:243-51.

15. **Cochran SD, Mays VM, Bowen D, et al.** Cancer-related risk indicators and preventive screening behaviors among lesbians and bisexual women. Am J Public Health. 2001;91:591-7.

16. **Fredriksen-Goldsen KI, Kim H, Emlet CA, Muraco A, Erosheva EA, Hoy-Ellis CP, et al.** The Aging and Health Report: Disparities and Resilience Among Lesbian, Gay, Bisexual, and Transgender Older Adults. Institute for Multigenerational Health; 2011. Available at: www.lgbtagingcenter.org/resources/pdfs/LGBT%20Aging%20and%20Health%20Report_final.pdf.

17. **Ryan H, Wortley PM, Easton A, Pederson L, Greenwood G.** Smoking among lesbians, gays, and bisexuals: a review of the literature. Am J Prev Med. 2001;21:142-9.

18. **Boehmer U, Miao X, Linkletter C, et al.** Adult health behaviors over the life course by sexual orientation. Am J Public Health 2012;102:292-300.

19. **Gritz ER, Vidrine DJ, Fingeret MC.** Smoking cessation a critical component of medical management in chronic disease populations. Am J Prev Med. 2007;33(6 Suppl):S414-22.

20. **Crothers K, Griffith TA, McGinnis KA, et al.** The impact of cigarette smoking on mortality, quality of life, and comorbid illness among HIV-positive veterans. J Gen Intern Med. 2005; 20:1142-5.

21. **Stein JH, Hadigan CM, Brown TT, et al.** Prevention strategies for cardiovascular disease in HIV-infected patients. Circulation. 2008;118:e54-60.

22. **Helleberg M, Afzal S, Kronborg G, et al.** Mortality attributable to smoking among hiv-1-infected individuals: a nationwide, population-based cohort study. Clin Infect Dis. 2012;2013; 56:727-34.

23. **Ulstad VK.** Coronary health issues for lesbians. J Gay Lesbian Med Assoc. 1999;3:59-66.

24. **Valanis BG, Bowen DJ, Bassford T, et al.** Sexual orientation and health: comparisons in the women's health initiative sample. Arch Fam Med. 2000;9:843-53.

25. **Bradford J, Ryan C, Rothblum ED.** National Lesbian Health Care Survey: implications for mental health care. J Consult Clin Psychol. 1994;62:228-42.

26. **Struble CB, Lindley LL, Montgomery K, et al.** Overweight and obesity in lesbian and bisexual college women. J Am College Health. 2011;59:51-6.

27. **Manson JE, Colditz GA, Stampfer MJ, et al.** A prospective study of obesity and risk of coronary heart disease in women. N Engl J Med. 1990;322:882-9.

28. **California Department of Health Services, Tobacco Control Section.** California Lesbians, Gays, Bisexuals, and Transgender Tobacco Use Survey 2004. Available at: www.cdph.ca.gov/programs/tobacco/Documents/CTCP-LGBTTobaccoStudy.pdf.

29. **Asscheman H, Giltay EJ, Megens JA, et al.** A long-term follow-up study of mortality in transsexuals receiving treatment with cross-sex hormones. Eur J Endocrinol. 2011;164:635-42.

30. **Gooren LJ.** Clinical practice. Care of transsexual persons. N Engl J Med. 2011;364:1251-1257.

31. **Park IU, Palefsky JM.** Evaluation and management of anal intraepithelial neoplasia in HIV-negative and HIV-positive men who have sex with men. Curr Infect Dis Rep. 2010;12:126-33.

32. **Guiguet M, Boue F, Cadranel J, et al.** Effect of immunodeficiency, HIV viral load, and antiretroviral therapy on the risk of individual malignancies (FHDH-ANRS CO4): a prospective cohort study. Lancet Oncol. 2009;10:1152-9.

33. **Perlman G, Drescher J.** A Gay Man's Guide to Prostate Cancer. Binghamton, NY: Haworth Medical Press; 2005.

34. **Tracy JK, Lydecker AD, Ireland L.** Barriers to cervical cancer screening among lesbians. J Womens Health (Larchmt). 2010;19:229-37.

35. **Roberts SJ, Patsdaughter CA, Grindel CG,** Tarmina MS. Health related behaviors and cancer screening of lesbians: results of the Boston Lesbian Health Project II. Women Health. 2004; 39:41-55.

36. **Diamant AL, Wold C, Spritzer K, Gelberg L.** Health behaviors, health status, and access to and use of health care: a population-based study of lesbian, bisexual, and heterosexual women. Arch Fam Med. 2000;9:1043-51.

37. **Moyer VA, U.S. Preventive Services Task Force.** Screening for cervical cancer: U.S. Preventive Services Task Force recommendation statement. Ann Intern Med. 2012;156:880-91, W312.

38. **Cochran SD, Mays VM.** Risk of breast cancer mortality among women cohabiting with same sex partners: findings from the National Health Interview Survey, 1997-2003. J Womens Health (Larchmt). 2012;21:528-33.

39. **Zaritsky E, Dibble SL.** Risk factors for reproductive and breast cancers among older lesbians. J Womens Health (Larchmt). 2010;19:125-31.

40. **U.S. Preventive Services Task Force.** Screening for breast cancer. July 2010. www.uspreventiveservicestaskforce.org/uspstf/uspsbrca.htm.

41. **Moyer VA, U.S. Preventive Services Task Force.** Screening for ovarian cancer: U.S. Preventive Services Task Force reaffirmation recommendation statement. Ann Intern Med. 2012;157:900-4.

42. **Antiretroviral Therapy Cohort Collaboration.** Causes of death in HIV-1-infected patients treated with antiretroviral therapy, 1996-2006: collaborative analysis of 13 HIV cohort studies. Clin Infect Dis. 2010;50:1387-96.

43. **Witt MD, Seaberg EC, Darilay A, Young S, Badri S, Rinaldo CR, et al.** Incident hepatitis C virus infection in men who have sex with men: a prospective cohort analysis, 1984-2011. Clin Infect Dis. 2013;57:77-84.

44. **Kahn J.** Preventing hepatitis A and hepatitis B virus infections among men who have sex with men. Clin Infect Dis. 2002;35:1382-7.

45. **Miksad RA, Bubley G, Church P, et al.** Prostate cancer in a transgender woman 41 years after initiation of feminization. JAMA. 2006;296:2316-7.

46. **Lindau ST, Schumm L, Laumann E, et al.** A study of sexuality and health among older adults in the United States. N Engl J Med. 2007;357:762-74.

47. **Stall R, Catania J.** AIDS risk behaviors among late middle-aged and elderly Americans. The National AIDS Behavioral Surveys. Arch Intern Med 1994;154:57-63.

48. **Lindau ST, Leitsch SA, Lundberg KL, Jerome J.** Older women's attitudes, behavior, and communication about sex and HIV: a community-based study. J Womens Health. 2006;15:747-53.

49. **Gott CM.** Sexual activity and risk-taking in later life. Health Social Care Community. 2001; 9:72-8.

50. **Jameson M.** Seniors sex lives are up—and so are STD cases around the country. Orlando Sentinel. May 17, 2011. Available at: http://articles.orlandosentinel.com/2011-04-18/health/os-seniors-stds-rise-20110416_1_std-cases-syphilis-and-chlamydia-seniors.

51. **Henderson SJ, Bernstein LB, George DM, et al.** Older women and HIV: how much do they know and where are they getting their information? J Am Geriatr Soc 2004;52:1549-53.

52. **Pratt G, Gascoyne K, Cunningham K, Tunbridge A.** Human immunodeficiency virus (HIV) in older people. Age Ageing. 2010;39:289-94.

53. **Centers for Disease Control and Prevention.** HIV among older Americans. Available at: www.cdc.gov/hiv/risk/age/olderamericans/index.html.

54. **Skiest D, Keiser P.** Human immunodeficiency virus infection in patients older than 50 years. Arch Fam Med 1997;6:289-94.

55. **Lekas H, Schrimshaw E, Siegel K.** Pathways to HIV testing among adults aged fifty and older with HIV/AIDS. AIDS Care 2005;17:674-87.

56. **Grossman AH.** At risk, infected, and invisible: older gay men and HIV/AIDS. J Assoc Nurses AIDS Care. 1995;6:13-9.

57. **Centers for Disease Control and Prevention.** HIV Surveillance Report. Volume 21, 2009. Available at: www.cdc.gov/hiv/surveillance/resources/reports/2009report/.

58. **Centers for Disease Control and Prevention.** Sexually transmitted diseases (STDs). Available at: www.cdc.gov/std.

59. **Branson BM, Handsfield HH, Lampe MA, et al.** Revised recommendations for HIV testing of adults, adolescents, and pregnant women in health-care settings. MMWR Recomm Rep. 2006;55(RR-14):1-17.

60. **U.S. Preventive Services Task Force.** Screening for HIV. April 2013. Available at: www.uspreventiveservicestaskforce.org/uspstf13/hiv/hivfinalrs.htm#summary.

61. **Rosen RC, Catania JA, Ehrhardt, Burnett AL, Lue TF, McKenna K, et al.** The Bolger conference on PDE-5 inhibition and HIV risk: implications for healthy policy and prevention. J Sex Med. 2006;3:960-75.

62. **Centers for AIDS Prevention Studies.** What are HIV prevention needs of adults over 50? September 1997. Available at: http://caps.ucsf.edu/uploads/pubs/FS/over50.php.

63. **Clements-Nolle K, Marx R, Guzman R, Katz M.** HIV prevalence, risk behaviors, health care use, and mental health status of transgender persons: implications for public health intervention. Am J Public Health. 2001;91:915-21.

64. **Centers for Disease Control and Prevention.** HIV among transgender people. 2012. Available at: www.cdc.gov/hiv/transgender/index.htm.

65. **Data Collection on Adverse Events of Anti-HIV drugs (D:A:D) Study Group; Smith C, Sabin CA, Lundgren JD, Thiebaut R, Weber R, Law M, et al.** Factors associated with specific causes of death amongst HIV-positive individuals in the D:A:D Study. AIDS. 2010;24: 1537-48.

66. **Simone MJ, Appelbaum J.** HIV in older adults. Geriatrics. 2008;63:6-12.

67. **Working Group for the HIV and Aging Consensus Project.** Recommended treatment strategies for clinicians managing older patients with HIV. 2012. Available at: www.hiv-age.org.

68. **Panel on Antiretroviral Guidelines for Adults and Adolescents.** Guidelines for the use of antiretroviral agents in HIV-1-infected adults and adolescents. Department of Health and Human Services. May 2014. Available at: http://aidsinfo.nih.gov/guidelines/.

69. **Mills TC, Paul J, Stall R, et al.** Distress and depression in men who have sex with men: the Urban Men's Health Study. Am J Psychiatry. 2004;161:278-85.

70. **D'Augelli AR, Grossman AH, Starks MT.** Childhood gender atypicality, victimization, and PTSD among lesbian, gay, and bisexual youth. J Interpers Violence. 2006;21:1462-82.

71. **Fredriksen-Goldsen KI, Kim HJ, Barkan SE.** Disability among lesbian, gay, and bisexual adults: disparities in prevalence and risk. Am J Public Health. 2012;102:e16-21.

72. **D'Augelli AR, Grossman AH, Hershberger SL, O'Connell TS. Aspects of mental health among older lesbian, gay, and bisexual adults.** Aging Mental Health. 2001;5:149-58.

73. **UCSF Center of Excellence for Transgender Health.** Mental Health. Available at: www.transhealth.ucsf.edu/trans?page=protocol-mental-health.

74. **Dean L Meyer IH, Robinson K, Sell RL, Sember R, Silenzio VM, et al.** Lesbian, gay, bisexual and transgender health: findings and concerns. J Gay Lesbian Med Assoc. 2000;4: 101-50.

75. **Grant JM, Mottet LA, Tanis J.** Injustice at every turn: a report of the national transgender discrimination survey. Washington, DC: National Center for Transgender Equality and National Gay and Lesbian Task Force; 2011. Available at: www.thetaskforce.org/reports_and_research/ntds.

76. **Quam JK, Whitford GS.** Adaptation and age-related expectations of older gay and lesbian adults. Gerontologist. 1992;32:367-74.

77. **MetLife Mature Market Institute.** Out and aging: The MetLife Study of Lesbian and Gay Baby Boomers. Lesbian and Gay Aging Issues Network of the American Society on Aging and Zogby International. November 2006. Available at: https://www.metlife.com/assets/cao/mmi/publications/studies/mmi-out-aging-lesbian-gay-retirement.pdf.

78. **Schope RD.** Who's afraid of growing old? Gay and lesbian perceptions of aging. J Gerontol Soc Work. 2005;45:23-38.

79. **Simone MJ, Appelbaum J.** Addressing the needs of older gay, lesbian, bisexual and transgender adults. Clin Geriatr. 2011;19:38-45.

80. Assistive Housing for Elderly Gays and Lesbians in New York City: Extent of Need and the Preferences of Elderly Gays and Lesbians. New York: Brookdale Center on Aging of Hunter College and Senior Action in a Gay Environment; 1999.

81. **Rosenfeld D.** Identity work among the homosexual elderly. J Aging Studies. 1999;13:121-44.

82. **Brennan-Ing M, Karpiak SE, Seidel L.** Health and psychosocial needs of LGBT older adults. Available from the AIDS Community Research Initiative of America (ACRIA) at: www.lgbtagingcenter.org/resources/pdfs/COH%20Study%20Final%20Report%20091911.pdf.

83. **Grant JM.** Outing Age 2010: Public policy issues affecting lesbian, gay, bisexual and transgender elders. National Gay and Lesbian Task Force Policy Institute. 2009. Available at: www.thetaskforce.org/reports_and_research/outing_age_2010.

84. **Kuyper L, Fokkeman T.** Loneliness among older lesbian, gay and bisexual adults: the role of minority stress. Arch Sexual Behav. 2009;39:1171-80.

85. **Cornwell EY, Waite LJ.** Social disconnectedness, perceived isolation, and health among older adults. J Health Social Behav. 2009;50:31-48.

86. **Kimmel D, Rose T, David S, eds.** Lesbian, Gay, Bisexual and Transgender Aging: Research and Clinical Perspectives. 6th ed. New York: Columbia University Press; 2006:233.

87. **National Resource Center on LGBT Aging.** LGBT Caregiving Facts. Available at: www.lgbtagingcenter.org/resources/resource.cfm?r=2.

88. **Goldberg NG.** The impact of inequality for same-sex partners in employer-sponsored retirement plans. The Williams Institute. 2009. Available at: http://williamsinstitute.law.ucla.edu/wp-content/uploads/Goldberg-Retirement-Plans-Report-Oct-2009.pdf.

89. **U.S. Department of Health and Human Services.** HHS announces first guidance implementing Supreme Court's decision on the Defense of Marriage Act. August 29, 2013. Available at: www.hhs.gov/news/press/2013pres/08/20130829a.html.

90. **Harding R, Epiphaniou E, Chidgey-Clark J.** Needs, experiences, and preferences of sexual minorities for end-of-life care and palliative care: a systematic review. J Palliat Med 2012;15:602-11.

91. **National Senior Citizens Law Center, National Center for Lesbian Rights, National Center for Transgender Equality, Lambda Legal, Services & Advocacy for GLBT Elders, National Gay and Lesbian Task Force.** Stories From the Field: LGBT Older Adults in Long-Term Care Facilities. Available at: www.lgbtagingcenter.org/resources/resource.cfm?r=54.

92. **Meyer H.** Safe spaces? The need for LGBT cultural competency in aging services. Public Policy Aging Rep. 2011;21:24-7.

93. **Zians J.** LGBT San Diego's Trailblazing generation: housing & related needs of LGBT seniors. 2011. Available at: www.thecentersd.org/pdf/programs/senior-needs-report.pdf.

94. **Silver J.** Language and LGBT housing: making models that fit all communities. Aging Today. 2011;32:1-2.

95. **Gay & Lesbian Elder Housing.** What we do. Available at: http://gleh.org/what-we-do.

96. **Meyer H.** Training day: National Resource Center teaches LGBT cultural competence. Aging Today. 2012;33:1-2.

97. **Parker-Pope T.** Kept from a dying partner's bedside. The New York Times. May 18, 2009. Available at: www.nytimes.com/2009/05/19/health/19well.html.

98. **Presendential Memorandum—Hospital Visitation.** Respecting the Rights of Hospital Patients to Receive Visitors and to Designate Surrogate Decision Makers for Medical Emergencies. Fed Reg. 2010;FR20511:20511-205.

Health Promotion and Disease Prevention

Chapter 8

Principles for Taking an LGBTQ-Inclusive Health History and Conducting a Culturally Competent Physical Exam

MARCY GELMAN, RN, MSN, MPH
AIMEE VAN WAGENEN, PhD
JENNIFER POTTER, MD

Introduction

Improving communication between lesbian, gay, bisexual, transgender, and queer/questioning (LGBTQ) patients and their providers is an important task. LGBTQ patients face substantial financial, structural, and cultural barriers in access to health care (1,2) and bring important concerns about discrimination and stigma to health care interactions. For many transgender patients, disrespectful conduct in health care is an everyday reality; in the largest national survey of transgender people to date, 19% had been refused medical care because of their transgender or gender-nonconforming status (3). While some cities offer health centers that specialize in providing comprehensive care for LGBTQ populations, most LGBTQ people do not have access to such specialized care. Furthermore, providers rarely receive enough training to meet the needs of their LGBTQ patients (4).

Voices from the LGBTQ community have long clamored for attention to their specific health care needs, and there are signs of change in recognizing the importance of cultural competency in the provision of care to LGBTQ people. For example, in its 2011 field guide, *Advancing Effective Communication, Cultural Competence, and Patient- and Family-Centered Care for the Lesbian, Gay, Bisexual, and Transgender Community*, the Joint Commission (formerly the Joint Commission on Accreditation of Healthcare Organizations, or JCAHO) provides checklists for health care organizations committed to equitable, appropriate care for sexual and gender minorities (5). The field guide is an example of increased efforts to promote improvement at a systems level. Such efforts, including published LGBTQ-specific learning objectives and clinical guidelines for care, provide a roadmap for what we need to learn and do as providers. These and other systems efforts are described in more detail in Chapter 1.

The goal of this chapter is to provide a framework to enable providers, with practice, to enhance the quality of interactions with LGBTQ patients by establishing and building trusting relationships and by conducting the physical examination with respect for a patient's dignity and autonomy. The framework we present is rooted in what we know from research and practice about the uniqueness of LGBTQ health and life experience. We have organized the chapter around a pivotal moment in LGBTQ patient–provider interactions: the medical history. The medical history is one of the first opportunities that providers have to establish a foundation for trust in the relationship. Unfortunately, because most medical history frameworks are fraught with assumptions about sexuality and gender identity and are designed without LGBTQ patients in mind, the medical history can also be the moment when trust is broken.

In this chapter, we offer providers tools for taking a sensitive and complete medical history using questions free of bias with respect to all identities and behaviors. We also briefly introduce other key aspects of LGBTQ patient care, such as how to perform a sensitive exam; the importance of providing culturally relevant education/outreach/risk reduction counseling; where to find resources; and what constitutes population-specific effective health maintenance and anticipatory guidance. Other chapters in this book focus on these latter areas in greater detail on a topic-by-topic basis.

Providers use various information collection tools in taking a medical history, including intake forms and medical interview templates. This chapter presents questions specifically designed for each modality. Appendix D provides an abbreviated list of questions appropriate for an LGBTQ-inclusive medical history form, organized in a modular format. Where possible, we include questions that have been validated in sexual and gender minority populations (or we have derived questions from instruments that have been validated in populations that include LGBTQ people). We hope this will make it easy for providers to pick and choose questions relevant to their own practice to incorporate into their own intake forms. We recognize that, at best, a medical history form can only provide a mere snapshot of key areas that then need to be addressed in more detail during the interview. We therefore use the text to expand each area on the medical history form into a broader discussion of why it is important to ask particular questions of LGBTQ individuals and how to formulate in-person questions in an open-ended, colloquial style most likely to result in a complete history. We consider both information collection modalities—the medical history form and the face-to-face interview—essential tools for understanding the medical histories of LGBTQ patients and key opportunities for building trust in relationships. The modalities each have their strengths and limitations, as summarized in Table 8-1.

Table 8-1   Relative Merits and Limitations of Learning About LGBTQ Patients Using Medical History Forms as Compared to Face-to-Face Discussions

Medical History Forms	Face-to-Face Discussions
Can include well-crafted questions inclusive of LGBTQ life experiences that signal an explicit welcome to patients before interactions with clinicians take place.	Provide an opportunity for clinicians to build trust by demonstrating an open and accepting demeanor and asking LGBTQ-inclusive questions.
Permit capture of demographic data in a systematic and preferably electronic format for use in research, quality improvement, and design of population-relevant outreach and education.	Permit clinicians to shape and craft more nuanced questions than is possible on intake forms in order to zero in on each patient's unique concerns.
May provide a more accurate assessment strategy for some patients who may be more comfortable answering sensitive questions on a self-reported form.	Provide an opportunity to obtain much more fine-grained detail than is possible on intake forms and permit capture of information that lies "outside the box"
Provide an opportunity to incorporate brief screening questions that flag important areas for follow-up during the face-to-face interview.	Allow clinicians to respond on the spot to patients' concerns by arranging time-sensitive follow-up and/or referrals as appropriate.

Organization of the topic sections on both the medical history form and corresponding in-depth discussion follows the usual medical history flow with which readers who are providers will be familiar. We start with initial rapport-building, then proceed to elucidating the patient's presenting concerns, documenting the medical history, performing a review of systems pertinent to the patient's presenting symptoms, and taking a family and social history. Where we digress from the usual flow, we explain the reasons for that digression. It is not our intent to outline basic details, such as how to elicit a medical history or obtain a list of a patient's medications and allergies; rather, this chapter concentrates on correcting inaccuracies and filling the gaps that persist with respect to obtaining accurate and relevant information from LGBTQ individuals. Not surprisingly, most of these inaccuracies and gaps fall in the realm of psychosocial stressors, relationships, and lifestyle behaviors. Comprehensive reviews of the basic principles of medical history-taking may be found elsewhere (6,7).

We want to emphasize the importance of experience and practice in challenging old attitudes and in acquiring new knowledge and skills. There is simply no substitute for getting out there and "walking the walk," however unfamiliar it seems to be at first, and learning bit by bit to "talk the talk." We therefore encourage you to challenge your assumptions about gender identity and sexual orientation by asking all of your patients—no matter what gender or sexual orientation you think they may be—questions in our recommended format. Each one of us harbors hidden biases, assumptions, and stereotypes about LGBTQ people—even those of us who define along the

LGBTQ spectrum. We encourage you to ask these questions of all patients, no matter their age, race/ethnicity, immigrant status, income/educational level, or whether they reside in a rural or urban area. We encourage you to ask these questions of patients who have a current or past history of opposite-sex relationships and who appear to be gender conforming or gender normative. Each of these groups is often incorrectly assumed not to include LGBTQ people among them. We also encourage you to seek out training experiences that will increase your exposure to LGBTQ patients and to view each interaction as an opportunity to not only practice new communication strategies but also to notice and attend to your own internal reactions. Regularly performing this type of internal inquiry is integral to the process of becoming a more sensitive and effective provider for LGBTQ (and indeed *all*) patients, and is addressed in detail in Chapter 15.

While this chapter focuses on the ways in which LGBTQ patients are different from non-LGBTQ patients, it is important to remember the myriad ways in which LGBTQ patients are similar to all patients. Each person in the LGBTQ community experiences life and goes about daily activities in much the same ways as their heterosexual peers. LGBTQ people share other statuses in common with non-LGBTQ people; they are students, parents, brothers, sisters, farmers, lawyers, service workers, business professionals, young, middle-aged, old, and live in urban, suburban, and rural communities. They have most of the same health care concerns as those of the general population. One unifying motive all people share when employing a health care organization or provider is the desire for a compassionate, knowledgeable, and nonjudgmental provider whom they can trust.

Laying the Foundation for Trust

Environment of Care

Providers can improve communication with LGBTQ patients by creating a welcoming environment. A patient's first impression of the clinical environment is a critical moment that can influence the remainder of their interaction with the institution, the provider, and other health care personnel. Health care providers can take positive steps to promote the health of their patients by examining their office and other practice environments, institutional policies, and staff training procedures for opportunities to improve access to quality health care for LGBTQ people. Both health care organizations and providers are often unaware of the degree of discrimination an LGBTQ person may have experienced during prior interactions in other health care settings. These experiences are formative and will influence the patient's current comfort or discomfort in health care settings even before they walk in the provider's door. Patients who have experienced bias in health care settings in the past may be highly attuned to even small and subtle signs and may arrive with the expectation that that they will be judged and discriminated against once more. When entering a new practice, an LGBTQ patient will often scan the environment for signs of inclusion or exclusion. The information they gather may help them determine whether they will feel comfortable in the practice and what information they will choose to share with their health care provider. The tone set with your LGBTQ patients will be established from their first encounter, whether by phone when scheduling the first appointment, during the registration and check-in process, while completing the medical history questionnaire, and while taking in the ambience of the environment they are waiting in. Some suggestions for creating a welcoming environment can be found in Appendix A; please refer to Chapter 1 for a more thorough discussion of this topic.

Confidentiality

Prior experiences of bias and discrimination may make LGBTQ patients particularly concerned about the confidentiality of information they provide regarding their sexual orientation and gender identity. We suggest encouraging openness by explaining that the patient–provider discussion is confidential and that complete and accurate information is essential to guide appropriate care. It is important to specify what, if any, information will be documented in the medical record and under what circumstances this information may be shared with third parties. We recommend developing and prominently displaying a confidentiality statement and providing it in writing to every patient along with registration and medical intake forms. An example privacy policy can be found on the Fenway Health website (8). Key elements of such a policy include an explanation of what information will be recorded, who will have access to the medical record, how test results will be kept confidential, the organization's policy on sharing information with insurance companies and other outside facilities, and instances when maintaining confidentiality will not be possible. Providers must also make sure that all staff members understand the importance of maintaining strict confidentiality and receive training on regulations that mandate protection of personal health information.

Inclusive Registration and Medical History Forms

Registration and medical history forms give patients one of their first and most memorable impressions of your approach to clinical practice. This experience sets the tone for how comfortable patients will feel about disclosing their sexual orientation and/or gender identity/expression. The medical history form also provides an opportunity to introduce the idea of a working partnership between patient and provider. We encourage including an explicit statement on the form that asks for input on how the patient feels things are going from the start.

Registration and medical history forms should be reviewed and revised to ensure LGBTQ inclusivity. For example, "marital status" should be replaced with the phrase "relationship status" or something similar to signal that same-sex relationships are recognized as legitimate and are part of what you are interested in learning about from your patients. We suggest adding *partner* wherever the words *spouse, husband,* or *wife* are typically used and using gender-neutral or inclusive language whenever asking about sexual or intimate partners. One might also consider including open-ended response choices to questions to avoid assumptions of heterosexuality and normative family structure. In addition, we strongly recommend including questions about sexual orientation and gender identity on patient registration forms. Including such questions alongside other demographic variables sends a message to patients that the provider considers sexual orientation and gender identity to be routine characteristics, much like veteran status or race/ethnicity, and that providers are interested in and comfortable with learning this information. Systematic collection of this information also allows organizations to characterize the sexual orientation and gender identity distribution of the patient population they serve, with the ultimate goal of monitoring and improving the health outcomes and quality of care of their LGBTQ patients. Finally, patients may be more likely to disclose minority sexual orientation or gender identity in response to a question on a form than they are to spontaneously come out in a clinical encounter or to answer truthfully to a face-to-face question from a provider. Recommendations on how to ask sexual orientation and gender identity questions are provided in Appendix B and in the "Registration Form" section below.

Communication During the Face-to-Face Medical Interview

As with all patient contacts, the approach to the face-to-face medical interview should demonstrate empathy, open-mindedness, and absence of judgment. Eliciting information about sexual orientation, gender identity and sexual practices—even when your patient may be reluctant to share the information—is important to avoid misdiagnosis and improper care and treatment. When you identify an LGBTQ patient, consider asking about experiences with health care providers and be aware that experiences of bias or discrimination underscore the need for careful rebuilding of trust. Additional barriers to open communication may be related to differences in socioeconomic status, cultural norms, racial/ethnic discrimination, age, physical ability, and geography. Similarly, it is important not to make assumptions about literacy, language capacity, and comfort with direct communication. Table 8-2 includes a list of common pitfalls to avoid when treating LGBTQ patients. Remember that it is impossible to avoid all assumptions and that you will inevitably make mistakes. Always apologize right away when you make a mistake, such as an incorrect assumption about a patient's

---

Table 8-2   Common Assumptions to Avoid

Assumptions about Identity and Sexual Orientation

Don't assume that all patients are heterosexual and nontransgender.

Don't assume that all transgender people have opposite- or same-sex partners; transgender people have diverse sexual orientations and may be straight, gay, lesbian, or bisexual or may identify as queer or with another orientation.

Don't assume that a person exploring their sexual orientation has an immediate need to establish a gay, straight, or bisexual orientation.

Don't assume that people who are exploring their gender identity have an immediate need to establish a male or female gender identity.

Don't assume that bisexual people are "confused" about their identity or that bisexuality is a stage in sexual orientation development that will likely resolve itself to a gay or lesbian identity.

Don't assume that the sexual/gender minority aspect of a person's identity is preeminent. For many people, other aspects of their identity, e.g. their race/ethnicity, may take precedence.

Don't assume that being LGBT or Q is always hard. Many LGBTQ people are well adjusted and face the same stresses in their lives as do heterosexual peers.

Assumptions about Relationships, Family, and Children

Don't assume that a self-identified lesbian cannot be pregnant.

Don't assume that interpersonal violence does not occur in LGBTQ couples.

Don't assume that LGBTQ patients do not have children or do not wish to have children.

Don't assume that a patient with children is heterosexual. LGBTQ people often have children.

Don't assume that adults of reproductive age have an interest in parenting; some do and some don't.

Don't assume that LGBTQ patients do not have strong family ties.

Assumptions about Sexual Behavior

Don't assume that LGBTQ people are all sexually active. Some are abstinent.

Don't assume that self-identified gay men do not have sex with women or that lesbians never have sex with men.

Don't assume that all gay men have sex with multiple partners or engage in high-risk activities.

Don't assume that sexual behavior will remain stable over time, and do not assume that a patient's sexual orientation identity tells you everything you need to know about their sexual behavior now or in the future.

Don't assume that lesbians are not at risk for HPV or other STIs.

Don't assume the presence of defined sex roles in any relationship. Sex roles can be fluid and interchangeable.

Don't assume that bisexually identified people are promiscuous or that they have or are seeking partners of both genders.

Don't assume that transgender women engage in sex work or risky sex or that all transgender people are "bottoms" sexually.

Assumptions about Transgender People's Anatomy

Don't assume that transgender people all want to change their bodies with hormones and surgeries.

Don't assume *anything* about the body of a transgender person (e.g., do not assume that transgender women do not have or use a penis or that transgender men do not have a uterus, cervix, or ovaries even after genital reconstruction surgery).

HPV = human papillomavirus; STI = sexually transmitted infection.

sexual orientation or gender identity, or using an incorrect term to which your patient does not relate.

Listen to your patients and how they describe their own gender, sexual orientation, partner(s), and relationship(s) and reflect their choice of language. Be aware that although some LGBTQ people may use words such as *queer*, *dyke*, and *fag* to describe themselves, these and other words have been used in a derogatory manner against LGBTQ individuals. Although some individuals may have reclaimed these terms for themselves, they are not appropriate for use by health care providers who have not yet established a trusting and respectful rapport with LGBTQ patients. If you are in doubt as to what words to use, ask your patient what terms they prefer. Avoid using the term *gay* with patients even if they have indicated a same-sex or same-gender sexual partner, unless they have used the term themselves. If patients themselves have not indicated a particular identity or have indicated a sexual orientation other than *gay*, using this term may cause alienation and mistrust that will interfere with information gathering and appropriate care. While some may identify as *queer*, others may not choose any label at all. Young people as well as adults may be unlikely to self-identify using traditional sexual orientation labels such as gay, lesbian, or bisexual. With transgender patients, indicate respect by making sure all staff members are trained to use preferred pronouns and names (9). Clearly indicate this information on their medical record in a manner that allows you to easily reference it for future visits. The key is to follow each patient's lead about self-description while exploring how this relates to current and potential medical needs.

Topics in the Registration Form and Medical History

In this section, we review the modular sections of the sample registration form and medical history form included in Appendix D. As you move through this section of the chapter, we encourage you to refer to these forms for a list of standardized questions that can be used to elicit information in each of the domains discussed. In the text of the chapter, we supplement these standardized questions with suggestions for prompts that can be used during the medical interview. We also highlight several LGBTQ-specific concerns to be addressed when performing the medical exam. Note that we do not include a separate section of the history form for transgender individuals but instead craft each topic section to be inclusive of transgender patients and to include transgender-specific concerns.

Registration Form

Information obtained at the time of registration is typically entered into an electronic health record by reception staff and used for billing and/or federal or state reporting purposes. We have included a registration form separate from the medical history form, as many practices do, and encourage providers to consider using this form as part of the process of improving communication with LGBTQ patients. As previously described, if your registration form includes demographic information such as race and ethnicity, we encourage you to consider adding sexual orientation and transgender-inclusive gender identity options. There are no universally agreed upon or standardized questions about sexual orientation and gender identity (10,11); however, Appendix B presents some suggestions based on identified best practices (12,13) and modified from questions tested for national population-based surveys (14). We have incorporated these methods into the patient registration and medical history forms presented in this chapter. Registration forms can be particularly difficult for transgender patients because most forms include only 2 categories for sex (male and female). Because health insurance coverage is sometimes sex-specific, providers need to collect sex and name information from patients as it is recorded with the insurer. This is a difficult experience for transgender patients, many of whom have not yet and may not ever change their sex designation or name with their health insurer. It may not be possible to eliminate all discomfort for transgender patients, but registration forms should be crafted to minimize discomfort. We therefore suggest that you include a section on your form that asks for name and sex information as they are listed on the patients' health insurance or government documents, as well as gender information that is concordant with the patients' preferences. We encourage inclusion of questions that also ask about preferred gender pronouns (e.g., *he, she, they, zie*). Once you ascertain information about gender and terminology preferences, it is important that this information is flagged in medical records and that all staff—from the front line to the provider—are trained to identify preferred names and pronouns from the chart and to use them during all future visits (9).

Biographical Information

The medical history begins by obtaining biographical information. Our sample form repeats some of the questions asked on the registration form in recognition of the fact that providers may not have immediate access to information elicited during the registration process, and demographic information provides important background about patients as individuals. Appendix D lists a few different sexual orientation and gender identity question options. We encourage providers to frame questions in the sample medical history form to include write-in options. Write-in options allow providers to learn about and record the terms that patients use for themselves; unlike the data obtained via a registration form, answers to questions asked during the medical history can be entered into free text fields in the electronic health record. The alternative gender identity question included in our sample medical history form is one recommended by the Center for Excellence in Transgender

Health at the University of California, San Francisco. In addition to the ability to write-in, it includes the option to "check all that apply." This enables transgender patients to identify with their current gender (e.g., by checking off the option "male") and also with a transgender-related term (e.g., by also checking the option "transmale").

Current Health

We suggest including general questions about any pressing health concerns early in the medical history form and clinical history. By asking patients about their own goals for their health, you will communicate interest in establishing a working partnership in which the patients' concerns are at the center. However, remain aware that presenting concerns might not actually be the major reason for an LGBTQ person's visit. It may require several visits before LGBTQ patients feel safe enough to reveal their true concerns and reasons for seeking medical evaluation.

Personal and Family Medical History and Preventive Screenings

The personal and family history section of the medical history form includes a standard set of questions that are pertinent to all patients no matter their sexual orientation or gender identity. These questions elicit information about the patient's history of present illness, review of systems, medical history, medications and allergies, and family history and provide valuable information about the person's past and current experience with illness, risk for inherited diseases, and preventive screenings.

As detailed in other chapters of this text, a limited but growing number of studies to date show that LGBTQ people are at greater risk for certain medical and behavioral health problems compared with the general population. Most of these health disparities are believed to be the consequences of high levels of exposure to societal stigma and discrimination, which can predispose LGBTQ people to isolation, homelessness, poverty, substance use, sexual risk behavior, depression, and other mental health problems and can hamper access to appropriate health care and community-based programs (3,15–22). It is therefore vital for providers to be aware of these issues, to assess patients thoroughly with sensitive questioning and probing, and to encourage them to receive all recommended preventive screenings.

Medical Risks Specific to Lesbian and Bisexual Women

Research on lesbian and bisexual women strongly suggests that they have a higher likelihood of being overweight or obese (23), using tobacco and alcohol (10,20,21,24,25) and having significant stress in their lives (26). These factors potentially put lesbian and bisexual women at higher risk for developing heart disease (10,27) and certain types of cancer (28), although currently there is not enough research on whether lesbians and bisexual women actually experience higher rates of these health conditions (10). On average, lesbians also have fewer pregnancies and live births and have a decreased probability of breastfeeding, meaning they are less likely to benefit from certain factors that may protect against breast, uterine, and ovarian cancers (27,29). Compounding the problem further, lesbians and bisexual women may be at risk for putting off or avoiding cancer screenings (30). For example, lesbians and bisexual women are less likely to undergo cervical Papanicolaou (Pap) tests (31). One explanation for this is the misconception on the part of some lesbians and health care professionals that lesbians are not at risk for cervical cancer (32). It is important for providers to be aware that human papillomavirus (HPV)—the chief cause of cervical cancer—can be sexually transmitted between women. In addition, many women who identify as lesbian have had male sex partners in the past or continue to have male sex partners periodically (32).

Medical Risks Specific to Gay and Bisexual Men

There is a disproportionate rate of and risk for sexually transmitted infections (STIs) among gay and bisexual men and other men who have sex with men (MSM) compared with heterosexual men (33). These infections include bacterial STIs, such as syphilis, gonorrhea, and chlamydia (pharyngeal, urethral, and anal), as well as viral STIs, such as HIV, HPV, herpes simplex virus infections, and hepatitis A, B, and C. MSM are more severely affected by HIV than any other group in the United States. While MSM of all races and ethnicities are affected, black MSM are particularly impacted (34). Because MSM have an increased risk for HIV and STIs, the Centers for Disease Control and Prevention provides screening guidelines specific to MSM, which can be found at www.cdc.gov.

All men, including MSM, are at risk for prostate, testicular, and colon cancer. However, among MSM, and especially HIV-infected MSM, the incidence of anal cancer is significantly more prevalent than in the general population and is increasing in prevalence annually (35). Anal cancer is caused by the same high-risk strains of HPV that cause cervical cancer in women; thus, MSM who engage in anal receptive sex at any point in their lives are at increased risk for contracting anal mucosal infection. Anal Pap tests can be considered as a screening test for anal intraepithelial neoplasia, although there is no consensus on whether screening is cost-effective (36–38). Please refer to Chapters 12 and 13 for more information on screening for HIV and STIs.

Medical Risks Specific to Transgender People

It is especially important for providers to ask transgender patients about their current anatomy because it is only possible to offer appropriate screening and treatment when one knows what organs are present. Transgender men (female-to-male) who still have a uterine cervix need to have regular

Pap tests in accordance with screening recommendations for natal women. Transgender women (male-to-female) retain prostate tissue even after genital reconstruction surgery and therefore need to have prostate screening in accordance with risk-based screening recommendations for natal men (39). With respect to breast cancer screening for transgender men and women, recommendations for breast examinations and mammography depend on the present anatomy, the type and duration of hormones they are using, and whether they have other breast cancer risk factors (39). Performance of some of these exams/procedures can be a difficult experience for transgender patients whose gender is not concordant with remaining anatomic structures and must be done sensitively, as discussed in the section on physical examination below. However, in some cases, as for transgender women advised to have breast examinations and mammography, these experiences can be validating and may be welcomed.

Additionally, lack of access to medical care or a history of negative encounters with health professionals has lead some transgender people to pursue gender affirmation via use of street hormones, silicone injections, and other methods potentially harmful to their health (40). It is therefore very important to ask questions about all of these areas. Hormone treatment may also be associated with a higher risk for various medical conditions (e.g., estrogen with cardiovascular disease, stroke, and venous thromboembolism; testosterone with adverse effects on lipids); however, more research is needed to elucidate the precise risks and outline appropriate surveillance strategies. Please refer to Chapter 18 for additional information.

Supporting Patients in Accessing Preventive Health Services

In summary, we want to stress the importance of asking all LGBTQ patients about their experiences accessing preventive health screenings such as mammograms, Pap tests, and colon cancer screening procedures. This line of questioning will provide information about any misconceptions and negative experiences that might serve as barriers to future screening, and will give you an opportunity to provide education and to construct a future screening plan that is acceptable to and appropriate for each individual patient. A detailed immunization history should also be obtained from all LGBTQ patients, and vaccinations should be updated in accordance with Advisory Committee on Immunization Practices recommendations. Particularly important vaccines include HPV for all LGBTQ youth until age 26 and hepatitis A and B for all MSM and other patients who engage in high-risk sexual activities or injection drug use.

Advance Health Directives

As part of this section of the medical history form, we have also included questions about advance health directives, which should be asked of all

LGBTQ patients. A health care proxy is an agent (a person) appointed to make a patient's medical decisions if the patient becomes unable to do so. Generally, patients assign someone they know well and trust to represent their preferences. Because LGBTQ individuals may be more likely to choose a friend or non-legally recognized partner to serve in this capacity, rather than a family member or legally recognized spouse, it is particularly important to document their choice so it will be upheld under the law if and when a healthy proxy is needed.

Lifestyle, Wellness, and Body Image

When creating a picture of your patient though the medical history, it is important to examine 3 major areas that contribute to the wellness of an individual: nutrition, exercise, and sleep. People can get into trouble when their behaviors with respect to eating, exercising, and sleeping are out of balance. For example, some people indulge too much, as in compulsive overeating or bingeing, over-exercising, or pushing their bodies beyond healthy limits. Conversely, some people restrict food intake and undereat, or engage in activities designed to mitigate behavioral extremes such as purging to avoid weight gain caused by compulsively overeating. Body image is an issue for everyone living in Western society, given our bombardment with messages about what we should look like (e.g. young, thin, sexy, and buff). However, issues surrounding body image and weight affect members of the LGBTQ community differentially. For instance, as a result of growing up with images of slender and effeminate gay men or "perfect" buff bodies in the media, some gay/bisexual men may worry that they are too thin or too fat, resulting in body image problems. Therefore, they may be more likely than heterosexual men to experience eating disorders, engage in excessive exercise, and use various substances to develop a more stereotypically masculine and muscular appearance (41).

At the other end of the spectrum, many lesbians reject traditional cultural norms regarding beauty and thinness (42). Although this may achieve a more positive body image than that of many heterosexual women, lesbians are more likely to be overweight (23), placing them at risk for certain medical problems. Broaching the topics of eating and exercise may therefore trigger strong emotional responses, including avoidance and overt denial, and should be done with compassion and care.

Based on how people feel about their body, they may treat it with care, attempt to hide it, openly flaunt it, become intently focused on changing or altering it, or either unintentionally or intentionally cause harm to it. As noted on the medical history form, it is important to ask nonjudgmental questions about attempts patients have already made to alter their bodies, such as getting tattoos, piercings, plastic surgery, or using steroids to bulk up, both to get a sense of how important it is to them to adorn or change their bodies and also because some of these practices can have negative health consequences. This lifestyle portion of the history is also a key place where providers can begin a discussion about medical transition with their transgender patients and support those who wish to begin or continue the transition of their bodies to affirm gender identity.

Once you have a sense of a patient's relationship to their body, you can ask additional questions about specific self-care behaviors, such as relationship to food, exercise, sleep, and other forms of relaxation/stress reduction. Questions about these areas are very often neglected in medical history taking because providers may not know how to ask them well; however, they are clearly crucial to address if we hope to successfully partner with patients to truly optimize their health. A good way to start is with general questions, such as "Tell me about your eating," "How are things going with exercise?" and "How are you doing with respect to sleep?", since they do not imply any judgment about the patient's body weight or any "should" about exercising regularly or maintaining a healthy sleep pattern.

If patients reveal that they are engaging in unhealthy patterns of behavior, such as compulsive overeating, restricting food intake, excessive exercise, use of purgatives such as diuretics/laxatives, or self-induced vomiting, it is important to unpack the context in which the behavior is occurring, what the behavior is doing for them, and what they don't like about it. Because extreme behaviors are most often an attempt to manage intolerable feelings, the context of the behavior is crucial to understand. To probe for context, maintain a stance of nonjudgmental curiosity, asking questions such as "Under what circumstances do you . . . ?", "What is (the behavior) doing for you?", "How is this strategy working for you?", as well as questions exploring what the patient doesn't like about it. A complete discussion of motivational interviewing and lifestyle behavioral counseling techniques is beyond the scope of this chapter, but useful questions to get you started are listed in Table 8-3 (just replace the word *drinking* with *eating* or *purging*).

Interventions to achieve a healthy weight meet with less than ideal success in the general population; the same is true among sexual minority populations, where it may be particularly important to use LGBTQ-sensitive methods and to provide culturally relevant support and connection (43). For patients who are not engaging in compulsive behaviors but who are eating poorly, leading a sedentary lifestyle, or not getting enough restful sleep, it is important to ask about barriers that get in the way. Examples of barriers include financial difficulty, living in an unsafe or noisy neighborhood, experiencing sexual minority harassment, or having a prohibitive work schedule. In the case of sleep, it is also important to ask about use of interfering substances, such as caffeine/other stimulants, a rebound effect after use of alcohol/other depressants, as well as symptoms of depression/anxiety/PTSD or a primary sleep disorder.

Provision of basic education, such as a recommendation to follow published nutrition/physical activity guidelines such as those outlined by the

World Health Organization (44) and the Centers for Disease Control and Prevention (45), may be all that is needed to get some patients started, whereas brainstorming ways to surmount specific barriers may be needed in other cases. A series of LGBTQ-sensitive health promotion brochures is available free of charge at the Fenway Health website (www.fenwayhealth.org).

It is also important to encourage LGBTQ patients to develop healthy ways to relax. To that end, we suggest asking patients about their school/work-life balance, what brings them joy, and what strategies they use to cope with stress. It is important to encourage regular use of healthy strategies, such as spending time with friends, listening to music, reading a book, taking a walk, or participating in a weekly LGBTQ square dance event. Use of integrative methods with proven health benefits, such as tai chi, yoga, or meditation, may also be encouraged; LGBTQ-specific classes may be available in many cities.

Finally, we recommend asking all patients about the role of spirituality in their lives. Spirituality may take different forms with different patients and represents an internal ability to find meaning and connectedness in life. Many LGBTQ people derive (or may have derived in the past) significant strength and hope from spiritual practice. While it is true that some traditional religious organizations reject LGBTQ people, many welcome people of any sexual orientation or gender identity, such that it is possible to guide patients who desire but have not yet found a spiritual home toward appropriate resources.

Family and Relationships

As is true for all people, the health of LGBTQ people is shaped by social contexts, including family, intimate and other close relationships. For LGBTQ people, as for all people, relationships can serve as a major source of social support, a major stressor, or both.

LGBTQ people as a group are at risk of being alienated from families of origin and biological kin. Many LGBTQ people have faced past or continue to experience ongoing family rejection that takes a toll on mental health. Accordingly, the medical history form includes several questions designed to identify potential family rejection, including questions that probe for satisfaction with social support. One question asks whether the patient has children under 18 who live elsewhere because some LGBTQ people have had the experience of having their children removed from their care because of their LGBTQ status. Providers may want to elicit additional information about support from biological family and make referrals to LGBTQ-friendly mental health and family counseling services. Providers should also screen for experiences of loss of family (including partners, biological family, and other chosen family) and have on hand LGBTQ-supportive bereavement groups and services.

It is important to be especially attentive to social support needs when working with LGBTQ youth. LGBTQ youth who come out to their families and friends risk disrupting social support networks. Research has shown that among LGBTQ youth, social support from family and friends fosters resilience and protects against negative mental health outcomes such as suicide ideation and attempts (10). Parental acceptance of an adolescent's LGBTQ identity is also an important protective factor (46). In addition to families and friends, schools and communities are potential sources of social support for LGBTQ youth. The supportiveness of school and community contexts varies geographically and seems to affect mental health outcomes for LGBTQ youth (47). Providers should therefore explore social support and family acceptance with young LGBTQ patients and be prepared with referrals to organizations that promote family acceptance, such as local gay-straight alliances in schools, community-based organizations that support LGBTQ youth, and chapters of Parents, Families, and Friends of Lesbians and Gays (PFLAG). For more on LGBTQ youth, see Chapter 5.

Social support is also important to LGBTQ adults, who may be more likely than heterosexual peers to create non-traditional structures of social support through relationships that can be described as "families of choice" (48–50). Families of choice are networks of support and care that are not related by blood or marriage yet function similarly to normative heterosexual families. While families of choice may include intimate partners, they may also comprise former partners, networks of friends (usually not exclusively LGBTQ), and adopted or biological children. When exploring sources of social support with patients, we encourage providers to look beyond the traditional normative family and to include and recognize the role that families of choice play for many patients. In the medical history form, we open the section on families and relationships with the question: "Who are the major support persons in your life?" This open-ended question is designed with a diversity of relationship structures in mind and makes no presumptions about what social support structures should look like in the lives of patients. We encourage providers to follow up in the clinical interview. A question such as "Who do you consider to be your family?" might elicit important information.

Many LGBTQ people are parents or are interested in becoming parents, and we encourage providers to ask their LGBTQ patients about parenting and parenting intentions. Providers should have on hand LGBTQ-friendly resources and referrals for those who seek to become parents through adoption, surrogacy, or alternative insemination. Note that a generic list of referrals is not adequate because some family service agencies have explicit policies that discriminate against LGBT people (e.g., some religiously affiliated adoption agencies) and others may overtly refuse to work with LGBTQ clients or otherwise be unwelcoming to them. For more on LGBTQ relationships and families, see Chapter 6.

While social isolation is a potential concern for older adults of all sexual orientations, LGBTQ older adults may face unique concerns. As LGBTQ people age and lose friends and partners, they may have more difficulty than their heterosexual counterparts in establishing new relationships. LGBTQ community spaces and organizations are typically youth-oriented and community spaces and organizations designed for older adults may not be perceived as welcoming of LGBTQ people. Several research studies have shown that LGB older adults are less likely be partnered than heterosexuals and more likely to live alone (10). LGBTQ older adults are less likely than heterosexuals to have adult children that they can rely upon for later life care (10). As with older adults of all orientations, most LGBTQ people prefer to "age in place" and remain in their own homes as they grow older. Aging in place may be especially important for LGBTQ people, who may fear discrimination in senior housing, assisted living, or nursing home facilities (51). For more on LGBTQ older adults, see Chapter 7.

Mental Health

Sexual and gender minorities experience a high burden of depression, anxiety, and self-harm behaviors—including suicide—because of the cumulative negative impact of social minority stressors (10,18,19,52). Asking specifically about any family or personal history of depression, anxiety, or other mental health problems is therefore exceedingly important, as is screening for currently worrisome symptoms and assessing carefully for the presence of self-harm thoughts or behaviors, whether covert (e.g., substance abuse and other addictions) or overt (e.g., suicidal ideation/having a suicide plan) (53).

Many of the screening questions included in the mental health portion of the sample intake form will be familiar to the reader and are adapted from validated questionnaires, such as the Patient Health Questionnaire-9 (54). Because of the high incidence of trauma among sexual and gender minority populations, we also recommend asking a screening question specific to post-traumatic stress disorder (PTSD), such as, "Have you ever had any experience that was so frightening, horrible, or upsetting that you had nightmares, thought about it when you did not want to, were constantly on guard, or felt numb/detached?" This question is adapted from a validated screening tool for PTSD (55).

Whenever patients screen positive for emotional distress of any kind, detailed follow-up questions need to be asked to determine how well they are coping, whether they need or are willing to accept behavioral health interventions, and whether they are at imminent risk for harming themselves or others. Please refer to Chapter 9 for additional insight into addressing mental health concerns among LGBTQ patients, including recommendations for appropriate urgent and non-urgent intervention and support.

Overall, the approach to the mental health portion of the history is the same for LGBTQ-identified patients as for any patient. Of crucial importance for providers when caring for LGBTQ people is to establish trust because many sexual and gender minority patients, particularly youth and the elderly, are especially isolated, hiding aspects of their lives, and are disconnected from family/other support systems. Traditionally, the mental health system has taken a pathologizing attitude toward sexual and gender minority people (56). The history of reparative therapies for homosexuality and the *Diagnostic and Statistical Manual of Mental Disorder*'s only recently discarded diagnosis of *gender identity disorder* are 2 examples. This historical stance has further compounded the internalized stigma of "something being wrong with me" expressed by many LGBTQ individuals. Therefore, we recommend particular emphasis on validating the patient's emotional experience, avoidance of medical jargon rife with illness-based diagnostic terminology, and creating a partnership focused on enhancing coping, healing, and resilience. To facilitate timely and appropriate referral, it is very helpful to have a resource list of LGBTQ-friendly mental providers and other behavioral health services at your fingertips.

Substance Use

Studies have shown that compared with the general population, LGBTQ individuals are more likely to use alcohol and drugs, have higher rates of substance abuse, and are more likely to continue heavy drinking into later life (10,21). In addition, smoking among LGBTQ persons has been documented to be 2.0 to 2.5 times more likely than among heterosexual peers (20). Long-term use of alcohol and other drugs can cause serious health complications affecting almost every organ in the body, including the brain. It can also damage emotional stability, finances, and career and affect family, friends, and the entire community. While this chapter will not address the details of why there is an increased use of substances among the LBGTQ populations (please refer to Chapter 10), note that substances are often used as a means to relieve, soothe, and manage the loneliness, sadness, and anxiety that can be caused by social minority stress. In addition, cultural norms around LGBTQ substance use have been reinforced by targeted marketing by the alcohol and tobacco industry, and by historical factors that have led LGBTQ people to socialize primarily in clubs and bars. While alcohol use can be an acceptable activity during socialization, the use and possible misuse of alcohol and drugs in LGBTQ populations may also be related to a desire for social acceptance or a wish to avoid feeling rejection or shame when in a sexually charged environment. In addition, some drugs (e.g., poppers and crystal methamphetamine) are popular among gay and bisexual men because they intensify sexual desire and pleasure while decreasing inhibitions. Crystal methamphetamine also helps people stay awake well into the night and prolongs penile erections. Whatever the reason for the use, the combination of drugs and/or alcohol with sex can be particularly detrimental because it is associated with an increased risk of exposure to various STIs, including HIV.

Given these complex motivations for substance use, it is vital for providers to assess LGBTQ patients for tobacco, alcohol, and drug use in a thorough and thoughtful manner. Although such a conversation can be challenging and may arouse shame and denial, broaching these topics communicates a willingness to address these issues with your patients and over time may encourage and support them to seek help and guidance.

As was true for the lifestyle behavior section, the questions about substance use that we have included on the intake form have been adapted from validated substance use assessment tools (see also Chapter 10 for a list of screening tools with strong psychometric ratings for identifying substance use problems). It is important to include questions about both illicit drugs and use of prescription drugs that are prone to misuse, given the growing prevalence of prescription drug diversion and addiction in the United States. It is also important to include questions about the mode and manner of use. Persons who use drugs may experiment with different modes of delivery. Often this experimentation is fueled by the desire to experience heightened sexual pleasure. One example—"booty bumping"—involves placing the drug (usually crystal methamphetamine) directly into the rectum so that rapid absorption results in central neurotransmitter effects and anal sphincter relaxation. All injection drug use carries risks for phlebitis and acquisition of infections such as hepatitis B and C and HIV infection, especially when users share their works/needles. Intranasal drug use (referred to as snorting or bumping) can also increase the risk for hepatitis C virus transmission when works are shared with others.

The interview provides an opportunity to discuss substance use at a deeper and more nuanced level. It is useful to start by asking nonjudgmental, open-ended questions (e.g., "Tell me about your drinking [drug use]"), then to proceed to more specific questions aimed at discovering what and how much the person uses, the circumstances of their use (when and where), and the consequences of their use (pleasure, relief from painful emotions) in motivational interviewing style, as outlined in Table 8-3. Many patients link drinking or drug use to positive social experiences. Therefore, it is useful to ask, "How does your drinking or drug use work for you?"

Table 8-3   Questions to Probe for Context and Consequences of Substance Use

When you drink or use drugs, are you usually alone or with other people?

Do you ever feel any guilt or remorse because of your drinking and/or drug use?

Do you drink or use drugs to influence your emotions or mood?

Have you failed to do what was expected of you because of your drinking or drug use?

Do you ever change your plans so you can drink or use drugs?

Have you or someone else been injured as a result of your drinking or drug use?

Have you ever tried to cut down on your drinking or drug use?

What happened when you tried to cut down?

Are you interested in cutting down, quitting, or getting support for alcohol or drug use?

before asking how it does not. Follow-up questions can then be asked to determine whether patients are using substances to self-medicate or are already experiencing harmful health consequences. Similar questions can also be used to probe for other behaviors that are prone to extremes/addiction, such as engaging in compulsive sexual behavior, shopping/spending in excess of one's means, or spending inordinate amount of time on the computer (e.g., Internet or video game addiction).

If the patient is disengaged but expresses any difficulty that appears to be connected to drinking or drug use, this contradiction can be discussed in an open and nonjudgmental way (e.g., "You say that you don't consider your drinking a problem, but you also say that you sometimes fight with your partner after drinking too much. What are your thoughts about that?"). If patients are not ready to contemplate making any changes in drinking or drug use, a useful next step is to discuss ways in which they might use their substance of choice more safely. This concept of harm reduction can be a productive approach that supports the patient to reduce the negative consequences of substance use while not yet eliminating it altogether. For example, one might say: "I hear you say you do not want to quit drinking, but you would like to be more focused at work. What do you think about stopping drinking by 9 pm instead of 11 pm?" Once you have identified alcohol or drugs as a health issue, it is crucial to schedule follow-up at regular intervals to continue the conversation and repeatedly check in about the substance use over time. Behavior change is a gradual process that may require regular check-ins over the course of many visits or years.

Safety and Social Stress

As discussed earlier and in other chapters, sexual and gender minorities experience stressors related to the social stigma of their sexual orientation and/or gender minority over and above the common, general stressors experienced by all people. This stress is chronic (not fleeting) and socially based (stemming from social institutions, structures, and processes, rather than internal characteristics) (57). Research reveals that sexual minority stress is experienced in several dimensions, including experiences of rejection and discrimination, expectations of future rejection and discrimination, and internalized homophobia (52). Recent literature on transgender health suggests that gender minorities may experience stress in a similarly patterned manner (58). The experience of such chronic added stress requires LGBTQ people to adapt their behaviors in order to cope or buffer the impact of the stress. The medical history provides an opportunity for the provider to assess the effect of current and past social stressors on a patient's health and to encourage development of healthy coping strategies during subsequent lifestyle behavior counseling.

Given the effect of social stress on health, we recommend screening all patients for minority stress related to their gender, physical appearance,

Table 8-4   Questions to Probe for Sexual and Gender Minority Stress
in the Clinical Encounter

Are you comfortable with your friends, family, or coworkers knowing about your sexual orientation or gender identity?

Have you experienced any harassment, discrimination, or stigma as a result of your sexual orientation, gender, or appearance or of being or coming out?

Has anyone ever threatened to out you?

Are you concerned that people will treat you differently, look down on you, or think less of you because of your sexual orientation or gender identity?

Do you conceal your sexual orientation or gender identity?

Do you ever feel depressed, anxious, upset, or stressed when you think about your sexual orientation, gender identity, or gender expression? What do you do to cope with that?

sexual orientation, race/ethnicity, and any other categorization that may be associated with stigma, using a general question such as appears in the Safety and Social Stress section of the sample medical history form. Follow-up questions can then be asked to probe for experiences of sexual and gender minority stress in particular, especially when patients answer affirmatively to initial screening questions. Table 8-4 lists several suggested questions that may be used during the interview to address each of these dimensions in greater detail.

Several of the questions in Table 8-4 specifically address the degree to which LGBTQ patients are "out" to their family, friends, coworkers, employers, and/or the extent of their social support or participation in community. While outness and identification with LGBTQ communities paradoxically bring LGBTQ people in contact with both sources of stress and sources of resilience (57), an individual's connectedness and level of identification with community support networks may correlate with health outcomes. For example, higher levels of outness have been associated with decreased sexual risk behaviors (59) and improved mental health (60).

The Safety and Social Stress section includes several gender-neutral screening questions about safety that will be familiar to the reader because they do not differ from the usual questions about safety that are recommended for use in any patient encounter. In addition, we suggest including a question, "Do you avoid people, places, or situations because you think something unpleasant might happen?" to address possible experiences of teasing, bullying, and harassment that are especially common in the lives of LGBTQ youth. When assessing safety, it is also important for providers to be aware that intimate partner abuse occurs in same-sex relationships. There is a tendency to consider conflict between same-sex partners less worrisome because of the belief that being of the same gender puts both partners on equal footing. Probing for safety is especially important in these situations, as is asking questions to ascertain the presence of a power differential (see Chapter 11 for specific approaches) that might imply that one person is being abused by the other. If unsure, and certainly when overt evidence of abuse is disclosed, patients should be referred for appropriate evaluation and support.

Sexual History

The sexual history is a critical element of a comprehensive health assessment. Information gathered during this part of the encounter will help identify problem areas that merit further evaluation or treatment. Many biopsychosocial problems can interfere with sexual satisfaction, including body image issues, a history of physical or sexual abuse, relationship problems, substance use, mental health conditions, overall poor physical health, and a high level of stress due to any cause. Taking a thorough sexual history communicates to the patient that you consider their sexuality and sexual function to be important and integral aspects of their health, and provides an invitation to discuss any sexual concerns and questions they may have at any time.

In general, creating a safe environment for taking a sexual history is similar for LGBTQ and heterosexual patients. With all patients, it is important to be open minded, nonjudgmental, patient, tactful, and respectful and to assure that privacy and confidentiality will be maintained. These principles are even more critical with LGBTQ patients, who may react to sexual history questions with greater anxiety and guardedness than their heterosexual counterparts. Many LGBTQ patients have had experiences with providers who were judgmental, made incorrect assumptions, or displayed discomfort discussing same-sex sexual practices. Some patients may expect to encounter such attitudes, even if this has never personally happened to them before. Some LGBTQ people internalize same-sex stigma and feel shame about their sexuality. Therefore, even providers who are experienced and feel at ease will occasionally encounter LGBTQ patients who are reluctant to discuss their sexual histories.

It is important to first build rapport and trust before beginning the sexual history. The manner in which sexual history questions are introduced, how they are framed and received, the provider's response to any discomfort expressed by the patient, and the body language exchanged throughout the interaction will together influence the success or challenges during this part of the encounter. It can be helpful to begin the discussion with an explanation such as: "Now I am going to take a few minutes to ask you some direct questions about your sex life. These questions are very personal, but it is important for me to know so I can help you be and stay healthy. I ask these questions to all of my patients regardless of age, gender or sexual orientation and they are just as important as other questions about your physical and mental health."

This kind of statement assures the patient that the questions are motivated by interest in understanding the patient's individual health care needs, rather than curiosity, voyeurism, or judgment. You can then go on to ask directed questions using phrasing that communicates an openness to hearing about all kinds of sexual practices between all genders and any number of partners.

Language on registration and medical history forms to gather information about relationship status sets the stage for sexual history-taking during the interview. For example, including options such as "single, married, widowed, or *partnered*" sends the message that you recognize all kinds of relationships. Open and inclusive language should continue to be used throughout the interview: A few starting questions to ask *all* patients include "Are you having sex?", followed by "Who are you having sex with?" Another way to ask is: "Are you sexually active with men, women, or both?", followed by "Does your sexual partner/Do any of your sexual partners consider themselves transgender?" These questions make no assumptions about heterosexuality or gender identity and open the door to further dialogue about sexual risk and other issues related to sexual health and identity. As the conversation continues, it is important to avoid gender stereotypes and discard assumptions about "masculine" and "feminine" roles in relationships and during sexual activity. Such assumptions and stereotypes can be stigmatizing and they may steer you away from engaging with your patient as a unique individual.

Several practices can help convey a nonjudgmental attitude and facilitate further dialogue. For example, attend to nonverbal cues such as body posture (e.g., use a relaxed stance) and room set up (e.g., don't sit behind your desk typing at the computer). Mirror patients' own language, using their terms to describe sexual practices, partners, and identities. Remember that not all patients who engage in sex with persons of their same sex or gender or with people of more than one sex or gender identify with sexual orientation labels such as gay, lesbian, or bisexual. If a patient acts offended or becomes anxious in response to a question or certain word, rather than avoiding the topic, explore the reaction, rephrase the question, or ask the patient what terminology would feel more comfortable. Remember that the patient may be flooded with anxiety-provoking thoughts, and the topic at hand may not necessarily be the cause of the observed reaction. Be prepared for your own uncomfortable feelings when hearing about sexual practices that are unfamiliar (e.g., fetishes, paraphernalia, or public sex) and try not to show your discomfort. It is okay to ask the patient to clarify any terms or behaviors with which you are unfamiliar, or to repeat a patient's term with your own understanding of its meaning to make sure you have no miscommunication. Table 8-5 includes some additional common pitfalls and best practices in taking a sexual history.

To assess sexual risk, a good place to begin is by determining the number and gender of a patient's sexual partners. Take care not to make assumptions about sexual behavior based on what you have learned about a person's sexual orientation. For example, do not assume that all gay men are at high

Table 8-5   Do's and Don'ts in Taking a Sexual History

Do begin with a statement explaining that you ask these questions of all your patients and that these questions are vital to your patient's overall health.

Do avoid language that presumes heterosexuality.

Do check yourself for judgmental facial expressions, body language, or tone of speech.

Don't make assumptions about past, current, and future sexual behavior.

Don't assume that a person who identifies as lesbian or gay has never had an opposite-sex partner.

Don't assume that an LGBT person does not have (or desire to have) children or has never been pregnant.

Do be prepared to answer questions about STI and HIV transmission risk for various sexual activities relevant to LGBTQ people.

Do note that MSM and transgender individuals who engage in high-risk sexual activities are at increased risk for contracting HIV and certain STIs. Screen and treat according to the CDC guidelines (www.cdc.gov/std/treatment/).

Do realize that although STIs are less common among lesbians, clinicians should still screen all women for STI risk, regardless of sexual orientation. The more sexual partners a woman has (female or male), the greater her risk. Bacterial vaginosis may be more common in women who have sex with women than in the general population.

Do consider the overall health of the patient who presents with sexual functioning concerns, including their psychological status, physical wellness, and relationship health.

CDC = Centers for Disease Control and Prevention; MSM = men who have sex with men; STI = sexually transmitted infection.

risk for STIs and HIV or that all lesbians do not have a history of sex with men. If the patient has one partner, ask about length of the relationship and potential sources of risk introduced by the sexual partner, such as history of STIs, other partners, and injection drug use. If the patient has multiple partners, explore for more specific risk factors, such as patterns of condom or other safer-sex barrier use and the risks introduced by other partners. To get at potential myths and misconceptions that your patients may have about sex and sexual risk, ask open-ended questions, such as "How do you protect yourself against STIs and HIV?" Table 8-6 includes some suggested questions for the clinical interview. Be sure to ask about specific types of sex practices. The answers will guide risk-reduction strategies and identify anatomic sites from which to collect specimens for STI testing.

When assessing the sexual history of transgender people, it is important to remember that gender identity is distinct from sexual orientation. In addition, it is important to understand that a person's transgender identity does not dictate their sexual orientation and that their sexual orientation may also change over time. For example, a married transgender woman who previously lived as a heterosexual man may now identify as a lesbian; her wife who previously lived as a heterosexual woman may also identify as a lesbian. Please refer to Chapter 17 for additional information on this topic. It is important to ask questions about the specific kinds of intimate contact a

Table 8-6   Suggested Sexual Health History Questions for the Face-to-Face Interview

Are you having sex?

Who are you having sex with? Anyone else? *or* Are you sexually active with men, women, or both? Does your sexual partner/Do any of your sexual partners consider themselves transgender?

What types of sex are you having? (Prompts: oral, vaginal, anal)

For each type of sex, are you using barriers or condoms? If yes, how often are you using them?

Do you have any questions about barriers?

What keeps you from using barriers?

transgender person engages in sexually, as this information will provide valuable information about what anatomic sites may require STI screening. For example, it is important not to assume that a transgender woman no longer has or uses a penis; however, at the same time it is important to keep in mind that some transgender patients may dissociate during discussion of genitals and sex acts that involve the use of parts of their body that are not gender concordant, and to be especially sensitive and respectful during these conversations, using the patient's preferred terminology to refer to anatomic parts.

Once you identify sexual risks, be prepared to discuss STI testing and risk reduction. For MSM and transgender individuals (or anyone else) who engage in high-risk sexual activities, an increasing number of strategies exist to reduce HIV risk. In addition to male and female condom use, discussion should include potential benefits of pre- and postexposure prophylaxis, frequent STI screening and prompt treatment, and avoiding use of disinhibiting substances during sex. For lesbian and bisexual women who have sex with men, and for transgender men who have vaginal sex with men, it is important to discuss contraception, including emergency contraception methods, because these individuals may be less knowledgeable and prepared than their heterosexual peers. Chapters 12, 13, and 14 provide more detail on assessing and addressing risk for STIs and HIV.

The sexual behavior of a bisexual person may not differ significantly from that of heterosexual or lesbian/gay people. Bisexual people may be monogamous for long periods of time and still identify as bisexual or they may be in multiple relationships with full knowledge and consent of their partners. Keep in mind that bisexuality is highly stigmatized, and bisexual patents may have been treated as confused, promiscuous, or even dangerous. They may be on guard against health care providers who assume that they are maladjusted or unstable simply because they have sexual relationships with people of more than one sex. Don't assume that bisexual patients are "experts" about contraception and/or safer sex methods: On the contrary, many may not have had access to comprehensive information that reflects their sexual practices and attitudes and may benefit from thorough discussions about sexual safety.

Several common factors can influence sexual satisfaction and fulfillment for LGBTQ people. For many, keeping and holding secrets about sexuality and gender is adaptive because it protects against experiencing
stigma, discrimination, and violence. However, secrets can easily drift to
the surface and create problems in a person's life. Nondisclosure of abuse
is often paired with self-blame, shame, confusion, and depression. Likewise, other personal secrets, such as infidelity (one's own, a partner's, or
both) or the nondisclosure of high-risk sexual activities (or simply the act
of having sex with an unknown or anonymous person) may also affect
patients' sex lives. Inquiring about childhood sexual abuse or any current
or past history of abuse or harassment is therefore an essential element of
the sexual history. If a patient reports such a history, it is important to
assess the effect of the abuse on their current relationships and functioning and to consider a referral for behavioral health services. Clinicians
must also be aware of local and state laws and regulations about mandatory reporting of abuse.

Cultural factors, including religious background, gender role expectations, and messages about sex and sexuality from both the familial context
and the broader culture can contribute significantly to the sexual satisfaction
and fulfillment of your patients. Further, sexual function, including the
extreme of absent libido, impotence, or anorgasmia on the one hand and
hyperarousal on the other can be greatly influenced by a patient's body image
as well as their perception of how others see their body. For example, many
MSM experience an intense social desirability to achieve a "perfect" body. For
transgender patients, hormonal treatment can have a significant impact on
sexual function, with testosterone fueling libido and responsiveness and
estrogen causing a decrease in both desire and overall sexual satisfaction.

Stress can also substantially affect sexual expression and sexual health.
Increased stressors can diminish the desire for physical intimacy and interfere with sexual responsiveness and sexual pleasure. As stress increases, so
can fatigue, and when tired, many people tend to prioritize sleep over sex.
For all of these reasons, it is important for providers to explore the effect of
stress on LGBTQ patients' sexuality and, conversely, ascertain and address
when it appears that their sexual activities or a lack of sexual engagement
are causing additional distress.

The Physical Examination

Physical examinations are intrinsically intrusive, and examination of the
private parts of the body—e.g., breasts, genitals, and anus—can be particularly threatening. Examination of these parts can be especially challenging
for people who experience shame about their bodies because of general
body image issues (e.g., people with obesity) or dysphoria specific to the
existence of organs that are discordant with gender identity. Intrusive exams

are also very difficult for people who have experienced mistreatment from medical providers in the past (61). Such mistreatment can take many forms, including showing disrespect for a patient's body by being voyeuristic or expressing contempt, failing to obtain a patient's permission before touching or instrumenting their body, failing to heed a patient's request to halt or stop an exam or procedure, or causing a patient pain while performing an exam or procedure. In addition, intrusive exams can reawaken posttraumatic stress reactions in any patient who has experienced emotional or physical trauma of any kind outside the medical arena.

Because mistreatment in medical settings is so commonplace among LGBTQ patients, it is not surprising that adherence to health screenings that involve intrusive exams or procedures (e.g., cervical Pap tests, mammography, colonoscopy) is not optimal in these populations. Because it is human to want to avoid situations that feel uncomfortable or awkward, providers may find themselves colluding with reticent or apprehensive patients in avoiding needed parts of the physical exam. It is important to resist this temptation because the risk for certain diseases for which screening is available is at least as high (e.g., cervical cancer in sexual minority women [31]) and potentially higher (e.g., breast cancer in lesbians [27]) compared with heterosexual populations. A cautious and gently persuasive approach over time can often be supremely successful.

It is, however, important to avoid doing unnecessary exams, particularly when such exams will violate trust and make patients feel that they are on display. Curiosity about the appearance of a postoperative transgender person's genitalia, while normal, is not a bona fide reason to perform a genital exam if the exam is not relevant to the evaluation of a patient's presenting symptoms. The decision to perform a particular exam or procedure should be based on presenting symptoms, behavioral risk factors, and (with respect to screening for asymptomatic disease) the presence of reproductive or other organs that require screening.

The first step is to establish trust; only then can one begin to gradually work with a reluctant patient toward eventually doing the exam at a pace that feels comfortable and right to the patient and with as much support and respect for the patient's autonomy and control as possible. Table 8-7 outlines steps providers can take to ease this process with LGBTQ patients (and indeed all patients) who express reticence or apprehension about any aspect of the physical exam.

For patients with clear PTSD, it is appropriate to offer referral to LGBTQ-sensitive behavioral health counseling, which can help normalize their experience (e.g., reassure them that they are not "crazy"), offer a safe and nonjudgmental place to reflect on and understand their traumatic experience, and increase coping skills to deal with traumatic symptoms. It is important for providers to understand that certain aspects of otherwise intrusive exams may be welcomed by LGBTQ patients under certain circumstances. For example, breast examination and mammography may be

Table 8–7   Recommendations on How to Approach Performance of Intrusive Parts of the Physical Examination in LGBTQ Patients Who Express Reticence or Apprehension

Before the Exam

Ask about and validate the patients' experiences with the exam in question and normalize any anxiety they express. It makes complete sense that they might wish to avoid undergoing an exam that has caused them physical and emotional distress in the past.

Educate patients about the reasons you believe it is important to perform the exam and exactly what the exam will entail if they choose to proceed.

Ask patients what language they prefer for you to use to refer to parts of the anatomy, and adhere to their preferences during the encounter (e.g., some patients may prefer gender-neutral terms such as "pelvic opening" to an anatomically correct term such as "vagina").

If feasible, explore means other than doing an exam to obtain the information (e.g., sending a self-collected vaginal swab or urine sample for gonorrhea and chlamydia testing, rather than collecting swab specimens during a pelvic exam).

Ask patients what they think might make them feel more comfortable. It is often useful to provide a menu of possible options from which they may choose, for example:
Having a provider other than you—e.g., of a different gender—perform the exam
Asking if they want to bring their own support person to the appointment when the exam will be performed
(For a pelvic exam): Maximizing comfort by using a very small speculum and topical lidocaine as the lubricant
(For a pelvic exam): Allowing patients to self-insert the speculum (or have their partner insert the speculum) in private before you enter the room
(For a pelvic exam): Offering positioning alternatives other than traditional footrests and the dorsal lithotomy position. Be sure to avoid potentially offensive terms (e.g., *stirrups*) and to avoid language that has sexual or violent connotations (e.g., "you will feel a prick right now" or "blades" of the speculum)
Offering draping alternatives. Some patients may wish to use an extra drape to assure modesty, while others may prefer to dispense with the drape completely and position themselves such that they can see everything that is going on.

If a medical assistant/chaperone is required to be present during the exam, be sure to explain why so patients do not view this person as a voyeur, and ask if patients have a preference regarding the chaperone's gender.

Assure patients that they will be able to stop the exam at any time and that as soon as they ask, you will stop immediately.

On the Day of the Exam

Explicitly obtain permission to proceed with the exam, even if the patient already gave consent at the last appointment.

Reiterate that the patient has ultimate control and can ask to stop the exam at any time.

Negotiate what will happen if the patient experiences physical or emotional distress during the exam. It may be acceptable to some patients to halt the exam and to try readjusting the technique (e.g., in the event of physical discomfort occurring during a speculum exam) or to try grounding techniques (e.g., if the patient manifests a post-traumatic distress reaction), before abandoning the exam altogether.

Clarify the role of everyone in the room. If the patient brought a support person, decide together where that person will sit/stand, and what that person's job will be during the exam.

(continued)

Table 8–7   Recommendations on How to Approach Performance of Intrusive Parts of the Physical Examination in LGBTQ Patients Who Express Reticence or Apprehension (*Continued*)

Position the chaperone in a way that does not give a bird's eye view of the patient's genitalia—this will reduce the likelihood of the patient perceiving the chaperone as a voyeur.

Ask the patient to assume the position for the exam on which you have previously agreed, providing adequate drapes as appropriate. Make sure you will be able to maintain eye contact with the patient throughout the exam.

Warn the patient before performing all exam maneuvers so there are no surprises (e.g., "First you'll feel the glove on your left thigh" . . . "Now you may feel some pressure as I insert the speculum . . . ")

Speak in a calm voice—if you talk too fast, it will make the patient feel more anxious.

When examining transgender individuals, if the need to use a pronoun comes up (e.g., while referring to the patient while addressing the patient's support person or the chaperone), be sure to use the pronoun appropriate to the patient's expressed gender identity and not to the genitalia you are examining. When possible, avoid use of language (e.g., *labia, vagina, penis*) that draws unnecessary attention to unwanted body parts.

Check in frequently during the exam to see how the patient is doing.

Adhere exactly to what was negotiated prior to starting the exam.

After the Exam

Help patients sit up, permit time to dress in private and generally to reconstitute themselves, then return to finalize the encounter.

If the examination was successful, congratulate the patient on achieving a successful exam, and make plans for follow-up.

If the exam is aborted because the patient develops distress, it is crucial to validate the importance of having stopped to avoid having a retraumatizing experience, since many patients will view lack of completion of the exam as a failure. Ask about support systems, what the patient has done in the past to cope in situations like this, and how the patient might use those skills to cope now. Make sure patients have a plan for what they will do to take care of themselves immediately after leaving the office. Be sure to also schedule routine follow-up with you.

affirming experiences for a transgender woman who is proud of the chest she has attained via use of estrogen and breast implants.

The experience of partnering with a patient in successfully performing a previously dreaded exam helps create a deep sense of trust in which the patient may truly feel safe and respected for the first time. Providers can thereby provide an invaluable corrective and healing experience.

Responding to Patients Productively and Maintaining an Enduring Connection Over Time

We recognize that providers seldom have the time necessary to take a complete medical history in one sitting that contains all of the elements mentioned above. As long as the provider is careful to extend a true welcome and sense of acceptance to all patients, including LGBTQ patients specifically, the initial meeting lays the foundation for trust, and additional information can be gathered gradually at subsequent encounters.

Some providers may be reluctant to ask certain questions during the history because those questions touch on culturally taboo topics that may arouse embarrassment/shame on the one hand and fascination/titillation on the other (sexual topics are a prime example). Other providers may find themselves loathe to delve into certain topics (e.g., unhealthy eating or problem drinking) that strike uncomfortably close to home—that is, they touch on personal "hot button" areas of unresolved conflict that providers themselves are grappling with internally. Chapter 15 explores techniques providers can use to recognize when this is going on, particularly around issues that come up commonly when interacting with LGBTQ patients, and provides resources to support ongoing personal growth of the provider, while making room to continue to offer appropriate care to the patient.

It is common for providers, especially trainees, to feel hesitant to ask certain questions because they are unsure how to respond productively (e.g., merely asking the question feels like opening Pandora's box). At times a patient's needs seem overwhelming; for example, when a patient presents who is homeless, is involved in a battering relationship but not yet ready to leave, or is actively abusing substances. In such situations it is okay not to be an expert and to ask for consultation and assistance from professionals who have more experience with LGBTQ populations or to ask your patients themselves. It is important for us to remember that it is not our responsibility as providers (and not possible) to provide an immediate solution, even when a patient expresses the hope that we will.

In our view, the provider's major role is to engage the patient in care and to form a partnership in which both parties work together to optimize the patient's health gradually over a series of successive visits. In concluding the initial encounter with any patient, it is therefore important to review what has just been discussed, which provides an additional opportunity to validate the patients' experiences and concerns—to let them know they have been heard—and to decide together what the next steps will be. This lets patients know they are not alone, which is of particular importance for many LGBTQ patients, and sets the stage for maintenance of an enduring connection—for some, a lifeline—over time.

Summary Points

- Many LGBTQ people face considerable financial, structural, and cultural barriers to accessing health care, including past negative experiences with health care providers. It is therefore critical for providers to build trusting relationships with their LGBTQ patients.

- The medical history (including face-to-face interviews and intake forms) is a key opportunity to establish a foundation for a trusting patient–provider relationship. However, most medical history frameworks assume heterosexual, non-transgender identities and miss opportunities for obtaining accurate and relevant information from LGBTQ individuals.

- An LGBTQ-inclusive and sensitive medical history includes questions about sexual orientation and gender identity; uses language that includes all identities, relationships, and behaviors; and clearly explains confidentiality policies in your practice.

- Eliciting information about sexual orientation, gender identity, and sexual practices is important not only to show awareness and acceptance but also to avoid misdiagnosis and improper care and treatment.

- Strategies to help facilitate effective communication during the face-to-face interview include: demonstrating empathy and open-mindedness without judgment or assumptions; mirroring the patient's language about identity and partners as much as feels comfortable; asking questions when a term the patient uses is unknown or unclear; using the patient's preferred name, pronoun, and terms to refer to anatomic structures; and apologizing promptly when a mistake is made.

- It is vital for providers to be aware of health disparities among LGBTQ people so they can assess patients thoroughly with sensitive questioning and probing, and encourage them to receive all recommended preventive screenings.

- LGBTQ-specific concerns to be addressed when performing the medical history include mental health (depression, anxiety, and suicidal ideation), substance use, preventive screenings, weight/nutrition/ body image, sexual health and risk, safety and history of trauma, family and peer support/rejection, stress related to stigma and shame, and sources of social support.

- Patients on the transgender spectrum should receive screenings and treatment based on their current anatomy and hormone status; however, some exams/procedures can be a difficult experience for a transgender patient whose gender is not concordant with anatomical structures. Exams should be done with particular sensitivity and only after a foundation of trust is formed.

- At times a patient's needs seem overwhelming. In such situations it is okay not to be an expert and to ask for consultation and assistance from professionals who have more experience with LGBTQ populations or to ask your patients themselves.

References

1. **Buchmueller T, Carpenter CS**. Disparities in health insurance coverage, access, and outcomes for individuals in same-sex versus different-sex relationships, 2000-2007. Am J Public Health. 2010;100:489-95.

2. **Khan L**. Transgender health at the crossroads: legal norms, insurance markets, and the threat of healthcare reform. Yale J Health Policy Law Ethics. 2011;11:375-418.

3. **Grant J, Mottet L, Tanis J, et al**. Injustice at Every Turn: A Report of the National Transgender Discrimination Survey. Washington, DC: National Center for Transgender Equality and National Gay and Lesbian Task Force; 2011.

4. **Obedin-Maliver J, Goldsmith ES, et al**. Lesbian, gay, bisexual, and transgender-related content in undergraduate medical education. JAMA. 2011;306:971-7.

5. **Joint Commission**. Advancing Effective Communication, Cultural Competence, and Patient- and Family-Centered Care for the Lesbian, Gay, Bisexual, and Transgender Community. Oak Brook, IL: The Joint Commission; 2011.

6. **Bickley LS, Szilagyi PG, Bates B**. Bates' Guide to Physical Examination and History Taking. Philadelphia: Wolters Kluwer Health/Lippincott Williams & Wilkins; 2009.

7. **Fortin AH, Smith RC, Dwamena FC, Frankel RM**. Smith's Patient Centered Interviewing: An Evidence-Based Method . 3rd ed. New York: McGraw-Hill Education; 2012.

8. **Fenway Health**. Patient privacy policy. 2009. Available at: www.fenwayhealth.org/site/PageServer?pagename=FCHC_abt_about_patientprivacy.

9. **National LGBT Health Education Center**. Affirmative care for transgender and gender non-conforming people: best practices for front-line health care staff. Boston: Fenway Health; 2013. Available at: www.lgbthealtheducation.org/wp-content/uploads/13-017_TransBestPracticesforFrontlineStaff_v9_04-30-13.pdf.

10. **Institute of Medicine**. The Health of Lesbian, Gay, Bisexual, and Transgender People: Building a Foundation for Better Understanding. Washington, D.C.: The National Academies Press; 2011.

11. **Alper J, Feit M, Sanders J**. Sexual Orientation and Gender Identity Data Collection in Electronic Health Records: A Workshop. Washington, DC: National Academies Press; 2013.

12. **Bradford J, Cahill S, Grasso C, Makadon H**. How to gather data on sexual orientation and gender identity in clinical settings. Boston: Fenway Health; 2012.

13. **Sausa LA, Sevelius J, Keatley J, Iñiguez JR, Reyes M**. Policy Recommendations for Inclusive Data Collection of Trans People in HIV Prevention, Care & Services. San Francisco: UCSF Center of Excellence for Transgender HIV Prevention; 2009.

14. **Miller K, Ryan J**. Design, Development and Testing of the NHIS Sexual Identity Question. National Center for Health Statistics; 2011 October.

15. **Garofalo R, Wolf RC, Wissow LS, Woods ER, Goodman E**. Sexual orientation and risk of suicide attempts among a representative sample of youth. Arch Pediatr Adolesc Med. 1999; 153:487-93.

16. **Coker TR, Austin SB, Schuster MA**. Health and healthcare for lesbian, gay, bisexual, and transgender youth: reducing disparities through research, education, and practice. J Adolesc Health. 2009;45:213-5.

17. **Haas AP, Eliason M, Mays VM, et al**. Suicide and suicide risk in lesbian, gay, bisexual, and transgender populations: review and recommendations. J Homosex. 2011;58:10-51.

18. **King M, Semlyen J, Tai SS, et al**. A systematic review of mental disorder, suicide, and deliberate self harm in lesbian, gay and bisexual people. BMC Psychiatry. 2008;8:70.

19. **Cochran SD, Mays VM**. Burden of psychiatric morbidity among lesbian, gay, and bisexual individuals in the California Quality of Life Survey. J Abnorm Psychol. 2009;118:647-58.

20. **Lee JG, Griffin GK, Melvin CL**. Tobacco use among sexual minorities in the USA, 1987 to May 2007: a systematic review. Tob Control. 2009;18:275-82.

21. **Hughes TL.** Alcohol use and alcohol-related problems among lesbians and gay men. Ann Rev Nurs Res. 2005;23:283-325.
22. **Cahill S, South K, Spade J.** Outing Age: Public Policy Issues Affecting Gay, Lesbian and Transgender Elders. Washington, DC: National Gay and Lesbian Task Force; 2009.
23. **Boehmer U, Bowen DJ, Bauer GR.** Overweight and obesity in sexual-minority women: evidence from population-based data. Am J Public Health. 2007;97:1134-40.
24. **Gruskin EP, Greenwood GL, Matevia M, Pollack LM, Bye LL.** Disparities in smoking between the lesbian, gay, and bisexual population and the general population in California. Am J Public Health. 2007;97:1496-502.
25. **Conron KJ, Mimiaga MJ, Landers SJ.** A population-based study of sexual orientation identity and gender differences in adult health. Am J Public Health. 2010;100:1953-60.
26. **Lewis RJ, Kholodkov T, Derlega VJ.** Still stressful after all these years: a review of lesbians' and bisexual women's minority stress. J Lesbian Stud. 2012;16:30-44.
27. **Case P, Austin SB, Hunter DJ, et al.** Sexual orientation, health risk factors, and physical functioning in the Nurses' Health Study II. J Womens Health (Larchmt). 2004;13:1033-47.
28. **Bradford J, Van Wagenen A.** Research on the Health of Sexual Minority Women. In: Goldman M, Troisi R, Rexrode K, eds. Women and Health. London: Elsevier; 2012:77-91.
29. **Zaritsky E, Dibble SL.** Risk factors for reproductive and breast cancers among older lesbians. J Womens Health (Larchmt). 2010;19:125-31.
30. **Clark MA, Rogers ML, Armstrong GF, et al.** Comprehensive cancer screening among unmarried women aged 40-75 years: results from the cancer screening project for women. J Womens Health (Larchmt). 2009;18:451-9.
31. **Peitzmeier S.** Promoting Cervical Cancer Screening Among Lesbians and Bisexual Women. Boston: Fenway Health; 2013. Available at: www.fenwayhealth.org/site/DocServer/PolicyFocus_cervicalcancer_web.pdf?docID=10661.
32. **Price JH, Easton AN, Telljohann SK, Wallace PB.** Perceptions of cervical cancer and Pap smear screening behavior by women's sexual orientation. J Comm Health. 1996;21:89-105.
33. **Wolitski RJ, Fenton KA.** Sexual health, HIV, and sexually transmitted infections among gay, bisexual, and other men who have sex with men in the United States. AIDS Behav. 2011;15 Suppl 1:S9-17.
34. **Sullivan PS, Wolitski RJ.** HIV infection among gay and bisexual men. In: Unequal Opportunity: Health Disparities Affecting Gay and Bisexual Men in the United States. Oxford: Oxford University Press; 2008:220-50.
35. **Dietz CA, Nyberg CR.** Genital, oral, and anal human papillomavirus infection in men who have sex with men. J Am Osteopath Assoc. 2011;111(3 Suppl 2):S19-25.
36. **Czoski-Murray C1, Karnon J, Jones R, Smith K, Kinghorn G.** Cost-effectiveness of screening high-risk HIV-positive men who have sex with men (MSM) and HIV-positive women for anal cancer. Health Technol Assess. 2010;14:iii-iv, ix-x, 1-101.
37. **Goldie SJ, Kuntz KM, Weinstein MC, Freedberg KA, Palefsky JM.** Cost-effectiveness of screening for anal squamous intraepithelial lesions and anal cancer in human immunodeficiency virus-negative homosexual and bisexual men. Am J Med. 2000;108:634-41.
38. **Goldie SJ, Kuntz KM, Weinstein MC, et al.** The clinical effectiveness and cost-effectiveness of screening for anal squamous intraepithelial lesions in homosexual and bisexual HIV-positive men. JAMA. 1999;281:1822-29.
39. **Center of Excellence for Transgender Health.** Primary Care Protocol for Transgender Patient Care. San Francisco: UCSF Center of Excellence for Transgender Health; 2011. Available at: http://transhealth.ucsf.edu/trans?page=protocol-00-00.
40. **Grossman AH, D'Augelli AR.** Transgender youth: invisible and vulnerable. J Homosex. 2006; 51:111-28.
41. **French SA, Story M, Remafedi G, Resnick MD, Blum RW.** Sexual orientation and prevalence of body dissatisfaction and eating disordered behaviors: a population-based study of adolescents. Int J Eating Disorders. 1996;19:119-26.

42. **Siever MD.** Sexual orientation and gender as factors in socioculturally acquired vulnerability to body dissatisfaction and eating disorders. J Consulting Clin Psych. 1994;62:252-60.

43. **Gay and Lesbian Medical Association.** Healthy People 2010 Companion Document for Lesbian, Gay, Bisexual, and Transgender (LGBT) Health. San Francisco, CA: Gay and Lesbian Medical Association; 2001.

44. **World Health Organization.** WHO guidelines on nutrition. Available at: www.who.int/publications/guidelines/nutrition/en/.

45. **Centers for Disease Control and Prevention.** Physical activity guidelines. Available at: www.cdc.gov/physicalactivity/everyone/guidelines/index.html?s_cid=govD_dnpao_004.

46. **Ryan C, Russell ST, Huebner D, Diaz R, Sanchez J.** Family acceptance in adolescence and the health of LGBT young adults. J Child Adolesc Psychiatr Nurs. 2010;23:205-13.

47. **Goodenow C, Szalacha L, Westheimer K.** School support groups, other school factors, and the safety of sexual minority adolescents. Psychol Schools. 2006;43:573-89.

48. **Weston K.** Families We Choose: Lesbians, Gays, Kinship. New York: Columbia University Press; 1991.

49. **Weeks J, Heaphy B, Donovan C.** Same Sex Intimacies: Families of Choice and Other Life Experiments. New York: Columbia University Press; 2001.

50. **Metlife Mature Market Institute.** Out and Aging: The MetLife Study of Lesbian and Gay Baby Boomers. J GLBT Fam Studies. 2010;6:40-57.

51. **Johnson MJ, Jackson NC, Arnette JK, Koffman SD.** Gay and lesbian perceptions of discrimination in retirement care facilities. J Homosex. 2005;49:83-102.

52. **Meyer IH.** Prejudice, social stress, and mental health in lesbian, gay, and bisexual populations: conceptual issues and research evidence. Psych Bull. 2003;129:674-97.

53. **Bolton SL, Sareen J.** Sexual orientation and its relation to mental disorders and suicide attempts: findings from a nationally representative sample. Can J Psychiatry. 2011;56:35-43.

54. **Kroenke K, Spitzer RL.** The PHQ-9: a new depression diagnostic and severity measure. Psychiatr Ann. 2002;32:509-15.

55. **Prins A, Ouimette P, Kimerling R, et al.** The primary care PTSD screen (PC-PTSD): development and operating characteristics. Int J Psychiatry Clin Pract. 2004;9:9-14.

56. **Cochran SD.** Emerging issues in research on lesbians' and gay men's mental health: does sexual orientation really matter. Am Psychologist. 2001;56:931-47.

57. **Meyer IH.** Prejudice and discrimination as social stressors. In: Meyer IH, Northridge ME, eds. The Health of Sexual Minorities: Public Health Perspectives on Lesbian, Gay, Bisexual and Transgender Populations. New York: Springer; 2007:242-67.

58. **Hendricks ML, Testa RJ.** A conceptual framework for clinical work with transgender and gender nonconforming clients: an adaptation of the Minority Stress Model. Prof Psychol Res Pract. 2012;43:460-7.

59. **White D, Stephenson R.** Identity formation, outness, and sexual risk among gay and bisexual men. Am J Mens Health. 2014;8:98-109.

60. **Feldman SE.** The Impact of Outness and Lesbian, Gay, and Bisexual Identity Formation on Mental Health [dissertation]. New York: Columbia University; 2012.

61. **Bates CK, Carroll N, Potter J.** The challenging pelvic examination. J Gen Intern Med. 2011; 26:651-7.

Chapter 9

Mental Health Care for LGBT People

KEVIN KAPILA, MD

Introduction

This chapter explores the mental and behavioral health challenges of lesbian, gay, bisexual, and transgender (LGBT) people. These challenges include how stigma and discrimination attached to LGBT identity can have serious mental health consequences and how negative life experiences, such as familial and peer rejection, homophobic violence, and other stressors, can affect the presentation of common psychiatric conditions. The chapter is written to be of relevance to both primary care providers and mental health professionals (the term *clinicians* is used here to refer to both medical and mental health providers) and discusses the elements of a comprehensive mental health evaluation, using a case study approach to illustrate key points. Throughout, clinicians should keep in mind that the key to providing effective treatment of LGBT people is to be informed, affirming, and supportive. By learning about the unique mental health needs of LGBT people, and by looking honestly at how internalized beliefs and culturally based biases may affect delivery of care, clinicians can optimize the care they provide to their LGBT patients.

History of Homosexuality and Gender Nonconformity in Psychiatry

The field of psychiatry has a long history of conceptualizing homosexuality and gender nonconformity as abnormalities. To this day, many LGBT people hold a residual distrust of psychiatry, hampering the community's ability to trust and seek care from mental health professionals. Clinicians who understand this history, however, will be better able to validate their clients' concerns, educate them about changes in the field, and, if indicated, refer them to LGBT-sensitive mental health resources.

Before the 20th century, the general understanding of sexual orientation was primarily based in religious beliefs which held that homosexuality should be viewed as a sin and a temptation to be avoided. Starting in the early 20th century, the professional view of sexual orientation began to change as it became grounded in the newly developed field of psychiatry. Early psychiatric theory, however, conceived same-sex attraction as a pathologic response to early life events. This may now seem antiquated, but for the times, it was a positive shift to view homosexuality as pathologic rather than immoral because this change validated homosexuality as a human behavior rather than as a sin based on a failed choice.

Toward the middle of the century, a debate began about whether homosexual behavior should be considered pathologic. Freud believed that all humans were essentially bisexual and that they developed as heterosexual or homosexual based on parental and environmental factors. In his 1935 "Letter to an American Mother," he wrote that homosexuality is a "variation of sexual function" and not pathologic (1). Charles Socarides, among some other analysts, disputed this and saw homosexuality as a pathology that could possibly be repaired (2). In his 1962 work, *Homosexuality: A Psychoanalytic Study* (3), Irving Bieber promoted the theory that homosexuality in men was due to a detached father and domineering mother.

Subsequently, nonpsychoanalytic behavioral health researchers challenged some of the core beliefs of psychoanalysis with more structured research. Evelyn Hooker, a psychologist in the 1950s, challenged the idea that homosexuality was always associated with psychopathology. She compared psychological test results of gay and heterosexual men and showed that analysts could not discern differences between the 2 groups. Where prior studies had recruited participants who sought treatment—indicating they were experiencing some type of psychological distress—Hooker recruited participants functioning normally in society (4).

Alfred Kinsey, who was a trained as a zoologist and tried to avoid culturally laden interpretations of human behavior, gained wide attention for his work that showed much higher rates of same-sex behaviors in Americans than previously appreciated (5). While some of his methodologic approaches were criticized later, Kinsey's work demonstrated that homosexuality was not a rare behavior practiced by a small minority of the population; this supported the notion of homosexuality as a normal variation of sexual behavior.

In the 1960s, LGBT people continued to be viewed as abnormal, and even as a threat to society. The year 1969 became a turning point, however, when patrons at the Stonewall bar in Greenwich Village, New York City, rioted in protest against a police raid (raids of gay bars were a common occurrence). Over the next weeks and months the gay community began mobilizing for their rights. As part of this growing movement, gay activists clashed with the American Psychiatric Association (APA) over the inclusion of homosexuality as a psychiatric diagnosis in the *Diagnostic and Statistical Manual of Mental Disorders (DSM)*. There was also opposition within the psychiatric community to the pathologic classification of homosexuality. In 1973, the APA responded by replacing homosexuality in the *DSM* with the designation of "sexual orientation disturbance" that set forth that not all homosexuals were mentally ill—only those who were in conflict with their sexual orientation.

Three decades passed before the APA made a complete shift in accepting same-sex attraction by putting out their position against the practice of conversion therapy. Conversion therapy is a form of psychotherapy that attempts to change the sexual orientation of an LGB person to heterosexual. Although some still practice this type of therapy, it is widely dismissed as ineffective and potentially destructive to a person's mental health.

The representation of transgender people in the *DSM* has also been a source of controversy. Issues surrounding gender identity were first addressed in the *DSM-III* in 1980, which introduced the terms *transexualism* and *gender identity disorder of adolescence or adulthood nontranssexual type or gender identity disorder not otherwise specified* (6). The 1994 publication of the *DSM-IV* attempted to be more inclusive of the spectrum of gender identity by removing transexualism and using only *gender identity disorder* (7). During the development of the *DSM-5*, many community members and professionals advocated in favor of removing a diagnosis altogether, believing that it continued to pathologize the transgender community. Just as the removal of homosexuality from the *DSM* was seen as a critical step toward reducing stigma and advancing the civil rights of the LGB community, there was hope that transgender people would experience similar benefits. In the end, however, the *DSM-5* changed the diagnostic category to *gender dysphoria*, which focuses on the distress that may accompany incongruence between gender identity and assigned sex at birth (8). For more discussion of the *DSM* classification of gender dysphoria, see Chapters 16 and 17.

General Considerations in LGBT Mental Health

Many of the mental health concerns of LGBT people are similar to those of the general population. However, LGBT people may also present with issues that are specific to being a sexual or gender minority. There is no "one-size-fits-all" approach that should be taken. Nonetheless, it is important to keep some general considerations in mind when meeting with an LGBT client. The following section provides insights into issues that are specific to LGBT people that may affect the client–clinician relationship, as well as the approach to care. The effect of these issues will vary by individual, especially because some people may have grown up in a supportive environment where issues around their sexuality did not have as much of an impact, while others grew up in less supportive situations. In all cases, the clinical interaction should be led by the client, with the clinician assessing how sexual orientation or gender identity affects the individual.

Coming Out

Coming out is the process by which an LGBT person accepts and discloses his or her sexual orientation or gender identity. This process is often nonlinear and can be a life-long process. For example, a person who is out about their sexuality in one work situation may have to go through this process again if he or she changes jobs. Some may come out to a few friends and then deny or hide their sexuality—termed "going back into the closet." Others may come out before they are completely sure about their sexual orientation or gender identity, not realizing how their disclosure might affect their relationships with others. The decision is not invariably all or nothing but may be a process of evolution. For example, a man may come out as gay but realize over time that he is bisexual; others may marry opposite-sex partners, raise a family, and then recognize and/or act upon same-sex attraction. For a more detailed discussion of the coming out process, see Chapter 4.

A clinician can be an important mentor who helps the client navigate the coming out experience in a safe and emotionally healthy way. There should be an evaluation of the possible risks or negative consequences of coming out, such as the potential for discrimination, rejection by friends and family, and anti-LGBT violence. The clinician should assess whether the client has the coping skills and supports needed to deal with rejection and whether the client is living in a situation where he or she may be in danger of violence if sexual orientation or gender identity is disclosed. In some cases, it may be necessary to help identify community supports or assist the client in moving to a safer situation before coming out. If the clinician assesses that the person may lack some coping skills—and the stress of coming out may put his or her emotional safety at risk—there should be a period of therapy to help the person stabilize first. Slowing the client down in the coming out process can be very difficult, and it must be done with extreme sensitivity, helping the client focus on safety first.

The clinician should also help the client see the positive aspects of coming out. Namely, the person no longer has to hide a major part of his or her identity from family and friends. Self-acceptance can start the process of leading a more fulfilling and authentic life and of healing from shame-based thinking. A person who comes out is free to look inward, addressing his or her own internalized homophobia or transphobia that may arrest optimal development. This positive change can also allow someone to have more honest relationships with friends and family since they are now able to share all aspects of his or her life. People who come out can also more readily engage with community and social groups and develop support networks. Helping a client through this process can be a very rewarding experience for a clinician.

Families of Choice

In some instances, LGBT people face rejection by their families after they come out and may choose to end relationships with their biological families if they are not accepting. A family of choice develops when clients find others with shared experiences—people who accept them and take on the family role. These families can include friends, partners, ex-partners, and older friends with more established life experience who take on a mentoring or parenting role in their lives. Families of choice may be the primary supports for LGBT clients; they may celebrate the holidays and other life events together and serve as lifelong supports for each other. When obtaining a history from a client, keep in mind that the family structure for these clients may not include their biological families or may be a combination of biological family and family of choice. Clinicians should validate families of choice and should educate clients about legal issues around health care that often involve families, such as choosing a health care proxy and writing a living will.

Aging

Aging in the LGBT community can present unique challenges. The current generation of seniors has lived through high levels of discrimination, the birth of the gay rights movement, and the AIDS epidemic. These life experiences may make older LGBT people more distrustful of medical professionals and less likely to be open about their sexual or gender identity. LGBT older adults who are not open about their sexual orientation may have concerns about receiving home health care services when they are infirm and may avoid congregate living because of fear of disclosure. Older gay men may also no longer feel comfortable at gay community and social events, as some perceive the gay male culture as placing too much value on youth and physical beauty. Bisexual seniors have higher rates of depression, anxiety, and suicidal ideation than not only heterosexuals but also gay men and lesbians (9). It becomes the responsibility of the clinician, then, to ensure they are sensitive to, and educated about, the needs of their older LGBT clients. The clinician can acknowledge the mistakes of the past by simply asking a client how homophobia has affected them. This can help the client perceive the clinician as a safe person, allowing the client to be more apt to share major concerns. A clinician should also educate LGBT older adults about having a health care proxy and should know whom the clients have for support. Social support and social network size are protective factors and decrease the odds of poorer health outcomes (10). For more information and resources on caring for older LGBT adults, see Chapter 7.

Dual Stigma

While there has been some progress in general society to be more understanding and accepting of mental illness, it is still often a source of shame for many. Concerns about the stigma of having a mental illness often results in the avoidance of treatment (11). Similarly, the shame sometimes associated with being LGBT could lead some people to deny their true sexual or gender identity, especially if they are already dealing with the stigma of having a mental illness, as demonstrated in the following vignette:

Ron is a 25-year-old man diagnosed with bipolar disorder at age 21. He had a tumultuous time for the first 2 years after he received his diagnosis. Since then, he has been stable on medication for 3 years, with a job, his own apartment, and a group of friends in the small town where he lives. Ron recently presented to his primary care doctor with rectal pain and discharge and was diagnosed with rectal gonorrhea. He admitted to having unprotected receptive intercourse with men but denied being gay, stating that he was manic and did not know what he was doing. However, there were no other manic behaviors, and the client appeared neither manic nor depressed. He later stated to his primary care doctor, "I can't be bipolar and gay, that is too much for me to handle."

Having a psychiatric diagnosis while also being gay can create what is called *dual stigma*. Dual stigma can also apply to an LGBT person who is a racial/ethnic minority, a person with a disability, or who belongs to another stigmatized group. In all cases, clinicians should be aware of the ways LGBT clients may hold and negotiate multiple identities that influence their health (see Chapter 3 for more on this topic), and how they may feel marginalized by the LGBT community, which itself is not immune from prejudice based on race, ethnicity, gender, socioeconomic status, psychiatric condition, or having a disability. Clinicians who assume, for example, that an LGBT client of color will not face racism within the LGBT community will be unable to appreciate their clients' life experiences and may not provide them the appropriate mental health care. When clinicians are aware of and validate the existence of multiple stigmas that may affect their clients, they create an environment where the clients will be more comfortable and more likely to have their needs met.

Case Studies of LGBT Mental Health Challenges

The following section consists of cases that introduce mental health challenges sometimes found in different subgroups of LGBT people. Please note that these cases are not meant to represent all LGBT people. Rather, they are written to inform clinicians of realistic situations they may encounter in their practice, to highlight the specific mental health disparities found in research on LGBT populations, and to demonstrate the potential effects of stigma and discrimination on LGBT mental health.

Case: Robert, a Young Gay Man

Robert is a 23-year-old gay graduate student who presents to the clinic to establish health care. He grew up in a rural community where he was not open about his sexual orientation. He came out his first year in a college that was located in a metropolitan area with a large gay community. He initially had a lot of anxiety about interacting with other gay men and going to clubs. He would consume large amounts of alcohol to get up the courage to go out to a gay bar. Through the use of Ecstasy, he felt for the first time like he was "part of the tribe." Then his Ecstasy use spiked to almost every weekend, and the after-effects began causing problems in school. He presents to his university health clinic for HIV testing because he is very afraid of contracting HIV. Robert is also very concerned about his muscle mass and wonders if his testosterone is low.

Robert's case illustrates the difficulties many gay men encounter in their first years after coming out, particularly in the context of the HIV/AIDS epidemic. Over the past 30 years, gay men have had to deal with coming out and exploring their sexuality, along with the fear of contracting HIV. Early in the HIV/AIDS epidemic, when there was no effective treatment, exploring sexual intimacy could mean contracting a deadly disease. Improvements in treatment have lessened this fear, but the fear is still present for many, affecting their ability to experience sexual intimacy. Conversely, some gay men have developed a sense of denial around AIDS and may engage in high-risk sexual behaviors. Gay men who are HIV infected often have to deal with issues of rejection when they disclose their HIV status. This can affect their self-esteem, worsen depression, and increase isolation. To avoid these adverse consequences, some HIV-infected men may not disclose their HIV status to potential sexual partners, putting their partners at risk.

HIV is not the only sexually transmitted infection (STI) that gay men have to contend with. Herpes, chlamydia, gonorrhea, and syphilis are also prevalent (12,13). STIs carry their own stigma and may bring about feelings of shame. A person who has recently come out as gay may have internalized self-hatred and feel that the STI is a punishment for being sexually active. Providers must be sensitive to these feelings when obtaining a medical history, providing STI screenings, and giving sexual risk-reduction counseling.

Robert's case also illustrates the clinician's need to have a basic understanding of the popular use of "club drugs" and alcohol among gay and bisexual men at clubs and "circuit parties." The most common club drugs are Ecstasy, crystal methamphetamine, ketamine, and gamma-hydroxybutyrate. Like their heterosexual counterparts, some gay men go through a phase of experimentation with club drugs. For most men, the use is transient; only a subset of men will develop problems with these drugs, especially if they are part of the club scene. Robert's story is common among gay men who have just come out. They may experience anxiety around meeting other gay men and going to gay clubs. Drugs like Ecstasy provide a sense of euphoria and of feeling very connected to others. A clinician must be able to understand why someone would use these drugs (essentially the benefits for the client) instead of immediately saying why the client should not use it. The use of illicit drugs in the gay community is discussed in greater detail in Chapter 10.

The desire of gay men to attract new partners can also create pressures to conform to physical ideals that many cannot achieve. This may cause dissatisfaction with body shape and overall appearance. Images in fitness magazines and gay male pornography may exacerbate dissatisfaction with body image (14–17). Gay men diet more and have more fear of becoming overweight then heterosexual men (17). The dissatisfaction with body image puts gay men at risk for eating disorders, anabolic steroid use, and human growth hormone abuse. Abuse of anabolic steroids can adversely affect mental health (18). In severe cases, steroid use can cause uncontrolled rage or psychosis. A gay man who is overweight may feel like an outsider—not fitting in with the gay community because of his weight. He may also feel like an outsider to the heterosexual community as a result of his sexual orientation. When excessive behaviors are noted, the clinician should assess how a client feels about his body image and evaluate possible eating disorders.

The evaluation of gay men should therefore include screening questions about body image, substance use, and sexual behavior. The clinician should not only ask whether the client engages in safer sex but also have the client explain his understanding of safer sexual practices. When a clinician is asking about drug use, the questions should not just be about whether the client uses drugs but also about why and for what the client uses them. Do they alleviate anxiety? Help him fit in? Allow him to have sex without guilt or shame? The issues around body image may not be as simple as concerns about being too fat or too thin; they may also be about wanting more muscle mass. The clinician may want to ask the client what the goal or ideal body would be. Chapter 8 provides suggestions for ways to interview patients about these concerns.

Case: Karin, a Bisexual Woman

Karin presents to her primary care doctor with trouble sleeping. She was in a relationship with a man that recently ended and feels that she has no one she can talk to about this. Karin, who is currently 28, first came out as a lesbian when she was 20 years old. Most of her closest friends are lesbian identified. She feels comfortable with her current bisexual identity but has found that both the heterosexual and lesbian/gay communities are less comfortable with it. When she started to have a relationship with a man a year ago, she found she lost the support of many of her lesbian friends. Karin started mental health treatment with a therapist that advertised as being "LBGT friendly," but Karin felt that the therapist did not really understand the bisexual community.

Bisexuality is the capacity for emotional, romantic, and/or physical attraction to more than one gender. That capacity for attraction may or may not manifest itself in terms of sexual interaction (19). Karin's case shows that bisexuals often have to contend with not being accepted by either the heterosexual or the lesbian and gay communities. Bisexuality challenges the binary view that many have regarding sexual orientation: the view that people are either heterosexual or gay. A man and woman holding hands are seen as heterosexual. Two men holding hands are seen as gay. The thought that any of these individuals may be bisexual does not occur to many people. Bisexuals have been a part of the LGBT movement, but their needs often go unaddressed, with negative consequences to their health care and well-being (20).

The lack of understanding about the bisexual community is associated with many myths and negative beliefs. Some believe that bisexuality is a phase that one goes through on the way to becoming gay or lesbian. This myth is supported by the fact that some people do identify as bisexual before they come out as gay or lesbian, but in no way does this apply to all people who identify as bisexual. Negative stereotypes of bisexuals as promiscuous and more likely to be unfaithful to their partners are common. The idea that one would have to worry about their partner cheating with both men and women speaks more to issues of trust in a relationship than it does to bisexual identity. One of the most negative beliefs is that bisexual men have been a major source for spreading HIV from the gay male community to the heterosexual community. A study from San Francisco, California, showed that bisexual men were not the primary cause of HIV spreading from male to female partners (21).

The negative stereotypes and misinformation about bisexuality adversely affects their physical and mental health. Studies have shown that bisexuals have higher rates of mental health problems, including depression, anxiety, suicidal ideation, and eating disorders, compared with gays and lesbians (19,22-24). A 2010 study looking at health issues of lesbian and bisexual woman showed that women who identified as bisexual had lower levels of education, were living below the federal poverty level, and had higher rates of poor general health and frequent mental distress (25). Bisexuals were also found to have survived higher rates of physical and sexual abuse than lesbians or gay men (26). These studies show that bisexual men and woman have specific mental health needs different from those of gay men and lesbians. At the same time, few resources are put toward addressing bisexual health directly, and general LGBT interventions may not reach bisexual populations (20).

Clinicians assessing the mental health needs of bisexual clients should be aware of how their own feelings and beliefs about the bisexual community may be influenced by negative stereotypes. They should understand that, while the bisexual client shares some issues with the lesbian and gay community, she or he has unique mental health needs that should be assessed because life experiences are different. It should not be assumed that the community and clinical resources for gay and lesbian people are appropriate or available for the bisexual client.

Case: Linda, a Lesbian Woman

Linda is a 36-year-old woman who identifies as a lesbian. She presents to the clinic for follow-up of high blood pressure. She has not been able to follow the program of diet and exercise that was discussed at the last visit, and although overweight, before now she has never attempted to lose weight. She and her partner have 2 children, and both work full-time. Linda puts the needs of her children and partner above her own. This structure leaves little time for exercise and the preparation of healthy meals. She feels torn between the needs of her family and the demands of her job, and she has turned down opportunities for career advancement that would take her away from her family. Her partner is willing to help, but Linda feels since she earns a much smaller salary, she should make up for it by doing more at home. Although her parents live nearby and help out with the grandchildren on occasion, she feels her parents are less supportive than they are of her heterosexual sister's family. She feels like she is failing at home and work and feels overwhelmed. She reports that her mood has been low and that she sometimes feels anxious. Overall, Linda experiences life as a number of tasks she completes on autopilot and does not really enjoy anything.

Much of this case could easily be describing a heterosexually identified woman. While many issues are unique to the mental health of lesbians, many more overlap with all women's health issues. As committed lesbian couples start families, they have the same struggles all women (and many men) do in balancing work and home life. Nonetheless, some research indicates that LGBT people have mood disorders and use mental health services at higher rates than the general population (22,23,27–32). Some of these data are limited, however, by a lack of adequate control groups and by grouping of lesbians, gay men, and bisexuals into 1 research group (rather than looking at subgroups). One study, in fact, found that higher mental health utilization rates among lesbians compared with heterosexual women may have to do with having more trust in psychotherapy and placing greater value on personal growth and introspection (33) rather than on having higher morbidity.

A study comparing mental health issues between lesbians, bisexual women, and heterosexual women (23) found that psychiatric disorders were associated with stigmatization of sexual orientation. Lesbians who were not out were more likely to have suicidal ideation, have attempted suicide, and have experienced more mental stress (23). Studies have also found that lesbians who are more out about their sexual orientation tend to have fewer depressive symptoms (23,27). For Linda, it is possible that her depression is triggered by current work-life stressors that may or may not be rooted in experiences of discrimination and stigma based on her sexual orientation (such as her parents' favoring time with her heterosexual sister's family).

Linda also is struggling with her weight. Obesity carries implications for both physical and mental health. Being overweight can negatively affect one's self-image, which is compounded by how society views obesity. Studies have shown that lesbians have higher rates of obesity than heterosexual women (34,35). This would be another stigmatizing issue that can affect the overall mental health of a lesbian woman. In addition, Linda, like all women, could be at risk for domestic abuse. The National Violence Against Women Survey showed that 11% of women in same-sex relationships have experienced violence (36). Clinicians should not assume that women in same-sex relationships do not suffer from partner abuse and should screen accordingly.

In summary, clinicians should understand that many of the issues that affect the mental health of lesbians are issues that all women face but are potentially exacerbated by societal stigmatization. Lesbian clients, like all clients, should be routinely screened for depression and anxiety. If a lesbian client is struggling with obesity, clinicians should be sensitive that this is another layer of stigma faced by the client. The studies showing increased utilization of mental health services indicate that lesbians are open to psychotherapy to deal with stressors in their lives, and that supportive clinicians can play a vital role in facilitating successful adaptation.

Case: Rex, a Transgender Man

Rex is a 42-year-old married transgender man who is the father of 2 children, stable on testosterone, with no active medical issues. He has lived full-time as a man for 2 years, with the full support of his family. He presents to the clinic with an upset stomach. During the history, Rex explains that because of cut backs in the school district, he has to move from the small elementary school where he has taught for 15 years to a much larger high school. He feels lucky to get another job but is very worried about the move. When he transitioned, the younger children were very accepting of the change, and while some staff made insensitive comments, he felt the personal relationships he had with them helped them be more accepting. Several teachers he will be working with at the high school knew him when he had lived as a woman, and he is worried that these colleagues will out him by gossiping to others or by referring to him as "she." He has also heard from some friends who work at the high school that some students are already talking about him. He feels that on top of being a working father of 2 small children, he does not have the energy to go through the challenges he knows are ahead of him.

Rex's situation shows how the mental health support needs of a transgender person may have nothing to do with gender dysphoria or transitioning but can be related to the stigma and everyday stressors attached to being transgender in our society. It is understandable that Rex is concerned about the possibility of gossip, not to mention verbal or physical harassment, in his new position at the high school. In the National Transgender Discrimination survey, *Injustice at Every Turn*, 90% of the 6450 transgender respondents reported having been harassed, mistreated, or discriminated against on the job or had taken steps to hide their identity in order to avoid these outcomes (37). It is also reasonable that Rex is worried about having to come out to new colleagues, which can be very stressful given the range of reactions people have to this information. Coming out might also make Rex feel obliged to educate others about his transition—something he is not interested in doing. Moreover, Rex desires for others to see him as male, rather than as transgender; his feelings and sense of identity can be deeply affected by witnessing others looking at him oddly or by hearing others accidentally or purposefully use the wrong pronouns.

Although Rex's family and employer were very supportive of his transition that occurred 2 years ago, clinicians should be aware that this is not always the case. Many transgender people have to deal with the loss of family, friends, housing, and/or employment when they transition. Employers may not allow time off for gender-affirming surgical procedures. When the changes of hormones or surgical procedures become evident, transgender people may face harassment or violence by others. Clinicians should be aware of these challenges, be careful to use the preferred pronouns and names of their clients, and recognize that binary constructs of gender may not apply to a client. Knowing about transgender support groups (online or local, if available) and other referrals that clients can be referred to is ideal. Chapters 16 and 17 offer more detailed discussions about ways to offer trans-affirming care. For detailed information on mental health care for transgender people, see the World Professional Association for Transgender Health's Standards of Care (www.wpath.org).

Psychiatric Conditions: Considerations for LGBT Clients

The next section uses case studies to discuss certain psychiatric conditions that could potentially manifest differently in LGBT people because of their unique life experiences as sexual or gender minorities.

Case: Adjustment Disorder

Lawrence is a 21-year-old gay man who presents to his primary care physician with depressed mood, feeling anxious, poor sleep, and decreased appetite. The symptoms started about 3 weeks ago when he came out to some close friends and his family. His announcement was met with mixed reactions, and he fears he is going to lose some of the people closest to him. He is having problems functioning at work and has found himself isolating in his apartment. The physician refers Rick to a therapist and asks that he follow up in 2 weeks. When the physician is documenting the case and submitting the billing, she is not sure if she should report this as an adjustment disorder with mixed anxiety and depressed mood or a major depressive episode.

The diagnosis of adjustment disorder is often used when people are presenting with mood and anxiety issues related to coming out. A study of patients in a large LGB mental health practice found that adjustment disorders were the most common presentation (32). The preceding case presents a situation where a clinician could misdiagnose a client as having a major depressive disorder, when the client more accurately meets the criteria for an adjustment disorder. The criteria for an adjustment disorder are as follows:

A. The development of emotional or behavior symptoms in response to an identifiable stressor(s) occurring within 3 months of onset of the stressor(s).
B. These symptoms or behaviors are clinically significant as evidenced by either of the following:
   1. Marked distress in excess of what would be expected from exposure to the stressor.
   2. Significant impairment in social or occupational functioning.
C. The stress-related disturbance does not meet the criteria for another specific Axis I disorder and is not merely an exacerbation of a preexisting Axis I or Axis II disorder.
D. The symptoms do represent bereavement.
E. Once the stressor (or its consequences) has terminated, the symptoms do not persist for more than an additional 6 months (8).

Looking at these criteria, Rick clearly meets the diagnosis for an adjustment disorder over the diagnosis of major depression. If the case had portrayed a client struggling with symptoms of panic and anxiety while undergoing the stress of coming out, the physician would have faced a similar dilemma of choosing a diagnosis of adjustment disorder over a diagnosis of generalized anxiety disorder or panic disorder. The difference in diagnosis is important because major depressive disorder and anxiety disorder may be recurrent. The diagnosis of an adjustment disorder is less stigmatizing because it is transient. Making a correct diagnosis can have implications for maintenance of treatment with pharmacologic agents.

An issue with using the diagnosis of adjustment disorder is that the diagnostic criteria are somewhat vague. The criteria require that there is distress "in excess of what would be expected." But one could argue that the stressful reactions of coming out are a normal response to societal homophobia. Again, the coming out experience of the LGBT client is wide and varied. Some clients are lucky enough to grow up in a very accepting environment and may experience very little distress in the coming out process. Others may not be as lucky and find they are rejected by friends and family. There is no standard coming out experience that can be qualified as the norm by which others can be measured. The closest way to be sure of the diagnosis of adjustment disorder is to follow the client over time and monitor if the symptoms resolve as the client becomes more comfortable with his/her sexual orientation.

The reality of modern medicine is that clinicians need to provide a diagnosis for billing purposes. The diagnosis of an adjustment disorder provides a billable diagnosis that is less stigmatizing to the client.

Case: Depression and Suicide Risk

Mary is a 36-year-old bisexual transgender woman who presents for her annual physical. She reports she is having problems with sleep. When questioned further, she reports she has been depressed, waking up early in the morning, worrying, and not enjoying anything anymore. She finds herself backing out of her commitments. Mary feels guilty that her wife is taking on most of the household responsibilities. More and more she feels like everyone would be better off without her around. Her ex-boyfriend, with whom she is still good friends, reminded her of a similar episode she had when they were together, which improved with a brief course of psychotherapy and medication. She is diagnosed with major depression, most likely a recurrent episode.

The preceding case raises some questions about the diagnosis of recurrent depression—and whether this is really her first episode. The clinician may want to inquire further if the prior episode could have been better classified as an adjustment disorder—and what may have been some issues surrounding episode. It is possible that she may truly have a recurrent depressive episode, and it has nothing to do with her sexual orientation or gender identity. Clearly, the clinician would not want to make that automatic assumption. The clinician could explore the issues surrounding her first episode and whether there were any indications that sexual orientation or gender identity was a factor.

The diagnosis of depression can be difficult to make in any patient. Shame, self-loathing, and doubt can keep a client from presenting for help or accurately reporting symptoms. The situation only worsens if the client fears being judged by a clinician. The causes of depression are multifactorial, with environmental stressors being a possible trigger or exacerbating factor for sexual and gender minority clients, who often have to deal with the stresses of a homo/transphobic society that bombards them with negative messages. If a client has grown up in a religious community, he or she may believe they are committing a sin and condemned to hell. They may have to contend with overt verbal, physical, and sexual abuse. They may worry about being disowned by family and friends if their sexual orientation or gender identity is discovered. These fears may be especially intense during the time a client is coming out.

Given all of these stressors, it is not surprising that strong evidence supports elevated risk for suicidal behavior in the LGBT population (22,29,38,39). In Mary's case, her remark that she feels that everyone would be better off without her could be a signal of suicidal ideation. The clinician should be aware of Mary's potential fears and ask directly if she has thought about hurting herself. Such clients should be asked directly if they have the means to harm themselves, such as a stockpile of pills or a weapon. There should also be an assessment of future orientation. Are there events or goals that Mary is looking forward to? A client that lacks any future orientation should raise concern for imminent risk of harm. If the client is abusing substances, he or she may also be at risk for impulsively making an attempt while intoxicated. Past suicide attempts should be evaluated for lethality. The client who previously attempted to overdose using 10 aspirin (and who called an ambulance right after taking the pills), while concerning, is less so than a client who attempted an overdose when he or she knew the family would be away. A client with active suicidal ideation with means and a plan should have an urgent psychiatric evaluation.

When treating an LGBT client with depression, the clinician should be aware of how sexual orientation or being transgender can affect the client's symptoms, but at the same time not assume these factors manifest the same way for all clients. A therapist who is educated and aware about the specific concerns of LGBT people can incorporate this knowledge into the therapeutic process. Appropriate interventional modalities include psychodynamic therapy, cognitive behavioral therapy, and relational therapy, as well as medication, which all work with the LGBT client dealing with depression. However, there is no specific medication or type of therapy that works better with LGBT clients than non-LGBT patients with similar levels of depression and associated clinical conditions. Depressed LGBT patients will respond best if they have a therapist who understands their issues and can create a safe space for them to engage in a plan to mitigate their depression, or other dysthymic disorder.

Case: Anxiety

Matt is a 45-year-old gay man who presents to the clinic for HIV testing. When reviewing the chart, the physician notices he has been tested 8 times in the past 3 months, despite reporting very-low-risk sexual activity, including periods of abstinence. Most recently, he went out to a gay bar with some friends and kissed a man he met. When he woke up, he was overcome with anxiety that he had contracted HIV. He spent most of the morning on the computer looking up information about HIV transmission. He went to an HIV testing clinic earlier in the day and had an oral secretion rapid HIV test whose result was negative. This provided momentary relief, but he then worried the rapid test was not reliable and came to the clinic to get a blood HIV test.

Matt admits to full-blown panic attacks when he has been tested in the past. The patient understands on a "logical" level that he is at very low risk but feels compelled to get tested. He admits when he was younger he had some problems with pulling his hair, needing order, and having to count things. He saw a therapist and these problems were better controlled, but flared up again 2 years ago when he came out.

Psychiatric disorders on the anxiety spectrum include obsessive-compulsive disorder, social phobia (social anxiety disorder), generalized anxiety disorder, and panic disorder. Before the recent publication of the *DSM-5*, post-traumatic stress disorder had been grouped with the anxiety disorders. Any one of these conditions can predominate, but patients can also show traits of the other conditions on the anxiety spectrum. For example, in the preceding case, the client had a flare-up of obsessive-compulsive disorder, but also had symptoms of panic and generalized anxiety. One of the core issues around all the anxiety disorders is the client's experience of a loss of control. This case illustrates the fear of HIV that is common in many gay men, and that may be especially evident when they come out and are sexually active. Some gay men self-medicate their anxiety by consuming alcohol and using drugs, which impair their judgment and may promote high-risk behavior.

Studies have shown higher rates of anxiety disorders in LGBT populations than other populations (22,28–30,32,39). The risks for developing an anxiety disorder may be multifactorial, but it is generally accepted that emotional stresses are triggers for anxiety. The LGBT community may face many stressors and, depending on their life experience and social supports, will experience homophobic stressors, which include bullying, fears of physical or verbal attack, discrimination at work, loss of family support, and fear of disease. If a person deals with internalized oppression by using drugs or alcohol, the substance abuse and consequences of substance use will become another stressor.

A client who is affected by homophobia and does not have the support or the coping skills to deal with this can feel a loss of control that puts him or her at risk for developing an anxiety disorder. Anxiety disorders start with dysfunctional behaviors that provide someone with a false sense of control. Matt's case provides an example where he logically knew his risk was low, but he felt compelled to get tested multiple times, which only transiently relieved his anxiety.

LGBT clients may also be at risk for post-traumatic stress disorder because of greater exposure to harassment, violence, childhood abuse, and other potentially traumatic events (40). It is therefore important to obtain a trauma history and consider that when treating a client. If Matt had disclosed an episode of prior sexual violence, the clinician may want to consider current symptoms as a trauma response that would influence the treatment recommendation.

Clinicians should understand the stressors that LGBT clients contend with in a homophobic society and how they fuel development of anxiety disorders. A clinician dealing with Matt may initially want to assess his understanding of HIV risk factors. If it is clear that Matt is well informed, it is not necessary to spend time educating him or debating what is high risk and what is low risk. A better approach would be to understand the stress factors in Matt's life, understand his coming out experience, and learn whether he is facing any current, or previous, discrimination. Matt would benefit from a course of therapy that focused on accepting his sexual orientation and understanding how it affects his obsessive-compulsive disorder, as well as skills-based therapy to help deal with acute symptoms. If therapy alone does not relieve symptoms, a trial of psychiatric medication could be considered.

Case: Bipolar Disorder

Jon is a 33-year-old gay man who was sent in by his psychiatrist for medical evaluation prior to having a trial of lithium for bipolar disorder. He had been having symptoms of depression after the loss of his job and a recent break-up. The medical provider asked about manic behavior and how the diagnosis of bipolar disorder was made. Matt grew up in a conservative family and had always repressed his sexual orientation. He describes himself as "exploding" out of the closet at 25. He was not educated about safer sex, and that first year was very sexually active and not always safe. He was active in the club scene and would sometimes stay up for days with little sleep, using crystal methamphetamine to help keep up his energy. He also had some financial problems related to his spending money at the clubs. This behavior lasted about a year, and he sought out counseling to help with his own internalized homophobia and accepting his sexual orientation. Later, he met his partner, stopped using drugs and maintained a monogamous relationship. The psychiatrist believed this period in his life was consistent with a manic episode, and his current episode was related to bipolar depression.

The preceding case illustrates the risk for misdiagnosing bipolar disorder when a clinician lacks knowledge about LGBT experiences, especially regarding the coming out process. A bipolar diagnosis must be made with careful considerations of the person's life experiences and the effect this may have on that person's mood and coping strategies. For example, a person such as Jon who had been repressing his sexual orientation may feel euphoric over finally understanding and acting on his repressed sexual feelings. At the same time, he may feel sadness and guilt due to the stigma that comes with this behavior. This fluctuation in mood is part of the normal journey that some people go through in accepting their sexual orientation.

In the case presented, Jon also immersed himself in the club scene and used crystal methamphetamine, which produces behaviors commonly seen in mania, such as impulsivity, poor judgment, the lack of need for sleep, and increased sexual behavior. While a clinician would keep the diagnosis of bipolar disorder in the differential, he or she would want to recognize whether the manic behaviors were primarily related solely to the stimulant drug use and should explore whether there were other manic periods in Jon's life other than the time when he came out, or when he was using stimulant drugs.

In cases such as Jon's, clinicians will also want to reflect on any personal biases that may lead them to label sexual behaviors they are not comfortable with as pathologic. Well-adjusted persons may choose to have more than one sexual partner and possibly many sexual partners. This does not necessarily mean they are engaging in hypersexual behavior. A clinician's own bias or lack of understanding about sexual diversity may label behavior they are not comfortable with as hypersexual and lead to misdiagnosis of a person as bipolar. No data clearly show LGBT people have a higher incidence of bipolar disorder. Some of this misconception comes from a very limited study of men who engaged in any same-sex behavior (41) but who did not necessarily identify as gay or bisexual. Hypersexuality is a manifestation of mania; in this state, people who identify as heterosexual may engage in same-sex activity as a symptom of their mania rather than as an expression of their sexual orientation.

This is not to say that LGBT people are immune from the diagnosis of bipolar disorder. LGBT clients who are diagnosed with bipolar disorder have some unique risks. For example, because the prevalence of some STIs is higher among men who have sex with men than among heterosexual men (12,13), a gay or bisexual man who is hypersexual during a manic period will be at increased risk for these STIs. Furthermore, bipolar LGBT people who live in areas or situations where it is not safe for them to be open about their sexual orientation may not be able to navigate complex issues during periods when their mood fluctuates. Clinicians should be aware of these safety concerns so they can identify resources for the client to help reduce risk for unintended consequences as they treat the affective disorder.

Case: Sexual Compulsivity

Doug is a 52-year-old man who presents to the clinic with penile discharge of 2 days' duration. He admits to feeling out of control with his sexual behavior, starting with periods of looking at pornography on the computer. This behavior progressed to meeting new partners online or at a cruising area. He has a primary partner who works the evening shift, and Doug will spend hours looking at cruising sites online. He has had problems at work when he twice left for 2 hours in the middle of the day to meet a sex partner. He finds the hunt for sex more exciting than the actual encounter and usually feels guilt and shame afterwards. He admits that when he gets caught up in this cycle, he may not always engage in safer sex practices. Doug feels he is telling so many lies all the time that he is not really sure what is true.

Sexual compulsivity is not listed as a formal diagnosis in the *DSM*, but it is a problem seen among some gay and bisexual men (42,43). The core symptoms that define sexual compulsivity are similar to those seen in other addictions. Specifically, it is a lack of control over one's sexual behavior despite the negative effect on relationships, work, health, and self-esteem. Unsuccessful attempts are often made to limit, control, or stop the behaviors. The manifestations of compulsive behavior can vary. Some people's compulsions are limited to sexually explicit websites. Others spend hours looking for sex and having multiple sexual encounters. The sexual behaviors or fantasies become a coping mechanism to deal with feeling of sadness, boredom, fear, frustration, or loss. Patients find they are engaging in more intense and frequent sexual behavior to meet their needs (44–46). As with Doug's case, the actual sexual encounter and achievement of orgasm is often not the goal of the activity, and is often accompanied by guilt and shame. The reinforcing aspects are the rituals and the heightened emotional state around looking for sex. Some describe the experience as a dissociative state where they can see what they are doing but are out of control and not connected.

Clients engaging in sexually compulsive behavior may be at increased risk for unsafe sexual activity. The use of drugs and alcohol can accompany the compulsive behavior and impair judgment. The sexual activity often becomes more intense or high risk as the addiction progresses. A study using the Sexual Compulsivity Scale showed sexual compulsivity was associated with sex under the influence of drugs, engaging in unprotected anal sex, higher number of sex partners, and desire to have unsafe sex without regard of the partner's HIV status (47).

When screening for sexual compulsivity, clinicians should take into account whether the client is first coming out as gay or bisexual. If so, he may not be comfortable meeting others in routine social venues. Some men may look online or in public cruising areas, which then may be followed by feelings of guilt. In this case, the guilt is more related to internalized homophobia and shame, and has less to do with an established compulsive behavior.

Clinicians should also recognize that some men who have multiple sexual partners function well in society. They do not see their behavior as out of control and do not put themselves at risk. Because the behavior does not have a negative effect on these men's lives, they should not be considered sexually compulsive.

For clients who do show signs of sexual compulsivity, clinicians should be aware of issues in the clients' lives that fuel the propensity to engage in sexually compulsive behaviors. Clients should be assessed for other addictive behaviors in their lives and for a family history of addiction. Did they overcome an addiction to drugs or alcohol? Is their sexual compulsivity another manifestation of their addiction? Providers should also explore the initial and continued benefits that clients gain from their behavior, including regulation of their emotions, validation of their self-esteem, or avoidance of painful issues in their life they do not want to address. Because internalized homophobia can affect a person's self-esteem and feelings about same-sex relationships, some clients may feel they do not deserve a fulfilling relationship and may engage in sexually compulsive behaviors that are degrading as way to decrease their engagement in an open same-sex relationship.

Clinicians can help clients start the process of recovery by helping them accept and understand their behaviors. Clients must first be able to understand and express what their problems are and which behaviors they see as unhealthy, and to determine what is normal sexual behavior for them and their partners. They should then commit to a plan to help address these issues. Connecting with an LGBT-sensitive counselor or therapist who understands that sexual compulsivity is an important first step. There are also 12-step groups that deal with sexual addiction, including SLAA (Sex and Love Addicts Anonymous) and SCA (Sexual Compulsives Anonymous).

Mental Health Assessment and Treatment

Self-Assessment of Attitudes and Beliefs

Caring for LGBT clients with mental health concerns requires that clinicians first take an honest look at their own feelings and attitudes towards LGBT people. Clinicians who lack insight about their personal feelings and biases regarding sexual and gender minorities can have a negative effect on patient care. This can be manifested by body language, how a medical and social history is obtained, and even options for care that are offered. For example, a clinician who is uncomfortable with bisexuality may create a situation in which a female client who is currently in a same-sex relationship is not comfortable talking about her history of relationships with men. The clinician may not obtain critical information about risk factors for HIV or may not provide education about birth control. Awareness of personal feelings may not change beliefs, but it will increase awareness of biases that can affect interactions with clients. In understanding biases, clinicians can assess how they affect the clinical interaction and adjust behavior accordingly so that ethical obligations to provide optimal health care are fulfilled.

Below are some questions that clinicians should consider asking themselves:

- Do I feel same-sex relationships are as valid as heterosexual relationships?
- Do I feel nervous when clients talk about their same-sex relationship?
- How do I feel about gay marriage?
- Do I feel more comfortable with lesbians than gay men or vice versa?
- Do I think all gay men are promiscuous?
- Do I think all lesbians dislike men?
- How do I feel about clients who identify as bisexual?
- How do I feel about clients who identify as transgender?
- How do I feel when I see a person whose gender is not clearly male or female?
- Do I feel sorry for people who identify as LGBT?

It is important to think about the answers you have to those questions. The next step would be to think about how you came to those answers. It may be based on images from the media or TV, friends or family members who are LGBT, religious beliefs, political beliefs, or limited interactions with LGBT people. Then, think about how these feelings and beliefs might affect your interactions with sexual or gender minority clients.

Sometimes just being aware of situations that cause discomfort helps clinicians in their interactions with clients. We can be more aware of questions that are relevant and can make sure to ask them in a sensitive manner, with appropriate body language. Self-education is important, and hopefully textbooks like this one will be helpful. See also Chapter 15 for more on ways to explore personal attitudes and beliefs.

Communicating About Sexual Orientation and Gender Identity

The ways that individuals describe their sexual orientation and gender identity are diverse and do not always provide all the information a clinician needs to understand the client's sexual behavior, relationships, and family structure. Social stigma around sexual orientation and gender identity may prevent some people who engage in same-sex behavior or who experience gender discordance from identifying as LGBT. A woman may identify as lesbian with strong ties to the lesbian community, but may also occasionally have sex with men. This has implications for health care screening. A clinician should feel comfortable asking, "Do you have sex with men? Women? Or both men and women?" The simple act of asking these questions signals to the client that you are open to a discussion of sexual orientation, identity, and behavior.

The use of gender-neutral terminology is very helpful in setting up an open and accepting clinical relationship. Imagine being a lesbian and having the following interaction:

Provider: Are you married?
Client: Yes.
Provider: What does your husband do?

The heterosexual presumption can create an intimidating and nonproductive clinical encounter. If the clinician presumes that marriage is only between a man and a woman, or that same-sex couples cannot have committed relationships, he or she will send a negative message to the client that the relationship is not valid. If the clinician had just changed *husband* to *spouse*, a welcome message would have been sent. There are other ways a clinician may ask about a relationship:

• Tell me about the person you are involved with.
• Do you have a partner?
• Are you in a relationship?

When gender is not assumed, it opens the door to more honest communication. If a lesbian tells a clinician that she is involved with a woman and they are married, it would then be appropriate to be gender-specific and use the term *wife*. A clinician should think about gender-neutral terminology when talking to all clients. For more on communicating with patients in an affirming and welcoming manner, see Chapter 8.

An LGBT client may be curious about the sexual orientation of his or her clinician, which may raise issues around self-disclosure. Some openly gay clinicians are out about their sexual orientation, and the disclosure happens before the clinical interaction. In a psychotherapeutic relationship, the clinician may want to first explore with the client what it would mean if the clinician were LGBT-identified, as this may be a critical part of the therapeutic process. The timing of this is also important. A client who is asking at the start of treatment may be looking to make sure the provider is a safe and understanding person. A client who does not ask early in the treatment but a year later could be less concerned about the clinician's homophobia, and may be manifesting transference with the clinician. A clinician should think about how he or she will answer questions about sexual orientation prior to the visit with the client, and how to do it in a way that is not alienating to a client. Clinicians should be able to answer questions a client has about their experiences working with the LGBT community and how they feel about same-sex relationships or transgender identities.

Exploring what it would mean to the client if the clinician were *or were not* LGBT-identified will provide some insights into what concerns the client may have and what answers or disclosures may be helpful. Clients may worry that they have to "educate" a clinician about being

LGBT and assume an LGBT clinician may be more qualified. This is not always the case. LGBT clinicians may have common experiences with an LGBT client, but it is not a substitute for clinical training and supervision. A heterosexual, nontransgender clinician can respond to the concern by a client of having to "educate" their clinician by stating, "I do not assume the experiences of all LGBT clients are the same. I am interested in what your experience is."

Mental Health Assessment: Case Example

The mental health assessment of an LGBT client is not structurally different from that of non-LGBT clients, but some special considerations need to be taken into account. The next section will go through parts of the assessment with a sample case, bringing together many of the major themes around LGBT mental health that were detailed earlier in this chapter.

History of Present Illness

Colin is a 34-year-old gay male lawyer who presents with increasing symptoms of depression. He has recently ended a relationship with his male partner of 2 years. His work environment is conservative, and there are high demands for billable hours. Colin cannot rely on his family for support, and he lost touch with some friends when he started his relationship. He denies any thoughts of harming himself and has goals for the future including making partner in the firm, meeting a new man, and having children.

In assessing the chief complaint/history of present illness, it is important to keep the client's sexual orientation or transgender identity in mind but not to assume these are the most important factors. A clinician can sometimes overemphasize or underemphasize the role of sexual orientation or gender identity. LGBT clients come into treatment with many similar mental health concerns as the general population. In the preceding case study, Colin presents with symptoms of depression after the end of a relationship and faces significant job stress, which are situations that any person may face. The clinician has assessed for safety and there is no suicidal ideation, with the patient being future-oriented.

There are some clues that Colin's sexual orientation may also be affecting his depression. He describes his work environment as conservative, so the clinician should inquire whether he is out about his sexual orientation at work and whether there is fear of discrimination. He also mentions he cannot rely on his family for support. At this point, more information should be obtained about his relationship with his family. Is he out to his family? How does his family feel about his sexual orientation? The clues given in the chief complaint should direct the clinician on how to explore the effect of sexual orientation.

Past Psychiatric History

Colin had a prior episode of depression when he was 23 and in law school. He had ended a relationship with a woman when she wanted to be sexually active. Colin had grown up in a very religious family and dated women from the same church where premarital sex was not accepted. His girlfriend in law school was not religious and felt rejected by his reluctance to have sex. Colin started to face his denial and realized he was not interested in sex with any woman and always felt more sexually drawn to his male friends. He became seriously depressed and took a leave from law school. He had a course of therapy to support him in coming out and his symptoms improved over the next 6 months. Colin was able to restart law school.

The clinician should evaluate how sexual orientation affected Colin's past psychiatric history. In this case, Colin's prior episode would be best characterized as an adjustment disorder with depressed mood. The clear stressor was his coming out experience, which resolved with supportive therapy.

The evaluation of past psychiatric history should include an assessment of the client's experience with the mental health system, including community supports and the client's willingness to utilize these resources. More specifically, was his sexual orientation affirmed by the clinician or seen as pathologic? How does that affect his feelings about the mental health care system now? Did the client have concerns in prior treatment that his confidentiality would be violated? If so, it is important to reassure the client of the ethical standards for the confidential nature of medical records. Did the client have positive or negative experiences with community supports? How willing is he to use these resources again? Clinicians should know whether the programs they refer the patient to are sensitive to the needs of LGBT people.

Substance Abuse History

Colin had a brief period of weekend binge drinking when he started college. Then, when he came out in law school and started to go out with friends to bars and clubs, he experimented with Ecstasy a few times. He tried crystal methamphetamine once and, realizing he liked it very much, was scared to use it again. The clinician asked Colin what he liked so much about crystal methamphetamine. Colin remembers when he used the drug his troubles seemed less relevant, and his mood improved. Since he has been depressed lately, he sometimes thinks about using it again. The clinician questions Colin further about his desire to use drugs and his ability to access them. Colin admits it would not be difficult to obtain drugs, but he has seen what they have done to several friends. It is clear to the clinician that Colin will not use drugs.

The clinician thanks him for his honesty and validates that with his depression it would be tempting to use drugs. He invites Colin to keep this line of communication open if he ever thinks about or uses drugs again.

The overt and subtle manifestations of homophobia can trigger and fuel the use of drugs and alcohol in the LGBT community. The psychiatric history should include a detailed substance abuse history. Clinicians should assess what drugs the client uses/has used, the degree of their use, and the potential reasons behind the use. For example, LGBT clients could use drugs to deal with the pain of rejection by friends and family. They could self-medicate anxiety caused by not being out about their sexuality, or by bullying and other forms of harassment. Drugs and alcohol are sometimes used as a way of fitting into the bar or club scene, or to alleviate the anxiety around going to an openly LGBT venue.

The clinician in the case example asked Colin what he liked about crystal meth. That is a very important question. Clients can often use an office session as a confessional about the bad things drugs do to them, but then go out and use again. People would not continue to use drugs that made them horribly ill or that did not produce any positive effect. When the benefits of the drugs are understood, it provides an opportunity to deal with the root causes of drug use.

When obtaining the substance use history, the clinician should assess the client's readiness to change. If Colin were not ready to stop his use, might he be willing to discuss and/or reduce his use? Harm reduction is the practice of meeting clients where they are at with their substance use and trying to reduce the impact. Simply asking the client, "How will you know when you have a problem?" can help you better understand the issue. For example, if the client says he knows he has a problem if he uses drugs and misses work, and later tells the clinician he has missed work due to drug use, the clinician may then reflect back to the client, "You mentioned before that you would consider your substance use a problem if you missed work, and now that it has happened, let's put our heads together and think of some ways we can prevent this from happening again."

Domestic Violence and Other Abuse History

Colin often ruminates to his clinician about the end of his relationship and the mistakes he made. The last few months of the relationship he and his partner fought a lot. The fights were about money, working too much, and his partner's jealousy of Colin's friendships with other men. Colin feels like he overreacts to any expressed anger and admits he easily feels bullied. He had several experiences when he was younger where he was a target of bullying; as an adult, he has occasionally been the target of homophobic slurs spoken by strangers who witnessed him leaving gay clubs.

Colin has given several clues that should trigger the clinician to screen further for domestic violence and past abuse. Abuse can be in the form of bullying, hate crimes, domestic violence, and sexual assault. Domestic violence occurs when an abusive partner attempts to exert power and control over his or her partner. Same-sex couples have the same risk for domestic violence as opposite-sex couples (48), despite the myths that women are not capable of abuse or that men cannot be victims of abuse. The clinician should screen for domestic abuse (but never with a partner present) and assess for safety needs and referrals.

Colin also gives a history of bullying and harassment that should be further explored and evaluated. While bullying has recently received more attention in the media, it is a term that has often been used to minimize a hate crime. LGBT hate crimes occur when people are victimized because of their sexual orientation and/or gender expression. When clients confide events to a clinician about a hate crime, the clinician should assess their safety, including whether they are at risk for being victimized again. Clients may try to minimize the incident because of fear or shame. It is very important to validate the experience and the serious nature of hate crimes. Clients who have been victimized by a hate crime can have their sense of identity shattered, and they are left feeling vulnerable. This, in turn, puts them at risk for symptoms of anxiety, depression, and, potentially, post-traumatic stress disorder. Abuse survivors may lose their ability to trust others, including health care professionals. In taking the clinical history, the clinician should assess the effect of violence and harassment on the client and how they may affect the ability to trust the health care system. Chapter 11 discusses screening and evaluation of hate crimes and domestic violence in LGBT clients.

Social History

Colin grew up outside a small city and was the youngest of 3 boys in a conservative Christian family. Much of the family's social life revolved around church life. His father owned a plumbing supply company. His mother was a high school principal. He did well in school and had a group of friends, although sometimes he was bullied for not being good at sports. This happened until high school when he played soccer. He graduated at the top of his class and did well in college and law school. He was recruited into a prestigious law firm. Colin always felt loved by his parents but at times worried their love was contingent on him doing the right thing and being a good Christian. His parents expressed their love for him but also disappointment when he came out, and he feels there has been distance from them since then. He has friends, but they are not as close because he had put so much time into his relationship and work. Colin is not out about his sexual orientation at work because he feels the culture is too conservative for him to come out.

The social history of the LGBT client should address how the client's sexual orientation and/or gender identity affected his or her education, vocation, family, and social relationships. The clinician can ask when clients became aware of their sexual orientation or transgender identity, how it was self-perceived, and whether others knew there was something different about them even before they did. The family's beliefs about the LGBT community should also be explored. If they were not accepting, did this change when the client came out? Some families may not express overt homophobia but instead have no awareness of same-sex relationships or transgender identity, resulting in covert oppression.

In the preceding case, the experience of the client in school and how he interacted with peers and friends should be assessed. Did he did fit in with others? Did he feel isolated? How much was he bullied? How did this affect his sense of identity and self-esteem?

The clinicians should also inquire about his experiences at work. Has he ever lost a job or been discriminated against on the basis of his sexual orientation? Why has he chosen not to come out at work? Living a double life in which a person is open about his or her sexual orientation in their personal life but hides it at work is a common experience in the LGBT community. It is also a significant source of stress. LGBT people may not feel comfortable bringing their partner to a work event or having a picture at their desk. In general, they may feel they need to put up an emotional barrier with work colleagues, being vague about details of their personal lives. Some LGBT people may also lead dual social lives in which they have a group of friends they are out to and a group to whom they are not.

The clients' social and family supports are critical for many LGBT people in helping them deal with internal and external homophobia. The families may be biological families, families of choice, or a combination of both. The clinician should ask about LGBT community supports such sports teams, social groups, and political groups. An LGBT person who has the support of friends and family and is involved in community organizations that empower them to enact change is better equipped to deal with the stresses of societal oppression.

Sexual History

Colin has never been sexually active with women. His first sexual activity was with same-sex peers at camp when he was 13. His first adult sexual experience was at age 24 with a male law school classmate. He felt it was a positive experience. He practices safer sex, except when he has been in a relationship (he has had 2 long-term relationships). He does not generally have sex on a first date, anonymous sex, or sex while intoxicated or under the influence of drugs. Colin also has regular testing for STIs. He reports a "healthy fear" of HIV but does not feel it has inhibited his sex life. He has been satisfied with his sex life and feels that sexual compatibility was a not a factor in his recent break-up. There is no history of sexual abuse.

Obtaining an accurate and complete sexual history is facilitated when a clinician can create an open, nonjudgmental environment that puts the client at ease. If the client is anxious, the clinician may want to normalize this by telling him this is an important part of the history that sometimes makes people uncomfortable. While eliciting the client's early sexual desires, fantasies, and experiences, feelings of shame may emerge—especially if the client grew up in a homophobic environment.

The mental health of LGBT people can affect their sexual health. A depressed person may lack desire for sex, while an anxious one may have problems with sexual performance. The medications used to treat psychiatric conditions can affect sexual function, and the clinician should ask about this if a client is on medication. Some clients may use sex to self-medicate their psychiatric symptoms and use sex as a way to temporarily feel better. Internalized trans/homophobia may interfere with sexual function and enjoyment. LGBT clients may feel that they can have sex only while using alcohol and drugs as way to deal with their internalized trans/homophobia. Finally, clinicians should consider the client's understanding of sexually transmitted infections and the associated risks and offer appropriate screening and counseling. In some cases, the clinician may not be able to obtain all this sensitive information early in the treatment relationship and may need to come back to the sexual history as the treatment alliance with the client develops over time. For more details on promoting the sexual health of LGBT clients, see Chapter 12.

Summary of Assessment

Colin realizes that he needs help with his symptoms and asks the clinician what he should do. The clinician thanks Colin for being so open about his history and acknowledges this is not always easy to do. The clinician feels sufficient information has been obtained to make some recommendations. The clinician does not feel Colin is in acute danger and does not need hospitalization or an intensive outpatient program. The clinician directly addresses safety concerns and, if they were to occur, tells Colin he should call their crisis line or go to the emergency department. They discuss options for treatment, including a therapy referral, and possibly medication if symptoms do not improve.

As has been shown in Colin's case, the mental health assessment of an LGBT person is similar to the assessment for the heterosexual client, in that the primary goal is to first assess safety and acuity and then to recommend appropriate treatment options for the primary complaint. The differences in the assessment come from how the client has experienced and navigated societal stigma that is still prevalent today. The experience of each client is unique, and the suggestions given are meant to be a guide to clinicians so they can obtain relevant information that will affect the care of the client.

Treatment for Mental Health Issues

The mental health treatment of LGBT clients uses the same modalities as for heterosexual clients, including psychotherapy, medication, or a combination of both. When an appropriate and culturally sensitive history is obtained, the client should feel comfortable relating the relevant information that will assist the clinician in obtaining a working diagnosis and developing a treatment plan.

As noted earlier in this chapter, conversion therapy is the attempt to change sexual orientation through different forms of cognitive behavioral therapy or psychodynamic therapy. This type of therapy by its very nature assumes that same-sex attraction is pathologic and needs to be repaired. Conversion therapies are not acceptable forms of mental health treatment. They work to exploit the client's own internalized homophobia and deepen their self-hatred and shame. The American Psychiatric Association and the American Psychological Association both recommend against the use of conversion therapy (49,50).

Affirming therapy assumes that LGBT identities are normal and focuses on helping clients accept and gain comfort with their sexual orientation and gender identity. The treatment should address whether internalized trans/homophobia contributes to the client's distress and whether/how negative experiences have affected the client's development. The experience of every client will be different, and individual experiences should be explored, with an understanding of the general issues facing LGBT patients. Some resources on providing affirming care and treatment to LGBT clients can be found in Table 9-1.

When assisting the patient in the coming out process, affirming therapy does not imply that the therapist takes a passive supportive role, allowing

Table 9-1   LGBT Mental Health Resources

Guidelines for Psychological Practice with Lesbian, Gay, and Bisexual Clients (American Psychological Association): www.apa.org/pi/lgbt/resources/guidelines.aspx

LGBT Training Curricula for Behavioral Health and Primary Care Practitioners: http://www.samhsa.gov/behavioral-health-equity/lgbt/curricula

National Alliance on Mental Illness's LGBT Resources: www.nami.org/Content/NavigationMenu/Find_Support/Multicultural_Support/Resources/GLBT_Resources.htm

Association of Gay and Lesbian Psychiatrists: www.aglp.org

Sex and Love Addicts Anonymous: www.slaafws.org

Sexual Compulsives Anonymous: www.sca-recovery.org

Pride Institute Treatment Center: http://pride-institute.com

the client to believe everything will be okay. The therapist should help clients build the skills to deal with challenges they may face when they come out. Having clients come out before they are ready or have needed supports in place would not be beneficial. As with any therapeutic treatment modality, the process will include addressing cognitive distortion and issues of transference. Therapists, regardless of their own sexual orientation or gender identity, need to address their own beliefs and assumptions about LGBT people and to recognize that same-sex attraction and transgender identity are normal variations of sexual behavior and gender.

The treatment of LGBT clients with psychiatric medications should follow the same principles that are used with the general population. For clients with HIV infection, consideration must be taken in prescribing psychiatric medications with HIV medications, especially protease inhibitors. The ability to review these interactions is beyond the scope of this chapter. Clinicians can use drug interaction software or refer to the AIDS Education and Training Centers website (www.aidsetc.org).

Summary Points

- The fields of medicine and psychology have evolved to be more accepting of LGBT identities and behaviors; nonetheless, clinicians should be aware that this was not always the case, and that LGBT clients (particularly those who are older) may have a lingering distrust of the medical professions.
- The coming out process for LGBT clients is a fluid, nonlinear lifelong process; helping the client safely navigate this process can be beneficial for the client and rewarding for the clinician.
- The stress caused by societal bias, stigma, and discrimination can negatively affect the mental health of LGBT people.
- Current research suggests that LGBT people are at higher risk for depression, anxiety, substance use, and suicidal ideation.
- LGBT clients with a mental health diagnosis have to manage the dual stigma of mental illness and societal homophobia and transphobia.
- Gay men should be evaluated for the use of club drugs, safer sex practices, and issues related to body image.
- Bisexual clients are often not accepted by the heterosexual or LGBT communities, which presents them with unique mental health challenges.
- Lesbians' mental health issues have many things in common with general women's health issues, but lesbians are also may be at increased risk for mood disorders and anxiety.
- Transgender people must deal with pervasive transphobia that puts them that at additional risk for violence, harassment, and job discrimination.

- Mental health conditions may have unique presentations in LGBT clients. For example, some LGBT people who show signs of depression or anxiety may actually be experiencing adjustment disorder.
- Clinicians should assess their own attitudes and beliefs about LGBT people because these beliefs may affect the treatment they provide to these clients.
- Conversion therapy should never be used with LGBT clients; this form of treatment is harmful and unethical.
- Clinicians who work with LGBT clients should provide therapy that affirms their client's identities, relationships, and life goals.

References

1. **Freud S.** A letter from Freud. Am J of Psychiatry. 1951;107:786-7.
2. **Bayer R.** Homosexuality and American Psychiatry: The Politics of Diagnosis. Princeton: Princeton University Press; 1987.
3. **Bieber R, Dain HJ, Dince PR, Drellich MP, et al.** Homosexuality: A Psychoanalytic Study. New York: Basic Books; 1962.
4. **Hooker E.** The adjustment of the male overt homosexual. J Projective Techniques. 1957;21: 18-31.
5. **Kinsey AC, Pomeroy WB, Martin CE.** Sexual Hehavior in the Human Male. Philadelphia: W.B. Saunders; 1948.
6. **American Psychiatric Association.** Diagnostic and Statistical Manual of Mental Disorders. 3rd ed. Arlington, VA: American Psychiatric Publishing; 1980.
7. **American Psychiatric Association.** Diagnostic and Statistical Manual of Mental Disorders. 4th ed, text revision. Washington, DC: American Psychiatric Association; 2000.
8. **American Psychiatric Association.** Diagnostic and Statistical Manual of Mental Disorders. 5th Ed. Arlington, VA: American Psychiatric Publishing; 2013.
9. **Jessup MA, Dibble SL.** Unmet mental health and substance abuse treatment needs of sexual minority elders. J Homosexual. 2012;59:656-74.
10. **Fredriksen-Goldsen KI, Emlet CA, et al.** The physical and mental health of lesbian, gay male and bisexual (LGB) older adults: the role of key health indicators and risk and protective factors. Gerontologist. 2013;53:664-75.
11. **Corrigan P.** How stigma interferes with mental health care. Am Psychol. 2004;59:614-25.
12. **Mayer KH.** Sexually transmitted diseases in men who have sex with men. Clin Infect Dis. 2011;53:S79-S83.
13. **Bohl DD, Katz KA, Bernstein K, et al.** Prevalence and correlates of herpes simplex virus type-2 infection among men who have sex with men, San Francisco, 2008. Sex Transm Dis. 2011;38:617-21.
14. **Duggan SJ, McCreary DR.** Body image, eating disorders and the drive for muscularity in gay and heterosexual men: the influence of media images. J Homosexual. 2004;47: 45-58.
15. **Siever MD.** Sexual orientation and gender as factors in socioculturally acquired vulnerability to body dissatisfaction and eating disorders. J Consult Clin Psychol. 1994;62:252-60.
16. **Silberstein LR, Mishkind ME, Striegel-Moore RH, Timko C, Rodin J.** Men and their bodies: a comparison of homosexual and heterosexual men. Psychosom Med. 1989;51:337-46.
17. **Kaminski PL, Chapman BP, Haynes SD, Own L.** Body image, eating behaviors and attitudes towards exercise among gay and straight men. Eating Behav. 2005;6:179-87.
18. **Ip EJ, Lu DH, Barnett MJ, Tenerowicz MJ, Vo JC, Perry PJ.** Psychological and physical impact of anabolic-androgenic steroid dependence. Pharmacotherapy. 2012;32:910-9.

19. **Miller M, Andre A, Ebin J, Bessonova L.** Bisexual Health: An Introduction and Model Practices for HIV/STI Prevention Programing. Boston: National Gay and Lesbian Policy Institute, The Fenway Institute, BiNet USA; 2007:2.

20. **San Francisco Human Rights Commission.** Bisexual Invisibility: Impacts and Recommendations. San Francisco: LBT Advisory Committee; 2011.

21. **Ekstrand ML, Coates TJ, Hauck WW, Collette L, Hulley SB.** Are bisexually identified men in San Francisco a common vector for spreading HIV to women? Am J Public Health. 1994;84: 915-9.

22. **King M, Semlyen J, Tai SS, et al.** A systematic review of mental disorder, suicide, and deliberate self-harm in lesbian, gay and bisexual people. BMC Psychiatry. 2008;70.

23. **Koh AS, Ross LK.** Mental health issues: a comparison of lesbian, bisexual and heterosexual women. J Homosexual. 2006;51:33-57.

24. **Brennan DJ, Ross LE, Dobinson C, Veldhuizen S, Steele LS.** Men's sexual orientation and health in Canada. Can J Public Health. 2010;101:255-8.

25. **Fredriksen-Goldsen KI, Kim H, Barakan SE, Balsam KF, Mincer SL.** Disparities in health-related quality of life: a comparison of lesbians and bisexual women. Am J Public Health. 2010;100:2255-61.

26. **McCabe S, Bostwick WB, Hughes TL, West BT, Boyd CJ.** The relationship between discrimination and substance use disorders among lesbian, gay and bisexual adults in the United States. Am J Public Health. 2010;100:1946-52.

27. **Bradford J, Ryan C, Rothblum E.** National Lesbian Health Care Survey: implications for mental health. J Consult Clin Psychol. 1994;62:228-42.

28. **Cochran SD, Mays VM.** Burden of psychiatric morbidity among lesbian, gay, and bisexual individuals in the California Quality of Life Survey. J Abnormal Psychol. 2009;118:647-58.

29. **Gilman SE, Cochran SD, Mays VM, Hughes M, Ostrow D, Kessler RC.** Risk of psychiatric disorders among individuals reporting same-sex sexual partners in the National Comorbidity Survey. Am J Public Health. 2001;91:933-9.

30. **Cochran SD, Mays VM, Sullivan JG.** Prevalence of mental disorders, psychological distress, and mental health services use among lesbian, gay, and bisexual adults in the United States. J Consult Clin Psychol. 2003;71:53-61.

31. **Cochran SD, Mays VM.** Relationship between psychiatric syndromes and behaviorally defined sexual orientation in a sample of the US population. Am J Epidemiol. 2001;151:516-23.

32. **Berg M, Mimiaga MJ, Safren S.** Mental health concerns of gay and bisexual men seeking mental health services. J Homosexual. 2008;54:293-306.

33. **Morgan KS.** Caucasian lesbians' use of psychotherapy: a matter of attitude? Psychol Women Q. 1992;16:127-30.

34. **Valanis BG, Bowen DJ, Bassford T, et al.** Sexual orientation and health: comparisons in the Women's Health Initiative sample. Arch Fam Med. 2000;9:843-53.

35. **Cochran SD, Mays VM, Bowen D, Gage S, Bybee D, Roberts SJ, et al.** Cancer-related risk indicators and preventive screening behaviors among lesbians and bisexual women. Am J Public Health. 2001;91:591-7.

36. **Tjaden PG, Thoennes N.** Extent, nature and consequences of intimate partner violence: findings from the National Violence Against Women Survey. Washington, DC: National Institute of Justice; 2000.

37. **Grant JM, Mottet LA, Tanis J, et al.** Injustice at Every Turn: A Report of the National Transgender Discrimination Survey. Washington, DC: The National Center for Transgender Equality and National Gay and Lesbian Task Force; 2011.

38. **Haas AP, Eliason M, Mays VM, et al.** Suicide and suicide risk in lesbian, gay, bisexual, and transgender populations: review and recommendation. J Homosexual. 2011;58:10-51.

39. **Conron KJ, Mimiaga MJ, Landers SJ.** A population-based study of sexual orientation identity and gender difference in adult health. Am J Public Health. 2010;100:1953-60.

40. **Roberts AL, Austin SB, Corliss HL, Vandermorris AK, Koenen KC.** Pervasive trauma exposure among US sexual orientation minority adults and risk of posttraumatic stress disorder. Am J Public Health. 2010;100:2433-41.

41. **Sandfort TM, De Graaf R, Bijl RV, Schnabel P.** Same-sex sexual behavior and psychiatric disorders: finding from the Netherlands Mental Health Survey and Incidence Study (NEMESIS). Arch Gen Psychiatry. 2001;58:85-91.

42. **Kelly BC, Bimbi DS, Nanin JE, Izienicki H, Parsons JT.** Sexual compulsivity and sexual behaviors among gay and bisexual men and lesbian and bisexual women. J Sex Res. 2009;46: 301-8.

43. **Parsons JT, Kelly BC, Bimbi DS, DiMaria L, Wainberg ML, Morgenstern J.** Explanations for the origins of sexual compulsivity among gay and bisexual men. Arch Sex Behav. 2008;37: 817-26.

44. **Sexual Compulsives Anonymous.** Available at: http://www.sca-recovery.org.

45. **Kafka MP.** Hypersexual disorder: a proposed diagnosis for DSM-V. Arch Sex Behav. 2010; 39:377-400.

46. **Weiss RE.** Cruise Control: Understanding Sex Addiction in Gay Men. New York: Alyson Books; 2005.

47. **Grove C, Parsons JT, Bimbi DS.** Sexual compulsivity and sexual risk in gay and bisexual men. Arch Sexual Behav. 2010;39:940-9.

48. **Walters ML, Chen J, Breiding MJ.** The National Intimate Partner and Sexual Violence Survey (NISVS): 2010 findings on victimization by sexual orientation. Atlanta, GA: National Center for Injury Prevention and Control, Centers for Disease Control and Prevention; 2013.

49. **American Psychological Association.** Orientation, APA Task Force on Appropriate Responses to Sexual. Report of the Task Force on Appropriate Therapeutic Responses to Sexual Orientation. Washington, DC: American Psychological Association; 2009.

50. **American Psychiatric Association.** COPP Position Statement: Therapies Focused on Attempts to Change Sexual Orientation. Washington, DC: American Psychiatric Association; 2000.

Chapter 10

Clinical Management of Substance Use and Substance Use Disorders Among LGBT Individuals

TIMOTHY M. HALL, MD, PhD, Dip ABPN, Dip ABAM
CATHY J. REBACK, PhD
STEVEN SHOPTAW, PhD

Introduction

Perhaps no topic engenders more stereotypes and stigma than that of substance use and addiction among lesbian, gay, bisexual, or transgender (LGBT) individuals. Many LGBT individuals have experienced discriminatory attitudes from clinicians, clinical staff, and community members regarding use of addictive substances. It is imperative that clinicians understand the research regarding the specific substances, the use and role of substances in diverse LGBT cultures, and the clinical evidence to guide selection of treatments for substance use disorders.

In this chapter, we address the following: 1) the history and social context of substance use in relation to LGBT health; 2) distinguishing *substance use* from *substance use disorder* (SUD) or addiction; 3) current epidemiology of substance use and addiction in LGBT populations; 4) links between substance use or SUD and high-risk sexual behaviors; and 5) evidence-based treatments for SUD. Throughout, *substance use* designates consumption that does not necessarily present problems for the individual, whereas *SUD* and its synonym *addiction* describe consumption that is clinically significant and carries negative consequences.

A note on language: Recent scholarship in public health has tended to use behaviorally based terms, such as *men who have sex with men* (MSM), which recognize that sexual behavior is not fully determined by one's sexual orientation and that sexual identity is not necessarily determined by one's behavior. One clinically relevant group comprises individuals who may have sex with nonpreferred partners in exchange for drugs or money. Others may feel a "gay" or "lesbian" identity does not fit their self-understanding, or carries political or cultural associations that they do not embrace. Some clinically relevant factors are more associated with behavior per se, while others are more associated with a lesbian, gay, bisexual, or transgender identity, or with participation in an LGBT community. For simplicity, we use the identity-based terms throughout this chapter.

Transgender individuals may understand and express gender identities in multiple ways. For the purposes of this chapter, we discuss male-to-female transgender persons as *trans women* and female-to-male persons as *trans men*, independent of their anatomic sex, although the presence or absence of functioning gonads and the anatomic sex at birth are highly relevant to possible adverse effects of hormone therapies and drug interactions. Chapter 17 provides definitions of terms related to transgender identities that the reader may find helpful. We use *LGBT* as the broadest term and preferable here to "sexual and gender minorities."

History and Context of Substance Use in Relation to LGBT Health

Multiple, possibly complementary, contextual explanations have been proposed with varying degrees of evidence regarding perceived elevated rates of substance use and addiction in LGBT populations. Some LGBT individuals use alcohol or other substances as a way of coping prior to coming out or to self-medicate conflicts in relation to perceived unsupportive family, religious, or other social relationships. Some LGBT persons use alcohol and, to a lesser extent, other intoxicating substances to decrease anxiety in social and sexual situations. LGBT-friendly bars and nightclubs have a long history in Western societies as critical sites for LGBT individuals to meet similarly LGBT friends and to find romantic or sexual partners (1–3). In this context, the social acts of drinking and smoking cigarettes have historically mediated many interactions among LGBT persons. Finally, certain drugs—particularly alkyl nitrite "poppers" and cocaine since the 1970s, "club drugs" (such as ketamine, gamma hydroxybutyrate (GHB), and 3,4-methylenedioxy-N-methylamphetamine [MDMA]) since the 1980s, and methamphetamine (often freebased as crystal meth) since the 1990s—have been used by some gay and bisexual (GB) men to reduce sexual inhibitions and enhance sexual experiences (4).

All of these contribute to a generally greater tolerance of the recreational use of drugs and of heavy or problematic alcohol use among LGBT communities than in the larger society (5). In turn, this prevalence and tolerance may place LGBT persons at greater risk for exposure to potentially addicting substance through their social networks. For persons in recovery from addiction, triggers, cues, and access to substances may be more prevalent than in non-LGBT communities. The use of intoxicating substances may also be deeply embedded in some LGBT people's networks of social support or their experience of sexuality. There may be few (or no) options for "sober" social events that are equivalent in perceived impact and value to those where substances are used (e.g., Halloween). The addiction itself and the precipitating and maintaining psychosocial dynamics must be addressed as part of successful recovery, yet treatment providers often have inadequate understanding of, and limited tolerance for, the cultural linkages among substance use, sexuality, and personal meaning that present challenges for LGBT individuals maintaining abstinence. In the section that follows, we discuss relations between substance use and overall health in the context of different LGBT subcultures.

Syndemics

Ron Stall and colleagues have applied the concept of *syndemics* (6) to explain the development and effect of substance use and addictions, particularly on the health of GB men. The syndemic concept interprets substance use and SUD as part of an interconnected web of health concerns that collectively affect health more negatively than any individual element of the syndemic. According to syndemic theory, intertwining epidemics of substance use, HIV, other sexually transmitted infections (STIs), depression, childhood abuse, and sexual compulsivity sustain poor health outcomes among GB men (7), likely exacerbated by minority stress (8,9) originating from the effect of societal homophobia, violence victimization, and other marginalization experiences (10). Syndemic effects may be greatest among LGBT individuals who are persons of color, so-called double minorities (11).

For clinicians, this implies that focusing intervention on one or a few aspects of the syndemic—say a SUD—is likely to be insufficient because GB men who receive treatment for a SUD may become substance abstinent yet continue to face health risks due to other syndemic conditions (e.g., mental illness, childhood abuse, discrimination, victimization, or internalized homophobia [11]). The related concept of *intersectionality* describes how different social statuses, such as "African-American bisexual woman," may intersect to produce challenges that are qualitatively distinct, for example, from those experienced by heterosexual African Americans, bisexual men, or Latina women (12). Attending to syndemics and intersectionality reminds us that patients may face multiple reinforcing challenges simultaneously. Treatment of addiction needs to address internalized or institutionalized homophobia or transphobia. A well-adjusted LGBT person in recovery from addiction will need to develop satisfying social networks that are not centered on bars and clubs. An LGBT person of color may have greater difficulties in accessing culturally appropriate, non-substance-involved LGBT-specific resources, simply because fewer of these venues are probably available.

Personal Resilience

Despite the potential challenges of addiction and related syndemic conditions, many LGBT individuals have learned to manage some or all of these with resiliency. Much of the literature on SUDs and mental health issues in LGBT populations before the 1980s pathologized homosexuality; research since then has often focused on pathologic aspects of same-sex sexuality as mediators of risk for HIV infection and STIs (13). Nonetheless, most LGBT persons do not have SUDs or HIV infection despite greater potential exposures to both. LGBT communities have shown strength in mobilizing against social discrimination, addiction, and HIV/AIDS. LGBT cultures can buffer against sexual minority stress (14) and foster healthier perspectives toward substance use. The process of coming out often aids in developing skills in self-awareness and in communication, with corresponding benefits that include a secure sense of self and access to networks of social support (15): friends, partners, ex-lovers, and others that can be as supportive as close-knit families of origin (16).

Cultural Resilience

It is also important to attend to changes over the lifespan and cultural changes experienced by successive generations of LGBT individuals regarding substance use (17). Ritch Savin-Williams and others have documented the resilience and successful adjustment of many contemporary LGBT youth and have critiqued the existing literature for focusing on subgroups that are most likely to be experiencing problems, such as clinical populations or those attending LGBT youth drop-in centers (18). Qualitative and mixed-methods studies suggest that the social context and developmental experiences of LGBT persons in Western countries since the 1960s have been changing with each cohort, such that LGBT persons born in different decades or coming out at different ages face very different sets of challenges and resources (19,20). The systematic study of resilience and psychosocial strengths among LGBT populations, particularly relevant to substance use, is still in its infancy. A symposium convened at Fenway Health in 2011 summarized understandings of how resilience offers supportive coping for syndemic conditions, including substance use, and identified key areas for future study. These include shamelessness (comfort and pride in one's sexual orientation, identity, and gender expression), adaptability, social bonding and relationship-building, queer family-building, and connection to an LGBT community (21).

Substance Use, Substance Use Disorder

Perceptions of a unique vulnerability among LGBT individuals to addiction or misuse of alcohol and other intoxicating substances likely stem from early views in psychiatry that homosexuality itself was a marker or result of mental illness (22) and clinical experience in which LGBT persons seeking therapy were likely to have an SUD (23,24). These impressions were reinforced by early studies that found an SUD in about a third of LGBT persons surveyed (25). However, these studies were based on convenience samples, often from settings that served alcohol (e.g., gay bars). Better definitions of SUD, better sampling frames, and better survey methods have yielded estimates of prevalence among LGBT persons closer to those in the general population (26). Nonetheless, as discussed below, some LGBT populations experience elevated risk for SUD and may also be at greater risk for exposure to HIV, hepatitis B and C viruses, and other STI pathogens.

It is important for clinicians not to pathologize their LGBT patients by attributing all substance-related problems to their sexual and/or gender identities. LGBT individuals use intoxicating substances for many of the same reasons as heterosexuals. Nonetheless, the use of substances can also take on unique functions for LGBT individuals, such as helping cope with stigma, discrimination, and other prejudices. Alcohol and cigarettes have historically been highly prevalent in LGBT social settings. LGBT-friendly bars (along with bathhouses) were historically among the few social institutions open to LGBT persons. More recently, stimulants, nitrite poppers, and the so-called club drugs have been a significant aspect of the "dance party" or "circuit party" scene, described below. The slang terms "to party," "party & play," or simply "PnP" have come to signify sexual encounters under the influence of drugs—particularly stimulants, dissociatives/hallucinogens (e.g., phencyclidine [PCP], lysergic acid diethylamide [LSD]), poppers, and empathogens like MDMA, which all reduce inhibitions and enhance the sexual experience (4). This is doubly problematic. First, the decreased inhibitions and increased stamina (with stimulants) may predispose to sexual behaviors with high risks for HIV infection and other STIs (27). Second, the incorporation of drug-altered consciousness with extreme sexual experiences in a context of facilitated community can be powerful and mutually reinforcing. Intense emotional linkages among drug use, sex, and experience of community can complicate efforts to become substance abstinent. Sexual or emotional intimacy may be seen as a trigger for drug use, and there may be no opportunities for drug-free experiences of similarly intense emotional connections.

Classifying Substance Use Disorders

During the 1980s, a consensus emerged in classification systems on distinguishing between addictions with and without evidence of physiologic dependence (28). The fourth edition of the American Psychiatric Association's *Diagnostic and Statistical Manual of Mental Disorders*, (29) and World Health Organization's International Classification of Diseases, 10th Revision (ICD-10) (30), codified this as a distinction between *abuse* (or *harmful use,*

F.1x.1 in ICD-10), designating a pattern of significantly problematic behavior and health problems related to use of a substance, versus *substance dependence*, a syndrome of adverse psychosocial or physical consequences in conjunction with physiologic dependence. Dependence is evidenced by *tolerance*, experiencing reduced intoxicating effects from a given dose or requiring a higher dose to achieve the same intoxicating effects, and *withdrawal*, a distinctive pattern of physiologic responses to the discontinuation of a substance. Neither occasional use nor temporary intoxication is sufficient to merit either diagnosis. The concept of *at-risk use* has been advanced to designate behavior that does not yet meet criteria for abuse or dependence but may elevate one's risk for abuse or dependence. Men who consume more than 4 drinks per day or more than 14 drinks per week and women who consume more than 3 drinks per day or more than 12 drinks per week are considered to be at elevated risk to develop a SUD (31).

The abuse/dependence distinction failed to resolve some conceptual problems, however. For one, abuse is not a milder form of dependence, though it is often perceived as such. One may meet criteria for physiologic dependence along with cravings but still not meet full criteria for the problematic behaviors that define abuse. Controversy has long existed over whether there is a clinically meaningful distinction between physiologic dependence and "psychological dependence," as both present problems. Some drugs, such as hallucinogens and nitrite inhalants, are used intermittently rather than chronically and lack defined withdrawal syndromes. Cannabinoid withdrawal has only recently been widely recognized. In response, the new fifth edition of the *Diagnostic and Statistical Manual of Mental Disorders* (32) collapses the criteria defining abuse and dependence into a single *substance use disorder* with a rating for severity and adds "craving or a strong desire to use" (Table 10-1).

Commonly Used Substances

The sections that follow provide information about the substances and the effects they produce. As this guide may be used in many primary care or general mental health settings that are not primarily oriented toward assessment and treatment of SUD, we briefly discuss some technical information that may not be familiar to providers in these settings. A brief overview of mechanisms is given in Table 10-2; for more detailed consideration, clinicians should consult a guide such as *Principles of Addiction Medicine* (33) from the American Society of Addiction Medicine (ASAM).

Alcohol

One of the oldest and most widely used intoxicating substances, alcohol (ethyl alcohol or ethanol) is legally available for adult use throughout the

Table 10–1   Criteria for Abuse, Dependence, and Substance Use Disorder

DSM-IV-TR	DSM-5
Abuse	*SUD*
A pattern of substance use leading to *significant impairment or distress*, as manifested by 1 or more of the following *within a 12-month period:*	A pattern of substance use leading to *significant impairment or distress*, as manifested by 2 or more of the following *within a 12-month period:*
1. Failure to fulfill major role obligations (work, school, home), such as repeated absences or poor work performance related to substance use; substance-related absences, suspensions, or expulsions from school; neglect of children or household	Severity of the substance use disorder is defined by the number of criteria endorsed, with 2–3 criteria endorsed being a mild SUD; 4–5 criteria endorsed being a moderate SUD; and 6+ criteria endorsed being a severe SUD
2. Frequent use of substances in situations that are physically hazardous (e.g., driving automobile, operating machinery under the influence)	1. Tolerance or markedly increased amounts of the substance to achieve intoxication or desired effect or markedly diminished effect with continued use of the same amount of substance
3. Frequent legal problems (e.g., arrests, disorderly conduct) for substance abuse	2. Withdrawal symptoms or the use of substances to avoid withdrawal
4. Continued use despite having persistent social or interpersonal problems (e.g., arguments about consequences of intoxication)	3. Use of a substance in larger amounts or over a longer period than was intended
Dependence	4. Persistent desire or unsuccessful efforts to cut down or control substance use
A maladaptive pattern of use leading to *significant impairment or distress*, as manifested by 3 or more of the following *occurring during the same 12-month period:*	5. Involvement in chronic behavior to obtain the substance, use the substance, or recover from its effects
1. Tolerance or markedly increased amounts of the substance to achieve intoxication or desired effect or markedly diminished effect with continued use of the same amount of substance	6. Reduction or abandonment of social, occupational or recreational activities because of substance use
2. Withdrawal symptoms or the use of substances to avoid withdrawal	7. Use of substances even though there are persistent or recurrent physical or psychological problems that are likely to have been caused or exacerbated by the substance
3. Use of a substance in larger amounts or over a longer period than was intended	8. Craving or a strong desire or urge to use a substance
4. Persistent desire or unsuccessful efforts to cut down or control substance use	9. Failure to fulfill major role obligations (work, school, home), such as repeated absences or poor work performance related to substance use; substance-related absences, suspensions, or expulsions from school; neglect of children or household

(continued)

Table 10-1   Criteria for Abuse, Dependence, and Substance Use Disorder (*Continued*)

DSM-IV-TR	*DSM-5*
5. Involvement in chronic behavior to obtain the substance, use the substance, or recover from its effects 6. Reduction or abandonment of social, occupational or recreational activities because of substance use 7. Use of substances even though there is a persistent or recurrent physical or psychological problem that is likely to have been caused or exacerbated by the substance	10. Frequent use of substances in situations that are physically hazardous (e.g., driving automobile, operating machinery under the influence) 11. Continued use despite having persistent social or interpersonal problems (e.g., arguments about consequences of intoxication)

*Criteria for abuse and dependence from fourth edition of *Diagnostic and Statistical Manual of Mental Disorders* (*DSM-IV-TR*). Criteria for substance use disorder from fifth edition of *DSM* (*DSM-5*).

SUD = substance use disorder.

United States and in most parts of the world. Alcohol is embedded in many social interactions, although it has particular significance in some LGBT subcultures. As discussed earlier, for decades "gay" bars were the only place for LGBT people to meet and socialize. Early political organizing for LGBT rights and mobilizing against HIV often occurred in and around bars and clubs (34). LGBT-friendly bars remain among the most visible and accessible LGBT institutions and are still a common point of entry and socialization in LGBT cultures.

Alcohol acts synergistically with other central nervous system (CNS) depressants, particularly benzodiazepines, barbiturates, opiates, and GHB, with risk for coma, respiratory suppression, and death. Alcohol and cocaine are often abused together, forming coca-ethylene, which may enhance cocaine's euphoria while decreasing alcohol's sedation, but likely with increased cardiotoxicity (35). Alcohol itself is uniquely hepatotoxic and interacts with hepatotoxins, such as acetaminophen, to increase risk for liver damage. This presents a risk to individuals who may treat a hangover with medications containing acetaminophen, such as Vicodin or Tylenol PM. Excessive alcohol consumption remains a leading cause of cirrhosis worldwide (36).

The withdrawal syndrome for alcohol, along with other CNS depressants such as benzodiazepines and GHB, is among the few that are potentially lethal. Heavy-using alcoholic patients should therefore be detoxified only under medical supervision. Withdrawal may begin up to 72 hours after the last ingestion of alcohol. Early symptoms are subjective anxiety, elevated heart rate and blood pressure, and increased perspiration, which may progress to tremulousness, hallucinations (delirium tremens or "DTs"), seizure, and sometimes death.

Table 10–2 Mechanisms and Effects of Substances of Abuse

Substance	Mechanism	Intoxication Symptoms	Withdrawal Symptoms
Ethanol, ethyl alcohol	↑ GABA$_A$ inhibition, blocks NMDA excitation	↓ Anxiety, disinhibits, impairs memory, impairs coordination, ↓ respiratory drive	↑ Anxiety, ↑ heart rate, tremors, risk of seizure
Benzodiazepines	↑ Frequency of GABA channel opening	↓ Anxiety, disinhibits, impairs memory, impairs coordination, interacts with other depressants	↑ Anxiety, ↑ heart rate, tremors, risk of seizure
GHB	GHB receptors	Euphoria, dizziness, ↑ salivation, hypotonia, amnesia; overdose: seizures, coma, death	↑ Anxiety, ↑ heart rate, tremors, risk of seizure
Cocaine	blocks DAT, NAT , SERT	↑ Heart rate, ↑ temperature, ↑ blood pressure, euphoria, disinhibition, ↑ anxiety, mydriasis, ↓ appetite	Fatigue, hypersomnolence, depressed mood, ↑ appetite
Amphetamine, methamphetamine	Blocks DAT, increases DA release	↑ Heart rate, ↑ temperature, ↑ blood pressure, euphoria, disinhibition, ↑ anxiety, mydriasis, ↓ appetite; lasts longer than equivalent amount of cocaine	Fatigue, hypersomnolence, depressed mood, ↑ appetite
Khat (*Catba edulis*, cathinones, "bath salts")	Triggers presynaptic DA release	Loss of appetite, irritability, insomnia, hallucinations, ↑ anxiety, panic attacks, hyperverbal, mydriasis	Fatigue, hypersomnolence, depressed mood, ↑ appetite
Opiates	Agonist at μ-opioid receptors, also at δ and κ receptors	↓ pain, ↓ GI motility, constipation, nausea, miosis	↑ GI motility, diarrhea, nausea, piloerection

(continued)

Table 10–2   Mechanisms and Effects of Substances of Abuse (Continued)

Substance	Mechanism	Intoxication Symptoms	Withdrawal Symptoms
Ketamine ("special K")	NMDA receptor antagonist; increases DAT, NAT, SERT	K-hole: black-out/"out of body experience" K-cramps: abdominal cramps	Nausea, dizziness, diarrhea, mental confusion
MDMA (Ecstasy, "molly")	Blocks NAT>DAT>SERT MAO-I; ↑ADH	Euphoria, entactogen (desire for physical contact), ↑ perspiration, ↑ temperature, ↑ heart rate	Dysphoria, lethargy
Cannabis (marijuana) delta-9-tetrahydrocannabinol, cannabidiol	CB_1 partial agonist CB_1 antagonist partial agonist at $5HT_{1A}$	Euphoria, relaxation, intensified sensory experiences, cognitive impairment, delayed reaction time, vasodilation, ↑ appetite	Withdrawal seen only with very heavy use; insomnia, irritability, ↓ appetite
Nitrite inhalants, poppers: amyl, butyl, isobutyl, isopentyl, and isopropyl nitrites	Nitric oxide, also known as endothelium-derived relaxing factor, is synthesized endogenously from L-arginine, oxygen and NADPH by nitric oxide synthases	Relaxes smooth muscles, especially blood vessel walls and anal sphincter; vasodilation leads to ↓ blood pressure, headache, flushing, lightheadedness, reactive ↑ heart rate; ↑ intraocular pressure, contraindicated in glaucoma; overdose: nausea, vomiting, hypotension, hypoventilation, dyspnea, syncope	No defined withdrawal symptoms; headache common after use

ADH = antidiuretic hormone; DA = dopamine; DAT = dopamine transporter; GABA = gamma-aminobutyric acid; GHB = gamma hydroxybutyrate; GI = gastrointestinal; MAO-I = monoamine oxidase inhibitor; NADPH = nicotinamide adenine dinucleotide phosphate-oxidase; NAT = norepinephrine transporter; NMDA = noncompetitive N-methyl-D-aspartate; SERT = serotonin transporter.

Benzodiazepines and Other CNS Depressants

Benzodiazepines, a class of synthetic molecules that enhance the inhibitory effects of the neurotransmitter gamma-aminobutyric acid (GABA), are used medically as sedatives, anxiolytics, and anticonvulsants. Benzodiazepines have amnestic effects, both acutely preventing encoding of memory (contributing to "blackout" states) (37), and causing diffuse, though reversible, memory problems in chronic users (38,39). In general, the main clinical differences relate to half-life, with greater abuse potential and dependence seen in shorter-acting benzodiazepines. Benzodiazepines such as flunitrazepam (Rohypnol or "roofies") have been used for their amnestic, sedating, and disinhibiting effects as date-rape drugs—surreptitiously slipped into a drink or given under false pretenses to make someone more likely to acquiesce to sexual intercourse or to forget it afterward.

GHB

Commonly included among club drugs, GHB ("G," "liquid Ecstasy" [see Table 10-3 for slang terms and their definitions]) occurs naturally in the body as a neurotransmitter. It acts on specific GHB receptors as well as having indirect effects at $GABA_B$ receptors that resemble those of benzodiazepines (40). While tightly regulated, GHB is legal in the United States to treat narcolepsy. Metabolic precursors of GHB such as gamma-butyrolactone and 1,4-butanediol may be purchased over the Internet. Bodybuilders and GB men involved in the gym culture sometimes take GHB or its precursors in hopes of enhancing muscle mass, as it increases endogenous release of human growth hormone. GHB has also been used by GB men at circuit parties and to enhance sexual experiences, reportedly by decreasing inhibitions. Physical tolerance and dependence can develop rapidly.

Opiate and Opioid Narcotics

Natural opiates, such as morphine, are derivatives of the resin of the opium poppy, which has been used in Europe and Asia since antiquity to treat pain. Various opiates are used medically for pain, for cough suppression, or as antidiarrheals. Codeine and heroin are semisynthetic opiates. Synthetic opioids, such as hydrocodone (in Vicodin and Norco), oxycodone (in extended-release OxyContin), and hydromorphone (Dilaudid), can cause seizures in overdose. Opioid compounds such as Vicodin and Percocet that contain acetaminophen can be unintentionally lethal if opioid-tolerant persons take high doses for the opioid effect without realizing the danger of acetaminophen poisoning.

All opioids have similar qualities in intoxication and withdrawal, differing mainly in their speed of onset and duration. Intoxication is characterized by feelings of euphoria, analgesia, sedation, constricted pupils (miosis), and

Table 10–3   Common Drug-Related Slang in LGBT Contexts

Slang	Definition
Crystal, Tina, Tina Turner, clouds, blowing clouds, broken windows, glass, ice, shards, shit, stuff, mojo, go-fast, peanut butter, candy	Terms for methamphetamine
Cri-cri, chispique	Spanish language terms for methamphetamine
Pookie, glass dick	Pipe used to smoke methamphetamine
Pinga, pipa	Spanish language for methamphetamine pipe
Chasing (the) dragon	Smoking methamphetamine or heroin from foil
Hot rail	Methamphetamine or cocaine placed on a creased sheet of foil with flame underneath; vapor inhaled with a straw
K-hole	Ketamine blackout
Booty bump, butt shot, turkey basting	Use of methamphetamine or another substance, typically administered rectally for fast absorption, to enhance sexual experience
Alkie	Booty bump with alcohol
Champagne douche	Methamphetamine dissolved in champagne with contents administered anally
Orange caps, needle nose, to the point	Injecting, or looking to inject
Tina and her evil sister	Tina = methamphetamine Evil sister = ketamine
420, 4:20, 4/20, or 420-friendly	Used in personal ads by individuals looking to party with marijuana
Trail mix	Mixture of club drugs usually with cocaine or methamphetamine as the base
Gacked, tweaked, tweaking, twacked, up in the attic	Really high on stimulants, usually methamphetamine
Bullet	Refers to getting high very quickly
Rush, jungle juice, other brand names	Nitrite inhalant "poppers"
Party and play, party, PnP	Using methamphetamines or other drugs in the context of sex.
Party favors, favors, favs	Drugs to use for PnP with stimulants, including erectile dysfunction drugs.
Peeking, peeping	Drug-induced paranoia
Disco me	Slang term used when a situation goes wrong involving drugs (e.g., "She discoed me" could mean "She sold me poor quality of drugs" or "she got me very high to take advantage of me.")

suppression of hunger and libido. Constipation is common with even short-term use, and long-term use can suppress normal cycling of sex hormones (hypogonadism), causing infertility. At high doses and when opiates are combined with alcohol or other sedatives, respiration is suppressed, sometimes causing death. Withdrawal is characterized by increased sensitivity to pain, yawning, piloerection ("goose bumps"), rhinorrhea, diarrhea, diaphoresis, and agitation. Unlike withdrawal from alcohol and benzodiazepines, withdrawal from opiates is not life-threatening in otherwise healthy individuals; however, it is extremely uncomfortable and often motivates those in withdrawal to return to opiate use for immediate relief.

Heroin and other injected opiates carry the most significant long-term risks, both from sharing needles that can transmit HIV and hepatitis B and C viruses, and from overdose. Taking opiates together with stimulants, such as cocaine or amphetamines, is called a "speedball." Among other effects, the combination may result in administering higher than usual doses of opiates. The stimulant usually has a briefer physiologic effect, which may wear off and leave the user with a potentially lethal dose of opiate still in their system. LGBT persons appear to use injected heroin at much lower rates than other populations (41), although they use prescription opiate analgesics at similar levels (42).

Marijuana

Various parts and derivatives of the *Cannabis* plant have been smoked or eaten as intoxicants for millennia. Marijuana is the most common illicit drug used in the United States and worldwide (43). As of 2014, "medical" use of marijuana was approved by 23 states and the District of Columbia, with the states of Washington and Colorado having entirely decriminalized marijuana possession and use in 2012. Currently there are no formal guidelines for medical marijuana use. Patients who use marijuana medically mention its capacity for reducing nausea and vomiting (including that associated with AIDS-related gastrointestinal infections and antiretroviral medications, and from chemotherapy), increasing appetite, and dampening chronic pain, such as HIV-related neuropathy, or muscle spasticity (44). Marijuana is commonly used among individuals with anxiety and insomnia, although among those with anxiety disorders, marijuana use may worsen symptoms related to social functioning and mental health (45).

Cannabinoid withdrawal has only recently been recognized as a clinical phenomenon (46). Heavy marijuana use among adolescents has been associated with precipitating psychotic syndromes, which may persist even after discontinuing marijuana use. An uncommon but serious risk of smoking marijuana for persons with HIV infection or other immune compromise is aspergillosis, a potentially lethal fungal infection (47,48). The *Aspergillus fumigatus* mold is widespread in the environment and is generally harmless; however, high doses of spores from smoking infected cannabis plants can develop into a potentially lethal fungal infection in immune-compromised persons.

Cocaine

Cocaine is a potent stimulant derived from the leaves of the Andean coca plant, *Erythroxylum coca*. While cocaine can be injected, it is more commonly insufflated ("snorted") in powder form, often with the aid of a straw or a tube made of rolled paper. Freebase cocaine ("crack"), which has been combined with an alkali to facilitate absorption, is most commonly vaporized in a glass pipe and inhaled, with very rapid onset and offset of effects. The subjective effects of cocaine are quite similar to those of other stimulants. Larger or repeated doses may cause anxiety, paranoia, hallucinations, tremors, and muscle spasms, with individual effects being highly variable. Cocaine is cardiotoxic, particularly in combination with alcohol; long-term use can cause arrhythmias and myocardial infarction.

Indirect evidence suggests that blood-borne diseases such as hepatitis B and C may be transmitted via shared coke straws (49), but there is currently no clear data to assess the likelihood of HIV transmission by this means. More reliably demonstrated are the ways in which cocaine is associated with significantly elevated rates of unprotected anal sex and heightened risks for HIV transmission among GB men, particularly among GB men of color (50). Trans women and GB men with stimulant dependence may be motivated to exchange sex for drugs. In this situation, they may feel less able to insist on safer sex practices, particularly if they receive higher compensation for unprotected intercourse or are disinhibited while using or in withdrawal.

Amphetamine-Type Stimulants

Amphetamine, methamphetamine, and several related drugs collectively called *amphetamine-type stimulants* are synthetic substances that share chemical structures with dopamine. They act as potent stimulants with subjective and physiologic effects similar to those of cocaine, but typically with a longer duration. Amphetamine-type stimulants (ATS) can be snorted as a powder, smoked, inhaled in a freebase form (crystal methamphetamine), inserted anally ("booty bump"), or injected. Methamphetamine in particular has been increasingly associated with risky sexual behaviors (51,52). It has displaced cocaine in many populations, including white and Latino GB men, because its longer half-life (more than 9 to 12 hours) provides much longer subjective effect from a single dose than for a similarly priced amount of cocaine.

Several ATS are approved for medical use in narcolepsy and attention-deficit/hyperactivity disorder (ADHD). Methylphenidate (Ritalin, Concerta), dextroamphetamine (Dexedrine, Benzedrine), and mixed amphetamine salts (Adderall) are among the best known. Since the 1990s, concern has grown over possible diversion of these medications for recreational use (53). This must be balanced clinically against a growing awareness of the complications of untreated ADHD—including elevated risk for SUD (54).

Club Drugs

MDMA is chemically related to amphetamine, has a short half-life (1 to 2 hours), and has distinct subjective effects, particularly empathogenic properties that facilitate subjective feelings of closeness to others, accounting for its popularity at raves and circuit parties. Long-term use of MDMA and some closely related compounds has been associated with neurotoxic effects. More acutely, individuals taking MDMA in the context of a circuit party may experience dehydration (related to continued dancing or moving about without rehydrating), hyponatremia (from excessive water intake because of fear of dehydration, without repleting electrolytes), bruxism (grinding teeth), and sexual disinhibition (with corresponding incident HIV infection/STIs). While MDMA is colloquially known as "Ecstasy" or "E," in practice Ecstasy purchased from dealers may contain anything from caffeine to methamphetamine. Any given dose of so-called Ecstasy may carry the risks for adverse effects of substances quite unlike MDMA.

Hallucinogens

Ketamine ("K," "Special K") is a synthetic chemical that is medically classed as a dissociative anesthetic. It is most commonly used in veterinary medicine, and most illicitly used ketamine in the United States is diverted from veterinary suppliers. Ketamine is commonly used at the circuit party and rave scenes. Subjective effects last about an hour and may include derealization or hallucinations, sometimes called a "K-hole." Other potential adverse effects include abdominal cramps ("K-cramps") and inflammation of the bladder and urinary tract that can occur with long-term use, sometimes causing incontinence. Ketamine can be insufflated or injected intravenously.

Various hallucinogens such as psilocybin mushrooms, mescaline, LSD, *Salvia divinorum*, dextromethorphan, and others may be used occasionally by GB men in conjunction with other club drugs or marijuana. Besides their use with other club drugs, there does not appear to be an LGBT-specific use of hallucinogens.

Alkyl Nitrites (Poppers)

Amyl nitrite is used medically to alleviate angina and to treat acute cyanide poisoning. It causes production of nitric oxide (NO) in endothelial cells of blood vessels, acting as a local vasodilator. Initially produced in glass ampules that were broken or "popped" and the vapors inhaled, it became popular as a club drug among both heterosexual and LGBT club-goers during the 1970s. Since the end of the disco era, poppers have been used predominantly by GB men. Amyl nitrite has been illegal to sell without a prescription in the United States since 1988, but congeners including cyclohexyl nitrite, butyl nitrite, isobutyl nitrite, and isopropyl nitrite are sold over the counter in "head shops" and sex shops under a number of brand names as "room odorizer" or "videohead cleaner." Poppers are typically sold in small bottles of dark glass to slow the breakdown of the nitrites from exposure to light and are administered by inhaling or sniffing from the bottle. Subjective effects last a few minutes per inhalation include warmth, mild to substantial behavioral disinhibition, and relaxation of muscles including anal sphincter muscles. For this last reason, they are commonly used as an adjunct to anal sex (55). Use of poppers was once implicated as a specific risk factor for HIV/AIDS, but consensus now sees them primarily as a marker for other risk behaviors.

The common health problems from popper use are largely related to the solvent in which the nitrites are suspended, which can cause chemical burns if spilled or inhaled. Poppers can also cause headaches, trigger migraines, and temporarily impair erectile function. Poppers can cause clinically significant hemolysis or rupture of red blood cells among some persons with a genetic illness called G6PD deficiency, more common in those with ancestry in the Mediterranean, Southeast Asia, and sub-Saharan Africa, including about 10% of African Americans (56). Although rare, visual changes ranging from temporary bright spots in the visual field (phosphenes) to permanent retinal damage have been reported with chronic use.

Many addiction texts group alkyl nitrites with other inhalants; however, most of these others are organic solvents or propellants that are inhaled after being poured or sprayed onto a rag ("huffing") or into a bag ("bagging"). They act in fairly nonspecific ways to produce a "high" through some combination of hypoxia (by displacing air from the lungs) and generalized disruption of neuronal transmission. Potential consequences of inhalant use include arrhythmias, liver and kidney damage, and cognitive impairment. In the last few years, some non-nitrite inhalants have been marketed as a "new kind of poppers" that are huffed rather than inhaled from a bottle. Because many clinicians do not recognize the difference between alkyl nitrite poppers and other inhalants, and because other inhalants have not commonly been used by American GB men, there is the possibility that GB men could use the potentially much more dangerous non-nitrite inhalants without realizing it.

Pro-erectile Drugs

Sildenafil, tadalafil, and vardenafil act by inhibiting phosphodiesterase type 5 (PDE-5) and thereby increasing blood flow to a number of body parts, which can enhance erectile function in males. The first of these to be approved by the U.S. Food and Drug Administration, sildenafil (Viagra), has been available by prescription since 1998 for treatment of erectile dysfunction.

Among GB men in particular, PDE-5 inhibitors have been used to overcome the negative effects of stimulants or depressants on male erections. This practice has been implicated in risk behavior for HIV infection and other STIs by promoting continuing sexual activity while in a disinhibited state (57). The PDE-5 inhibitors were initially developed to lower blood pressure and can have catastrophic effects if combined with potent vasodilators, such as nitrite inhalants. PDE-5 inhibitors are frequently integrated with stimulant use among GB men in order to ensure erectile adequacy for long sex sessions; the tablets are sometimes even included with paper invitations for selected sex parties.

Sex Hormones

Sex hormones are natural or synthetic androgens (testosterone and other male hormones), estrogens, and progesterones, taken to enhance or alter secondary sexual physiognomy and sexual function. All sex hormones are steroids. Estrogens and progesterone are readily available in pill forms, often as oral contraceptives. Some forms of testosterone are available in a topical gel, but many are administered as either depot or immediate-release injections. Illicit use of injected sex hormones carries the same risks of other injection drugs if needles are shared or reused: transmission of blood-borne pathogens like HIV and hepatitis B and C viruses, or local infections with skin flora, such as methicillin-resistant *Staphylococcus aureus*.

Exogenously administered sex hormones have 4 main uses in an LGBT context: androgen supplementation for treatment of HIV-related hypogonadism and wasting in men, attempts by GB men to gain a more muscular physique from bodybuilding with anabolic steroids, use by trans women to achieve or maintain female secondary sexual characteristics, and use by trans men to achieve or maintain male secondary sexual characteristics.

Androgen Supplementation: Hypogonadism and Bodybuilding

Some gay and bisexual men misuse exogenous androgens to accelerate development of muscle mass (when integrated with intense physical workouts), to increase energy, and/or to counter reductions in natural androgen production due to aging or HIV-related issues. Deleterious effects of exogenous androgens include acne, cholestatic jaundice, dyslipidemia (particularly increased low-density lipoprotein cholesterol levels), gynecomastia, testicular atrophy, mood instability (58), and cardiovascular problems (59).

Hormone Supplementation in Transgender Persons

Trans women may take estrogens or estrogens and progesterones as part of the process of feminizing their physical characteristics to better match their gender identity. For reasons of cost or difficulty in accessing medical care, some purchase these over the Internet or other illicit sources, often in the form of oral contraceptives. In the presence of functioning testes, trans women may take estrogens up to several times normal physiologic doses. Estrogens promote blood clotting and raise the risk for stroke, myocardial infarction, and pulmonary embolism; this is greatly exacerbated in tobacco smokers. Sudden discontinuation of high-dose estrogens produces symptoms similar to menopause: hot flashes, mood swings, diaphoresis, and dysphoria.

Trans men may take testosterone ("T") as part of the process of masculinizing their bodies to match their gender identity. In addition to the virilizing effects (lowering voice, growing body and facial hair in a male pattern, amenorrhea, and increasing muscle mass), exogenous androgens can cause the effects noted above, including male pattern baldness, acne, and mood swings.

Transgender persons who no longer have functioning ovaries or testes— whether due to surgical removal or the effects of exogenous hormones— need to take lifelong sex hormone supplementation. This is not only to maintain their appearance in matching their gender identity but also to protect against wasting and loss of muscle mass, cardiac problems, and osteoporosis. It is important that their care be managed by competent clinicians. See Chapters 17 and 18 for more on the care of transgender persons.

Emerging Trends in Substance Use and New Drugs of Abuse

Shifting patterns of substance use and the ways in which they are used continue to present new concerns and potential health consequences, particularly among GB men. New compounds are being derived from parent substances of abuse, altered sufficiently to avoid laws on drug possession and distribution. Their use is on the rise.

Synthetic Cannabis

Synthetic cannabinoids are made in liquid form, then sprayed onto dried plant materials that are packaged and sold in head shops and over the Internet as "spice," "synthetic marijuana," "K-2," and "herbal incense." The dried plant materials are smoked, resulting in an acute rush/high favored by youth and adults, particularly those who know they will be drug tested (many agencies do not yet test urine samples for synthetic cannabis and the drug is not identified by standard cannabis tests).

Cathinone

Khat, *Catha edulis*, is a plant native to East Africa and the Arabian Peninsula that has been used for centuries as a mild stimulant. Its most active alkaloid, cathinone, is chemically unstable and breaks down quickly once the plant is harvested. In recent years a number of synthetic derivatives of cathinone have become available. Circulating primarily as club drugs, they have also been sold under the names "bath salts," "herbal ecstasy," and other names (55).

Current Epidemiology

In understanding estimates of SUD among LGBT individuals, it is important to recognize that substance use in the United States is normative. In 2012, 22.2 million or 8.5% of U.S. persons older than age 12 years met criteria for substance abuse or dependence during the preceding year (60). The most common substance of abuse was marijuana, followed by nonprescription use of opiates and stimulants (60). Recognizing that substance use and addiction are common phenomena in general can reduce biases among clinicians who work with LGBT individuals.

Lesbians and Bisexual Women

In a recent review of epidemiologic studies published between 2000 and 2009 on the prevalence of SUD among LGBT persons (26), 6 of 8 studies on substance use and SUD found that LB women had significantly higher rates of alcohol use; 4 of the 8 reported higher rates of alcohol use disorders compared with rates in heterosexual women; and 2 studies found no differences. Rates of drug use and drug use disorders were more complex. Six of 7 studies reported higher rates of use of at least 1 drug or drug class (marijuana, club drugs, cocaine) among LB women as compared with heterosexual women, but findings were inconsistent across studies. Of 3 studies that reported on drug use disorder diagnoses, LB women had a higher prevalence than heterosexual women, but differences in sampling and methods preclude making broad generalizations about SUD in LB women.

In the National Epidemiological Survey on Alcohol and Related Conditions (NESARC) (n = 34,653), women who identified as LB reported significantly higher rates of alcohol use, alcohol dependence, and other drug dependence compared with women who identified as heterosexuals (Table 10-4) (61,62). Yet it is important to remember that despite higher prevalence rates, most LB women did not report substance use and did not meet criteria for dependence in the past year (61). In a probability sample of 2272 Californians, women who reported a lesbian or bisexual sexual identity had a threefold greater risk for likely alcohol dependence disorder compared with heterosexual women. In contrast to the NESARC sample, having a lesbian sexual identity in the California sample did not significantly raise relative risks for a likely drug dependency disorder compared to heterosexual women (63).

Among youth, rates of substance use are higher among LB girls than heterosexual girls. In a meta-analysis of 18 studies of substance use prevalence in LB youth, odds of substance (combined alcohol and drug) use were tripled or quadrupled for LB youth compared with heterosexually identified youth (64). Two large representational samples of female youth replicated this finding, particularly for cigarette smoking and alcohol use among LB young women (65,66). Although adolescence is a developmental period marked for

Table 10-4   Lifetime and Past Year Prevalence of Alcohol and Drug Use Disorders in the National Epidemiological Survey of Alcohol and Related Conditions by Reported Sexual Identities ($n = 34,653$)

Variable	Lifetime (%)			Past Year (%)		
Females*	Alcohol Use Disorder	Drug Use Disorder	Heavy Drinking	Alcohol Use Disorder	Other Drug Use	Drug Use Disorder
Lesbian	58.6[†]	24.5[†]	20.1	13.3[†]	12.6[†]	5.7[‡]
Bisexual	53.5[†]	40.4[†]	25.0[‡]	15.6[†]	14.1[†]	3.0[‡]
Heterosexual	22.0	8.0	8.4	2.5	3.1	0.4
Males[§]						
Gay	58.7	32.7[†]	18.1	16.8[†]	16.8[†]	3.2[‡]
Bisexual	52.1	25.0[‖]	16.4	19.5[†]	17.7[†]	5.1[‡]
Heterosexual	47.7	15.7	13.7	6.1	4.5	0.5

For lifetime, data obtained from reference 62. For past year, data obtained from reference 61.

*Comparisons are between lesbian/bisexual and heterosexual females.

[†]$P < 0.001$.[‡]$P < 0.05$.

[§]Comparisons are between gay/bisexual and heterosexual males.

[‖]$P < 0.01$.

many by sexual and substance use exploration, these rates are remarkable and suggest that these experiences may be linked to escaping stigma, discrimination, bullying, and other experiences all too common for LB youth.

Limited data exist to describe treatment experiences among LB women, but one study found that among 69,525 individuals admitted to publicly funded substance abuse treatment programs in Washington State, identifying as lesbian significantly correlated with having a co-occurring psychiatric condition, though it had no association with completion of treatment compared with heterosexually identified women (67).

Gay and Bisexual Men

Among GB men, a similarly complex picture emerges regarding prevalence of substance use and addiction. In a review of 13 studies published between 2000 and 2009 (26), no consistent pattern of results was identified to distinguish different rates of substance use for GB men compared with heterosexually identified men. A landmark study of 2184 GB men interviewed by telephone and living in ZIP codes populated by GB men in 4 U.S. cities (68), GB men reported high rates of alcohol use (87.7%), marijuana (42.4%), poppers (19.8%), cocaine (15.2%), Ecstasy/MDMA (11.7%), ATS (9.5%), and "downers" (8.8%) in the prior 6 months compared with household survey data. The prevalence of tobacco smoking among GB men (31.4%) was higher than among heterosexual men (24.7%) (69). Similar high rates of substance use (not misuse) by GB men were reported in a Chicago household survey (70).

In the NESARC, men who identified as GB had higher rates of lifetime drug use disorders than did heterosexually identified males (Table 10-4), with no differences in alcohol use disorders (62). The past year prevalence of any SUD was higher for men who identified as GB than for heterosexual men (61). Most GB men in the sample, however, neither used substances nor met criteria for any SUD. In a probability sample of 2272 Californians, GB men had more than double the risk for a probable alcohol dependence disorder in the past year compared with heterosexual men, although the rates of probable drug dependency disorders did not differ by type of sexual orientation or behavior (63). As with LB young women, substance use is higher among GB young men than heterosexual youth, but the association is not as strong as that observed among young LB women, particularly regarding alcohol use (64,66).

In sum, while there is moderate agreement in epidemiologic reports showing higher prevalence of alcohol use and alcohol use disorders among LGB individuals (more so for young LGB persons), the overall picture of substance use is complex. Prevalence reports of substance use vary by whether respondents are queried according to their identity (as an LGB person), to their sexual attraction to people of the same gender, or to having had sexual experiences with people of the same gender. Additionally, identified rates of substance use and SUD also vary substantially across different kinds of venues. Significantly higher percentages of GB men interviewed at bars and clubs reported recent cocaine use and more frequent alcohol drinking compared with GB men interviewed at bathhouses or on Internet-based dating venues such as Craigslist; more GB men at bathhouses reported recent use of erectile dysfunction drugs than those at bars and clubs or on Craigslist (71). In addition, rates of substance use change over time among GB men. For example, according to street-based surveys of GB men in both Los Angeles during 1999–2007 (72) and in New York during 2002–2007 (73), alcohol was the most consistently reported substance used (~90%), with reported use of all substances, including marijuana and ATS, decreasing throughout the period.

Transgender Individuals

The stigma and discrimination faced by transgender individuals can be overwhelming and may contribute to the higher rates of alcohol and other substance use reported in this group, especially as many trans women engage in sex work for basic survival needs. In what stands as the best systematic review of substance use and other HIV risk behaviors among trans women (74), estimated means for substance use combined across 13 studies were 26.7% for crack/other illicit drug use, 43.7% for alcohol use, and 20.2% for marijuana use. Trans women also reported high rates of drug injection across 16 studies, particularly for street drugs (12.0%), hormones (27.0%), and silicone (24.7%), with relatively few reporting needle sharing when injecting street drugs (2.0%) or hormones/silicone (6.0%). A study of trans women recruited on the streets and from high-risk venues (e.g., bars, clubs) in Los Angeles ($n = 2136$) from 2005 to 2011 found substance use to be common (75), with the rate of methamphetamine use (22%) similar to that reported by GB men; however, alcohol (58%) and marijuana (26%) use were both lower than that reported by GB men in Los Angeles (76). Fewer studies were available for trans men, but it was estimated that 13.7% reported problems with alcohol and other substances, which is relatively low (74).

Sex and Substance Use: Special Considerations

Discussions of drug and alcohol use among LGBT persons have focused on intoxication as a mediator of sexual risk behaviors in relation to HIV and other STIs, although interpretation of the relationship between substance use and concomitant sex remains complex. Most studies rely on correlational data showing that use of illicit drugs (particularly methamphetamine and poppers) among GB men is associated with sexual risk behaviors (77) or with being HIV-infected (78). These associations have been documented among GB men from most minority ethnic/racial groups, including African Americans (79), Latinos (80) and Asian Pacific Islanders (81). Yet there is a methodologic problem: Studies frequently test global measures of substance use with global measures of sexual risk behaviors, while failing to assess the question of whether substance use is interrelated with high-risk sexual behaviors. Some prospective studies that ask about instances of substance use proximal to high-risk sexual behaviors have suggested that some GB men will engage in certain sexual behaviors regardless of substance use (82), while others have suggested that substance use may be a form of self-medication to alleviate anxiety around high-risk sex, such as "barebacking" (having intentional or planned anal sex without a condom) (83).

Notwithstanding caveats about the issue of causality, substance use in the context of sex or of seeking sexual partners marks potentially high-risk behavior in relation to HIV and other STI transmission. In particular, there is a robust association between use of ATS, cocaine, and/or poppers, with HIV transmission (78,84). Subjectively, many users of stimulants, club drugs, and poppers report increased libido, decreased anxiety, and increased sexual pleasure (including access to extreme sexual behaviors) that are possible only when using these drugs. Some users report increased anxiety, while long-term use can cause erectile dysfunction (85). Colloquially called "crystal dick," this is now commonly treated with erectile dysfunction medications, which are also associated with riskier sexual behavior (41).

A particular phenomenon among GB men has been the "circuit" of large, elaborate events called "circuit parties." Typically lasting several days over a long weekend, these events comprise round-the-clock festivities in multiple locations in a given city in the United States or internationally. Some parties draw thousands of attendees, mostly men in their 20s to 40s, who may travel long distances to experience the event. Use of stimulants and club drugs is common at circuit parties.

While some date the origins of the party circuit to gay events of the 1970s, the contemporary circuit largely developed over the course of the 1990s at the height of the AIDS epidemic. It has been described by some commentators as a reaction to and defiance of the fear of AIDS, as well as a celebration of LGBT communities (4). Attendance at circuit parties has declined over the last decade, for unclear reasons. While the circuit scene only involves a subgroup of GB men in Western countries, it is significant both for its symbolic position within gay subcultures and for the high rates of substance use and STI transmission among attendees.

What To Do? Evidence-Supported Recommendations to Providers

In this section, we review assessments for substance use and addiction, from self-report to biomarkers. Evidence-based recommendations for screening techniques and brief interventions are presented. We then list resources and guidance for referrals and conclude with a review of the evidence-based treatments for SUDs.

Screening, Brief Intervention, Referral to Treatment

The most important step in addressing substance use in patients in general care settings is simply to ask about it. An emerging consensus advises primary care and mental health providers to incorporate assessment of substance use behaviors into their practice at regular intervals. Normalizing inquiries about substance use as part of ongoing basic health assessment reduces potential defensiveness on the part of the patient and recognizes that prevalence of substance use is normative for all Americans. Periodic reassessment is useful. Patients may feel more comfortable discussing substance use as they develop a relationship with a provider; patterns of substance use may change over time.

The emerging model for primary care providers is called SBIRT: Screening, Brief Intervention, and Referral to Treatment. SBIRT involves using brief screening questions to query possible substance use problems, more standardized measures to assess likely severity if present, and brief interventions combining psycho-education with motivational techniques. SBIRT can substantially reduce self-reported drug and alcohol use when implemented in general care settings. If SUDs appear to be present and severe, or if they do not respond to brief interventions, then referral to an addiction or dual diagnosis specialist is indicated (86).

Screening tools with strong psychometric ratings for identifying substance use problems in general settings are described in Table 10-5. For alcohol use,

Table 10–5 Validated Screening Instruments for Substance Use Disorders

Measure (Reference)	Length/Time	Utility/Metrics	Item Examples
CAGE (71)	4 questions 1 min	Screening clinical populations for alcohol abuse Cutoff score: 2 Sensitivity: 0.78 Specificity: 0.81	1. Have you ever felt you should cut down on your drinking? 2. Have people annoyed you by criticizing your drinking? 3. Have you ever felt bad or guilty about your drinking? 4. Have you ever had a drink first thing in the morning to steady your nerves or get rid of a hang-over (eye-opener)?
Alcohol, Smoking, and Substance Involvement Screening Tool (WHO ASSIST) and NIDA-modified ASSIST (72)	10 questions 5–15 min depending on responses	Screening in primary care for problem use of alcohol, tobacco and other substances Cutoff score: 14.5 Sensitivity: 0.80 Specificity: 0.71	1. Reported ever and past 3 mo use of tobacco, alcohol, marijuana, cocaine/crack, amphetamine-methamphetamine, inhalants, sedatives/sleeping pills, hallucinogens, opioids 1a. EVER injected drugs? 2. For each drug used in the past 3 mo: • How often have you used the drug? • How often have you had an urge to use the drug? • How often has your drug use led to health, social, legal, or financial problems? • How often have you failed to do what is normally expected of you due to your use of the drug? • Has a friend or relative or anyone else expressed concern about your use of the drug? • Have you tried and failed to control, cut down or stop using your drug? WHO ASSIST available at: www.who.int/substance_abuse/activities/assist/en/index.html NIDA Modified ASSIST: www.drugabuse.gov/nmassist/ (continued)

Table 10–5   Validated Screening Instruments for Substance Use Disorders *(Continued)*

Measure (Reference)	Length/Time	Utility/Metrics	Item Examples
Current Opioid Misuse Measure (COMM) (74)	17 behavioral items with 5-point Likert scales for responses. 10 min	Screening for potential opioid abuse (aberrant behaviors) in patients with chronic pain Cutoff score: 9 Sensitivity: 0.77 Specificity: 0.66	Available at: www.inflexxion.com/COMM
Alcohol Use Disorders Identification Test (AUDIT) (73)	10 multiple-choice questions with behavioral responses; 2–5 min	Alcohol screening to identify patients who are hazardous drinkers or have active alcohol use disorders Cutoff score: 9 Sensitivity: 0.88 Specificity: 0.87	Measure available at: http://whqlibdoc.who.int/2001/who_msd_msb_01.6a.pdf
Alcohol Use Disorders Identification Test-C (AUDIT-C) (73)	First 3 questions from the AUDIT 1–2 min	Brief alcohol screening to identify patients who are hazardous drinkers or have active alcohol use disorders Cutoff score: 6 Sensitivity: 0.90 Specificity: 0.83	1. How often do you have a drink containing alcohol? 2. How many standard drinks containing alcohol do you have on a typical day? 3. How often do you have 6 or more drinks on 1 occasion?
Alcohol Use Disorders Identification Test-3 (AUDIT-3) (73)	The third multiple-choice question on the AUDIT 30 sec	Very brief alcohol screening to identify patients who are hazardous drinkers. Cutoff score: 2 Sensitivity: 0.84 Specificity: 0.84	How often do you have 6 or more drinks on 1 occasion?

this includes the CAGE (87) and the Alcohol Use Disorders Identification Test (AUDIT) (88). Broader substance use involvement can be assessed using the Alcohol, Smoking and Substance Involvement Screening Test (ASSIST) (89). The Current Opioid Misuse Measure (COMM) (90) is a validated measure designed to detect opioid misuse, the leading cause of accidental deaths among adults. See also Chapter 8 for strategies on interviewing patients about substance use and abuse in the primary care setting and Chapter 9 for information on assessing and addressing substance use in mental health care settings.

Biomarkers

No reliable biomarkers conclusively diagnose SUD. Abnormal results on liver function tests, particularly aspartate aminotransferase (AST), alanine aminotransferase (ALT), and gamma-glutamyltransferase (GGT), suggest heavy drinking in the absence of viral hepatitis or other medical conditions. Reliable biomarkers of recent substance use include testing of urine, breath, hair, and blood samples for the presence of the substances or their metabolites. Tests range in method, cost, and specificity from radioimmune assays (portable, fast, and reliable enough for most clinical purposes) to spectroscopy methods that can be moderate to expensive in cost and can meet scrutiny required for forensic purposes.

Limitations related to the use of biomarkers for substance use in health care settings relate to the short time it takes the body to completely excrete the substance and its metabolites. Alcohol has the shortest window of detection at 12 hours or less. Urine screens of other drugs can detect use during the preceding 48 to 72 hours for cocaine (including crack), amphetamine, methamphetamine, MDMA, most opiates, and a single use of cannabis. The following drugs can be detected over longer intervals: benzodiazepines (3 to 7 days), phencyclidine (8 days), methadone (7 to 9 days), and heavy use of cannabis (3 to 21 days) (91).

When using a biomarker with a patient, it is important to anticipate how to respond to a positive result. In most instances, a positive biomarker result will lead to a discussion between the provider and the patient on the type and extent of substance use. It is not appropriate to refer all people who provide drug-positive samples to treatment. In drug treatment settings, however, use of biomarkers is considered standard of care, as one or more positive urine drug screens describes a treatment approach that is insufficient to reach the patient's goals. Self-reports of substance use are often sufficient for assessing drug use within general care settings (92,93). Clinicians should inquire about lifetime, past year, and past month (recent use) for each substance.

Brief Interventions

Brief interventions have long been used by clinicians with remarkable success when advising patients whom they suspect of hazardous alcohol use to

Table 10–6   Brief Interventions Using the 5 A's and 5 R's

Ask	...about smoking, now, and lifetime	Relevance	Encourage the patient to indicate why quitting is personally relevant
Advise	...it is your medical/professional opinion that the person quit now or in the next 30 days	Risks	Ask the patient to identify potential negative consequences of tobacco use
Assess	...if the person is willing to quit (now/next 30 days) using clear, personalized messages	Rewards	Ask the patient to identify potential benefits of stopping tobacco use
Assist	...in quitting by providing brief intervention or referring to available resources (e.g., pharmacotherapy, behavioral support, telephone quit lines)	Roadblocks	Ask the patient to identify barriers or impediments to quitting
Arrange	...follow-up and support by scheduling check-in with the person in the next 30 days to see how things are going	Repetition	For smokers who were unsuccessful with a quit attempt, advise that most fail multiple quit attempts before quitting for good. Encourage the patient to try again!

"knock it off." Brief interventions also have been used with success in reducing tobacco smoking. Table 10–6 presents the 5 A's, an effective way of screening and conducting brief intervention on tobacco smoking status in primary care settings (94). A parallel set of brief interventions are used for smokers who tried to quit and failed (the 5 R's). Both sets of interventions can be easily adapted to address other SUDs and as a way to encourage consideration of more intensive treatment. A range of evidence-based programs have been modified to address problems in quitting specific to LGBT persons. Many of these are available at the website of the National LGBT Tobacco Control Network (www.lgbttobacco.org/resources.php).

Treatment

Referring LGBT individuals to treatment raises challenges, as most providers would prefer culturally competent therapists and agencies that not only deliver evidence-based treatments but also recognize LGBT-specific concerns. Yet, some evidence shows mainstream providers rarely discuss issues related to sexual and/or gender identity with their LGBT clients, even though they believe these to be important (95,96), nor do they discuss concerns related to legal and family issues that can affect treatment, including gay marriage (and divorce), domestic partnership, power of attorney, and issues related to family of origin and one's current family. Discrimination may be common among mainstream SUD counselors, with about half admitting negative or ambivalent attitudes toward LGBT clients (95–97). Finally, only a minority of agencies outside major cities provide specialized addiction services for LGBT clients (98). A manual published in 2001 provides guidelines for tailoring SUD treatment approaches specifically for GLBT clients (www.nalgap.org/PDF/Resources/ProvidersGuide-SAMSHA.pdf).

While the goal for treatments of SUD is to increase the individual's ability to inhibit impulses for getting and using substances, the central underlying psychological construct for SUD is ambivalence. Most individuals with SUD have 2 opposing thoughts about their use of substances, often held simultaneously: It is a problem, and it is not a problem. Even after years of abstinence, ambivalence toward substance use often remains unresolved. For many, the inability to control substance use requires sustained abstinence during treatment and afterward as their goal. A few are able to return to controlled levels of use through techniques such as moderation management (99,100), although this carries controversy in the treatment community and potential risks for patients. Data are consistent in not recommending return to alcohol or marijuana use following a formal treatment episode, as this is often is a first step toward relapse.

Considerations When Referring Individuals to Treatment

The American Society of Addiction Medicine has published consensus criteria to match patient needs with appropriate levels of care for SUD treatment. These consider the severity of current substance use, need for medically supervised detoxification if actively using and at risk of withdrawal, and the presence and type of comorbid psychiatric disorders (*dual diagnosis*). Patients who require medical care will need facilities that can provide it, such as a licensed medical detox facility or an inpatient setting. Most programs treating SUDs are not equipped to optimally treat patients with active psychiatric illnesses other than mild to moderate depression and anxiety. Patients with comorbid bipolar disorder, ADHD, severe anxiety disorders, or psychotic disorders need medication management or management by a psychiatrist.

Pharmacotherapies

Pharmacotherapies are approved by the Food and Drug Administration for treatment of alcohol, nicotine, and opioid dependence (Table 10-7). There are no pharmacologic treatments for stimulants, cannabis, or hallucinogen use disorders. Behavioral interventions comprise individual and group psychotherapies as well as support groups and are effective alone or can enhance efficacy of pharmacologic interventions. This is perhaps best demonstrated for nicotine-replacement therapies for smoking cessation (101) and opioid-agonist maintenance therapies (102).

Table 10–7   U.S. Food and Drug Administration–Approved Medications for Substance Use Disorders

Drug/Medication	Mechanism	Efficacy/Limitations
Opioids		
Methadone	Full agonist–replacement	Very effective, but can only be dispensed from licensed clinics. Needs daily or near-daily visit to clinic for observed dosing. Impractical for full-time employed. More effective in conjunction with behavioral therapies.
Buprenorphine	Partial agonist–replacement	Effective, useful in patients who cannot attend narcotic treatment clinics. Can be prescribed in outpatient settings with refills. Requires special waiver for prescribing physician. More effective in conjunction with behavioral therapies.
Naltrexone	Full antagonist–relapse prevention	Requires motivated patient; impractical in patients with chronic pain because of opiate blockade.
Nicotine		
NRT: lozenges, gum, patch, spray	Full agonist–replacement	High acceptability; different modalities largely dependent on patient preference. NRT is tapered off over weeks, but some patients continue for months. Original recommendation was full nicotine withdrawal before starting; now clinicians start NRT 1–2 days before full cessation to ensure steady state.
Varenicline	Partial agonist at $\alpha_4\beta_2$ nicotine receptors and competitive antagonist with nicotine	Highly effective in clinical trials. Can cause nausea. Not recommended in combination with nicotine replacement. Since 2008, FDA warning for risk for suicidal thoughts.
Bupropion (Zyban)	Unknown, but presumed increase in dopamine	Effective, though less so than varenicline. May be maintained indefinitely, especially in patient with comorbid depression or ADHD.

(continued)

Table 10-7   U.S. Food and Drug Administration–Approved Medications for Substance Use Disorders (*Continued*)

Drug/Medication	Mechanism	Efficacy/Limitations
Alcohol		
Disulfiram	Blocks metabolism of acetaldehyde by acetaldehyde dehydrogenase; causes severe nausea and vomiting ("Antabuse reaction")	Effective in motivated patients. Needs to be taken daily; can be skipped if patient plans to drink alcohol.
Acamprosate	Unknown	More effective in European trials; may be more useful in daily drinkers than binge drinkers. FDA approved for abstinent drinkers who are engaged in a behavioral intervention.
Naltrexone–oral	Opiate antagonist, presumed decrease in reward of alcohol	Reduces frequency and amount of binge drinking; most useful in highly motivated patients. Needs to be taken daily; adherence often is poor. Risk for hepatotoxicity.
Naltrexone–depot injection		Administered by injection every 2–3 weeks.

ADHD = attention-deficit/hyperactivity disorder; FDA = Food and Drug Administration; NRT = nicotine replacement therapy.

Pharmacologic treatment of SUDs falls into 3 broad categories: *Agonist or partial-agonist therapy* has been very successful. Methadone is a synthetic full μ-opioid agonist that can be prescribed for chronic pain as a Schedule II medication. It can also be dispensed from federally licensed clinics for opioid maintenance therapy, usually with daily, directly observed administration. Buprenorphine is a partial-agonist at mu-receptors; this has the benefit that almost no patients escalate their dose above 24 mg per day. One formulation combines buprenorphine with the opiate blocker naloxone to reduce risk for abuse, as any route of administration other than sublingual absorption (such as injection) will introduce the opiate blocker and precipitate opiate withdrawal. Pure buprenorphine is also available for patients in whom naloxone is contraindicated.

Nicotine replacement therapy is available as lozenges, gum, and transdermal patches. Varenicline, an agonist on a particular nicotine receptor subtype, can also be effective in smoking cessation. Both opioid and nicotine replacement therapies are more effective in conjunction with behavioral interventions. Multiple attempts have been made to find a viable agonist or partial-agonist therapy for stimulants, depressants, and cannabinoids, but so far without success.

Antagonist therapy involves regular administration of a medication that blocks the effects of a substance. Examples include the use of opiate blockers for opiates. Treating alcohol addiction with disulfiram (Antabuse) may be considered a variation on this. Ethanol is normally converted in the body to acetaldehyde and then to acetic acid. Disulfiram blocks the enzyme acetaldehyde dehydrogenase and causes a rapid buildup of the toxic chemical acetaldehyde, with usual effects of severe nausea and vomiting. Current attempts to develop vaccines for substances such as cocaine and nicotine are a variation on this strategy, although again without successful results as yet.

A third strategy is medications that seem to *reduce the reinforcing effects* of substances, often through unclear mechanisms. Naltrexone, an opiate-blocker, is available in oral or long-acting injection for alcohol dependence. In clinical trials it reduces frequency and intensity of binge drinking. Acamprosate helps with cravings and maintaining abstinence in alcohol dependence through an unclear mechanism, possibly antagonism at NMDA receptors and agonism at GABA receptors. It has performed better in European trials than in the United States (103). Like most of the pharmacotherapies, acamprosate works best in context of psychosocial support.

Bupropion, an antidepressant that blocks dopamine reuptake, has been effective in trials for smoking cessation. It has shown inconsistent benefits in clinical trials for stimulant dependence, but may have utility as a harm-reduction strategy. Bupropion and mirtazapine have been evaluated as treatments for stimulant use disorders in randomized, placebo-controlled trials among GB men in San Francisco. One of these studies found statistically significant reductions in methamphetamine use and concomitant high-risk sexual behaviors in a 12-week trial of mirtazapine at 30 mg daily (104). Replication of this finding is underway, but initial results are encouraging.

Behavioral Therapies

Evidence-based behavioral therapies for treating SUD are from 3 broad areas: cognitive behavioral therapy (CBT), motivational interviewing, and contingency management (again, these are not specific to LGBT populations; see Table 10-8). In addition, the table describes community-based self-help approaches, including 12-step (e.g., Alcoholics Anonymous, Narcotics Anonymous) and SMART Recovery groups.

Cognitive Behavioral Therapy

CBT approaches are didactic: teaching skills and information necessary to initiate abstinence and prevent relapse. Techniques are closely related to CBT used for major depressive disorders. Meta-analyses show CBT has small but significant effects in reducing substance use compared to standard of care (105). CBT shows few effects when compared with low-intensity interventions for amphetamine-dependent individuals but substantial benefit when compared with high-intensity interventions among GB men (106). CBT requires trained therapists when delivering the intervention. The model is easily adapted to incorporate cultural or behavioral specifics that can enhance acceptability. One example of this is "Getting Off," a behavioral intervention for GB men who use methamphetamine (107). The adaptation of this model began with a mainstream CBT approach to stimulant dependence, called the Matrix Model. Using a consultative approach, it was tailored to retain key CBT elements while integrating cultural and behavioral referents to enhance its acceptability. In this treatment approach, links among methamphetamine use, concomitant sexual risk behaviors, and HIV were addressed. Effects in reductions in methamphetamine and high-risk sexual behaviors were demonstrated for up to 1 year (108).

Motivational Interviewing

Motivational Interviewing is a client-centered, directive approach to treatment that helps clinicians identify the factors that work for ("pros") and against ("cons") continued substance use (109). Program materials often involve a balance (or scale) that asks patients to reconcile the pros and cons of substance use to understand their contributions to the ambivalence that supports use or abstinence. Therapists provide information that relates to the patient's substance use so the individual can accurately perceive their use of substances compared to national (household survey, National Institutes of Health) and local (convenience samples) data. Techniques to deliver motivational interviewing include OARS-E: open-ended questions, affirmations, reflective listening, summarizing, and eliciting "change talk" (client statements that recognize the need for change). In meta-analyses, motivational

Table 10-8   Efficacious Behavioral Therapies for Substance Use Disorders

Therapy	Approach/Skills

Cognitive behavioral therapy	• Based on social learning model
	• Substance use problems are a result of learning experiences and cognitive beliefs
	• Teaches skills and presents education to help patients establish abstinence and avoid relapse:
	  • Encourage and reinforce behavior change
	  • Use structure and schedule to scaffold return to premorbid functioning
	  • Recognize and avoid high-risk settings and triggers (persons, places, things linked to drug use)
	  • Avoid abstinence violation effect
	  • Recognize thinking styles that support drug use and challenge these with new thinking
	  • Replace drug use with prosocial activities, especially moderately reinforcing social activities
	• Manual driven and available on-line; can be delivered in individual or group therapy settings

Contingency management	• Derived from operant conditioning; understands drug use as a learned behavior • Therapy provides positive reinforcement (in the forms of money or prizes) in exchange for proof of drug abstinence (biological samples that document abstinence) • Highly efficacious with stimulant use disorders • Often a part of community reinforcement approach
Motivational interviewing Motivational enhancement therapy	• Brief counseling model that conceptualizes the psychological foundation of addiction as ambivalence • Intervention techniques are client centered and exaggerate ambivalences that support continued drug use and drug abstinence; avoids confrontation • Designed for primary care settings • Values reductions in drug use as well as abstinence as treatment goals
Network therapy	• Mobilizes and enhances existing social support (family, friends, spouse, coworkers) for maintaining abstinence • Very low cost; family and friends may be available in hours when professionals are not • Often implemented in conjunction with individual therapy and/or 12-step

(continued)

Table 10-8   Efficacious Behavioral Therapies for Substance Use Disorders (*Continued*)

Therapy	Approach/Skills
12-step (e.g., Alcoholics Anonymous, Narcotics Anonymous, Crystal Meth Anonymous)	• Not actually a therapy, but is a worldwide mutual-help group program that uses a structured 12-step approach to helping addicts and alcoholics establish and maintain sobriety • Highly effective as meetings are free and occur many times and places during the week • Groups for specific subgroups, such as LGBT individuals or specific substance users, are available • All groups organized and run by addicts/alcoholics (i.e., there are no professionals responsible for the groups)
12-Step Facilitation Therapy	• An individual therapy designed to facilitate use of 12-step support groups • Efficacious for use with alcoholic patients and among patients who find 12-step groups helpful
SMART Recovery: Self-Management and Recovery Training	• A secular alternative to 12-step programs • Draws on principles from cognitive behavioral therapy and 12-step • Attendance is donation-based, can be free.

LGBT-specific resources available at www.nalgap.org/.

interviewing produced 29% reduction in substance use compared to standard care (110). Meta-analyses of applications of motivational interviewing to substance use problems among GB men, however, showed no consistent findings (111).

Contingency Management

Contingency management is based on operant conditioning. Clients earn increasingly valuable reinforcers with consecutive biological samples (such as urine drug screens) that document abstinence. It remains one of the most effective forms of treatment for cocaine and amphetamine use disorders; meta-analyses show that contingency management has an effect size of about 0.6 (i.e., it is 60% better) compared with usual treatments (112). Contingency management can be easily incorporated with other standard substance use therapies, particularly CBT. One example is Azrin's Community Reinforcement Approach, which integrates community supports and resources (e.g., employers) into the delivery of the reinforcements.

Contingency management has been used with GB male methamphetamine users, alone and in combination with CBT, to significantly reduce drug use at 1-year follow-up evaluations (107). Lower-cost CM treatments also are effective for treating methamphetamine dependence among GB men (108). Despite strong efficacy, some complain that providing financial incentives to addicted individuals who achieve abstinence using the therapy is simply paying them to do what they should do anyway. There also appear to be limits for contingency management solely as a treatment for SUD because it shows no significant effects when implemented in public health settings in non–treatment-seeking, stimulant-using GB men (113).

Conclusions

At the intersection of substance use, addiction, and related conditions that affect the health of LGBT individuals, clinicians are challenged to understand the meanings of behaviors in clinical contexts that determine how to intervene in a culturally competent and caring fashion. Not all LGBT substance users need treatment, although some do; this requires cultural competence on the part of the clinician to understand the unique place substances occupy historically and currently in the lives of LGBT patients. Still, given the comparatively high prevalence of substance use and SUD among LGBT populations, an evidence-based approach should involve SBIRT for those who screen positive for potential problem use of substances. Recognizing the impact of syndemics, it is also appropriate to screen for comorbid mental illnesses or other trauma conditions when screening for SUDs and to treat or refer them appropriately. Culturally tailoring treatment responses can improve retention and acceptability for LGBT clients; behavioral and medical treatments for SUD work as well as but not better than treatments of SUD in other populations.

Summary Points

- Until very recently, individuals who engaged in same-sex romantic and sexual relationships, whether or not they self-identified as lesbian, gay, or bisexual, often experienced stress from threats to personal safety, to restrictions of rights and freedoms, and to being pathologized. Many of these threats have lessened, to some degree, particularly in major metropolitan areas. Transgender individuals, however, still disproportionately face these threats. This situation provides foundational contexts for understanding the role of substance use in the lives of LGBT individuals:
  - Some LGBT individuals use substances to medicate stress related to being a minority; these stresses are enhanced for LGBT individuals who also are members of racial/ethnic minority groups.
  - Substance use and SUD are interconnected with other threats to the health of LGBT individuals; focusing prevention and treatment only on substances will have poor outcomes because of the syndemic nature of substance use and concurrent health threats.
  - The historical role of substances in facilitating safety and familiarity in social and cultural contexts for LGBT individuals complicates understanding substance use and SUD. This role also complicates identifying

valued substance-free alternatives for LGBT individuals who complete substance use treatment and adopt abstinence as a goal.

• In the United States, substance use is normative—particularly use of alcohol, tobacco, and (increasingly) marijuana. SUDs are marked by a pattern of substance use over a substantial period that causes biological (withdrawal, tolerance, craving), interpersonal/familial, or workplace, problems that invoke clinical distress.

• Epidemiologic studies show LGBT individuals have higher, but not dramatically higher, rates of substance use (especially for alcohol and tobacco) than heterosexual individuals; less consistency is observed regarding drug use disorders.

• Among GB men, substance use—particularly of stimulants, erectile dysfunction drugs and poppers—is linked to transmission of HIV and other STI pathogens. Trans women face risks for using substances associated with engaging in survival sex.

• Screening for SUD in general and sexually transmitted infection clinical settings is recommended. Validated, brief tools can be used for this purpose.

• For LGBT individuals who screen positive in general clinical settings for problem levels of substance use, brief interventions are appropriate.

• For individuals who merit referral to treatment, effective pharmacotherapies exist for those with alcohol, nicotine, and opiate use disorders.

• Effective behavioral therapies exist for SUD as monotherapy and for use in conjunction with pharmacotherapies.

Acknowledgments

The authors gratefully acknowledge support from the National Institute of Mental Health (P30 MH58107), the National Institute on Drug Abuse (T32 DA 24600), and the assistance of Ms. Julia De Palma.

References

1. **Norton R.** Mother Clap's molly house: the gay subculture in England, 1700-1830. East Haven, CT: GMP; 1992.

2. **Newton E.** Cherry Grove, Fire Island: Sixty Years in America's First Gay and Lesbian Town. Boston: Beacon Press; 1993.

3. **Kennedy EL, Davis MD.** Boots of Leather, Slippers of Gold: The History of a Lesbian Community. New York: Routledge; 1993.

4. **Race K.** Pleasure Consuming Medicine: The Queer Politics of Drugs. Raleigh, NC: Duke University Press; 2009.

5. **Cochran S, Grella C, Mays V.** Do substance use norms and perceived drug availability mediate sexual orientation differences in patterns of substance use? Results from the California Quality of Life Survey II. J Studies Alcohol Drugs. 2012;73:675-85.

6. **Singer M.** Introducing Syndemics: A Critical Systems Approach to Public and Community Health. New York: Wiley; 2009.

7. **Stall R, Friedman M, Catania JA.** Intersecting epidemics and gay men's health: a theory of syndemic production among urban gay men. In: Wolitski RJ, Stall R, Valdiserri RO, eds. Unequal Opportunity: Health Disparities Affecting Gay and Bisexual Men in the United States. New York: Oxford; 2008:251-74.

8. **Goffman E.** Stigma: Notes on the Management of Spoiled Identity. New York: Simon & Schuster; 1963.

9. **Steele CM.** The psychology of self-affirmation: sustaining the integrity of the self. Advances Exp Social Psychol. 1988;21:261-302.

10. **Meyer IH, Oullette SS, Haile R, McFarlane TA.** "We'd be free": narratives of life without homophobia, racism, or sexism. Sex Res Social Policy. 2011;8:204-14.

11. **Dyer TP, Shoptaw S, Guadamuz TE, et al.** Application of syndemic theory to black men who have sex with men in the Multicenter AIDS Cohort Study. J Urban Health. 2012;89:697-708.

12. **Crenshaw KW.** Mapping the margins: intersectionality, identity politics, and violence against women of color. Stanford Law Rev. 1991;43:1241-99.

13. **Herrick AL, Lim SH, Wei C, et al.** Resilience as an untapped resource in behavioral intervention design for gay men. AIDS Behav. 2011;15 Suppl 1:S25-9.

14. **D'Augelli AR.** Identity development and sexual orientation: toward a model of lesbian, gay, and bisexual development. In: Trickett, EJ, Watts RJ, Birman D, eds. Human Diversity: Perspectives on People in Context. The Jossey-Bass Social and Behavioral Science Series. San Francisco, CA: Jossey-Bass; 1994:312-33.

15. **Nardi PM.** Gay Men's Friendships: Invincible Communities. Chicago: University of Chicago Press; 1999.

16. **Weston K.** Families We Choose: Lesbians, Gays, Kinship. New York: Columbia University Press; 1991.

17. **Cohler BJ, Galatzer-Levy RM.** The Course of Gay and Lesbian Lives: Social and Psychoanalytic Perspectives. Chicago: University of Chicago Press; 2000.

18. **Savin-Williams RC.** A critique of research on sexual-minority youths. J Adolesc. 2001;24:5-13.

19. **Grierson J, Smith AMA.** In From the Outer: Generational Differences in Coming Out and Gay Identity Formation. J Homosexual. 2005;50:53-70.

20. **Hall TM.** Stories from the Second World: narratives of sexual identity across three generations of Czech men who have sex with men. In: Cohler BJ, Hammack PL, eds. The Story of Sexual Identity: Narrative Perspectives on the Gay and Lesbian Life Course. New York: Oxford University Press; 2009:77-130.

21. **Herrick AL, Stall R, Goldhammer H, Egan JE, Mayer KH.** Resilience as a research framework and as a cornerstone of prevention research for gay and bisexual men: theory and evidence. AIDS Behav. 2014;18:1-9.

22. **Lewes K.** Psychoanalysis and Male Homosexuality. 20th anniversary ed. Lanham, MD: J. Aronson; 2009.

23. **Nardi PM.** Alcoholism and homosexuality: a theoretical perspective. In: Ziebold TO, Mongeon JE, eds. Alcoholism and Homosexuality. New York: Haworth Press; 1982. p. 9-25.

24. **Lolli G.** Alcoholism and homosexuality in Tennessee Williams' "Cat on a Hot Tin Roof." Q J Studies Alcohol. 1956;17:543-53.

25. **Bux DA.** The epidemiology of problem drinking in gay men and lesbians: a critical review. Clin Psychol Rev. 1996;16:277-98.

26. **Green KE, Feinstein BA.** Substance use in lesbian, gay and bisexual populations: an update on empirical research and implications for treatment. Psychol Addictive Behav. 2012;26:265-78.

27. **Frosch D, Shoptaw S, Huber A, Rawson RA, Ling W.** Sexual HIV risk among gay and bisexual male methamphetamine abusers. J Subst Abuse Treat. 1996;13:483-6.

28. **Schuckit MA, Smith TL, Daeppen JB, et al.** Clinical relevance of the distinction between alcohol dependence with and without a physiological component. Am J Psychiatry. 1998;155:733-40.

29. **American Psychiatric Association.** Diagnostic and Statistical Manual of Mental Disorders. 4th ed. Washington, DC: American Psychiatric Association; 1994.
30. **World Health Organization.** The ICD-10 Classification of Mental and Behavioural Disorders: Clinical Descriptions and Diagnostic Guidelines. Geneva, Switzerland: World Health Organization; 1992.
31. **WHO ASSIST Working Group.** The Alcohol, Smoking and Substance Involvement Screening Test (ASSIST): development, reliability and feasibility. Addiction. 2002;97:1183-94.
32. **American Psychiatric Association.** Diagnostic and Statistical Manual of Mental Disorders. 5th ed. Washington, DC: American Psychiatric Association; 2013.
33. **Ries RK, Fiellin DA, Miller SC, Saitz R, eds.** Principles of Addiction Medicine. 4th ed. Philadelphia: Lippincott Williams & Wilkins; 2009.
34. **D'Emilio J.** Sexual Politics, Sexual Communities: The Making of a Homosexual Minority in the United States, 1940-1970. 2nd ed. Chicago: University of Chicago Press; 1998.
35. **Farre M, de la Torre R, Gonzalez ML, et al.** Cocaine and alcohol interactions in humans: neuroendocrine effects and cocaethylene metabolism. J Pharmacol Exp Therap. 1997;283:164-76.
36. **World Health Organization.** Global Status Report on Alcohol and Health. Geneva: World Health Organization; 2011.
37. **Fisher J, Hirshman E, Henthorn T, Arndt J, Passannante A.** Midazolam amnesia and short-term/working memory processes. Conscious Cogn. 2006;15:54-63.
38. **Vermeeren A, Coenen AM.** Effects of the use of hypnotics on cognition. Progr Brain Res. 2011; 190:89-103.
39. **Deckersbach T, Moshier SJ, Tuschen-Caffier B, Otto MW.** Memory dysfunction in panic disorder: an investigation of the role of chronic benzodiazepine use. Depress Anxiety. 2011; 28:999-1007.
40. **Schep LJ, Knudsen K, Slaughter RJ, Vale JA, Megarbane B.** The clinical toxicology of gamma-hydroxybutyrate, gamma-butyrolactone and 1, 4-butanediol. Clin Toxicol. 2012;50:458-70.
41. **Lea T, Mao L, Bath N, et al.** Injecting drug use among gay and bisexual men in Sydney: prevalence and associations with sexual risk practices and HIV and hepatitis C infection. AIDS Behavior. 2013;17:1344-51.
42. **Cochran SD, Ackerman D, Mays VM, Ross MW.** Prevalence of non-medical drug use and dependence among homosexually active men and women in the US population. Addiction. 2004; 99:989-98.
43. **United Nations Office on Drugs and Crime.** World Drug Report 2012. Geneva, Switzerland: United Nations, 2012.
44. **Leung L.** Cannabis and its derivatives: review of medical use. J Am Board Intern Med. 2011;24:452-62.
45. **Lev-Ran S, Le Foll B, McKenzie K, Rehm J.** Cannabis use and mental health-related quality of life among individuals with anxiety disorders. J Anxiety Disord. 2012;26:799-810.
46. **Gorelick DA, Levin KH, Copersino ML, et al.** Diagnostic criteria for cannabis withdrawal syndrome. Drug Alcohol Depend. 2012;123(1-3):141-7.
47. **Johnson TE, Casiano RR, Kronish JW, Tse DT, Meldrum M, Chang W.** Sino-orbital aspergillosis in acquired immunodeficiency syndrome. Arch Ophthalmol. 1999;117:57-64.
48. **Walsh TJ, Anaissie EJ, Denning DW, et al.** Treatment of aspergillosis: clinical practice guidelines of the Infectious Diseases Society of America. Clin Infect Dis. 2008;46:327-60.
49. **Aaron S, McMahon JM, Milano D, et al.** Intranasal transmission of hepatitis C virus: virological and clinical evidence. Clin Infect Dis. 2008;47:931-4.
50. **Tobin KE, German D, Spikes P, Patterson J, Latkin C.** A comparison of the social and sexual networks of crack-using and non-crack using African American men who have sex with men. J Urban Health. 2011;88:1052-62.
51. **Colfax G, Shoptaw S.** The methamphetamine epidemic: implications for HIV prevention and treatment. Curr HIV/AIDS Rep. 2005;2:194-9.
52. **Shoptaw S, Reback CJ.** Methamphetamine use and infectious disease-related behaviors in men who have sex with men: implications for interventions. Addiction. 2007;102 Suppl 1: 130-5.

53. **Repantis D, Schlattmann P, Laisney O, Heuser I.** Modafinil and methylphenidate for neuroenhancement in healthy individuals: a systematic review. Pharmacol Res. 2010;62:187-206.

54. **Perez de Los Cobos J, Sinol N, Perez V, Trujols J.** Pharmacological and clinical dilemmas of prescribing in co-morbid adult attention-deficit/hyperactivity disorder and addiction. Br J Clin Pharmacol. 2014;77:337-56.

55. **Romanelli F, Smith KM, Thornton AC, Pomeroy C.** Poppers: epidemiology and clinical management of inhaled nitrite abuse. Pharmacotherapy. 2004;24:69-78.

56. **Nkhoma ET, Poole C, Vannappagari V, Hall SA, Beutler E.** The global prevalence of glucose-6-phosphate dehydrogenase deficiency: a systematic review and meta-analysis. Blood Cells Mol Dis. 2009;42:267-78.

57. **Rosen RC, Catania JA, Ehrhardt AA, et al.** The Bolger conference on PDE-5 inhibition and HIV risk: implications for health policy and prevention. J Sex MedThe journal of sexual medicine. 2006;3:960-75; discussion 73-5.

58. **Lumia AR, McGinnis MY.** Impact of anabolic androgenic steroids on adolescent males. Physiol Behav. 2010;100:199-204.

59. **Angell P, Chester N, Green D, et al.** Anabolic steroids and cardiovascular risk. Sports Med. 2012;42:119-34.

60. **Substance Abuse and Mental Health Services Administration.** Results from the 2012 National Survey on Drug Use and Health: mental health detailed tables Rockville, MD: Center for Behavioral Health Statistics and Quality; 2013.

61. **McCabe SE, Hughes TL, Bostwick W, West BT, Boyd CJ.** Sexual orientation, substance use behaviors and substance dependence in the United States. Addiction. 2009;104:1333-45.

62. **McCabe SE, West BT, Hughes TL, Boyd CJ.** Sexual orientation and substance abuse treatment utilization in the United States: results from a national survey. J Subst Abuse Treat. 2013;44:4-12.

63. **Cochran SD, Mays VM.** Burden of psychiatric morbidity among lesbian, gay and bisexual individuals in the California Quality of Life Survey. J Abnormal Psychol. 2009;118:647-58.

64. **Marshal MP, Friedman MS, Stall R, et al.** Sexual orientation and adolescent substance use: a meta-analysis and methodological review. Addiction. 2008;103:546-56.

65. **Marshal MP, King KM, Stepp SD, et al.** Trajectories of alcohol and cigarette use among sexual minority and heterosexual girls. J Adolesc Health. 2012;50:97-9.

66. **Brewster KL, Tillman KH.** Sexual orientation and substance use among adolescents and young adults. Am J Public Health. 2012;102:1168-76.

67. **Lipsky S, Krupski A, Roy-Byrne P, et al.** Impact of sexual orientation and co-occurring disorders on chemical dependency treatment outcomes. J Studies Alcohol Drugs. 2012;73:401-12.

68. **Stall R, Paul JP, Greenwood G, et al.** Alcohol use, drug use and alcohol-related problems among men who have sex with men: the Urban Men's Health Study. Addiction. 2001;96:1589-601.

69. **Greenwood GL, Paul JP, Pollack LM, et al.** Tobacco use and cessation among a household-based sample of US urban men who have sex with men. Am J Public Health. 2005;95:145-51.

70. **Mackesy-Amiti ME, Fendrich M, Johnson TP.** Symptoms of substance dependence and risky sexual behavior in a probability sample of HIV-negative men who have sex with men in Chicago. Drug Alcohol Depend. 2010;110:38-43.

71. **Grov C.** HIV risk and substance use in men who have sex with men surveyed in bathhouses, bars/clubs and on Craigslist.org: venue of recruitment matters. AIDS Behav. 2012;16:807-17.

72. **Reback CJ, Shoptaw S, Grella CE.** Methamphetamine use trends among street-recruited gay and bisexual males, from 1999 to 2007. J Urban Health. 2008;85:874-9.

73. **Pantalone DW, Bimbi DS, Holder CA, Golub SA, Parsons JT.** Consistency and change in club drug use by sexual minority men in New York City, 2002 to 2007. Am J Public Health. 2010;100:1892-5.

74. **Herbst JH, Jacobs ED, Finlayson TJ, McKleroy VS, Neumann MS, Crepaz N; HIV/AIDS Prevention Research Synthesis Team.** Estimating HIV prevalence and risk behaviors of transgender persons in the United States: a systematic review. AIDS Behav. 2008;12:1-17.

75. **Reback CJ, Fletcher JB.** HIV prevalence, substance use, and sexual risk behaviors among transgender women recruited through outreach. AIDS Behav. 2014;18:1359-67.

76. **Reback CJ, Fletcher JB, Shoptaw S, Grella CE.** Methamphetamine and other substance use trends among street-recruited men who have sex with men, from 2008 to 2011. Drug Alcohol Depend. 2013;133:262-5.

77. **Rajasingham R, Mimiaga MJ, White JM, et al.** A systematic review of behavioral and treatment outcome studies among HIV-infected men who have sex with men who abuse crystal methamphetamine. AIDS Patient Care STD. 2012;26:36-52.

78. **Plankey MW, Ostrow DG, Stall R, et al.** The relationship between methamphetamine and popper use and risk of HIV seroconversion in the multicenter AIDS cohort study. J Acquir Immune Defic Syndr. 2007;45:85-92.

79. **Mimiaga MJ, Reisner SL, Fontaine YM, et al.** Walking the line: stimulant use during sex and HIV risk behavior among black urban MSM. Drug Alcohol Depend. 2010;110:30-7.

80. **Bedoya CA, Mimiaga MJ, Beauchamp G, Donnell D, Mayer KH, Safren SA.** Predictors of HIV transmission risk behavior and seroconversion among Latino men who have sex with men in Project EXPLORE. AIDS Behav. 2012;16:608-17.

81. **Operario D, Choi KH, Chu PL, et al.** Prevalence and correlates of substance use among young Asian Pacific Islander men who have sex with men. Prev Sci. 2006;7:19-29.

82. **Halkitis PN, Shrem MT, Martin FW.** Sexual behavior patterns of methamphetamine-using gay and bisexual men. Subst Use Misuse. 2005;40:703-19.

83. **Rhodes T.** Culture, drugs and unsafe sex: confusion about causation. Addiction. 1996;91: 753-8.

84. **Koblin BA, Husnik MJ, Colfax G, et al.** Risk factors for HIV infection among men who have sex with men. AIDS. 2006;20:731-9.

85. **Bell DS, Trethowan WH.** Amphetamine addiction and disturbed sexuality. Arch Gen Psychiatry. 1961;4:74-8.

86. **Madras BK, Compton WM, Avula D, Stegbauer T, Stein JB, Clark HW.** Screening, brief interventions, referral to treatment (SBIRT) for illicit drug and alcohol use at multiple healthcare sites: comparison at intake and 6 months later. Drug Alcohol Depend. 2009;99:280-95.

87. **Mayfield D, McLeod G, Hall P.** The CAGE questionnaire: validation of a new alcoholism screening instrument. Am J Psychiatry. 1974;131:1121-3.

88. **Meneses-Gaya C, Zuardi AW, Loureiro SR, et al.** Is the full version of the AUDIT really necessary? Study of the validity and internal construct of its abbreviated versions. Alcohol Clin Exp Res. 2010;34:1417-24.

89. **Humeniuk R, Ali R; WHO ASSIST Phase II Study Group.** Validation of the Alcohol, Smoking and Substance Involvement Screening Test (ASSIST) and pilot brief intervention: a technical report of phase II findings of the WHO ASSIST Project. Geneva: World Health Organization; 2006.

90. **Butler SF, Budman SH, Fernandez KC, et al.** Development and validation of the Current Opioid Misuse Measure. Pain. 2007;130(1-2):144-56.

91. **Moller M, Gareri J, Koren G.** A review of substance abuse monitoring in a social services context: a primer for child protection workers. Can J Clin Pharmacol. 2010;17:e177-e93.

92. **Fendrich M, Mackesy-Amiti ME, Johnson TP.** Validity of self-reported substance use in men who have sex with men: comparisons with a general population sample. Ann Epidemiol. 2008;18:752-9.

93. **Schiller MJ, Shumway M, Batki SL.** Utility of routine drug screening in a psychiatric emergency setting. Psychiatr Serv. 2000;51:474-8.

94. **Fiore MC, Jaén CR, Baker TB, et al.** Clinical Practice Guideline: Treating Tobacco Use and Dependence: 2008 Update. Rockville, MD: U.S. Department of Health and Human Services; 2008.

95. **Hellman RE, Stanton M, Lee J, Tytun A, Vachon R.** Treatment of homosexual alcoholics in government-funded agencies: provider training and attitudes. Hosp Commun Psychiatry. 1989; 40:1163-8.

96. **Eliason MJ, Hughes T.** Treatment counselor's attitudes about lesbian, gay, bisexual, and transgendered clients: urban vs. rural settings. Subst Use Misuse. 2004;39:625-44.

97. **Eliason MJ.** Substance abuse counselors' attitudes about lesbian, gay, bisexual, and transgender clients. J Subst Abuse. 2000;12:311-28.

98. **Cochran BN, Peavy KM, Robohm JS.** Do specialized services exist for LGBT individuals seeking treatment for substance misuse? A study of available treatment programs. Subst Use Misuse. 2007;42:161-76.

99. **Humphreys K, Klaw E.** Can targeting nondependent problem drinkers and providing Internet-based services expand access to assistance for alcohol problems? A study of the moderation management self-help/mutual aid organization. J Stud Alcohol. 2001;62:528-32.

100. **Kishline A.** Moderate Drinking: The Moderation Management Guide for People Who Want to Reduce Their Drinking. New York: Crown Trade Paperbacks; 1994.

101. **Stead LF, Lancaster T.** Combined pharmacotherapy and behavioural interventions for smoking cessation. Cochrane Database Syst Rev. 2012;10:CD008286.

102. **Amato L, Minozzi S, Davoli M, Vecchi S, Ferri M, Mayet S.** Psychosocial combined with agonist maintenance treatments versus agonist maintenance treatments alone for treatment of opioid dependence. Cochrane Database Syst Rev. 2004:CD004147.

103. **Yahn SL, Watterson LR, Olive MF.** Safety and efficacy of acamprosate for the treatment of alcohol dependence. Subst Abuse: Res Treat. 2013;6:1-12.

104. **Colfax GN, Santos G-M, Das M, et al.** Mirtazapine to reduce methamphetamine use: a randomized controlled trial. Arch Gen Psychiatry. 2011;68:1168-75.

105. **McGill M, Ray LA.** Cognitive-behavioral treatment with adult alcohol and illicit drug users: a meta-analysis of randomized controlled trials. J Studies Alcohol Drugs. 2009;70:516-27.

106. **Colfax G, Santos GM, Chu P, et al.** Amphetamine-group substances and HIV. Lancet. 2010; 376:458-74.

107. **Shoptaw S, Reback CJ, Peck JA, et al.** Behavioral treatment approaches for methamphetamine dependence and HIV-related sexual risk behaviors among urban gay and bisexual men. Drug Alcohol Depend. 2005;78:125-34.

108. **Reback CJ, Shoptaw S.** Development of an evidence-based, gay-specific cognitive behavioral therapy intervention for methamphetamine-abusing gay and bisexual men. Addict Behav. 2014;39:1286-91.

109. **Miller W, Rollnick S.** Motivational Interviewing: Preparing People to Change Addictive Behavior. New York: Guilford; 1991.

110. **Smedslund G, Berg RC, Hammerstrøm KT, et al.** Motivational interviewing for substance abuse. Cochrane Database Syst Rev. 2011;11:CD008063.

111. **Berg RC, Ross MW, Tikkanen R.** The effectiveness of MI4MSM: how useful is motivational interviewing as an HIV risk prevention program for men who have sex with men? A systematic review. AIDS Educ Prev. 2011;23:533-49.

112. **Dutra L, Stathopoulou G, Basden SL, et al.** A meta-analytic review of psychosocial interventions for substance use disorders. Am J Psychiatry. 2008;165:179-87.

113. **Menza TW, Jameson DR, Hughes JP, Colfax GN, Shoptaw S, Golden MR.** Contingency management to reduce methamphetamine use and sexual risk among men who have sex with men: a randomized controlled trial. BMC Public Health. 2010;10:774.

Chapter 11

Intimate Partner Violence and Hate Crimes: Recognition, Care, and Prevention for LGBT People

KEVIN L. ARD, MD, MPH

Introduction

Violence and trauma are all too common occurrences in the lives of many lesbian, gay, bisexual, and transgender (LGBT) persons. Violence and trauma can take many forms, from rejection by one's family of origin, to bullying in school, to hate crimes, to sexual assault, to intimate partner violence between individuals in a current or former romantic relationship; all have been associated with negative health outcomes. Family rejection and bullying are addressed in Chapter 4. This chapter presents two case studies, one reflecting intimate partner violence and the other describing a hate crime. Each case is followed by a review of the epidemiology of violence and a description of how clinicians can assist survivors by understanding and diagnosing the problem, providing psychosocial support, treating the health effects of the violence, and taking steps to prevent future occurrences. Finally, specific recommendations for care are presented after each of the cases.

Intimate Partner Violence

Case

Michael is a 24-year-old man who presents to your clinic to establish primary care. Before his visit today, he had scheduled but missed 2 previous appointments. He appears depressed, anxious, and fatigued, and you initially have difficulty engaging him in conversation. Upon taking his sexual history, you learn that he lives with a male partner, John; is sexually active with men; and does not consistently use condoms. You explore his thoughts on condom use and discover that he would like to use condoms more but that John often coerces him into having unprotected receptive anal intercourse. You also learn that John occasionally pushes and shoves Michael, often because of anger at perceived infidelity on Michael's part. Moreover, John attempts to prevent Michael from spending time with friends as a result of jealously. Michael identifies as a gay man but has not yet revealed this to his parents and siblings because he anticipates they will respond negatively; when John is angry, he threatens to out Michael to his family unless Michael agrees to his demands. How would you respond to Michael's situation?

Overview

Michael is experiencing intimate partner violence, also called domestic violence or partner abuse. Intimate partner violence refers to psychological, physical, or sexual abuse in a current or former romantic relationship. Psychological abuse is most common and can take many forms, including threats, financial neglect, and social isolation. It may progress to physical abuse over time. Physical violence, in turn, tends to occur in cycles, with episodes of violence followed by apologies and promises to change on the part of the batterer and optimism on the part of the victim. Intimate partner violence was long considered to primarily affect heterosexual women; however, research now shows that LGBT persons experience intimate partner violence at least as commonly and that intimate partner violence may have unique characteristics in LGBT relationships. Here, we discuss the epidemiology, clinical presentation, diagnosis, treatment, and prevention of intimate partner violence in LGBT populations.

Epidemiology

Obtaining an accurate picture of intimate partner violence in LGBT individuals has historically been hampered by a lack of research on the subject. The few studies that were published tended to rely on small, convenience samples of gay or lesbian persons; bisexual or transgender individuals were rarely included. In addition, research methods varied, making generalizations problematic. Some studies defined sexual orientation behaviorally based on cohabitation or sexual contact with same-sex individuals, while others relied on self-report of sexual identity. Research has also differed with regard to whether prior, current, or lifetime violence was assessed.

Nevertheless, emerging evidence indicates that intimate partner violence is at least as common in lesbian, gay, and bisexual individuals as in heterosexual persons. The most recent and comprehensive data come from the 2010 National Intimate Partner and Sexual Violence Survey (NISVS), a telephone survey of more than 16,000 English- and Spanish-speaking persons across the United States. Sexual orientation in the survey was established by self-report at the time of the interview. The NISVS found that 61% of bisexual women had experienced intimate partner violence in their lifetimes, compared with 44% of lesbians and 35% of heterosexual women. The corresponding rates for gay, bisexual, and heterosexual men were 26%, 37%, and 29%, respectively (1). The perpetrators of the violence were predominantly male with the exception of violence reported by lesbians, in which case 67% of the perpetrators were female.

Some LGBT groups may be disproportionately affected by intimate partner violence. In the NISVS, bisexual women, and to a lesser extent bisexual men, reported more domestic violence than their gay-, lesbian-, or heterosexual-identified counterparts. Transgender individuals may also experience higher rates of partner abuse, although data are limited. In a convenience sample of nearly 1600 persons in Massachusetts, 34.6% of transgender respondents recounted a lifetime history of physical violence by a partner, compared with 13.6% of nontransgender respondents (2). Intimate partner violence is also more common among HIV-infected than non–HIV-infected men who have sex with men (MSM) (3).

Aside from bisexual orientation, transgender identity, and HIV infection, little is known about which demographic characteristics are associated with a higher risk for intimate partner violence among LGBT persons. One study of African-American men found that MSM who reported a history of childhood sexual abuse were more likely to be victims of intimate partner violence in adulthood than were non-MSM (4). Otherwise, in studies not focused on LGBT populations, higher rates of intimate partner violence have been observed among those who are younger, nonwhite, and poorer (5,6); it is not known whether these associations also apply to LGBT individuals. The effect on intimate partner violence of societal factors, such as norms around sexual orientation and gender identity, and the legal status of LGBT relationships, is also not known.

Taken together, the epidemiologic studies on LGBT partner abuse expose common misconceptions about intimate partner violence. In particular, they show that LGBT groups experience partner abuse at least as commonly as heterosexual women, who are typically considered to be at highest risk for intimate partner violence. These data also contradict the perception that women cannot perpetrate, and men cannot be victims of, intimate partner violence.

Distinctive Features of LGBT Intimate Partner Violence

Intimate partner violence in lesbian and gay relationships resembles that in heterosexual relationships with regard to the role of power dynamics (7); in both cases, the abusive partner maintains power and control through social isolation, humiliation, control of financial resources, and threatened or actual physical harm. However, LGBT intimate partner violence also differs from that in heterosexual relationships in important ways. For many survivors of LGBT partner abuse, the prospect of forced outing—the revealing of one's sexual orientation or gender identity to others—constitutes a form of psychological violence. Abusers may threaten victims with unwanted outing as a way to exert power in the relationship, as John does to Michael in the preceding case scenario. Concerns about coming out can also serve as a barrier to seeking help (8). For those in same-sex intimate relationships, reporting partner violence entails outing oneself; survivors may not seek help if they anticipate stigma and discrimination once they disclose the nature of their relationships (9).

LGBT intimate partner violence is also unique in that it occurs within the context of homo- and transphobia. Many LGBT individuals have been repeatedly traumatized on account of their sexual orientation or gender identity, in the form of family rejection, bullying, discrimination in the workplace, or hate crimes. Overall, LGBT individuals appear more likely to experience violence than non-LGBT persons. The violence often begins at a young age: One meta-analysis of 26 school-based studies in North America found that lesbian, gay, and bisexual youth were significantly more likely than their heterosexual counterparts to experience childhood sexual abuse, physical abuse by parents, and assault at school (10). Higher rates of violence victimization extend into adulthood for gay, lesbian, and bisexual individuals, as well as non–gay-identified individuals who have same-sex relationships (11). In addition, compared with nontransgender individuals, transgender men and women experience more harassment and discrimination (12). Such experiences may affect how, and whether, LGBT individuals seek help in the context of partner abuse. Inadequate responses on the part of authority figures or support personnel to experiences of violence may dissuade them from seeking help altogether.

Even if survivors of LGBT intimate partner violence do seek help, they may find that resources are lacking. Few temporary shelters cater specifically to the LGBT population, and some individuals—especially men and transgender women—may not be admitted to traditional shelters, which have primarily served women fleeing heterosexual relationships (13,14). In addition, a lack of cultural competence on the part of the police and other domestic violence personnel may create negative experiences for LGBT individuals fleeing abusive relationships. Research has shown that shelter workers perceive violence in LGBT relationships as less severe than that in heterosexual relationships; shelter staff are also less likely to consider women in same-sex relationships as victims compared with women in heterosexual relationships (15).

Intimate Partner Violence and Health

Intimate partner violence has been associated with detrimental effects on both physical and psychological well-being. The most visible health consequences of intimate partner violence are the physical injuries—fractures, stab wounds, burns, and lacerations—that result directly from violence. However, these are uncommon, and survivors of intimate partner violence are at risk for a range of other conditions that impair health, many of which stem from maladaptive responses to trauma (16). Compared with their peers lacking any history of partner abuse, gay and bisexual men who report intimate partner violence have higher rates of depression, substance abuse, and unprotected anal sex, thus placing them at increased risk for HIV and other sexually transmitted infections (STIs) (3,17,18). Among HIV-infected gay and bisexual men, partner abuse predicts lapses in care, more advanced disease, and HIV-related hospitalizations (19). The nature of the relationship between intimate partner violence and poorer HIV-related health outcomes is not clear but may result from perpetrators' direct interference with medication adherence or medical visits in an effort to exert control and/or isolate their partners (8).

Research on the association between health and intimate partner violence among lesbian and bisexual women and transgender individuals has been sparse. However, female survivors of opposite-sex intimate partner violence have been found to have increased rates of self-reported poor health, pain, memory impairment, gynecologic symptoms, emotional distress, and suicidal ideation (20). In addition, a community-based study in Los Angeles, California, demonstrated a correlation between sexual partner violence and depression in Latina male-to-female transgender persons (21).

The negative health effects of intimate partner violence also extend to bystanders. Exposure to intimate partner violence has been linked to a range of negative outcomes among children, including insomnia, self-harm, and pain; these associations remain even if the children are not directly abused (22). Negative health effects associated with witnessing intimate partner violence during childhood persist for decades. As adults, individuals who were exposed to intimate partner violence as children have higher rates of alcoholism, drug abuse, depression, suicide attempts, smoking, risky sexual behavior, and obesity (23). They are also more likely to perpetrate intimate partner violence in adulthood (4).

Screening and Diagnosis

Screening

Screening asymptomatic individuals for intimate partner violence has historically been controversial because of debate about the benefits of screening. However, screening does not appear to be harmful, and several organizations have issued screening guidelines. The American College of Obstetricians and Gynecologists (24) and the U.S. Preventive Services Task Force (25) recommend that asymptomatic women be screened for intimate partner violence. Other organizations, such as the American Medical Association (26), recommend screening for all individuals. However, no national guidelines specifically address screening in asymptomatic LGBT persons.

We recommend that all persons be screened for intimate partner violence regardless of sex, sexual orientation, or gender identity, consistent with guidelines from the American Medical Association. Screening may be particularly important for bisexual and transgender individuals, given the higher rates of lifetime intimate partner violence in these groups. While no large-scale, randomized controlled trials have assessed screening among LGBT persons, studies of women have shown that screening is generally well received (27). The potential benefits of screening are controversial but include opportunities to educate patients about healthy relationships, provide psychosocial support, and refer to domestic violence programs and other resources. Victimized patients may not report abuse because they are ashamed of the abuse, optimistic that their batterers will change, or fearful that their abusers will discover their disclosure and retaliate (8). However, even if affected individuals do not disclose intimate partner violence, simply asking about abuse in a routine way communicates that such violence is unacceptable and a source of concern to clinicians.

Screening can be accomplished at new patients visits and periodically thereafter, such as at routine follow-up appointments. No screening instruments have been validated in LGBT populations, but several tools have been developed and tested in other populations (28). One commonly used instrument, called the Partner Violence Screen, consists of 3 gender-neutral questions:

1. Have you been hit, kicked, punched, or otherwise hurt by someone in the past year? If so, by whom?
2. Do you feel safe in your current relationship?
3. Is there a partner from a previous relationship who is making you feel unsafe now?

The Partner Violence Screen and other screening instruments tend to be more specific than sensitive at identifying abuse (28). Directly questioning patients about intimate partner violence may also be effective; in a study of female orthopedic trauma patients, asking directly about physical, emotional, and sexual abuse was more sensitive than other screening instruments (29).

Perhaps more important than what words are used to screen is how the screen is performed. Patients should be asked about intimate partner violence alone; same-sex individuals who accompany patients to the visit should not be assumed to be friends or relatives, as they may be intimate partners. In addition, openly discussing sexual orientation or gender identity before screening for intimate partner violence may be important for LGBT individuals, as they may not be willing to discuss same-sex relationships without first being assured of providers' nonjudgmental attitudes (30). LGBT-themed pamphlets or posters can also help communicate that the clinic is accepting of LGBT relationships (31).

Diagnosis

While many survivors of intimate partner violence appear asymptomatic in routine clinical encounters, clinicians occasionally note signs or symptoms that raise suspicion for abuse. Clues to the presence of intimate partner violence include nonspecific or inconsistent symptoms, particularly fatigue, chronic pain, gastrointestinal symptoms, pelvic pain, and sexual dysfunction; unexplained injuries, especially if presentation to care is delayed; a history of missed appointments; and witnessing controlling or abusive behavior on the part of a partner during a clinic visit (32). The same questions used to screen for intimate partner violence can be employed to establish a diagnosis, but more direct questioning can also be appropriate. For instance, as part of the evaluation of injuries, clinicians can say, "In my experience, this type of injury is sometimes caused by other people; has anyone been hurting you?" (32).

Caring for Survivors of Intimate Partner Violence

Upon diagnosis of intimate partner violence, whether through routine screening or investigation of concerning symptoms or signs, health care providers should take crucial steps to support survivors, address their medical and psychological needs, and help ensure safety. Clinicians may be a particularly important source of support for LGBT survivors of intimate partner violence due to the paucity of other domestic violence services for these individuals. Table 11-1 lists recommendations for responding to the disclosure or diagnosis of intimate partner violence in health care settings.

Table 11-1   Responding to Intimate Partner Violence in Health Care Settings

Express empathy
Communicate that violence is not deserved; acknowledge patient's courage in disclosure

Assess safety
Inquire about real or threatened physical violence, the use and availability of weapons, and drug and alcohol abuse; assist patients in safety planning

Review resources
Offer referrals to LGBT advocacy programs and shelters; screen non-LGBT focused programs for their cultural competence in working with LGBT clients

Address health effects of intimate partner violence
Treat injuries, screen for depression and substance abuse; evaluate for HIV infection and other STIs and offer HIV postexposure prophylaxis, as needed

Clearly document findings in the medical record
Describe and photograph physical injuries, record a diagnosis of "suspected intimate partner violence," offer a SANE evaluation in cases of sexual assault

Report suspected violence as mandated by law
Become familiar with local mandatory reporting laws; inquire about involvement of children, disabled persons, and/or elders in the abuse

Ensure continuity of care
Arrange close interval follow-up; seek to address barriers to medical visits, including cost, transportation, and direct interference from the perpetrator

SANE = sexual assault nurse examiner; STI = sexually transmitted infection.

A multipronged approach is recommended for the care of those affected by intimate partner violence. First, clinicians should express empathy and support, assuring the survivor that the violence is unacceptable and is not his or her fault. Patients can be also praised for their strength in disclosing the abuse and, if applicable, coming out to the provider.

Assessing safety is a second key task; clinicians can begin by asking a simple question, such as "Is it safe for you to go home today?" Other factors to inquire about in the safety assessment include the presence of weapons in the house, the use of weapons to threaten the survivor, escalation in the abuse over time, and drug and alcohol abuse in the home (32,33). Providers should also inquire whether any other persons are involved in the abuse; depending on local laws, reporting of violence against children, disabled persons, or elders may be mandated.

Next, clinicians should discuss resources available to the patient. Providers should inform themselves ahead of time about LGBT-specific services, shelters, legal support, and counseling so that they can offer information about these options to patients when the need arises. However, in many areas, no LGBT-focused intimate partner violence services are available. With patients' permission, clinicians can, in these cases, initiate contact with standard domestic violence services to inquire about a program's ability to assist victims of LGBT intimate partner violence. Screening programs in this way may help the survivor avoid futile or discriminatory experiences while trying to seek help. Providers can also refer patients to national resources on LGBT intimate partner violence (see Table 11-2).

Additionally, clinicians can assist patients by helping them develop a safety plan. They may wish to ask patients, "Where is a safe place you could stay in an emergency?" and "How would you get there?" and then help brainstorm options (32). Clinicians should generally refrain from recommending that individuals leave an abusive relationship. Instead, patients should be allowed to make these decisions at their own pace; attempting to end a violent relationship often results in increased violence, and patients typically have greater insight into the dynamics of these situations than do clinicians.

In addition to treating any physical injuries that result from intimate partner violence, clinicians should also assess for and address the other health risks associated with partner abuse. All survivors should be evaluated for depression and suicidal ideation. Moreover, because some individuals cope with abusive relationships by using drugs and/or alcohol, providers should assess for these comorbidities. For MSM, intimate partner violence has been associated with sexual risk-taking and HIV infection. A thorough sexual history, along with screening for HIV infection and other STIs, may be indicated for these survivors. Prompt treatment with antiretrovirals (postexposure prophylaxis) may decrease the possibility of HIV infection after a sexual assault by an HIV-infected person and should be offered, when appropriate, if the patient presents for care within 72 hours of the assault (34). Interventions to prevent pregnancy and decrease transmission of other STIs are also available.

Table 11–2   Resources to Support LGBT Victims of Violence

Intimate Partner Violence: The Clinician's Guide to Identification, Assessment, Intervention, and Prevention, 5th edition
www.massmed.org/patient-care/health-topics/intimate-partner-violence-5th-edition-(pdf)
General guidelines from the Massachusetts Medical Society Committee on Violence Intervention and Prevention

GLBTQ Domestic Violence Project
www.glbtqdvp.org
Formerly the Gay Men's Domestic Violence Project, offers training, resources, and support services to individuals, community groups, service providers, and criminal justice professionals on domestic violence and sexual violence

National Coalition of Anti-Violence Programs (NCAVP)
www.avp.org/about-avp/national-coalition-of-anti-violence-programs
Provides training, technical assistance, support services, and resources on reducing violence and its impact on LGBTQ and HIV-affected communities

Federal Bureau of Investigation: Hate Crimes
www.fbi.gov/about-us/investigate/civilrights/hate_crimes
Explains how to report a hate crime and offers specific information on the Matthew Shepard and James Byrd, Jr., Hate Crimes Prevention Act of 2009

Southern Poverty Law Center
www.splcenter.org
Uses litigation, education, and other forms of advocacy to combat hate and bigotry against the most vulnerable populations, including LGBT people

Human Rights Campaign: Maps of State Laws & Policies
www.hrc.org/resources/entry/state-laws-policies
The largest civil rights organization working to achieve equality for LGBT Americans offers resources on state laws and policies pertaining to LGBT hate crimes, antibullying, and public accommodations discrimination

National Domestic Violence Hotline
1-800-799-SAFE (7233)
www.thehotline.org

National Sexual Assault Hotline
1-800-656-HOPE (4673)

At the same time that they are addressing the health correlates of intimate partner violence, health care providers should also recognize how medical documentation can help those who wish to pursue legal action against their abusers. Outside of the few states that explicitly exclude same-sex partner abuse from domestic violence laws (13), clear and detailed documentation in the medical chart may both assist persons seeking legal redress and facilitate longitudinal care. Drawings can be used to indicate the location of injuries; photographs—with a ruler showing the size of the injury and the patient's face, if possible—can also be used for this purpose (32). The history should be reported matter-of-factly, avoiding use of terms such as *claims* or *alleges*, which some interpret to indicate doubt of the patient's account. Clinicians can even note a diagnosis of *suspected intimate partner violence* in the patient's chart (16). In the setting of sexual assault, patients can be referred to a local emergency department for procurement of evidence by a sexual assault nurse examiner (SANE) (16). To maximize the likelihood of obtaining useful evidence, sexual assault survivors should not bathe before presenting to the emergency department and should bring any clothes involved in the assault with them (16).

Finally, clinicians should ensure continuity of care for survivors of intimate partner violence for their ongoing medical and psychosocial needs. Patients may not choose to avail themselves of any additional domestic violence services but may still benefit from the longitudinal support of their health care providers. The acronym RADAR has been used to summarize the steps in responding to intimate partner violence in health care settings; it stands for *r*outinely inquiring about violence, *a*sking direct questions, *d*ocumenting findings, *a*ssessing safety, and *r*eviewing options and referring, as necessary (8).

Identifying and Caring for Perpetrators of Intimate Partner Violence

Outside of the NISVS—which demonstrated that the perpetrators of intimate partner violence against gay and bisexual men and bisexual women were predominantly male, while the perpetrators of intimate partner violence against lesbians were predominantly female (1)—little is known about the demographic characteristics, physical and mental health, and trauma histories of perpetrators of LGBT partner abuse. One study found that abuse in early life predicted both intimate partner violence victimization and perpetration (4). Research outside of the LGBT setting has shown that men who abuse their female partners have higher rates of substance abuse, serious mental illness, and unmet mental health needs (35,36); perpetrators may also have higher rates of traumatic brain injury (37).

Patients rarely disclose intimate partner violence perpetration in clinical settings, and there are currently no recommendations to screen for perpetration of intimate partner violence, although a short, 3-question screening tool for perpetration of physical violence has been developed (38).

If patients do report violence perpetration in clinical settings, they can be referred to batterer intervention programs. Historically, treatment programs for batterers have often been court-mandated and consisted of cognitive behavioral therapy or education in feminist perspectives; neither approach has been more than modestly effective in reducing perpetration (39). Batterer interventions focused on the LGBT population are rare to nonexistent, and individuals who may otherwise be willing to attend such programs may be reluctant to do so because of concern about encountering homo- or transphobia.

Prevention

Clinicians can help prevent intimate partner violence in several ways. First, simply by screening for violence routinely, providers educate victims and perpetrators alike that such abuse is not acceptable. Second, to the extent that mental illness and substance abuse foster or perpetuate intimate partner violence, clinicians may help prevent abuse by rigorously identifying and treating these conditions in their patients. Health care providers—whose opinions are often afforded significant weight in public discussions—can also advocate for inclusion of LGBT populations in existing violence prevention efforts (16). One example in which the addition of an LGBT-focused approach has been advocated is bystander intervention programs, wherein community members are taught to recognize and intervene in situations of intimate partner violence (40). Although not yet formally studied, such an intervention may be particularly key for LGBT populations, which have historically been reluctant to recognize domestic violence in their ranks out of concern for further stigmatizing LGBT relationships (7,9). Finally, by framing intimate partner violence as a pressing public health issue, clinicians can lend their voices to those calling for a change in societal norms surrounding violence for all people, straight and LGBT alike.

Summary of Recommendations

In the case of Michael, the 24-year-old man who disclosed psychological, physical, and sexual abuse by his partner John, you should first express concern about his situation, assure him that such violence is unacceptable, offer support, and ensure safety. With his consent, you can refer him to a local domestic violence service organization catering to LGBT individuals, if available. In addition, Michael should be evaluated and treated for health problems related to abuse. If physical examination shows any signs of trauma, these should be photographed, if possible, and clearly described in the medical chart. His mood is depressed, and he appears anxious; these signs deserve further investigation. Treatment for depression and referral to a mental health provider may be necessary. In addition, he should be assessed for substance abuse. John has forced Michael to have unprotected anal sex; this places him at risk for HIV infection and other STIs for which testing and, in some cases, prophylactic treatment can be offered. Finally, arranging close interval follow-up for Michael will provide him with a longitudinal source of care and support.

Hate Crimes

Case

Juanita is a 35-year-old transgender woman who presents to your clinic with insomnia. Her insomnia began after she was attacked by a group of men upon leaving a bar approximately 1 month ago; the men hit and kicked her and told her that she deserved the beating because she was a "filthy cross-dresser." Now, Juanita has difficulty falling asleep. When she does sleep, she often experiences nightmares about the attack. She has avoided the bar, even though it was formerly one of her favorite places to meet friends, and has nearly stopped going out all together. She feels emotionally numb and isolated. Her alcohol use has increased; she used to drink 1 to 2 alcoholic beverages per day and now has 3 to 5. She did not seek legal assistance after the attack because she doubted that the police would be sympathetic. Examination discloses a flat affect and healing lacerations on her face, arms, and buttocks. How would you respond to Juanita's situation?

Overview

This case illustrates the consequences of a hate crime motivated by anti-transgender bias. Hate crimes are attacks on person or property that stem from bias against race, ethnicity, religion, disability, sexual orientation, or gender identity. Hate crimes vary in severity from threats, to vandalism, to physical or sexual assault, to homicide. They traumatize not only the victims but also others who belong to a targeted group but are not personally affected by the crime. In this section, we describe the epidemiology and characteristics of anti-LGBT hate crimes, the care of affected individuals, and legal protections for those victimized by hate crimes.

Epidemiology

In recent years, several anti-LGBT hate crimes have garnered significant public attention:

- In 1998, Matthew Shepard, a 21-year-old gay man, was abducted, tied to a fence, beaten, and killed by 2 men outside of Laramie, Wyoming.
- 25-year-old Ryan Skipper was stabbed to death in 2007 by 2 men in Florida who later boasted about murdering a homosexual (41).
- Duanna Johnson, a 43-year-old transgender woman, was beaten by law enforcement officials in 2008; the officials reportedly shouted antitransgender slurs during the abuse. Ms. Johnson was later found shot to death in Memphis, Tennessee (42).

These cases highlight the brutality of anti-LGBT hate crimes. The public outcry they prompted has led to positive developments, such as the passage of anti-LGBT hate crimes legislation. However, despite the widespread denunciation of these crimes and the increasing acceptance of LGBT individuals in society, more than 1000 anti-LGBT crimes are reported every year.

The Federal Bureau of Investigation (FBI) has maintained statistics on reported hate crimes since 1992. In 2011, the most recent year for which data are available, 7240 hate crime offenses were reported to the FBI, of which 1508 (20.8%) were motivated by sexual orientation bias. Sexual orientation bias was the second most common motivation for hate crimes after racial bias. More than half of the anti-LGBT offenses were directed against gay males, while 28%, 11%, 1.5%, and 1.1% were motivated by general antihomosexual, antilesbian, antibisexual, and antiheterosexual bias, respectively; the FBI does not report statistics on antitransgender crimes (43). For the same year, the National Coalition of Anti-Violence Programs (NCAVP), which collects data on hate violence from member programs around the country, reported 2092 incidents of violence against LGBT and HIV-infected individuals. As in the FBI report, gay men were the most common group to be targeted, representing 46% of all cases, followed by lesbians (24%), heterosexual persons (15%), and bisexual individuals (9%). Eighteen percent of survivors identified as transgender (44). The NCAVP report also concluded that people of color and transgender persons were more likely than others to be injured as a result of hate crimes (44). Both the FBI and NCAVP data probably underestimate the number of anti-LGBT hate crimes because many incidents may not be reported to authorities as a result of survivors' concerns about retaliation or doubts that reporting will be helpful, as in the case of Juanita above. In a national survey of 662 gay, lesbian, and bisexual adults, 20% reported experiencing a crime motivated by sexual orientation bias; this would correspond to significantly more cases than were reported to the FBI or the NCAVP (45).

Distinctive Features of Anti-LGBT Hate Crimes

Sexual orientation-based hate crimes differ from other hate crimes according to important characteristics. In a comparison of anti-LGBT and racially motivated offenses, the former were more likely to involve male victims, and both victims and perpetrators were more likely to be white (46). Sexual orientation-based crimes also more commonly occurred in schools than did racially based crimes and were more likely to involve weapons. Consistent with this finding, hate crimes based on sexual orientation and gender identity are often considered more violent than those affecting other groups.

Anti-LGBT Hate Crimes and Health

There are few data on the health consequences of hate crimes, but available evidence suggests that such violence exacts a toll on survivors' health. Death and disability may result directly from the crimes themselves, as in the cases of Matthew Shepard, Ryan Skipper, Duanna Johnson, and others. Indeed, at least 30 anti-LGBT homicides occurred nationwide in 2011 (44). In addition, as for intimate partner violence, hate crimes are linked to poor mental health. One survey found that lesbian, gay, and bisexual survivors of hate crimes were more likely than other crime victims to experience depression, anger, anxiety, and post-traumatic stress (47). Anti-LGBT violence has also been found to help account for the increased rates of depression and suicidality in LGBT adolescents (48). Because hate crimes, by their very nature, aim to intimidate a particular population of people, members of the targeted group may also experience depression, anxiety, and stress in the wake of a hate crime, even if they are not directly victimized by the crime (49). In the case of anti-LGBT hate crimes, the effects of this vicarious trauma may also include internalized homophobia and decreased willingness to be open about one's sexual orientation or gender identity for fear of experiencing violence oneself (16).

Caring for Persons Affected by Anti-LGBT Hate Crimes

Individuals affected by anti-LGBT hate crimes may come to medical attention in several ways. Survivors of physical or sexual assaults may present directly to hospitals or clinics for care of injuries sustained in a crime. Others may be identified when they present with psychological distress following a traumatic experience; in patients who seek care for depression, anxiety, or post traumatic stress disorder (PTSD), the provider may learn that the symptoms are tied to a hate crime only after in-depth questioning. Clinicians should be particularly alert to the presence of an antecedent hate crime in patients presenting with manifestations of PTSD, although other forms of trauma, such as intimate partner violence or natural disasters, can also lead to post-traumatic stress. Symptoms of PTSD include hypervigilance, emotional detachment, and intrusive thoughts or nightmares related to a traumatic event. Finally, hate crime survivors may also be identified by screening instruments for intimate partner violence that elicit information on experiences of violence but do not necessarily specify that the violence occurs in the context of an intimate relationship. Screening specifically for experience of hate crimes among LGBT patients is not currently recommended.

The care of hate crime survivors is similar to that of patients experiencing intimate partner violence. Survivors should first be assured of providers' empathy and support. Victim blaming may be particularly prominent in causes of anti-LGBT hate crimes (50); clinicians can help counteract this by assuring survivors that the violence is not deserved or the patients' fault. Next, survivors' safety should be assessed. If the crime has not yet been reported to law enforcement officials and the patient desires to do so, the police can be contacted directly from the health care setting. Individuals experiencing depression, anxiety, or PTSD may warrant referral to mental health professionals for treatment. As with intimate partner violence, physical injuries sustained in an attack should be thoroughly documented, both to facilitate ongoing medical care and to assist in potential legal proceedings. Survivors of sexual assault should be offered an examination by a SANE professional for evidence collection. It is important that such examinations be undertaken sensitively and with full explanation of their purpose, as survivors of sexual assault may experience invasive examinations as a repeated trauma.

Legal Considerations

Historically, sexual orientation and gender identity were not included in federal hate crimes legislation, which applied only to crimes related to race, religion, national origin, or federally protected activities such as voting (51). This changed with the passage of the Matthew Shepard and James Byrd, Jr., Hate Crimes Prevention Act of 2009. The Act created a new federal law criminalizing harm inflicted upon individuals because of their LGBT or disability status; it also allowed the federal government to assist local jurisdictions in prosecuting anti-LGBT hate crimes and to prosecute such cases if state or local authorities fail to do so. State laws vary with regard to the existence of hate crimes legislation and the groups to which they apply; currently, only 12 states and the District of Columbia include protections based on both sexual orientation and gender identity (52). Such state laws may be associated with improved health of LGBT populations; in one study, rates of generalized anxiety disorder, PTSD, dysthymia, and psychiatric comorbid conditions in lesbian, gay, and bisexual individuals were lower in states with such protections as compared with states without them (53).

Summary of Recommendations

In the case of Juanita, the 35-year-old transgender women who experienced a physical assault motivated by antitransgender bias, you should express empathy and concern and communicate that such violence is unacceptable. Her disrupted sleep, emotional detachment, and avoidant behaviors all suggest PTSD, for which prompt referral to a mental health professional is warranted. She may be using alcohol to address anxiety and should be counseled about appropriate use; you can also offer participation in an alcohol treatment program. Although it has been a month since the hate crime occurred, thorough documentation of her lacerations in the medical record may be beneficial should she choose to pursue legal action against her attackers. You should schedule a close interval follow-up appointment with Juanita to reassess her symptoms of PTSD and her alcohol use.

Conclusion

The cases of Michael and Juanita illustrate 2 forms of violence victimization—intimate partner violence and hate crimes—that affect a substantial proportion of LGBT individuals. Because of the prevalence of violence and trauma across the lifespan, clinicians must practice medicine in a trauma-informed manner: Antecedent violence should be considered in patients presenting with injuries, depression, substance abuse, and PTSD; conversely, in patients reporting violence, a sensitive evaluation for its health effects should be undertaken. Clinicians can assist survivors of violence not only by expressing empathy, ensuring safety, and addressing its health consequences but also by lending their voices to those calling for a safer and more humane society for people of all sexual orientations and gender identities.

Summary Points

- Intimate partner violence consists of psychological, sexual, and/or physical abuse. Psychological abuse occurs most commonly and may take the form of threats, social isolation, forced outing of one's sexual orientation or gender identity, or economic control.
- Gay and lesbian individuals report intimate partner violence at least as commonly as heterosexual men and women; the prevalence of intimate partner violence in bisexual persons, transgender individuals, and HIV-infected gay men is higher.
- Hate crimes based on sexual orientation bias are one of the most common types of hate crimes, tend to be more violent than hate crimes directed at other groups, and are more likely to occur at school.
- In addition to physical injuries, intimate partner violence and hate crimes can result in depression, substance abuse, PTSD, and high-risk sexual behavior. In the case of hate crimes, members of the targeted group who were not directly victimized may also experience psychological distress that brings them to medical attention.
- All patients should be asked about intimate partner violence, in a private setting. For LGBT patients, it may be important to first convey an open and nonjudgmental attitude about sexual orientation and gender identity before inquiring about abuse because patients may otherwise be reluctant to discuss their intimate relationships.
- Crucial first steps in responding to patients affected by intimate partner violence or hate crimes are to express empathy, assure survivors that the violence is not their fault, and assess safety.
- Any injuries sustained in violent acts should be clearly documented in the medical record with drawings and/or photographs. Survivors of sexual assault should be offered evaluation by a Sexual Assault Nurse Examiner (SANE) for evidence collection.
- Continuity of care for survivors of hate crimes and intimate partner violence should be ensured. Given the lack of LGBT-focused trauma services, clinicians may serve as the primary source of longitudinal support for LGBT individuals affected by violence.

References

1. **Walters ML, Chen J, Breiding MJ.** The National Intimate Partner and Sexual Violence Survey (NISVS): 2010 findings on victimization by sexual orientation. National Center for Injury Prevention and Control, CDC. 2013. Available at: www.cdc.gov/ViolencePrevention/pdf/ NISVS_SOfindings.pdf.

2. **Landers S, Gilsanz P.** The health of lesbian, gay, bisexual, and transgender (LGBT) persons in Massachusetts. Massachusetts Department of Public Health. 2009. Available at: www.mass. gov/eohhs/docs/dph/commissioner/lgbt-health-report.pdf.

3. **Li Y, Baker JJ, Korostyshevskiy VR, Slack RS, Plankey MW.** The association of intimate partner violence, recreational drug use with HIV seroprevalence among MSM. AIDS Behav. 2012; 16:491-8.

4. **Welles SL, Corbin TJ, Rich JA, Reed E, Raj A.** Intimate partner violence among men having sex with men, women, or both: early life sexual and physical abuse as antecedents. J Community Health. 2011;36:477-85.

5. **Mechem CC, Shofer FS, Reinhard SS, Hornig S, Datner E.** History of domestic violence among male patients presenting to an urban emergency department. Acad Emerg Med. 1999;6: 786-91.

6. **McCloskey LA, Lichter E, Ganz ML, et al.** Intimate partner violence and patient screening across medical specialties. Acad Emerg Med. 2005;12:712-22.

7. **McClennen JC.** Domestic violence between same-gender partners: recent findings and future research. J Interpers Violence. 2005;20:149-54.

8. **Alpert EJ.** Intimate partner violence: the clinician's guide to identification, assessment, intervention, and prevention. Massachusetts Medical Society. 2010. Available at: www. massmed.org/patient-care/health-topics/intimate-partner-violence-5th-edition-(pdf)/.

9. **Kulkin HS, Williams J, Borne HF, de la Bretonne D, Laurendine J.** A review of research on violence in same-gender couples: a resource for clinicians. J Homosex. 2007;53:71-87.

10. **Friedman MS, Marshal MP, Guadamuz TP, et al.** A meta-analysis of disparities in childhood sexual abuse, parental physical abuse, and peer victimization among sexual minority and sexual nonminority individuals. Am J Public Health. 2011;101:1481-94.

11. **Roberts AL, Austin SB, Corliss HL, et al.** Pervasive trauma exposure among US sexual orientation minority adults and risk of posttraumatic stress disorder. Am J Public Health. 2010; 100:2433-41.

12. **Factor RJ, Rothblum ED.** A study of transgender adults and their non-transgender siblings on demographic characteristics, social support, and experiences of violence. J LGBT Health Res. 2007;3:11-30.

13. **Pattavina A, Hirshel D, Buzawa E, Faggiani D, Bentley H.** A comparison of the police response to heterosexual versus same-sex intimate partner violence. Violence Women. 2007; 13:374-94.

14. **Hines DA, Douglas EM.** The reported availability of U.S. domestic violence services to victims who vary by age, sexual orientation, and gender. Partner Abuse. 2011;2:3-30.

15. **Basow SA, Thompson J.** Service providers' reactions to intimate partner violence as a function of victim sexual orientation and type of abuse. J Interpers Violence. 2012;27:1225-41.

16. **Pitt EL, Alpert EJ.** Violence and trauma: recognition, recovery, and prevention. In: Makadon HJ, Mayer KH, Potter J, Goldhammer H, eds. Fenway Guide to Lesbian, Gay, Bisexual, and Transgender Health. Philadelphia: American College of Physicians; 2008:249-70.

17. **Houston E, McKirnan DJ.** Intimate partner abuse among gay and bisexual men: risk correlates and health outcomes. J Urban Health. 2007;84:681-90.

18. **Parsons JT, Grov C, Golub SA.** Sexual compulsivity, co-occurring psychosocial health problems, and HIV risk among gay and bisexual men: further evidence of a syndemic. Am J Public Health. 2012;102:156-62.

19. **Siemieniuk R, Miller P, Woodman K, et al.** Prevalence, clinical associations, and impact of intimate partner violence among HIV-infected gay and bisexual men: a population-based study. HIV Med. 2013;14:293-302.

20. **Ellsberg M, Jansen HA, Heise L, et al.** Intimate partner violence and women's physical and mental health in the WHO multi-country study on women's health and domestic violence: an observational study. Lancet. 2008;371:1165-72.

21. **Bazargan M, Galvan F.** Perceived discrimination and depression among low-income Latina male-to-female transgender women. BMC Public Health. 2012;12:663.

22. **Lamers-Winkelman F, De Schipper JC, Oosterman M.** Children's physical health complaints after exposure to intimate partner violence. Br J Health Psychol. 2012;17:771-84.

23. **Felitti VJ, Anda RF, Nordenberg D, et al.** Relationship of childhood abuse and household dysfunction to many of the leading causes of death in adults. The Adverse Childhood Experiences (ACE) Study. Am J Prev Med. 1998;14:254-58.

24. **Intimate partner violence.** Committee Opinion No. 518. American College of Obstetricians and Gynecologists. Obstet Gynecol. 2012;119:412-7.

25. **Moyer VA, U.S. Preventive Services Task Force.** Screening for intimate partner violence and abuse of elderly and vulnerable adults: a U.S. Preventive Services Task Force recommendation statement. Ann Intern Med. 2013;158:478-86.

26. Opinion 2.02. Physicians' obligations in preventing, identifying, and treating violence and abuse. American Medical Association. 2008. Available at: www.ama-assn.org/ama/pub/physician-resources/medical-ethics/code-medical-ethics/opinion202.page.

27. **MacMillan HL, Wathen CN, Jamieson E, et al.** Screening for intimate partner violence in health care settings: a randomized trial. JAMA. 2009;302:493-501.

28. **Rabin RF, Jennings JM, Campbell JC, Bair-Merritt MH.** Intimate partner violence screenings tools: a systematic review. Am J Prev Med. 2009;36:439-45.

29. **Sprague S, Madden K, Dosanjh S, et al.** Screening for intimate partner violence in orthopedic patients: a comparison of three screening tools. J Interpers Violence. 2012;27:881-98.

30. **Ard KL, Makadon HJ.** Addressing intimate partner violence in lesbian, gay, bisexual, and transgender patients. J Gen Intern Med. 2011;26:930-3.

31. **The Joint Commission.** Advancing effective communication, cultural competence, and patient- and family-centered care for the lesbian, gay, bisexual, and transgender (LGBT) community: a field guide. October 2011. Available at: www.jointcommission.org/assets/1/18/LGBTFieldGuide_WEB_LINKED_VER.pdf.

32. **Cronholm PF, Fogarty CT, Ambuel B, Harrison SL.** Intimate partner violence. Am Fam Physician. 2011;83:1165-72.

33. **Hegarty K, O'Doherty L.** Intimate partner violence—identification and response in general practice. Aust Fam Physician. 2011;40:852-6.

34. **Smith DK, Grohskopf LA, Black RJ, et al.** Antiretroviral postexposure prophylaxis after sexual, injection-drug use, or other non-occupational exposure to HIV in the United States: recommendations from the U.S. Department of Health and Human Services. MMWR Recomm Rep. 2005;54(RR-2):1-20.

35. **Shorey RC, Febres J, Brasfield H, Stuart GL.** The prevalence of mental health problems in men arrested for domestic violence. J Fam Violence. 2012;27:741-8.

36. **Lipsky S, Caetano R, Roy-Byrne P.** Triple jeopardy: impact of intimate partner violence perpetration, mental health, substance abuse on perceived unmet need for mental health care among men. Soc Psychiatry Psychiatr Epidemiol. 2011;46:843-52.

37. **Farrer TJ, Frost RB, Hedges DW.** Prevalence of traumatic brain injury in intimate partner violence offenders compared to the general population: a meta-analysis. Trauma Violence Abuse. 2012;13:77-82.

38. **Ernst AA, Weiss SJ, Morgan-Edwards S, et al.** Derivation and validation of a short emergency department screening tool for perpetrators of intimate partner violence: the PErpetrator RaPid Scale (PERPS). J Emerg Med. 2012;42:206-17.

39. **Babcock JC, Green CE, Robie C.** Does batterers' treatment work? A meta-analytic review of domestic violence treatment. Clin Psychol Rev. 2004;23:1023-53.

40. **Potter SJ, Fountain K, Stapleton JG.** Addressing sexual and relationship violence in the LGBT community using a bystander framework. Harv Rev Psychiatry. 2012;20:201-8.

41. **Persall S.** Documentary spotlights gay victim Ryan Skipper's story. Tampa Bay Times. May 28, 2008. Available at: www.tampabay.com/features/movies/documentary-spotlights-gay-victim-ryan-skippers-story/529810.
42. **Brown R.** Murder of transgender woman revives scrutiny. New York Times. November 17, 2008. Available at: www.nytimes.com/2008/11/18/us/18memphis.html?_r=0.
43. **Federal Bureau of Investigation.** Hate crimes statistics 2011. 2011. Available at: www.fbi.gov/about-us/cjis/ucr/hate-crime/2011.
44. **Dixon E, Jindasurat C, Tobar V, et al.** Hate violence against lesbian, gay, bisexual, transgender, queer, and HIV-affected communities in the United States in 2011. National Coalition of Anti-Violence Programs. 2012. Available at www.cuav.org/wp-content/uploads/2012/08/4379_NCAVPHVReport2011Final_Updated.pdf
45. **Herek GM.** Hate crimes and stigma-related experiences among sexual minority adults in the United States: prevalence estimates from a national probability sample. J Interpers Violence. 2009;24:54-74.
46. **Stacey M.** Distinctive characteristics of sexual orientation bias crimes. J Interpers Violence. 2011;26:3013-32.
47. **Herek GM, Gillis JR, Cogan GC.** Psychological sequelae of hate-crime victimization among lesbian, gay, and bisexual adults. J Consult Clin Psychol. 1999;67:945-51.
48. **Burton CM, Marshal MP, Chisholm DJ, Sucato GS, Friedman MS.** Sexual minority-related victimization as a mediator of mental health disparities in sexual minority youth: a longitudinal analysis. J Youth Adolesc. 2013;42:394-402.
49. **American Psychological Association.** The psychology of hate crimes. Available at: www.apa.org/about/gr/issues/violence/hate-crimes-faq.pdf
50. **Plumm KM, Terrance CA, Henderson VR, Ellingson H.** Victim blame in a hate crime stimulated by sexual orientation. J Homosexual. 2010;57:267-86.
51. The Matthew Shepard and James Byrd, Jr., Hate Crimes Prevention Act of 2009. Department of Justice. Available at: www.justice.gov/crt/about/crm/matthewshepard.php.
52. **Human Rights Campaign.** State laws and policies. Available at: www.hrc.org/resources/entry/state-laws-policies.
53. **Hatzenbuehler ML, Keyes KM, Hasin DS.** State-level policies and psychiatric morbidity in lesbian, gay, and bisexual populations. Am J Public Health. 2009;99:2275-81.

Chapter 12

Sexual Health of LGBTQ People

DEMETRE C. DASKALAKIS, MD, MPH
ANITA RADIX, MD, MPH
GAL MAYER, MD

Introduction

This chapter explores sexual health issues, with a focus on how these issues differ or require further attention in lesbian, gay, bisexual, transgender, and queer/questioning (LGBTQ) populations. The sexual lives of LGBTQ individuals are diverse and heterogeneous. Nonetheless, the core tenets for the promotion of sexual health–that is, open discussion and recognition of personal bias on the part of the provider–remain consistent for all populations. This chapter discusses topics in sexual health throughout the very broad spectrum of the LGBTQ experience. Sexually transmitted infections (STIs), for instance, are addressed, with the assumption that the reader has access to basic information about these conditions. Because the U.S. Centers for Disease Control and Prevention (CDC) regularly updates treatment guidelines (available at www.cdc.gov/std/treatment), this chapter will only highlight key topics and new information that specifically affect the sexual health of LGBTQ people. Furthermore, rather than focusing on diseases as isolated entities, we focus on how LGBTQ patients' biology, behavior, and treatment might be improved by the implementation of guidelines and new medical data to enhance happiness, pleasure, and prevent/treat disease. Overall, the clinician's role in optimizing sexual health is to provide patients with the tools and knowledge necessary to not only prevent disease but to also engage in physically and emotionally gratifying safer sex.

A Framework for Providing Optimal Sexual Health Care to LGBTQ People

A central goal of the provision of care to LGBTQ patients is to support the patient's healthy self-concept of both their sexuality and sexual behaviors. Although this is not the only issue in a care encounter, this area tends to be the alliance maker or "deal breaker" between the LGBTQ patient and provider. Quality of care is often measured in disease screening statistics;

however, helping patients achieve a level of satisfaction with their sexual lives is also critical for the delivery of high-quality care. Discussing all of these aspects of sexual health (behavior, identity, function, and contentment) with LGBTQ patients requires an open-ended approach free of assumptions and judgments of how desire and sexuality can or should be expressed. The discussion should always be completed on the patients' terms to optimize their sexual health. Vocabulary should match that used by the patient, unless the provider is uncomfortable with the terms used.

It is also important for providers to address their own assumptions and limits. Providers uncomfortable with same-sex behaviors and gender issues are limited in their ability to care for this population and should have a low threshold to refer such patients to other caregivers (1,2).

Because social stigma and discrimination on the basis of sexual orientation and gender identity can have devastating effects on the health and well-being of LGBTQ persons, including their sexual health, it is important for providers to understand the effects of cultural, institutional, and internalized stigma as part of providing sensitive and culturally appropriate health care. Providers should also become better informed of the specific mental health, substance use, and violence victimization issues found in LGBTQ populations and understand how these factors can have a substantial influence on patient risk and sexual fulfillment. Other chapters explore these issues in detail; see especially Chapters 9, 10, and 11.

Obtaining a Sexual History

Benefits of the Sexual History

Caring for the whole patient, regardless of gender, gender identity, sexual orientation, or sexual or gender expression, includes having a frank and open discussion about sexual activity, desire, function, and satisfaction. Obtaining a thorough sexual history can help a medical provider assess risky behaviors and find opportunities for prevention, diagnose and evaluate sexual dysfunction, identify physical and mental health issues, and assist with family planning (3–12). Additionally, the sexual history can improve provider–patient communication and can provide the patient an opportunity to get information and answers to questions from a reliable source.

Despite these benefits, medical providers and patients often avoid conversations about sexuality for a multitude of reasons. Clinicians cite time constraints, inadequate training, reimbursement concerns, fear of offending patients, personal discomfort with sexual topics, and specific discomfort discussing sexuality with younger or older patients as barriers. Patients report the following reasons for not discussing sexual issues: lack of opportunity, societal taboos, embarrassment or shame, fear of judgment, fear around data confidentiality, and uncertainty about whether sexual concerns are part of health care. For LGBTQ patients, these obstacles are magnified and compounded by potential discrimination and discomfort on the provider side, and fear of disclosure and stigma on the patient side (5,6,12). To overcome these obstacles, it is important to provide the LGBTQ patient with a welcoming, affirming environment (see Appendix A) and to collect the sexual history in an open, nonjudgmental way.

Best Practices in Taking a Sexual History

It is appropriate to collect a comprehensive sexual history during the history and physical at the first encounter between a provider and a new patient, and then to periodically update the history. The components of a complete sexual history are listed in Table 12-1. (See also Chapters 7 and 8 for additional strategies on taking a sexual history with LGBTQ populations and Appendix D for sample sexual history questions for medical history forms.)

In initiating the sexual history, it is sometimes helpful to start with a more neutral topic (such as how the patient is experiencing school or work) before moving on to sexuality. Before talking about sex, you may want to reassure the patient that you are in a private space and that the patient's confidentiality will be respected and is protected by law, and that the questions that will be asked are intended to provide optimal patient care. As explained below, language choices can make a big difference in the patient's level of comfort and openness, but nonverbal cues are equally important.

Table 12-1   Components of a Complete Sexual History

Gender of partners

Number of current and lifetime partners

Relationship types (e.g., traditional monogamous relationship, open relationship, polyamorous relationship, casual partners, anonymous partners)

Frequency of sexual activity (may be important in exploring sexual compulsivity)

Age of sexual debut and effect of peer pressure (may be important in adolescents)

STI/HIV prevention practices including barriers (condoms, finger cots), vaccines (hepatitis A and B, HPV), and medications (HIV post- or pre-exposure prophylaxis, HSV suppression)

Use of drugs or alcohol during sex

Alternative sexual practices, such as sadomasochism, bondage, oral-anal contact ("rimming"), manual or digital anal manipulation ("fingering" or "fisting") or urine play ("water sports")

A history of exchanging sex for money, drugs, food, or shelter or paying for sex

Current and prior STIs; HIV and STI testing history

Problems related to sexual functioning or desire

History of sexual abuse

HPV = human papillomavirus; HSV = herpes simplex virus; STI = sexually transmitted infection.

The clinician should assure the space is comfortable and that his or her body language is open and inviting (e.g., limbs uncrossed, direct eye contact).

The clinician should normalize the collection of a sexual history and ask the patient for permission to open the discussion. A statement such as "I talk with all my patients about their sex life because sexuality is an important part of health. May I ask you some questions about your sex life now?" can help reassure the patient that the clinician is not asking sexual history questions because of a judgment or assumption the clinician has made. Asking for permission also gives the patient control over whether the conversation can move forward, which can help the patient feel more comfortable. If patients respond that they do not want to answer questions about their sexuality, it is wise to discontinue the line of questioning. Forced answers are less likely to be truthful. If the clinician feels that the information is critical for exploring a presenting complaint, the clinician should make it clear to the patient why the information is important and ask for permission again.

During the interview it is important to select language that makes no assumptions about the patient's sexuality. For example, asking patients about the gender(s) of their sexual partner(s) is preferable to asking "Do you have a girlfriend?" of a male patient. Similarly, asking a female patient about whether she has concerns or questions about pregnancy makes fewer assumptions than the question "What do you use for birth control?" In general, anatomic euphemisms and slang should be avoided, with some notable exceptions. When communicating with transgender patients about their anatomy, we recommend the clinician ask the patient what word(s) the patient prefers to use to describe anatomy and use those words. With other patients, using the correct anatomic terms is usually acceptable. But if patients wish to call their body part by another name and the clinician is comfortable with that name, using terms the patients prefer can increase the patients' comfort level.

Certain topics may elicit discomfort, agitation, silence, or awkwardness from the patient. Statements validating the patient's experience and gently exploring the topic may help the clinician gather more information. For example, "I noticed you became quiet when I mentioned oral sex. I find that talking about sex makes many patients uncomfortable. Is there something in particular that is bothering you now?" Individuals who have experienced childhood sexual abuse or sexual assault as adults may feel retraumatized when asked about sexual issues, so evasive or uncomfortable responses should heighten clinician sensitivity. Reassuring patients that the data they provide can help improve their care is important.

The sexual history may also elicit reactions in the clinician, especially when the patient's sexual orientation, behavior, or choices differ from that of the clinician. To continue helping the patient feel at ease with disclosing a sexual history, the clinician may need to be careful to avoid verbal and nonverbal reactions that convey judgment and may limit a patient's willingness to continue the interview.

Throughout the sexual history interview, it is good practice for the clinician to maintain transparency about the reasons for the questions. For example, the statement "Bladder infections are uncommon in men and may be related to anal sex. Have you had anal sex recently?" conveys to the patient the reason for the question. This technique may reassure the patient in the example that the clinician has asked him about anal sex not because of voyeurism or curiosity but because of the clinical correlation of the behavior to the diagnosis. Transparency can also help the clinician feel more at ease about asking potentially provocative questions.

In assessing disease risk, the primary focus of the sexual history should be on specific behaviors, including the types of sexual acts and the type of protection used, if any. Providers should avoid making assumptions about behaviors based on a person's sexual orientation or gender. To properly assess sexual risks, the clinician must understand which body parts were used by patients with their sexual partners. The risk of practices is closely tied to anatomy. For example, penile-anal contact may be more efficient in transmitting some pathogens (e.g., HIV) than penile-vaginal contact. Therefore, when assessing the risk of a transgender person or a cisgender (a person who is not transgender) person with a transgender sex partner, it is important to ask and understand whether the anatomy was surgically altered. Making the reasoning and goals of these intrusive questions transparent to the patient can help to alleviate some of the discomfort or awkwardness that sometimes accompanies the elicitation of specific sexual history information.

Distinguishing Orientation, Identity, and Behavior

Sexual orientation, identity, and behavior describe 3 separate but related concepts. Sexual orientation refers to the inclination to develop emotionally and sexually intimate relationships with people of the same and/or a different gender (e.g., homosexual, heterosexual, bisexual). Sexual identity is how individuals describe their sexuality (e.g., gay, bisexual, lesbian, straight), whereas sexual behavior refers to what one does and with whom (e.g., men who have sex with men [MSM], women who have sex with women [WSW], anal sex, oral sex). In evaluating patients it is important to differentiate among sexual orientation, identity, and behavior because these may not be concordant. Self-identification as a member of the LGBTQ community may differ across age, racial, and ethnic groups because of societal and cultural factors (13). MSM may have sex with women and may not identify as gay or bisexual. WSW may have sex with men and may not identify as lesbian or bisexual.

Gender identity refers to one's inner sense of being male, female, both, or neither. Transgender individuals have gender identities that do not match their assigned sex at birth (see more explanation of transgender identities in Chapter 17). Transgender individuals, like their nontransgender counterparts, may be sexually attracted to men, women, or both. There is considerable diversity and fluidity in how transgender persons define their sexual orientation during their life course. Although there are no long-term studies, some reports have indicated that changes in sexual attraction may occur after initiation of hormone therapy (14–16). For some patients, these changes in sexual attraction can be unwelcome and confusing, necessitating another "coming out" process. As with all patients, it is important for clinicians to maintain open communication and to continue to inquire about sexual behavior and the gender of sexual partners, in order to evaluate risk and provide appropriate health screenings as necessary.

Although the risk assessment portion of the sexual history should focus on behavior, rather than the sexual or gender identity of the patient, clarifying sexual and gender self-identity is important for treating the whole patient and for building rapport; in particular, it is important when counseling patients about sexual satisfaction, identifying identity-related issues, and helping to reduce institutional barriers to care. In fact, asking about sexual and gender identity may best be done earlier in the general history rather than during the sexual history. By doing so, you indicate to the patient that you understand that sexual and gender identity are related not just to sexual health but to all aspects of a person's life and health. For more on collecting sexual and gender identity information, see Chapters 1, 8, and 17.

Addressing HIV Infection and Other STIs in LGBTQ Populations

While it is critical to support the healthiness of LGBTQ sexual expression, it is also important to recognize the medical challenges associated with sexual risk behaviors. Rates of STIs and HIV infection among MSM and transwomen continue to increase and have led to specific screening recommendations for individuals in the LGBTQ community reporting this epidemiologic risk. Myths of the lack of STI transmission among LGBTQ WSW continue to abound and are often reflected in lost opportunities in the medical care setting. In this section, we review the evidence that supports CDC guidance on STI and HIV testing in these populations. To simplify the discussion, we use the terms *MSM* and *WSW* to reflect sexual behaviors, with the acknowledgment that LBGTQ sexuality is far more complex than these simple categories.

STI/HIV Screening: MSM

In the revised 2010 Sexually Transmitted Disease Guidelines (17), the CDC provides recommendations about appropriate screening of asymptomatic MSM who are sexually active. STI screening should include a review of symptoms associated with common STIs; however, specific laboratory testing for

STIs should be guided not just by symptoms but also by the patient's history of exposure to extragenital sites, such as the pharynx and anus. Although urethral infections in men are frequently symptomatic and will cause men to seek treatment, extragenital sites are frequently asymptomatic, leading to delays in detection. The lack of symptoms, coupled with the low rates of extragenital screening by providers, has resulted in many missed opportunities for diagnosis and treatment (18). Some experts, including the authors, recommend extragenital screening (i.e., obtaining oropharyngeal and anal samples) of MSM independent of specific exposure history; this is because the cultural stigma attached to such sexual practices may hinder patients from discussing them with their providers, even when asked.

STI screening for most MSM should be performed at least annually unless the patient engages in sex with multiple or anonymous partners, has sex in relation to illicit drug use, or has partners that participate in such activities. In such individuals, testing every 3 to 6 months may be more appropriate (17). At a minimum, testing should include HIV serology, syphilis serology, screening for urethral *Neisseria gonorrhoeae* and *Chlamydia trachomatis* infection in men who have participated in insertive anal intercourse within the prior year, screening for rectal *N. gonorrhoeae* and *C. trachomatis* in men who have been the receptive anal partner in the preceding year, and screening for pharyngeal *N. gonorrhoeae* infection in men who engaged in receptive oral intercourse within the prior year (17).

The 2010 CDC STI guidelines recommend that anal swabs be obtained for *N. gonorrhoeae* and *C. trachomatis* for sexually active MSM who have had receptive anal intercourse during the preceding year, while those with a history of oral receptive sex should be screened for *N. gonorrhoeae* (17). Some centers also screen for oral *C. trachomatis*; however, the CDC does not yet recommend this. Nucleic acid–based tests (NAATs) are the preferred modality for screening and for diagnosing these extragenital infections because of their increased sensitivity and specificity when compared to culture. Many laboratories have internally validated this test for extragenital samples, although the U.S. Food and Drug Administration (FDA) has not yet approved it for this indication. Although there are no guidelines for transgender persons, most centers extend the same guidelines to transgender persons who have sex with men.

Hepatitis A, B, and C are viruses that may be sexually transmitted, specifically in the context of male-to-male sexual contact. Hepatitis A virus is transmitted through fecal-oral routes, while hepatitis B and C viruses are traditionally thought of as blood-borne pathogens. Hepatitis A and B are vaccine preventable illnesses for which MSM should be screened and vaccinated against if nonimmune, as per the most recent Advisory Committee on Immunization Practices (19). Screening for hepatitis B should include a hepatitis B surface antigen at minimum, and vaccine should be offered to uninfected individuals without documented vaccination. Vaccination schedules may be found on the CDC website at www.cdc.gov/vaccines/schedules and may include stand-alone hepatitis A and B vaccinations or combination vaccines that cover both hepatitis A and B.

Increasing evidence supports the role of sexual transmission of hepatitis C virus in MSM, specifically those living with HIV, and screening is supported for this population (20,21). Hepatitis C antibody testing is adequate for most individuals at risk, but in cases where acute hepatitis C is suspected, plasma hepatitis C viral RNA screening might be considered; however, this test is not approved as a diagnostic. Testing for hepatitis C virus should be conducted at least annually for at-risk HIV-infected men and women and guided by history of relevant risk behaviors in others (22,23).

STI Screening: WSW

Although it is commonly thought that WSW are at very low risk for STIs, WSW can and do acquire bacterial, viral, and protozoal STIs from both female and male partners (24–27). STIs that have been reported as transmitted between female sex partners include trichomoniasis, chlamydia, syphilis, gonorrhea, hepatitis A, human papillomavirus (HPV), and herpes simplex virus (HSV) type 1 and 2 (24).

WSW are a diverse group with varied sexual and risk behaviors that may not be concordant with their stated sexual identity. Medical providers should be aware that some WSW (including women who self-identity as lesbians) have sex with men, increasing the potential for transmission of STI pathogens and HIV and for unwanted pregnancies (25). In addition, certain sexual practices among WSW can allow transmission of STI pathogens through exchange of vaginal fluids (e.g., unprotected oral sex, mutual masturbation, and sharing of insertive sex toys, especially if they are not washed between uses) (26,27).

For WSW, screening and prevention must include education and improving perceptions of risk for STI and HIV infection. Decreasing the marginalization of this population in the medical community is essential. Practitioners should facilitate open discussions about sexual preferences and practices. WSW should be encouraged to be HIV tested at least once, according to CDC guidelines (28), and to know the HIV status of their partners. The authors recommend that vaccination against hepatitis A and B should be offered to sexually active WSW, as should testing for hepatitis C. Syphilis screening should also be done routinely because oral transmission has been documented between women. Adequate mental health and substance abuse screening and referrals for harm reduction should be performed since intravenous drug use continues to be an important risk factor for HIV and bloodborne virus transmission in this population (29,30). WSW should be evaluated for *N. gonorrhoeae* and *C. trachomatis* and have screening for HPV-related disease using a Papanicolau (Pap) smear, according to current STI and cancer screening guidelines for women, regardless of the gender of their partners (17).

Screening Transgender Patients for STIs

Studies of STI rates among transgender men and women are very limited, but some have shown high rates of infection (31,32). HIV infection rates are extremely high in transgender women (see section below on HIV) (33,34). Reports have found that transgender MSM, particularly those who recently transitioned and are finding themselves attracted to men for the first time, frequently engage in high-risk sexual activity, including unprotected anal and vaginal sex with partners of unknown HIV status (15,16).

As with any population group, STI risk in transgender people is related to sexual behavior, including gender of sexual partners; therefore, providers should avoid making assumptions about their individual patients. The CDC provides no specific screening guidelines for transgender individuals; however, other organizations that specialize in transgender health offer recommendations for STI screening based on the limited evidence available (e.g., Center of Excellence for Transgender Health Primary Care Protocol, www. transhealth.ucsf.edu). In addition, some experts believe that transgender people who have sex with men should be screened according to the CDC's guidelines for MSM. Taking these recommendations together, transgender people with ongoing risk behaviors (e.g., unprotected intercourse, history of STIs, sharing needles for injection of hormones or illicit drugs), should be considered for HIV testing every 3 to 12 months depending on specific behaviors. Screening for gonorrhea, chlamydia, and syphilis should be a routine part of care and should be performed at least yearly (more often if the patient engages in high-risk sexual behavior). Specific interventions and screening tests should be based on the organs present, behaviors reported, or, alternatively, on a standardized protocol of multisite genital and extra-genital screening regardless of anatomy or reported behavior (35). Chapter 18 discusses more on preventive screening for transgender people.

STIs of Specific Concern for LGBTQ People

This section focuses on diseases of specific concern to LGBTQ people, either because prevalence rates are higher in certain populations or because means of transmission and acquisition differ. Further coverage of treatment and diagnostics can be explored by accessing the most recent CDC STD guidelines online at www.cdc.gov/std/treatment/2010.

HIV

HIV disease disproportionately affects MSM and transgender women. In 2011, the MSM risk category accounted for 62% of new HIV diagnoses (the majority occurring in men of African American and Latino descent) and over half of people living with HIV (36). Although the CDC does not collect separate data on transgender persons, several studies have highlighted the increased risk among transgender women, making this group possibly the most disproportionately affected in the United States and worldwide, with prevalence rates of almost 17% to 28% (33,34).

HIV infection among WSW is more commonly due to nonsexual risk factors (i.e., injection drug use); however, the potential for transmission through mucous membrane exposure to infectious vaginal secretions and menstrual blood exists, but evidence for this is only anecdotal or on the case report level (37). Because many WSW have had and may continue to have sex with men, providers should not ignore the potential for sexual transmission of HIV among their WSW clients (25).

Although HIV infection is too great a topic to cover in any detail here, it is important to remember the possibility of acute HIV infection in sexually active individuals. Acute HIV infection may present with fevers, rashes, genital ulcers, a sore throat, and swollen lymph nodes. Recognition of this syndrome is critical given studies that demonstrate substantial infectiousness during this stage of infection (38). Individuals with an undifferentiated viral syndrome in the context of sexual risk should be screened for acute HIV infection. Individuals suspected of having acute HIV infection should be tested with standard antibody tests coupled with viral detection assays, such as an HIV viral load, or be tested with a combined antigen/antibody serologic test for HIV using fourth-generation serology assays. Treatment during acute infection continues to be an area of debate, but most experts and guidelines encourage early initiation of antiretroviral therapy (39).

Resistant Gonorrhea

Increasing rates of resistance to multiple antibiotics have been observed in gonorrhea, with treatment failures reported in many countries (40). These increasing rates of resistance are being noted more frequently in MSM, with concern that they will spread beyond this population (41). N. gonorrhoeae has demonstrated increasing resistance to many oral agents, including fluoroquinolones and cephalosporins. Recent alarming surveillance data indicate that injectable drugs, such as ceftriaxone, may also be threatened by these resistance trends. In an environment where few new antibiotics are being developed, the implications for this alarming trend is that gonorrhea will eventually require more toxic, injectable therapies to treat a multidrug-resistant infection. Current recommendations are to treat gonorrhea with a combination of intramuscular ceftriaxone (250 mg) and either azithromycin (1 g in a single dose) or doxycycline (100 mg twice daily for 7 days) (40). Penicillin-allergic patients require treatment with alternative regimens and need a test of cure.

Hepatitis C

As discussed earlier, hepatitis C virus has traditionally been thought to be transmitted most efficiently through parenteral exposures, such as shared injection paraphernalia among intravenous drug users. Epidemiologic data indicate that MSM, especially those with HIV, might be at increased risk for sexually acquired hepatitis C (42–45). Although the overall prevalence of this infection is not high among MSM, it should be considered in the differential diagnosis of men presenting with liver function test abnormalities. Serologic testing cannot detect early HCV infection, so nucleic acid tests, such as viral load testing, might be used off-label to detect early infection. Individuals with acute hepatitis C should be observed for 12 to 20 weeks to see whether they clear their infection; if they have not, they should be offered therapy (46).

Syphilis

Syphilis is caused by *Treponema pallidum*. Disease manifestations are protean and often difficult to diagnose in the asymptomatic early stages and clinically variable later stages of infection. This infection can have long-term consequences that make it an important public health concern. In 2000, the CDC targeted *T. pallidum* for eradication. But since 2001, the rates of syphilis among MSM have been increasing. In 2012, the CDC estimated that 75% of all primary and secondary syphilis cases were among MSM (47). Oral sex, traditionally considered a safer activity, has been implicated in the ongoing MSM syphilis epidemic (48). Although the burden of disease appears to be less in WSW, oral-genital transmission of syphilis has been reported between women, and due vigilance should be paid for diagnostics and screening of this population (17). Disease manifestations of syphilis are not different in the LGBTQ population save for the possibility of some atypical presentations in HIV-infected MSM with increased neuroinvasiveness and disease that is more difficult to treat in individuals living with HIV infection (49,50).

A specific diagnostic question that causes substantial confusion for providers in the HIV-positive population is when to perform a lumbar puncture to evaluate a patient for central nervous system involvement with syphilis. The CDC recommends lumbar puncture of individuals with syphilis if there are neurologic or ocular signs or symptoms, in late latent or syphilis of unknown duration in HIV-infected individuals, in active tertiary syphilis, and in treatment failure of regimens that do not treat CNS involvement. Evidence exists to limit cerebrospinal fluid (CSF) evaluation of HIV-positive individuals with no neurologic symptoms to those with rapid plasma reagin titers of 1:32 or greater and T-cell counts < 350 cells/mm^3 (51). CSF should be tested for cell count, protein, and CSF VDRL and/or CSF fluorescent treponemal antibody test. There are no standardized guidelines to define a positive CSF result. A positive result on CSF VDRL or fluorescent treponemal antibody test is an absolute indication to treat for neurosyphilis. Five or more white cells on cell count or an elevated protein level > 45 mg/dL are also considered evidence of CNS involvement in HIV-negative individuals. Given the lymphocytic pleocytosis expected in the CSF of individuals with HIV, most experts will set a higher threshold for cell count, closer to 20 white cells (17).

Resistance to penicillin has not emerged in *T. pallidum* given the ongoing clinical success noted among treated individuals. Therapeutic decisions require a clear perspective of disease stage, timing, and symptoms. Follow-up of nontreponemal test titers are necessary after therapy to guide further diagnostics and treatment strategies. Patients being treated for syphilis should be warned about the Jarisch-Herxheimer reaction, a not uncommon febrile response to therapy that is often flu-like. It can occur as early as 2 hours after treatment, usually resolves within 12 to 24 hours, and may be treated with antipyretics and analgesics (52).

Follow-up nontreponemal tests should be checked in all patients treated for syphilis at 6 and 12 months after therapy. HIV-positive patients should also be tested at 3, 9, and 24 months given some evidence that treatment failure may be more common in this population. Between 5% and 11% of patients may require retreatment or treatment intensification because of inadequate serologic response to therapy. An appropriate response to therapy is defined as resolution of symptoms and a 4-fold (2-dilution) drop in VDRL or rapid plasma reagin titer at 6 months after treatment. The presence of clinical symptoms, less than a 4-fold dilution in nontreponemal test titer within 6 months of treatment, or persistent 4-fold increase at 6 months after therapy is considered a failure. Those in whom treatment fails should have their CSF evaluated and be treated for neurosyphilis or late latent disease, guided by these CSF results. Patients with neurosyphilis should have repeat lumbar punctures 3 to 6 months after therapy and every 6 months for 3 years or until CSF findings normalize (17).

Chlamydia: Focus on Lymphogranuloma Venereum

The prevalence of *C. trachomatis* infection among MSM was thought to be low, but with increasing concern that inflammatory genital tract diseases may increase risk for HIV transmission, renewed interest has emerged in screening for and preventing *C. trachomatis* infection among MSM (53,54). Chlamydia is a major cause of rectal infection among those engaging in receptive anal sex (55) with some more invasive strains requiring extended durations of antibiotics. Chlamydia cervicitis appears to be rare among WSW who do not have sex with men, although it might be more common than previously thought (17).

The most common strains causing human infection are serovars A through K; these are responsible for classic presentations such as trachoma and urethritis. Serovars L1, L2, and L3, which are responsible for lymphogranuloma venereum infection, lead to more systemic disease manifestations. Previously a disease of the developing world, LGV has re-emerged among sexually active MSM, primarily as proctitis (56).

In 2003, an outbreak of LGV caused by the L2 serovar of chlamydia occurred among MSM in the Netherlands presenting with proctitis (56). Despite limited surveillance data, LGV has become a common concern among providers caring for MSM in many urban areas. Classically, LGV is on the differential diagnosis of ulcerative genital disease and has a 3- to 30-day incubation period. Generally, after a subtle, nonpainful papule resolves, unilateral inguinal lymphadenopathy develops. Secondary LGV presents very differently in men inoculated rectally and in women inoculated vaginally. Because rectal lymphatics drain to retroperitoneal lymph nodes, MSM who engage in anal intercourse may not present with inguinal lymphadenopathy but rather proctitis due to retroperitoneal lymphatic congestion. After this second stage, untreated LGV can lead to lymphatic obstruction, genital lymphedema, rectal strictures, and fistulae (57).

The strains of *Chlamydia* responsible for LGV can be detected by using all the above techniques, but these testing strategies do not distinguish LGV from the more standard serovars of *Chlamydia*. Serovar-specific bacterial detection tests are often not available and may not be cost-effective. Therefore, many providers empirically treat for LGV using 21-day courses of doxycycline in cases of symptomatic proctitis in MSM. High-titer positive chlamydia blood serology (>1:256 on complement fixation or >1:128 on microimmune fluorescence) may also be used as supportive evidence for LGV infection beyond clinical and epidemiologic suspicion (17).

Azithromycin and doxycycline are the main drugs used for treating chlamydial infections. LGV requires a longer duration of therapy with appropriate antibiotics than does routine chlamydia, usually 3 weeks compared with 1 week. Current LGV recommendations are to treat with doxycycline 100 mg twice daily for 21 days. Second-line therapy that is less studied is 1 weekly dose of 1 g of azithromycin for 3 weeks. Partners of these cases should be evaluated and treated. Although resistance does not appear to be the driver of failure, some sources cite doxycycline as a superior drug for treating standard chlamydia; it remains the drug of choice for LGV (17,58).

HPV

HPV disease is a common health concern for all sexually active individuals, including LGBTQ people, and may be a preventable cause of cervical and anal cancer. HPV has been detected in WSW, even in the absence of a history of sex with men (59). Risk factors associated with HPV detection in WSW are an increased number of male partners and the use of insertive sex toys between female partners. Despite these risks, studies indicate that lesbians and bisexual women are much less likely to undergo cervical cancer screening (Pap testing) compared with heterosexual women, in part because of misconceptions about risk (60–62). Among MSM, anal cancer is 17 times higher than in heterosexual men, and is particularly prevalent among HIV-infected MSM (63). Given these disparities, a combined strategy of screening for HPV-related disease and vaccinating those at risk is a critical part of the sexual health assessment of LGBTQ patients.

WSW should undergo cervical Pap tests according to the same guidelines as all women; transgender men with a cervix should also follow the same screening guidelines as for natal females. Some experts and centers of excellence in MSM health care offer screening for anal squamous intraepithelial lesions in MSM using anal Pap smears and referral of patients with positive test results to specialists for high-resolution anoscopy. However, there are no official guidelines or recommendations, so the practice is center-dependent. Some experts recommend that HIV-infected MSM who engage in receptive anal intercourse be screened once a year and that HIV-uninfected MSM who engage in receptive anal sex be screened every 3 to 5 years. Screening should be performed only if a specialist is able to perform high-resolution anoscopy and a biopsy is available. It is unclear whether identification of anal dysplasia affects disease course, and surgical interventions for high-grade lesions are difficult and may not be definitive. Some evidence suggests that, unlike with other malignancies, antiretroviral medications may have little effect in modifying progression of dysplasia from lower- to higher-grade lesions in HIV-infected individuals (64–66).

Protective immunity against HPV has been demonstrated by 2 vaccine products: Gardasil and Cervarix. Gardasil is a quadrivalent vaccine that protects against HPV 6, 11, 16, and 18. HPV 16 and 18 are the strains responsible for most cervical cancer (70%) and may be the dominant strains responsible for anal dysplasia in MSM. HPV 6 and 11 are responsible for 90% of genital warts. Cervarix is a bivalent vaccine that targets only the more frequently oncogenic strains of HPV (16 and 18) (67,68). Current guidelines recommend vaccination of males age 11 to 26 years and females age 9 to 26 years. Ongoing studies are evaluating the use of vaccine beyond 26 in MSM and individuals with HIV infection (69).

The implications of HPV vaccination for LGBTQ people are significant. HPV vaccine joins hepatitis B vaccination as an intervention that can prevent a sexually transmitted infection that can lead to cancer. Ongoing studies will be needed to evaluate specific efficacy and indications in this population (70,71).

Bacterial Vaginosis

Bacterial vaginosis (BV) is a common cause of vaginal concerns in women. Several studies have reported higher prevalence of BV among WSW compared with women who have sex with men, in some cases a 2-fold increase (72). Supporting the idea of transmission of BV pathogens between women are studies that have identified concordant vaginal flora, including the presence of BV in lesbian couples (73,74). The risk for BV appears to correlate with an increased number of lifetime sexual partners, as well as sharing insertive sex toys and use of vaginal lubricant (74,75).

Many women with BV can be completely asymptomatic and are diagnosed during routine screening or in conjunction with another diagnosis. The predominant symptom of BV is by a copious gray-colored discharge and a distinct foul-smelling "fishy" odor that can become more pronounced after sexual intercourse or during menses. Vaginal irritation or pain, if it occurs, is usually mild (17).

The definitive bacterial agent of BV is disputed. The criteria for the diagnosis of BV in the presence of a vaginal discharge are a vaginal pH greater than 4.6; a positive result on a whiff test with 10% potassium hydroxide; and the microscopic presence of clue cells, known as Amsel criteria. Clue cells represent the abundant coccobacilli bacteria adhering to vaginal epithelial cells. New technologies include a DNA probe for detection of BV, including a 1-stop test that examines for 3 common vaginal pathogens: *Candida* species, *Gardnerella vaginalis,* and *Trichomonas vaginalis.* The treatment of BV is highly effective. The standard treatment is metronidazole, 500 mg orally twice a day for 7 days. The higher 2-g oral dose taken once has the advantage of witnessed adherence to treatment and coverage for trichomonas; however, it is less effective and has an increased incidence of gastrointestinal adverse effects. Tinidazole, either in one 2-g oral dose daily for 2 days or 1-g daily for 5 days, or intravaginal treatment with preparations containing metronidazole or clindamycin provides other options for treatment (17).

While asymptomatic women found to have BV are usually not treated, special considerations should be taken into account with WSW patients. Given BV's association with adverse outcomes in pregnancy, all pregnant women and those actively trying to become pregnant should be treated. Because some evidence supports that BV may represent an STI in WSW (73), it can be concluded that treatment of an asymptomatic carrier may decrease transmission. This may be more relevant in the case of recurrent or refractory disease in a female partner in a monogamous lesbian couple. To date no clinical data support treatment of asymptomatic partners.

Trichomonas

T. vaginalis is a protozoan parasite transmitted principally through vaginal intercourse. Trichomonads can also be spread through direct contact with infected material: underwear, wash cloths, or towels. Infection with the organism, while frequently asymptomatic, can cause vaginitis in women and urethritis in men. Symptoms include yellow-green, frothy, foul-smelling vaginal discharge; itching or tenderness in the vagina; pain during sex; or urinary frequency (17). Transmission of *T. vaginalis* has been reported among a lesbian couple (76). Studies suggests that trichomonas may play a role in facilitating HIV transmission (77,78). Although expensive polymerase chain reaction–based diagnostic testing has been developed, the infection can be diagnosed by visualization of the motile parasites on wet mount. *Trichomonas* infections are usually treated with a 1-time dose of metronidazole, 2 g orally. Studies have shown that at least 5% of clinical cases of trichomoniasis are caused by parasites resistant to the drug (79). Trichomonas among MSM is rare and should likely not be included in routine screening (80).

Herpes Simplex Virus Infection

HSV type 1 and type 2 (HSV-1 and HSV-2) are transmitted by skin-to-skin contact or contact with a mucus membrane and are the most common cause of genital ulcers. These viruses have the ability to generate latent infection in peripheral nerves after primary exposure and can lead to recurrent vesicular and ulcerative disease. This virus sheds with or without the presence of ulcerative or vesicular lesions and can be transmitted through intimate or sexual contact with a completely asymptomatic carrier (17).

The seroprevalence of genital HSV is on the rise, with seroepidemiologic surveys estimating that at least 50 million people in the United States have genital HSV infection (17,81). Traditionally, HSV-1 was thought to be restricted to orolabial herpes, with HSV-2 causing the preponderance of genital infections. More recently, increasing rates of HSV-1 genital infection have been detected among sexually active adults (17). MSM are one of the groups with the highest rates of HSV seroprevalence in the United States (82,83), and an increasing number of young MSM are developing anogenital herpes due to HSV-1 (84). Beyond being a clinical annoyance with recurrent and painful lesions, HSV disease may represent an important risk factor for HIV transmission among MSM whether or not the HSV infection is symptomatic (17,83).

HSV occurs in WSW. Marrazzo and colleagues found a prevalence of HSV-2 in WSW that was similar to that in non-WSW, although HSV-2 in WSW was associated with a history of having a male sexual partner with herpes. Among women reporting never having had a male sex partner, 3% were HSV-2 seropositive. The prevalence of antibodies to HSV-1 associated with oral lesions was higher in WSW than their heterosexual counterparts and was proportional to the number of lifetime female sexual partners (85). Because HSV can be transmitted in the absence of a detectable outbreak and the presence of open lesions facilitates transmission of other STI pathogens, WSW should be counseled on the possible increased asymptomatic carriage of the oral HSV type and encouraged to engage in protected sex.

HSV in LGBTQ people presents with clinical manifestations similar to those in other populations. These manifestations include vesicular skin eruptions, cervicitis, urethritis, and proctitis. In a series of 101 MSM with proctitis, 13% of cases were caused by HSV alone. An additional 3% of cases were caused by mixed infections, including with HSV (86).

Herpes diagnosis is primarily based on detecting virus through culture or other molecular tests of clinical samples from suspected lesions. In addition to these viral detection tests, serology may also be used to evaluate patients with atypical symptoms or to document exposure status to guide potential suppressive therapy.

Treatment and supression of herpes are well desribed in the CDC STD treatment guidelines and do not differ for LGBTQ people, save some differences in duration and dose based on HIV status (17).

Patients diagnosed with herpes need to be educated on the natural history of disease, specifically that recurrences are possible and that these events can be addressed with episodic or suppressive antivirals. Disclosure to sex partners should be encouraged, and patients should be reminded that asymptomatic shedding may lead to disease transmission. Individuals with prodromal or active symptoms should avoid sexual activity. Condoms may prevent transmission if they cover the lesions. Partners should be evaluated for previous HSV outbreaks and taught to recognize the symptoms.

Meningitis

A well-publicized outbreak of meningococcal meningitis in New York City from about 2010 to 2013 resulted in the deaths of several MSM, many of whom were living with HIV. The outbreak was associated with use of telephone applications and Internet "hook up" sites (87). This prompted a large vaccination effort and a change in local vaccination guidelines for MSM. Final national guidelines surrounding vaccination of MSM against meningococcal disease are being considered. To date there is no recommendation for a global MSM vaccination policy outside of an outbreak scenario.

Education and Counseling to Prevent HIV Infection and STIs

When providing education and counseling to prevent HIV and STIs in LGBTQ patients, it is important to do so in the context of promoting a healthy sexual life. Although sexual risk-taking can threaten health, so might unhappiness with one's sexuality. It is critical, then, that providers focus on sexual health rather than pathology, and that they have a plan to provide appropriate testing, vaccination, education, and counseling for patients in a "sex-positive" environment that encourages sexual expression.

Relative Risk of Sexual Practices

Many patients may not know the specific HIV and STI risks associated with certain behaviors. For example, patients may not be aware that STI pathogens can be transmitted through unprotected oral sex, sharing sex toys, digital manipulation, or body rubbing. Educating patients about the relative risks of different sexual practices allows them to make informed decisions about the level of risk they are willing to accept. The San Francisco City Clinic maintains a basic chart of risks that you can refer your patients to (www.sfcityclinic.org/stdbasics/stdchart.asp). Another STI relative risk chart can be found at SoTheyCanKnow (www.sotheycanknow.org/assess). The CDC also provides fact sheets for patients on certain STIs (www.cdc.gov/std/HealthComm/fact_sheets.htm).

For MSM, the highest-risk activity for HIV infection is receptive anal intercourse, followed by insertive anal intercourse, and followed distantly by receptive and insertive oral sex (88). Breeches in the oral mucosa, gingival inflammation, ejaculation in the mouth, STIs, trauma, and other oral infections appear to increase risk for oral transmission of HIV.

Activities such as mutual masturbation, body-to-body contact without fluid exchange, and role-play activities without fluid exchange do not transmit HIV, although transmission of syphilis, HPV, HSV, *Molluscum contagiosum*, and ectoparasites is still possible with these activities. "Rimming" (oral-anal contact), "water sports" (urine play), and "scat" (fecal play) present lower risk for HIV, although blood contamination is possible, increasing the chance for transmission of HIV and hepatitis viruses. Although a low-risk activity for HIV, fecal-oral contact may put individuals at risk for hepatitis A, bacterial STI, enteric infections, and intestinal parasites (89). Sex toys, such as dildos, that are inserted in mucous membranes and shared between partners can transmit HIV, hepatitis A or B virus, and other STI pathogens if not properly sterilized. It is recommended that dildos and other toys not be shared between partners or that they be cleaned with bleach (or at minimum with soap and water) and used with condoms. Needles for piercing or other play should not be shared or should be sterilized between uses.

Latex Barrier Use

Latex barrier use during activities where fluids may be exchanged is the cornerstone of safer sex. Although most patients are probably aware of the benefits of condoms to prevent HIV infection/STIs and pregnancy, providers should not hesitate to advise and instruct their patients on the consistent and correct use of male and female condoms and dental dams, including the use of adequate water-based lubrication to avoid malfunction, breakage, and minimize mucosal trauma. MSM should be advised to avoid even brief unprotected anal penetration, termed "dipping," given the presence of HIV in pre-ejaculate (pre-cum) (90). The phenomenon of "barebacking," or purposeful unprotected anal intercourse, is psychologically complex and often linked to drug-using behaviors (91). This behavior continues to be an important target for preventive interventions to reduce the risk for HIV infection and other STIs among MSM. Additionally, barriers should be encouraged even if both partners are HIV infected to prevent transmission of STIs, as well as to avoid the possibility of HIV superinfection with multiple strains of HIV of varying virulence and susceptibility to HIV medications. For oral sex, unlubricated condoms should be recommended and can be cut open to create a makeshift dental dam (as can plastic wrap).

Education and counseling on barrier use aimed at WSW should focus on minimizing the sexual transfer of vaginal fluids and menstrual blood between sexual partners. Methods include the use of latex gloves and other latex barriers, such as dental dams for vaginal-digital insertion, anal-digital insertion, and oral sex. Use of lubricants should be encouraged to decrease mucosal irritation and tearing, a potential portal of entry for viral infections. Condoms used with insertive objects should be changed between partners, and efforts should be made to avoid the introduction of fecal flora into the vagina. As noted above, patients should be encouraged to clean dildos and other sex toys with bleach before using or storing them.

Risk-Reduction Counseling

As discussed, a frank discussion of specific sexual activity is needed both to encourage a pleasurable sex life and to identify risk practices. When such behaviors are identified, it is important to work within the patient's sexual context and "comfort zone" to encourage mitigation of this risk. As mentioned previously, there is a wide spectrum of root causes of risk-taking behaviors, including mental health issues, drug and alcohol abuse, domestic/partner violence, history of child abuse, sexual compulsivity, and internalized homophobia/transphobia. The clinician should attempt to identify causes and make referrals to programs, providers, or interventions (see Chapter 9 for more on this topic).

Safer sex is a continuum and should be approached by using a harm reduction model. Some individuals are more willing to accept risk than others, and counseling should focus on optimizing individual risk rather than forcing an individual's sexuality into a series of guidelines or recommendations. Abstinence or mutual monogamy may be the correct approach for some individuals, while reducing the number of partners, even by a few, may be the best intervention for others. Individuals should be advised to have a pre-emptive plan rather than just react to certain situations that may occur. They should be advised to contemplate what risk they are willing to accept prior to an encounter as well as what preventive intentions they will operationalize in those settings. Rational decision-making, however, is less effective while under the influence of drugs and alcohol, so minimizing substance use and abuse when possible is critical to realizing the intention of safer sex.

When counseling patients about sexual behavior change, clinicians should also manage their own expectations regarding the speed and durability of behavioral changes and should approach the maintenance of their patients' sexual health as an ongoing process that requires revisiting during clinical interactions. Providers interested in enhancing their client-centered counseling skills can access training through the CDC STD/HIV National Network of Prevention Training Centers (nnptc.org). For high-risk patients, providers can consider referrals to evidence-based interventions, where available. The CDC hosts a website listing evidence-based biomedical, behavioral, and structural interventions for targeted populations, including MSM (www.effectiveinterventions.org). Because such interventions are not always available, it is also important to be familiar with the local landscape of referrals to providers and community-based organizations with resources and specialty in these areas.

Biomedical Interventions
Bioprophylaxis refers largely to the use of biologically active therapeutic agents to prevent HIV infection. This burgeoning field at the interface between prevention and treatment draws on expertise from both fields and holds both exciting promise and new challenges. It is certain that any biomedical intervention will have to be intimately tied to behavioral modification to be effective at reducing risk over the long term.

Pre- and postexposure prophylaxis are 2 interventions that use antiretroviral therapy to reduce the risk for HIV infection. Postexposure prophylaxis is broadly defined as the administration of antiretroviral agents to a patient after an exposure or potential exposure to HIV. Pre-exposure prophylaxis is a novel strategy in which antiretroviral agents are used in anticipation of an exposure to HIV in high-risk individuals. Chapters 13 and 14 discuss these topics and provide additional information on interventions for HIV risk reduction.

Addressing Sexual Dysfunction in LGBTQ Patients

LGBTQ individuals face many of the same issues regarding sexual dysfunction as heterosexuals, but they also have some unique challenges that an informed provider can address. Sexual dysfunction is complex and is affected by many factors, such as relationship status, psychological, social, cultural, and biological factors, as well as comorbid conditions (diabetes, cardiovascular disease), medications, and substance and alcohol use. The increased rates of comorbidities among LGBTQ individuals, such as anxiety, depression, tobacco and recreational drug use, along with negative self-image, may all contribute to sexual dysfunction. Clinical evaluation of sexual function begins with open-ended and frank history-taking supported by a shame-free clinical environment, and root causes of sexual dysfunction must be explored to create a plan for managing these issues.

Sexual Dysfunction in Men

Erectile Dysfunction
Erectile dysfunction is a common concern among all men and may be more prevalent in MSM (92–94). ED may be caused by psychogenic issues, medical disease (e.g., diabetes and other vasculopathies), medications, or a combination of factors. A thorough history, physical examination, and laboratory evaluation can usually pinpoint the cause.

The most important historical clue in the evaluation of ED is the rapidity of onset. Most rapid-onset ED is associated with a psychogenic etiology. ED caused by medical disease—most commonly endocrine, vascular, or neurologic etiology—is almost always gradual in onset or from obvious trauma or surgery. Organic causes of ED are also often associated with the lack of spontaneous nocturnal or morning erections. A complete review of prescription, recreational, and over-the-counter drug use, as well as alcohol use, should be performed to identify a reversible pharmacologic cause of ED.

The physical examination should focus on the causes of ED: endocrine, vascular, and neurologic. The testes should be examined for atrophy, masses, and asymmetry. Plaques in the penis may indicate Peyronie disease. Thyroid function should be examined. Visual fields should be tested to identify defects that may be caused by a pituitary adenoma. The chest should be examined for gynecomastia. Peripheral pulses should be assessed for any evidence of vascular insufficiency. The cremasteric reflex should be elicited to check the integrity of central erection function. Laboratory testing should include examination of thyroid function, glucose tolerance, lipids, prolactin, and testosterone levels. Nocturnal penile tumescence testing may be necessary if no obvious cause is identified as a gateway to more complex tests of penile vasculature.

Several treatment modalities are available to address ED beyond treating underlying organic and psychogenic causes. These include prostaglandin injections, vacuum devices, and implants. In the last several years, these have been eclipsed by the phosphodiesterase-5 (PDE-5) inhibitors, such as sildenafil, tadalafil, and vardenafil. These drugs have shown efficacy in treating ED of multiple causes and may be commonly prescribed for, and used by, MSM (95,96). Special attention should be paid to concurrent medications, such as protease inhibitors and nitrates (including amyl nitrate poppers), given known severe drug-to-drug interactions (97). In addition, these drugs may be associated with increased sexual risk-taking and the transmission of HIV and other STI pathogens alone or in combination with other drugs of abuse, so men should be reminded about safer sex and risk-reduction behaviors (98). ED in relation to condom use may also be a reason that some MSM, specifically those with HIV, engage in unprotected sex (99).

Ejaculatory Problems

Ejaculatory problems may include premature ejaculation, retrograde ejaculation, decreased volume of ejaculate, retarded ejaculation, and anorgasmia/anejaculation. A complete physical examination and history may uncover causes of these disorders. Premature ejaculation and inability to achieve orgasm are common concerns that more than one third of MSM have reported experiencing in the last year (93).

The most common problem, premature ejaculation, is not associated with any organic cause and may be treated with exercises to train the patient to better delay ejaculation, with topical anesthetics, or with medications such as daily or on-demand selective serotonin reuptake inhibitors (100). These antidepressants are, not surprisingly, among the drugs that cause retrograde and retarded ejaculation. Retarded and retrograde ejaculation may be associated with HIV, diabetes, and/or antiretroviral-associated neuropathy (99).

Disorders of delayed or absent ejaculation or orgasm are less well studied but may require evaluation if they interfere with sexual function and satisfaction. Causes include congenital or postsurgical anatomic issues, psychogenic causes, hypogonadism, hypothyroidism, neurologic disease, substance abuse, and medication adverse effects. Retrograde ejaculation may be identified if sperm are found in postorgasmic urine samples. Management of these conditions should focus on the cause identified (101).

Sexual Compulsivity

Sexual compulsivity, also called sexual addiction, is a state in which sexual fantasies and behaviors reach a frequency and intensity sufficient to interfere with normal functioning or personal, interpersonal, and vocational pursuits (102). The consequences of persistent sexual compulsivity may include conflict and stress in interpersonal relationships, social and work problems caused by the time spent on sexual activities, low self-esteem and other forms of psychological distress, and financial problems arising from excessive spending on pornography and paying for sex or from income lost by avoiding work responsibilities (103).

The prevalence of sexual compulsivity has been estimated at 3% to 6% of the general population, with a male:female predominance of approximately 4:1 (104). In LGBTQ populations, the focus of research on sexual compulsivity has been on gay and bisexual men and the condition's relationship to HIV acquisition risk (105). There are few data on sexual compulsivity in lesbian/ bisexual women or transgender people. In a study that applied a sexual compulsivity scale to LGB participants, mean scores among men were significantly higher than women, suggesting more sexual compulsivity in gay and bisexual men than lesbian and bisexual women (106). Researchers have suggested that prevalence of sexual compulsivity may be higher among gay and bisexual men than heterosexual men, perhaps because of increased access to sexual outlets and therefore more opportunity for men at risk to develop sexual compulsivity (107,108).

The lack of a universally accepted case definition of sexual compulsivity hampers the development of formal screening and diagnostic tools. In clinical primary care practice, most diagnoses are based on presenting symptoms of low self-esteem, loneliness, problems with intimacy, sexual thrill-seeking behavior, social anxiety, social skills impairment, guilt, and impulse control problems (103).

Importantly, sexual compulsivity has been associated with high rates of coprevalent mental health disorders, especially mood, anxiety, and substance use disorders (64% to 81% comorbidity) and personality disorders (41% to 46% comorbidity). A history of childhood sexual abuse has also been shown to correlate with sexual compulsivity, occurring in 30% to 78% of people with sexual compulsivity (105,109). In 1994, Kalichman developed the Sexual Compulsivity Scale (SCS) to evaluate the severity of sexual compulsivity in MSM (110). The SCS is more commonly used in research and mental health treatment settings than in primary care; however, the online, self-administered version may be helpful as a primary care tool for a patient to self-evaluate (www.chip.uconn.edu/chipweb/ documents/Research/K_SexualCompulsivityScale.pdf).

The most important component of treating sexual compulsivity in primary care is referring the patient to a mental health professional with experience in treating sexual compulsivity in LGBTQ populations. Limited data support the use of serotonin reuptake inhibitors and hormonal agents (111).

Psychotherapeutic approaches to sexual compulsivity vary. Many experts recommend an addiction approach using the 12-step model in addition to individual psychotherapy (103). Meetings of Sexual Compulsive Anonymous groups and the like can be found commonly in LGBTQ community centers and online (www.sca-recovery.org). Chapter 9 offers additional information on the manifestation and treatment of sexual compulsivity.

Anorectal Symptoms

History and Physical Examination

Anal symptoms and disorders are highly prevalent in adults, especially among people whose sexual behavior includes receptive anal sex, and among people with HIV (112). Despite this prevalence, many patients delay seeking evaluation for anal symptoms, perhaps because of shame or stigma associated with the anus in general and anal sex in particular (113).

Collecting a full history is critical to the evaluation of anorectal symptoms. Most anorectal problems begin with pain, bleeding, discharge, a palpated mass, or a combination of these symptoms. In addition to collecting the details about the presenting symptoms, it is important to note whether the patient has had a change in bowel habits and whether any constitutional symptoms are present.

The evaluation of most anorectal symptoms in LGBTQ people should include determining whether the patient is engaging in receptive anal sex. It is important to make no assumptions about the patient's anal sex history. Anyone with an anus, regardless of gender or self-identified sexual preference, may engage in anal sex, and many do; it is always prudent to ask. In anal sex history, as with all sexual history, the focus should be on behavior rather than identity. Some patients may say that they are not having anal sex because they are not having anal penetration with a partner, but may have fingers, sex toys, or other objects inserted into their anus.

The anal exam should begin with a visual and tactile examination of the perianal and external anal areas. The examination should pay particular attention to thickening, induration, tenderness, masses, ulceration, and abnormal vessels. The cause of many anal problems may be visible, including fissures, external hemorrhoids, ulcerative STIs (HIV infection, herpes, syphilis, chancroid) and proliferative STIs (HPV infection, molluscum), superficial fungal infections, chronic skin conditions such as eczema and psoriasis, and invasive anal cancer.

Anorectal laboratory specimens are best collected before the introduction of lubricant into the anal canal and therefore before the digital anorectal examination. Lubricant can interfere with optimal cell collection for an anal cytologic sample (anal Pap) and may interfere with both culture- and non-culture-based diagnostics. Most anal collection kits include small swabs that may be moistened with water for comfort before insertion. Lubricant is usually not necessary.

The anal examination should continue with the digital rectal examination. Most primary care providers are trained in a prostate-focused digital rectal examination for male bodies. While assessing the prostate remains an important part of an anal examination (as prostatitis and prostate cancer can cause anorectal symptoms), it is equally important to examine the walls of the anal canal. It may be helpful to think of the digital anorectal examination as akin to a cervicovaginal examination, especially in a patient who engages in receptive anal sex. The mucosa of the anal walls should be palpated circumferentially from the external sphincter to the distal anal canal and proximal rectum, feeling for masses, ulceration, fissures, thickening, induration, and tenderness. Extreme tenderness on digital rectal examination can be an important clue in the diagnosis of infectious proctitis.

After the digital examination, the anal canal should be visually examined using a standard anoscope with a good built-in or external light source. As in the cervicovaginal examination, direct visual inspection of the anal walls can reveal lesions, masses, fissures, and ulcerations that are more common among patients who engage in anal sex and may not be palpable upon digital examination.

Common Noninfectious Anal Conditions

Anal fissure is a tear in the anoderm distal to the dentate line, resulting from the mucosa stretching beyond its capacity (114). Anal fissures are an important cause of anal symptoms in MSM.

Primary anal fissures are usually caused by local trauma, such as anal sex, vaginal delivery, excessive wiping, prolonged diarrhea, or the passage of hard stools. Secondary anal fissures may occur in patients with a history of anal surgery or may result from STIs, malignancies, inflammatory bowel disease, or granulomatous diseases (115).

Patients with an acute anal fissure most commonly present with painful defecation that feels like a tearing sensation. Other symptoms that may accompany an acute anal fissure include small amounts of rectal bleeding and perianal pruritus. Chronic fissures are usually less painful.

Most anal fissures are readily apparent on physical examination of the external anus. The most common location for a fissure is the posterior midline, although lateral and anterior fissures may also occur (115). Acute fissures may look like a fresh laceration, while chronic fissures often have raised or heaped up edges and may be accompanied by external skin tags distally and hypertrophied anal papillae proximally. Some fissures may be internal, requiring an anoscopic view to make the diagnosis. Anal fissures, especially when they are small or nonlinear, may be difficult to distinguish from other types of anal ulceration.

Many patients do not seek care for acute fissures because they sometimes heal quickly and spontaneously without medical intervention. In fissures requiring treatment, there is often a cycle of sphincter spasm and continued tearing cause by the patient tensing while defecating in anticipation of the pain. The goal of treatment of acute anal fissures is to minimize the pain and promote healing. Fiber therapy, warm sitz baths, and using moist towelettes for wiping are useful for reducing the pain and trauma of defecation. Topical anesthetic creams may also be helpful. In more advanced cases, topical therapy with nitroglycerin, diltiazem, or nifedipine are helpful in promoting healing of the fissure. Studied medical interventions include oral nifedipine, oral diltiazem, and botulinum toxin (116–119). Fissures that do not improve with topical therapies are generally referred to a specialist (gastroenterologist or rectal surgeon). Anal fissures that do not heal within 6 weeks with conservative local management are considered chronic and should be referred for surgical management.

Hemorrhoids occur when the normal vascular cushions in the anal canal enlarge and bulge causing symptoms. Hemorrhoids are a very common condition, affecting millions of people worldwide. Despite the high prevalence of hemorrhoidal disease, its pathophysiology is poorly understood and data on risk factors are inconsistent (120).

While data are limited about the association of receptive anal sex and the formation of hemorrhoids, it is clear that receptive anal sex can aggravate and prolapse pre-existing hemorrhoids (121).

Hemorrhoids should be diagnosed by examination and visualization of the hemorrhoid. External hemorrhoids are usually easily seen on the external anal opening as dark (color of venous blood) bulges. Thrombosed external hemorrhoids may be very tender. Internal hemorrhoids are usually painless, except when strangulated. Visualizing internal hemorrhoids usually requires anoscopy, unless they have prolapsed externally. To avoid misdiagnosis, anal pain or bleeding should not be attributed to a hemorrhoid–if the hemorrhoid cannot be seen on physical examination, especially in a person who engages in anal sex. For example, the combination of rectal bleeding and painful defecation is uncommon with internal hemorrhoids, but can be a symptom of several STIs causing proctitis (122–124).

Anodysparunia (pain during anal sex) has not been well studied. Many people may infer from our cultural and artistic representations of receptive anal sex that it is inherently painful. However, many experts agree that with proper preparation, anal sex can be comfortable and pleasurable (125,126). Rosser, in a 1998 study, further found that 13% of MSM report frequent and severe pain during receptive anal intercourse, and referred to it as anodyspareunia (127). A similar prevalence was found in another study by Damon in 2005, which also found that men with anodyspareunia experienced significant disruption to their lives, manifesting as avoidance of receptive anal sex completely (82%), restriction to insertive anal sex only (49%), problems in an existing sexual relationship (31%) or finding a new one (15%), and less satisfaction with sexual relationships than men without anodyspareunia (128). The 3 most common factors associated with anodyspareunia were not feeling relaxed or otherwise psychologically prepared, having a partner with a large penis, and lack of foreplay, followed by lack of lubrication and lack of sexual arousal (128). A clinician managing a patient who reports anodyspareunia should review psychological preparation (relaxation), and the importance of foreplay and proper lubrication.

Sexual Dysfunction in Women

Sexuality is an important part of a woman's well-being; however, few studies have addressed sexual dysfunction among lesbians and bisexual women. A recent survey revealed that as many as 25% of WSW met criteria for high risk for female sexual dysfunction, although only 1 in 10 had sought medical advice, underscoring the need for health care providers to discuss sexual health concerns, sexual desire, and satisfaction with their clients (129). Sexual dysfunction in women is more complex than among men and is usually classified in 4 domains: problems with sexual desire (including hypoactive sexual desire disorder) or arousal, sexual pain, and anorgasmia.

If sexual dysfunction has been ascertained in a female patient, a comprehensive history and gynecological examination should be completed. Clinicians should be aware that a WSW patient may have avoided gynecologic care because of fear of discrimination; therefore, it is important to reassure the patient that sexual dysfunction is not a harbinger of more serious gynecologic issues. The gynecologic history should cover use of hormones, menstrual cycle, menopause, perimenopause, pregnancy and lactation, oophorectomy, and hysterectomy. The provider should obtain a full list of medications, including over-the-counter preparations, that may affect arousal and desire, such as antidepressants (especially selective serotonin reuptake inhibitors), antipsychotics, and antihypertensives (especially β-blockers).

The gynecologic examination should focus on obvious causes of genital pain, such as increased vaginal tone, vaginal atrophy, ulcerations (herpes simplex), vaginitis, STIs, cervical cancer, presence of ovarian masses, or tenderness and rectal disease. A detailed examination usually includes visualization of the external genitalia and bimanual, rectovaginal, and speculum examinations. Although there are no specific tests for sexual dysfunction, screening for cervical cancer and STIs may be indicated.

Sexual Pain

Sexual pain is often caused by vaginismus or dyspareunia. Vaginismus is an involuntary spasm of the perineal muscles surrounding the vagina resulting in difficult or painful vaginal penetration. This condition can often be detected during a routine gynecologic examination. Dyspareunia is genital pain associated with sexual activity and is usually based on the patient's self-report. Dyspareunia may commonly occur after menopause, often as a result of vulvovaginal atrophy, affecting about 35% to 45% of women (130). Declines in estrogen are associated with urogenital atrophy, vaginal dryness, and urinary incontinence. Over time vascular changes lead to changes in vaginal and clitoral tissues that decrease sensation, elasticity, and the ability to self-lubricate. These in combination may cause dyspareunia and create a cycle of anxiety and fear that makes sexual activity physically and mentally unpleasant. Other causes of dyspareunia include HSV infection, atrophic vulvitis, topical irritants, pelvic inflammatory disease, endometriosis, ovarian cysts, and bowel disease. Treatment relies on the underlying diagnosis. Sexual pain may be minimized through the use of lubricants, topical lidocaine, and complementary medicine (including biofeedback and acupuncture). Ospemifene and lasofoxifene are selective estrogen receptor modulators approved for the treatment of vulvovaginal atrophy associated with dyspareunia (131,132).

Anorgasmia

Anorgasmia is a very complex condition, affecting up to 1 in 4 women, that is categorized by the inability to achieve an orgasm (133). This problem may be situational or absolute. Women may have never experienced an orgasm or may have had orgasms successfully in the past. Although not formally studied in WSW, anorgasmia may be associated with sexual repression of sensations and emotions, a phenomenon that may accompany issues surrounding sexual identity. Nonpharmacologic treatment may involve cognitive behavioral therapy to reduce guilt or shame around sexuality or low self-esteem, self-exploration, and couples' counseling (133). Anorgasmia may be related to underlying conditions (including diabetes, renal failure) or present as an adverse effect of medications, especially selective serotonin reuptake inhibitors (133). Identifying and treating underlying causes may include androgen replacement in postmenopausal women. In sexual dysfunction associated with selective serotonin reuptake inhibitors, adding or switching to antidepressants with fewer sexual adverse effects (e.g., bupropion) may alleviate sexual dysfunction. Adjunctive therapy with sildenafil has had mixed results in clinical studies (133). A nonpharmaceutical option is a small portable vacuum applied to increase clitoral blood flow (the Eros-Clitoral Therapy Device) that is FDA approved for treatment of anorgasmia.

Hypoactive Sexual Desire Disorder

Hypoactive sexual desire disorder can be difficult to treat. Lack of desire may be related to both psychosocial and biologic factors. Historical evaluation should focus on a complete review of prescription, over-the-counter, and recreational drug use (134). Because sexual pain may affect desire, causes of dyspareunia should be pursued (135). Reduced sexual desire may be addressed through treatment of underling conditions, sex therapy, individual or couple counseling, changes in sexual routine, use of erotic material, and experimentation with sex toys such as vibrators. Although there are no FDA-approved treatments, estrogen and low-dose testosterone replacement have been used to increase sexual desire in post- and perimenopausal women (136).

Sexual Dysfunction in Transgender Individuals

Few studies have investigated sexual dysfunction in transgender persons; however, there is evidence that hormone therapy and genital surgery can affect sexual function and satisfaction (137,138). Before talking to transgender patients about their sexual function, medical providers should be sure they have built a rapport and have the trust of the patients, as some transgender patients may be uncomfortable discussing their sexual lives. Compounding the issue is the lack of trans-sensitive and inclusive language to describe transgender bodies, making it difficult to broach subjects of sexual dysfunction. History and physical examination should focus on the organ systems present and not the perceived gender of the patient. It is also important for providers to avoid assumptions about the patient's sexual identity, sexual activities, or the gender of the patient's partners.

Testosterone use in transgender men may result in vaginal atrophy and dyspareunia; however, it has also been shown to increase sexual desire (137). In transgender women, androgen blockers may result in ED disorders, which can be treated with modification of hormonal therapy and/or by prescribing erection-enhancing drugs, such as PDE-5 inhibitors. For transgender women who have undergone genital surgery, rates of hypoactive sexual desire disorder mirror those in the general female population. For transgender men, sexual desire may improve after surgery (138). For these reasons, medical providers should be aware of the possible effect of hormonal and surgical treatment on their transgender patients' sexual function and desire. By maintaining open communication and using respectful language (i.e., mirroring the language that transgender patients use to describe their anatomy), clinicians should be able to increase opportunities to discuss, identify, and treat sexual function issues in their transgender patients.

Fertility Goals/Children

The fertility goals of LGBTQ patients are often overlooked based on provider assumptions that these are not relevant concerns. It is important to ask LGBTQ patients about their interest in having children to better guide them in the medical, legal, and social process in achieving their goals. Several options exist to conceive or adopt children, although cost and social/provider bias may limit access to adoptive or conception services for LGBTQ patients. Chapter 6 provides comprehensive information on parenting options for LGBTQ families.

Hormonal therapy in transgender patients can affect fertility, but many transgender patients have successfully conceived. Chapter 18 provides more detail on fertility in transgender patients.

HIV can complicate efforts to conceive. Before pursuing pregnancy, HIV-infected patients may need help in accessing information about interventions, such as washing of sperm to remove HIV from infected ejaculate before insemination, or pre-exposure prophylaxis for HIV-negative partners in a serodiscordant couple. Data for both these interventions are promising but very limited (139).

Conclusion

Sex, however or with whomever it is performed, should be a joyous part of life. Understanding a patient's sexuality and sexual activities allows for troubleshooting to maintain sexual satisfaction and preventive interventions to maintain sexual health. LGBTQ sex should not focus solely on pathology, HIV, or STIs; rather, it is about satisfaction and good health. LGBTQ sex is normal sex. Omission of a sexual history from a medical assessment or minimization of sexual issues is not a neutral mistake. Not asking about sex implies a judgment that sex is not healthy or a part of health care. To marginalized people who may doubt the validity of their sexual feelings, taciturn responses are tantamount to invalidating the normalcy of their sexual selves. Asking about sexuality and sexual satisfaction affirms and validates patients sexual identity. Engaging patients to partner with them to enhance their sexual health is an important part of comprehensive medical care.

Summary Points

- Addressing the sexual health of LGBTQ patients should be a routine part of primary care.
- Asking about sexual and gender identity and behavior are critical in providing appropriate health care to all patients.
- Many patients do not know about the STI/HIV risks associated with certain behaviors. Educating them allows them to make informed decisions about the level of risk they are willing to accept.
- It is important to educate patients about safer sex, focusing on harm reduction advice to minimize personal risk for HIV. It is also important to point out that safer sex techniques to prevent HIV do not always prevent other STIs.
- Routine screening for HIV infection and STIs should be a standard part of the health care of LGBTQ clients.
- Routine and streamlined HIV testing should be offered in all health care settings, following CDC guidelines and local laws.
- The signs and symptoms of STIs should guide the choice of diagnostic tests and therapies. Keep in mind special treatment considerations among LGBTQ patients, such as the emergence of quinolone-resistant gonorrhea among MSM.

- LGBTQ clients should be vaccinated against sexually transmitted pathogens such as hepatitis A and B viruses.
- Sexual dysfunction is common among LGBTQ patients and should be discussed so appropriate interventions and therapies can be offered.

References

1. **Potter JE.** Do ask, do tell. Ann Intern Med. 2002;137:341-3.
2. **Bell R.** ABC of sexual health: homosexual men and women. BMJ. 1999;318:452-5.
3. **Broekman CP, van der Werff ten Bosch JJ, Slob AK.** An investigation into the management of patients with erection problems in general practice. Int J Impot Res. 1994;6:67-72.
4. **Hartmann U, Burkart M.** Erectile dysfunctions in patient-physician communication: optimized strategies for addressing sexual issues and the benefit of using a patient questionnaire. J Sex Med. 2007;4:38-46.
5. **Althof SE, Rosen RC, Perelman MA, Rubio-Aurioles E.** Standard operating procedures for taking a sexual history. J Sex Med. 2013;10:26-35.
6. **Gott M, Hinchliff S, Galena E.** General practitioner attitudes to discussing sexual health issues with older people. Soc Sci Med. 2004;58:2093-103.
7. **Kingsberg SA.** Taking a sexual history. Obstet Gynecol Clin North Am. 2006;33:535-47.
8. **Shifren JL, Johannes CB, Monz BU, Russo PA, Bennett L, Rosen R.** Help-seeking behavior of women with self-reported distressing sexual problems. J Womens Health (Larchmt). 2009;18:461-8.
9. **Fisher WA, Rosen RC, Eardley I, et al.** The multinational Men's Attitudes to Life Events and Sexuality (MALES) study phase II: understanding PDE5 inhibitor treatment seeking patterns, among men with erectile dysfunction. J Sex Med. 2004;1:150-60.
10. **Williamson C.** Providing care to transgender persons: a clinical approach to primary care, hormones, and HIV management. J Assoc Nurses AIDS Care. 2010;21:221-9.
11. **McNair R.** Lesbian and bisexual women's sexual health. Aust Fam Physician. 2009;38:388-93.
12. **Nusbaum MR, Hamilton CD.** The proactive sexual health history. Am Fam Phys. 2002;66:1705-12.
13. **Institute of Medicine.** The Health of Lesbian, Gay, Bisexual, and Transgender People: Building a Foundation for Better Understanding. Washington, DC: The National Academies Press; 2011.
14. **Daskalos CT.** Changes in the sexual orientation of six heterosexual male-to-female transsexuals. Arch Sex Behav. 1998;27:605-14.
15. **Reisner SL, Perkovich B, Mimiaga MJ.** A mixed methods study of the sexual health needs of New England transmen who have sex with nontransgender men. AIDS Patient Care STDS. 2010;24:501-13.
16. **Rowniak S, Chesla C.** Coming out for a third time: transmen, sexual orientation, and identity. Arch Sex Behav. 2013;42:449-61.
17. **Centers for Disease Control and Prevention.** Sexually transmitted treatment guidelines, 2010. MMWR Morb Mortal Wkly Rep. 2010;59(RR-12):1-110.
18. **Hoover KW, Butler M, Workowski K, et al.** STD screening of HIV-infected MSM in HIV clinics. Sex Transm Dis. 2010;37:77—1-6.
19. **Centers for Disease Control and Prevention.** Recommended adult immunization schedule—United States, 2012. MMWR Morb Mortal Wkly Rep. 2012;61:1-7.
20. **Bradshaw D, Matthews G, Danta M.** Sexually transmitted hepatitis C infection: the new epidemic in MSM? Curr Opin Infect Dis. 2013;26:66-72.

21. **Yaphe S, Bozinoff N, Kyle R, et al.** Incidence of acute hepatitis C virus infection among men who have sex with men with and without HIV infection: a systematic review. Sex Transm Infect. 2012;88:558-64.

22. **Aberg JA, Gallant JE, Ghanem KG, et al.** Primary care guidelines for the management of persons infected with HIV: 2013 update by the HIV Medicine Association of the Infectious Disease Society of America. Clin Infect Dis. 2013;58:1-10.

23. **American Association for the Study of Liver Disease and the Infectious Diseases Society of America.** Recommendations for testing, managing, and treating hepatitis C. Available at: http://hcvguidelines.org.

24. **Gorgos LM, Marrazzo JM.** Sexually transmitted infections among women who have sex with women. Clin Infect Dis. 2011;53 Suppl 3:S84-91.

25. **Diamant AL, Schuster MA, McGuigan K, Lever J.** Lesbians' sexual history with men: implications for taking a sexual history. Arch Intern Med. 1999;159:2730-6.

26. **Marrazzo J, Koutsky LA, Eschenbach DA, et al.** Characterization of vaginal flora and bacterial vaginosis in women who have sex with women. J Infect Dis. 2002;185:1307-13.

27. **Muzny CA, Sunesara IR, Martin DH, Mena LA.** Sexually transmitted infections and risk behaviors among African American women who have sex with women: does sex with men make a difference? Sex Transm Dis. 2011;38:1118-25.

28. **Centers for Disease Control and Prevention.** Revised recommendations for HIV testing of adults, adolescents, and pregnant women in health-care settings. MMWR Recomm Rep. 2006;55(RR14):1-17.

29. **Friedman SR, Ompad DC, Maslow C, et al.** HIV prevalence, risk behaviors, and high-risk sexual and injection networks among young women injectors whohave sex with women. Am J Public Health. 2003;93:902-6.

30. **Reisner SL, Mimiaga MJ, Case P, et al.** Sexually transmitted disease (STD) diagnoses and mental health disparities among women who have sex with women screened at an urban community health center, Boston, MA, 2007. Sex Transm Dis. 2010;37:5-12.

31. **Dos Ramos Farías MS, Garcia MN, et al.** First report on sexually transmitted infections among trans (male to female transvestites, transsexuals, or transgender) and male sex workers in Argentina: high HIV, HPV, HBV, and syphilis prevalence. Int J Infect Dis. 2011;15: e635-40.

32. **Toibaro JJ, Ebensrtejin JE, Parlante A, et al.** [Sexually transmitted infections among transgender individuals and other sexual identities]. Medicina (B Aires). 2009;69:327-30.

33. **Baral SD, Poteat T, Strömdahl S, et al.** Worldwide burden of HIV in transgender women: a systematic review and meta-analysis. Lancet Infect Dis. 2013;13:214-22.

34. **Herbst JH, Jacobs ED, Finlayson TJ, et al; HIV/AIDS Prevention Research Synthesis Team.** Estimating HIV prevalence and risk behaviors of transgender persons in the United States: a systematic review. AIDS Behav. 2008;12:1-17.

35. **Deutsch MB, Feldman JL.** Updated recommendations from the world professional association for transgender health standards of care. Am Fam Phys. 2013;87:89-93.

36. **Centers for Disease Control and Prevention.** HIV among gay, bisexual, and other men who have sex with men: Fact Sheet. Available at: www.cdc.gov/hiv/risk/gender/msm/facts/index.html.

37. **Chan SK, Thornton LR, Chornister KJ, et al.** Likely female-to-female sexual transmission of HIV—Texas, 2012. MMWR Morb Mortal Wkly Rep. 2014;63:209-12.

38. **Kahn JO, Walker BD.** Acute human immunodeficiency virus type 1 infection. N Engl J Med. 1998;339:33-9.

39. Guidelines for the use of antiretroviral agents in HIV-1-infected adults and adolescents: considerations for antiretroviral use in special patient populations, acute and recent (early*) HIV infection. AIDSinfo. Clinical Guidelines Portal. Available at: www.aidsinfo.nih.gov/guidelines/html/1/adult-and-adolescent-treatment-guidelines/20/acute-hiv-infection

40. **Centers for Disease Control and Prevention.** Grand Rounds: the growing threat of multi-drug-resistant gonorrhea. MMWR Morb Mortal Wkly Rep. 2013;62:103-6.

41. **Kirkcaldy RD, Zaidi A, Hook EW 3rd, et al.** Neisseria gonorrhoeae antimicrobial resistance among men who have sex with men and men who have sex exclusively with women: the gonococcal isolate surveillance project, 2005-2010. Ann Intern Med. 2013;158(5 Pt 1): 321-8.

42. **Fisher MJ, Richardson D.** Consider acute hepatitis C, syphilis, and HIV in MSM with hepatitis. BMJ. 2011;343:d5169.

43. **Garg S, Taylor LE, Grasso C, Mayer KH.** Prevalent and incident hepatitis C virus infection among HIV-infected men who have sex with men engaged in primary care in a Boston community health center. Clin Infect Dis. 2013;56:1480-7.

44. **van der Helm JJ, Prins M, del Amo J, et al.** The hepatitis C epidemic among HIV-positive MSM: incidence estimates from 1990 to 2007. AIDS. 2011;25:1083-91.

45. **Zhang L, Zhang D, Yu B, et al.** Prevalence of HIV infection and associated risk factors among men who have sex with men (MSM) in Harbin, P. R. China. PLoS One. 2013;8:e58440.

46. **Ghany MG, Strader DB, Thomas DL, Seeff LB; American Association for the Study of Liver Diseases.** Diagnosis, management, and treatment of hepatitis C: an update. Hepatology. 2009;49:1335-74.

47. **Centers for Disease Control and Prevention.** 2012 sexually transmitted disease surveillance: STDs in men who have sex with men. Available at: www.cdc.gov/std/stats12/msm.htm.

48. **Centers for Disease Control and Prevention.** Transmission of primary and secondary syphilis by oral sex—Chicago, Illinois, 1998-2002. MMWR Morb Mortal Wkly Rep. 2004;53: 966-8.

49. **Hofer K, Kreft B, Marsch WC.** Unusual cutaneous manifestations of syphilis II in an HIV-infected MSM. J Deutsch Dermatol Gesell. 2011;9:246-6.

50. **Kyriacou A, Kingston MA, Higgins SP.** The effect of concomitant HIV infection on the clinical manifestations of syphilis. Sex Transm Infect. 2006;82:A3-A3.

51. **Marra CM.** Deja vu all over again: when to perform a lumbar puncture in HIV-infected patients with syphilis. Sex Transm Dis. 2007;34:145-6.

52. **Belum GR, Belum VR, Chaitanya Arudra SK, Reddy BS.** The Jarisch-Herxheimer reaction: revisited. Travel Med Infect Dis. 2013;11:231-7.

53. **Ciemins EL, Flood J, Kent CK, et al.** Reexamining the prevalence of Chlamydia trachomatis infection among gay men with urethritis: implications for STD policy and HIV prevention activities. Sex Transm Dis. 2000;27:249-251.

54. **Cohen MS, Hoffman IF, Royce RA, et al.** Reduction of concentration of HIV-1 in semen after treatment of urethritis: implications for prevention of sexual transmission of HIV-1. AIDSCAP Malawi Research Group. Lancet. 1997;349:1868-73.

55. **van Liere GA, Hoebe CJ, Niekamp AM, Koedijk FD, Dukers-Muijrers NH.** Standard symptom- and sexual history-based testing misses anorectal Chlamydia trachomatis and neisseria gonorrhoeae infections in swingers and men who have sex with men. Sex Transm Dis. 2013;40:285-9.

56. **Nieuwenhuis RF, Ossewaarde JM, Götz HM, et al.** Resurgence of lymphogranuloma venereum in Western Europe: an outbreak of Chlamydia trachomatis serovar l2 proctitis in The Netherlands among men who have sex with men. Clin Infect Dis. 2004;39:996-1003.

57. **Stamm WE, Batteiger BE.** Chlamydia trachomatis (trachoma, perinatal infections, lymphogranuloma venereum, and other genital infections). In: Mandell GL, Bennett JE, Dolin R, eds. Principles and Practice of Infectious Diseases. 7th ed. Philadelphia: Elsevier Churchill Livingstone; 2009:180.

58. **Bhengraj AR, Vardhan H, Srivastava P, Salhan S, Mittal A.** Decreased susceptibility to azithromycin and doxycycline in clinical isolates of Chlamydia trachomatis obtained from recurrently infected female patients in India. Chemotherapy. 2010;56:371-7.

59. **Marrazzo JM, Koutsky LA, Kiviat NB, Kuypers JM, Stine K.** Papanicolaou test screening and prevalence of genital human papillomavirus among women who have sex with women. Am J Public Health. 2001;91:947-52.

60. **Cochran SD, Mays VM, Bowen D, et al.** Cancer-related risk indicators and preventive screening behaviors among lesbians and bisexual women. Am J Public Health. 2001;13:591-7.

61. **Roberts SJ, Patsdaughter CA, Grindel CG, Tarmina MS.** Health related behaviors and cancer screening of lesbians: results of the Boston Lesbian Health Project II. Women Health. 2004; 13:41-55.

62. **Tracy JK, Lydecker AD, Ireland L.** Barriers to cervical cancer screening among lesbians. J Womens Health (Larchmt). 2010;13:229-37.

63. **Dietz CA, Nyberg CR.** Genital, oral, and anal human papillomavirus infection in men who have sex with men. J Am Osteopath Assoc. 2011;111(3 Suppl 2):S19-25.

64. **Czoski-Murray C, Karnon J, Jones R, Smith K, Kinghorn G.** Cost-effectiveness of screening high-risk HIV-positive men who have sex with men (MSM) and HIV-positive women for anal cancer. Health Technol Assess. 2010;14:iii-iv, ix-x, 1-101.

65. **Palefsky J, Berry JM, Jay N.** Anal cancer screening. Lancet Oncol. 2012;13:e279-80; author rreply e280.

66. **Palefsky JM.** Antiretroviral therapy and anal cancer: the good, the bad, and the unknown. Sex Transm Dis. 2012;39:501-3.

67. **Rank C, Gilbert M, Ogilvie G, et al.** Acceptability of human papillomavirus vaccination and sexual experience prior to disclosure to health care providers among men who have sex with men in Vancouver, Canada: implications for targeted vaccination programs. Vaccine. 2012;30: 5755-60.

68. **Kim JJ.** Targeted human papillomavirus vaccination of men who have sex with men in the USA: a cost-effectiveness modelling analysis. Lancet Infect Dis. 2010;10:845-52.

69. Recommendations on the use of quadrivalent human papillomavirus vaccine in males—Advisory Committee on Immunization Practices (ACIP), 2011. MMWR Morb Mortal Wkly Rep. 2011;60:1705-8.

70. **Palefsky J.** Can HPV vaccination help to prevent anal cancer? Lancet Infect Dis. 2010;10: 815-6.

71. **van der Burg SH, Palefsky JM.** Human immunodeficiency virus and human papilloma virus—why HPV-induced lesions do not spontaneously resolve and why therapeutic vaccination can be successful. J Transl Med. 2009;7:108.

72. **Fethers KA, Fairley CK, Hocking JS, Gurrin LC, Bradshaw CS.** Sexual risk factors and bacterial vaginosis: a systematic review and meta-analysis. Clin Infect Dis. 2008;47:1426-35.

73. **Berger BJ, Kolton S, Zenilman JM, et al.** Bacterial vaginosis in lesbians: a sexually transmitted disease. Clin Infect Dis. 1995;21:1402-5.

74. **Marrazzo JM, Koutsky LA, Eschenbach DA, et al.** Characterization of vaginal flora and bacterial vaginosis in women who have sex with women. J Infect Dis. 2002;185:1307-13.

75. **Bailey JV, Farquhar C, Owen C.** Bacterial vaginosis in lesbians and bisexual women. Sex Transm Dis. 2004;31:691-4.

76. **Sivakumar K, De Silva AH, Roy RB.** Trichomonas vaginalis infection in a lesbian. Genitourin Med. 1989;65:399-400.

77. **Mavedzenge SN, Pol BV, Cheng H, et al.** Epidemiological synergy of Trichomonas vaginalis and HIV in Zimbabwean and South African women. Sex Transm Dis. 2010;37:460-6.

78. **Van Der Pol B, Kwok C, Pierre-Louis B, et al.** Trichomonas vaginalis infection and human immunodeficiency virus acquisition in African women. J Infect Dis. 2008;197:548-54.

79. **Schmid G, Narcisi E, Mosure D, Secor WE, Higgins J, Moreno H.** Prevalence of metronidazole-resistant Trichomonas vaginalis in a gynecology clinic. J Reprod Med. 2001;46: 545-9.

80. **Kelley CF, Rosenberg ES, O'Hara BM, Sanchez T, del Rio C, Sullivan PS.** Prevalence of urethral Trichomonas vaginalis in black and white men who have sex with men. Sex Transm Dis. 2012;39:739.

81. **Xu F, Sternberg MR, Kottiri BJ, et al.** Trends in herpes simplex virus type 1 and type 2 seroprevalence in the United States. JAMA. 2006;296:964-73.

82. **Xu F, Sternberg MR, Markowitz LE.** Men who have sex with men in the United States: demographic and behavioral characteristics and prevalence of HIV and HSV-2 infection: results from National Health and Nutrition Examination Survey 2001-2006. Sex Transm Dis. 2010; 37:399-405.

83. **Bohl DD, Katz KA, Bernstein K, et al.** Prevalence and correlates of herpes simplex virus type-2 infection among men who have sex with men, San Francisco, 2008. Sex Transm Dis. 2011;38:617-21.

84. **Ryder N, Jin F, McNulty AM, Grulich AE, Donovan B.** Increasing role of herpes simplex virus type 1 in first-episode anogenital herpes in heterosexual women and younger men who have sex with men, 1992-2006. Sex Transm Infect. 2009;85:416-9.

85. **Marrazzo JM, Stine K, Wald A.** Prevalence and risk factors for infection with herpes simplex virus type-1 and -2 among lesbians. Sex Transm Dis. 2003;30:890-5.

86. **Klausner JD, Kohn R, Kent C.** Etiology of clinical proctitis among men who have sex with men. Clin Infect Dis. 2004;38:300-2.

87. Notes from the Field: serogroup C invasive meningococcal disease among men who have sex with men—New York City, 2010-2012. MMWR Morb Mortal Wkly Rep. 2013;61:1048.

88. **Varghese B, Maher JE, Peterman TA, Branson BM, Steketee RW.** Reducing the risk of sexual transmission: quantifying the per-act risk for HIV infection based on choice of partner, sex act, and condom use. Sex Transm Dis. 2002;29:38-43.

89. **Gill SK, Loveday C, Gilson RJ.** Transmission of HIV-1 infection by oroanal intercourse. Genitourin Med. 1992;68:254-7.

90. **Pudney J, Oneta M, Mayer K, Seage G III, Anderson D.** Pre-ejaculatory fluid as potential vector for sexual transmission of HIV-1. Lancet. 1992;340:1470.

91. **Halkitis PN, Parsons JT, Wilton L.** Barebacking among gay and bisexual men in New York City: explanations for the emergence of intentional unsafe behavior. Arch Sex Behav. 2003; 32:351-7.

92. **Shamloul R, Ghanem H.** Erectile dysfunction. Lancet. 2013;381:153-65.

93. **Hirshfield S, Chiasson MA, Wagmiller RL Jr, et al.**, Sexual dysfunction in an Internet sample of U.S. men who have sex with men. J Sex Med. 2010;7:3104-14.

94. **Shindel AW, Horberg MA, Smith JF, Breyer BN.** Sexual dysfunction, HIV, and AIDS in men who have sex with men. AIDS Patient Care STDS. 2011;25:341-9.

95. **Briganti A, Salonia A, Deho' F, et al.** Clinical update on phosphodiesterase type-5 inhibitors for erectile dysfunction. World J Urol. 2005; 23:374-84.

96. **Swearingen SG, Klausner JD.** Sildenafil use, sexual risk behavior, and risk for sexually transmitted diseases, including HIV infection. Am J Med. 2005;118:571-7.

97. **Cove J, Petrak J.** Factors associated with sexual problems in HIV-positive gay men. Int J STD AIDS. 2004;15:732-6.

98. **Fisher DG, Reynolds GL, Napper LE.** Use of crystal methamphetamine, Viagra, and sexual behavior. Curr Opin Infect Dis. 2010;23:53-6.

99. **Richardson D, Lamba H, Goldmeier D, Nalabanda A, Harris JR.** Factors associated with sexual dysfunction in men with HIV infection. Int J STD AIDS. 2006;17:764-7.

100. **Balon R.** Antidepressants in the treatment of premature ejaculation. J Sex Marital Ther. 1996;22:85-96.

101. **McMahon CG, Jannini E, Waldinger M, Rowland D.** Standard operating procedures in the disorders of orgasm and ejaculation. J Sex Med. 2013;10:204-29.

102. **Grov C, Parsons JR, Bimbi DS.** Sexual compulsivity and sexual risk in gay and bisexual men. Arch Sex Behav. 2010;39:940-9.

103. **Muench F.** Sexual compulsivity and HIV: identification and treatment. Focus. 2004;19: 1-5.

104. **Kuzma JM, Black DW.** Epidemiology, prevalence, and natural history of compulsive sexual behavior. Psychiatr Clin North Am. 2008;31:603-11.

105. **Parsons JT, Grov C, Golub SA.** Sexual compulsivity, co-occurring psychosocial health problems, and HIV risk among gay and bisexual men: further evidence of a syndemic. Am J Public Health. 2012;102:156-62.

106. **Bimbi DS, Nanin JE, Izienicki H, Parsons JT.** Sexual compulsivity and sexual behaviors among gay and bisexual men and lesbian and bisexual women. J Sex Res, 2009;46:301-8.

107. **Daneback K, Cooper A, Mansson SA.** An Internet study of cybersex participants. Arch Sex Behav. 2005;34:321-8.

108. Parsons JT, Kelly BC, Bimbi DS, DiMaria L, Wainberg ML, Morgenstern J. Explanations for the origins of sexual compulsivity among gay and bisexual men. Arch Sex Behav. 2008;37: 817-26.

109. Raymond NC, Coleman E, Miner MH. Psychiatric comorbidity and compulsive/impulsive traits in compulsive sexual behavior. Compr Psychiatry. 2003;44:370-80.

110. Kalichman SC, Johnson JR, Adair V, Rompa D, Multhauf K, Kelly JA. Sexual sensation seeking: scale development and predicting AIDS-risk behavior among homosexually active men. J Pers Assess. 1994;62:385-97.

111. Kafka MP, Prentky R. Fluoxetine treatment of nonparaphilic sexual addictions and paraphilias in men. J Clin Psychiatry. 1992;53:351-8.

112. Abramowitz L, Benabderrahmane D, Baron G, Walker F, Yeni P, Duval X. Systematic evaluation and description of anal pathology in HIV-infected patients during the HAART era. Dis Colon Rectum. 2009;52:1130-6.

113. Sohn N, Robilotti JG. Gay bowel syndrome — review of colonic and rectal conditions in 200 male homosexuals. Am J Gastroenterol. 1977;67:478-84.

114. Zaghiyan KN, Fleshner P. Anal fissure. Clin Colon Rectal Surg. 2011;24:22-30.

115. Madalinski MH. Identifying the best therapy for chronic anal fissure. World J Gastrointest Pharmacol Ther. 2011;2:9-16.

116. Gorfine SR. Topical nitroglycerin therapy for anal fissures and ulcers. N Engl J Med. 1995; 333:1156-7.

117. Lund JN, Scholefield JH. A randomised, prospective, double-blind, placebo-controlled trial of glyceryl trinitrate ointment in treatment of anal fissure. Lancet. 1997;349:11-4.

118. Oettle GJ. Glyceryl trinitrate vs. sphincterotomy for treatment of chronic fissure-in-ano: a randomized, controlled trial. Dis Colon Rectum. 1997;40:1318-20.

119. Jonas M, Neal KR, Abercrombie JF, Scholefield JH. A randomized trial of oral vs. topical diltiazem for chronic anal fissures. Dis Colon Rectum. 2001;44:1074-8.

120. Lohsiriwat V. Hemorrhoids: from basic pathophysiology to clinical management. World J Gastroenterol. 2012;18:2009-17.

121. Sohn N. Anorectal disorders. Curr Probl Surg. 1983;20:1-66.

122. Moesgaard F, Nielsen ML, Hansen JB, Knudsen JT. High-fiber diet reduces bleeding and pain in patients with hemorrhoids: a double-blind trial of Vi-Siblin. Dis Colon Rectum. 1982; 25:454-6.

123. Rivadeneira DE, Steele SR, Ternent C, Chalasani S, Buie WD, Rafferty JL; Standards Practice Task Force of The American Society of Colon and Rectal Surgeons. Practice parameters for the management of hemorrhoids (revised 2010). Dis Colon Rectum. 2011;54: 1059-64.

124. Alonso-Coello P, Guyatt G, Heels-Ansdell D, Johanson JF, Lopez-Yarto M, Mills E, et al. Laxatives for the treatment of hemorrhoids. Cochrane Database Syst Rev. 2005:CD004649.

125. Goldstone S. The Ins and Outs of Gay Sex. New York: Random House; 1999.

126. Morin J. Anal Pleasure and Health: A Guide for Men, Women, and Couples Down There Press; 1998.

127. Rosser BR, Short BJ, Thurmes PJ, Coleman E. Anodyspareunia, the unacknowledged sexual dysfunction: a validation study of painful receptive anal intercourse and its psychosexual concomitants in homosexual men. Sex Marital Ther. 1998;24:281-92.

128. Damon W, Rosser BR. Anodyspareunia in men who have sex with men: prevalence, predictors, consequences and the development of DSM diagnostic criteria. J Sex Marital Ther. 2005; 31:129-41.

129. Shindel AW, Rowen TS, Lin TC, Li CS, Robertson PA, Breyer BN. An Internet survey of demographic and health factors associated with risk of sexual dysfunction in women who have sex with women. J Sex Med. 2012;9:1261-71.

130. Kao A, Binik YM, Kapuscinski A, Khalife S. Dyspareunia in postmenopausal women: a critical review. Pain Res Manag. 2008;13:243-54.

131. Tan O, Bradshaw K, Carr BR. Management of vulvovaginal atrophy-related sexual dysfunction in postmenopausal women: an up-to-date review. Menopause. 2012;19:109-17.

132. **Portman DJ, Bachmann GA, Simon JA.** Ospemifene, a novel selective estrogen receptor modulator for treating dyspareunia associated with postmenopausal vulvar and vaginal atrophy. Menopause. 2013;20:623-630.

133. **Ishak WW, Bokarius A, Jeffrey JK, Davis MC, Bakhta Y.** Disorders of orgasm in women: a literature review of etiology and current treatments. J Sex Med. 2010;7:3254-68.

134. **Butcher J.** ABC of sexual health: female sexual problems I: loss of desire-what about the fun? BMJ. 1999;318:41-3.

135. **Butcher J.** ABC of sexual health: female sexual problems II: sexual pain and sexual fears. BMJ. 1999;318:110-2.

136. **Phillips NA.** Female sexual dysfunction: evaluation and treatment. Am Fam Phys. 2000;62: 127-36,141-2.

137. **Costantino A, Cerpolini S, Alvisi S, Morselli PG, Venturoli S, Meriggiola MC.** A prospective study on sexual function and mood in female-to-male transsexuals during testosterone administration and after sex reassignment surgery. J Sex Marital Ther. 2013;39:321-35.

138. **Klein C, Gorzalka BB.** Sexual functioning in transsexuals following hormone therapy and genital surgery: a review. J Sex Med. 2009;6:2922-39; quiz 2940-1.

139. **Matthews LT, Smit JA, Cu-Uvin S, Cohan D.** Antiretrovirals and safer conception for HIV-serodiscordant couples. Curr Opin HIV AIDS. 2012;7:569-78.

Chapter 13

HIV/AIDS Prevention for Sexual and Gender Minority People

MATTHEW J. MIMIAGA, ScD, MPH
MICHAEL S. BOROUGHS, PhD, MA
CONALL O'CLEIRIGH, PhD
JON VINCENT, BA
STEVEN A. SAFREN, PhD, ABPP
KENNETH H. MAYER, MD

Introduction

With more than 2 million new HIV infections occurring worldwide each year (1), including approximately 50,000 new infections in the United States (2), the development of effective HIV prevention strategies remains a critical public health priority. Although many countries have noted decreases in HIV incidence and greater uptake of antiretrovirals in recent years (3), globally, every day nearly 6300 people contract HIV (1), creating a need for increased scaling up of evidence-based prevention interventions. Over the past few years, several groundbreaking advances in biomedical HIV prevention interventions have been achieved, creating optimism about the potential to implement effective strategies to successfully curtail the HIV epidemic (4). However, each biomedical advance requires strong social and behavioral components to be effective, including community engagement, promotion of individual willingness to use the new modalities, medication adherence, and minimization of risk compensation (i.e., increased sexual risk because of perceived protection). The ultimate success of these new technologies requires careful coordination with evidence-based behavioral interventions that have been developed over the first 3 decades of the epidemic.

Epidemiology of HIV in Sexual and Gender Minority Populations

More than 30 years after the beginning of the HIV epidemic, gay, bisexual, and other men who have sex with men (MSM), as well as transgender women, continue to be the most affected populations in the United States, not only because of biological and behavioral reasons but also because of sociocultural influences. Homophobia, transphobia, systemic racism and inequality, poverty, shame, and stigma continue to exact additional challenges that support unequal access to health care and education in the United States. As U.S. sexual and gender minorities continue to battle with these issues in all aspects of their lives, HIV epidemiology in the United States illustrates that there are still huge hurdles to overcome before reaching the much-discussed "end of AIDS."

MSM

According to the U.S. Centers for Disease Control and Prevention (CDC), MSM accounted for more than half (56%) of persons living with HIV in the United States—nearly 500,000 men in 2010 (5). Additionally, in the same year, MSM accounted for 63% of new HIV infections (5). The reasons for this exaggerated health disparity include biological factors (e.g., the increased efficiency of HIV transmission via unprotected anal intercourse) as well as social and structural factors (such as homophobia) that continue to act as barriers and impediments to HIV prevention efforts (6). Homophobia (also known as sexual prejudice), at its core, is a form of prejudice and discrimination based on what people do in their personal and private lives (7). Internalized homophobia, or negative feelings about one's same-sex attractions, has been associated with psychological distress, increased sexual risk behavior, hesitation to participate in risk reduction and HIV prevention services, and lack of concern, by those with internalized homophobia for their or their partner's health (8), especially among young MSM.

Young MSM

Perhaps one of the most concerning developments in recent years has been the dramatic increase in HIV incidence rates among young MSM. In 2010, young MSM (ages 13 to 24 years) made up 30% of all new HIV infections among MSM and accounted for 72% of all new HIV infections among people in the same age cohort (5). Adolescence is a time period characterized by identity formation, social and biological transition, decreased supervision, independent living, and first sexual relationships, during which young MSM are more likely to engage in risky behaviors that increase their chances of becoming infected with HIV (9). Some recent studies have noted the need for additional research on youth and HIV and the need for combined biomedical, behavioral, and structural interventions (9), while others have emphasized the subtleties of family life and its effect on the development of LGBT youth (10).

Black/African American MSM

Black/African-American (referred to in this chapter as *black*) MSM in general, and especially young black MSM ages 13 to 24 years, are at the highest risk for being HIV-infected relative to all other demographic groups. In 2010, black MSM accounted for almost the same number of new HIV infections as white MSM, despite the large difference in population size between the two groups (11). Also in 2010, young black MSM accounted for more new HIV infections than any other racial or age group of MSM (approximately 4800)— more than 50% of new infections in that age group (5,11). Much of the increase in HIV among all young MSM is due to a 20% increase of HIV diagnoses among young black MSM between 2008 and 2010 (5). Despite being the group with the highest concentration of HIV in the United States, studies have not found black MSM to engage in sexual risk-taking behaviors at higher levels compared with other MSM (12). A recent study highlighted the relationship between institutional racism and sexual risk-taking among black men as well as contextual factors surrounding HIV risk, including housing instability, incarceration, and unemployment, which disproportionately affect black men and have been documented as risk factors for HIV (13,14). Lower socioeconomic status can lead to less access to HIV education and risk prevention, as well as intervention services. Given the elevated HIV risk for black MSM, more research is needed to confirm the role of racism, prejudice, discrimination, and disproportionate poverty, as well as the notion of a higher prevalence pool of sexual partners, on sexual risk behaviors among this population (13).

Hispanic/Latino MSM

Hispanic/Latino (referred to in this chapter as Latino) MSM are also disproportionately affected by HIV relative to their proportion of the U.S. population, although the rates are not as elevated as those noted among Black MSM. According to the CDC, Latinos accounted for 22% of new HIV infections in 2011 in the United States while comprising only about 16% of the overall population (15). The same report notes that in 2011, 79% of new HIV infections in Latino men were attributed to male-to-male sexual contact (15). Similar to black MSM, more research is needed on HIV risk behaviors, as well as patterns of drug use and social contexts, in order to understand HIV disparities among Latinos. Some studies suggest that among intravenous drug users, Latinos were more likely to be HIV infected (16,17) and diagnosed later (16,18) and less likely to access HIV prevention/drug user services than non-Latino White intravenous drug users because of stigma surrounding HIV and drug use and associations of both with homosexuality (16,19,20). More research on Latino MSM is needed, as is the development of culturally tailored interventions that meet the specific needs of this population.

MSM Couples

A recent study using behavioral surveillance data from 5 U.S. cities found that a majority (68%) of new HIV infections among MSM were attributable to sex with main partners (21). The proportion was even higher among younger MSM (21). Several studies have found that MSM are more likely to have more frequent unprotected anal sex with their main partners than with other partners (22–26).

Transgender Women

Transgender women have long been characterized as a high-risk group for HIV (27). Although there are incomplete data for this population because of limited inclusion in national HIV surveillance systems (28), a 2008 meta-analysis of 29 studies that focused on transgender women found a prevalence of 27.7% laboratory-confirmed HIV infection (4 studies) and 11.8% self-reported (18 studies) (29). The CDC reports that in New York City, from 2005 to 2009, 206 new cases of HIV infection were diagnosed among transgender people, almost all of which were transgender women, and about 90% of whom were black or Latina (27). As seen with MSM, the main mode by which transgender women become infected with HIV is via unprotected receptive anal intercourse (28). Most of the published literature on HIV among transgender populations focuses on adults; however, the few published studies on younger transgender women suggest that they have rates of HIV infection similar to transgender adults of all ages. For example, in a study of 51 young racial/ethnic minority transgender women ages 16 to 24 years, Garofalo and colleagues found that 22% self-reported being HIV-infected (30). Discrimination, harassment, and rejection from friends, family, and others often become a central part of early adolescence and young adulthood for transgender youth (29,31–36), affecting their ability to secure housing, employment, social services, and health care (29,31,37). This basic struggle for survival undermines young transgender women's ability to prioritize and practice safer sexual behaviors (38,39). Transgender youth are disproportionately represented among homeless persons, which is often the result of rejection or estrangement from their families of origin (40).

HIV Transmission Factors and Behaviors That Potentiate Risk

HIV can be most readily transmitted via intimate contact with infected blood or anogenital secretions (41). Most humans have become infected via heterosexual contact, followed by male same-sex behavior, with fewer cases being detected via injection drug use and maternal-child transmission in most parts of the world because of harm reduction approaches (e.g., provision of clean syringes and opiate substitution therapy) and maternal antenatal use of antiretovirals.

HIV transmission is a high-consequence, low-probability event. At present, nearly all who are infected will be so for life, and the majority will need to take medication to prevent the development of immunodeficiency. Although the average per contact risk from sexual exposure to HIV is less than 1 per 100 contacts, specific factors can substantially alter the efficiency of HIV transmission (41). Because the colonic mucosal epithelia contain a high density of mononuclear cells that express the CCR5 receptor that HIV can bind to in order to gain cell entry, receptive anal intercourse is the most effective mode of HIV transmission. The male foreskin also contains many cells that can become infected by HIV, so men who are uncircumcised are more susceptible to HIV than circumcised males. Similarly, the female cervix is the most susceptible part of the female genital tract anatomy. The common link between the colon, foreskin, and cervix is that each tissue protects surrounding orifices that are in unsterile environments. Unfortunately, the same cells that are responsible for immune surveillance from many pathogens contain the largest number of receptors that can bind HIV, facilitating its "Trojan horse effect." Although individuals who are exposed to HIV through anal receptive sex are most at risk for HIV acquisition, men who are exclusively insertive in either anal or vaginal sex are still at moderate risk because both anal and cervicovaginal secretions may contain high concentrations of HIV. Although circumcised males are less susceptible to HIV infection than those who are uncircumcised, the distal urethra contains cells that can bind HIV, and the shaft of the penis can become HIV-infected in the presence of abrasions from sexual trauma and ulcerations from sexually transmitted infections (STIs). Similarly, women without a cervix, posthysterectomy can become HIV-infected, because the vaginal mucosa contain many cells that can bind HIV.

The efficiency of HIV transmission is not only a function of the density of cells that can bind HIV but the inoculum to which mucosa are exposed (41). The concentration of HIV in plasma is a reliable marker of the transmission efficiency (42,43). Thus, individuals who have longstanding untreated HIV infection are more likely to transmit HIV than those whose infection is controlled with antiretroviral therapy. Similarly, individuals who are acutely infected with HIV before the host immune response controlling viral replication (preventing rapid progression to AIDS) are more infectious to their partners (41). Most data that inform these observations come from studies of heterosexual HIV transmission; however, observational studies among MSM corroborate these findings. Although genital tract HIV concentrations tend to parallel those in plasma, the correspondence is not 100% because local events in the genital tract, such as STIs, may increase HIV expression even in a setting where HIV is not detectable in plasma secondary to effective antiretroviral therapy (44).

Sexually transmitted infections may potentiate both HIV susceptibility and infectiousness through a variety of mechanisms (41). Some infections, such as syphilis and herpes simplex virus infections, may produce anogenital ulcerations, which can facilitate mucosal access and recruit more HIV target cells to the site of the ulcer. Others, such as gonorrhea and chlamydia, primarily increase infectiousness and susceptibility through inflammation, which can increase local concentrations of cells that can transmit or acquire HIV, and by increasing genital tract cytokines, which may increase HIV replication (41). Other factors may also increase genital tract inflammation, such as the use of concentrated hypertonic lubricants (e.g., nonoxynyl-9), douching, abrasive sexual practices (e.g., having multiple sexual partners in a short time period), and "fisting" (insertion of digits into the rectum).

The role of hormonal contraception and HIV susceptibility remains unclear because women using contraception may be less likely to use barrier protection (45). However, animal studies have suggested that some hormonal combinations may be associated with increased susceptibility to HIV, and epidemiologic studies have found this association to be particularly true for progestins. The relevance of these findings for transgender women is not clear and warrants further study. There has been no biological association of increased susceptibility to HIV among individuals using exogenous androgens (e.g., MSM wanting to build muscle, or transgender men) if the injections use sterile techniques.

Although receptive anal intercourse is the most efficient means of HIV transmission, it is role versatility among MSM that particularly enhances HIV spread. Unlike other populations, MSM may acquire HIV efficiently through unprotected receptive anal sex, and then transmit to others through insertive unprotected anal sex. The increased efficiency of anal sex and role versatility can lead to more rapid spread of HIV in MSM than seen among heterosexual populations engaging in similar levels of unprotected penile-vaginal sex (46,47).

Being a member of a sexual and gender minority can also potentiate HIV transmission, given the limited choice of partners in any community. Thus, once HIV becomes established in a subpopulation, it can become concentrated within that community; as prevalence rises, any new partner can be associated with an increased risk for HIV transmission. This has been found to be particularly true for racial and ethnic minority populations in the United States, Canada, and the United Kingdom, where assortative mixing (i.e., preferentially choosing partners from within one's own subgroup) can be associated with enhanced risks for HIV acquisition, even in the face of less individual risk-taking compared with MSM from the majority population (48).

Psychosocial Factors and HIV Risk

Although biological and sexual behavioral factors are important for understanding HIV transmission, they do not function in isolation, and in fact interact with many factors, including psychosocial factors that influence the HIV epidemic among MSM and transgender women (49). This section explores how mental and behavioral health issues together with substance use disorders interact with sexual risk behaviors to produce greater risk for HIV infection and transmission among these populations. Like other populations of interest, substance use and comorbid mental health issues are relatively prevalent among LGBT people and are influenced, in part, by stress related to societal and internalized homophobia. These co-occurring problems are often underidentified and undertreated in HIV-infected populations (50–52). Therefore, clinicians who assess for and treat these common behavioral health issues among their gay, bisexual, other MSM, and transgender patients should also be helping to mitigate sexual risk taking associated with acquiring or transmitting HIV with these groups.

Depression

Moderate levels of unipolar depression are associated with increased levels of sexual risk for HIV-infected gay and bisexual men and for increased sexual risk for men without HIV infection (53,54). For those with bipolar disorder, research suggests that gay and bisexual men are at risk for "acting out sexually" and thus are at increased risk during manic and hypomanic episodes (55–58). Depression may be associated with increased HIV risk-taking because individuals who are depressed often experience decreased levels of self-efficacy (i.e., feeling that they are unable to safely negotiate safer sex). For example, feelings of helplessness or worthlessness may lead to an unwillingness or inability to insist on condom use during sexual interactions. These concerns may be compounded with the sexual side effect profile documented among many commonly prescribed antidepressant medications.

Trauma and Post-Traumatic Stress Disorder

Individuals who are sexually traumatized during their formative years may develop enduring disturbances of adult sexual behavior that may compromise adult sexual health (59–62). The most conspicuous result is increased risk for HIV following an experienced trauma, particularly sexual trauma, during this imperative developmental stage. Sexual violation, whether in childhood or early adolescence, and the companion psychological trauma create a psychosocial situation upon which LGBT patients are less likely to advocate explicitly, or even implicitly, on behalf of their sexual safety even after moving into adulthood. A variety of additional risk factors contribute to the clinical profile often found between childhood sexual abuse and adult sexual health. For example, individuals who experience childhood sexual abuse have earlier sexual debut, are more likely to have sex while abusing alcohol and/or other drugs, are more likely to have multiple sexual partners, have a greater incidence of exchanging sex for drugs or money, and are at greater risk for being retraumatized in adulthood. Patients may present with symptoms that have their foundation in the various clusters of post-traumatic stress disorder (PTSD), such as troubled sleep, triggered anger or irritability, difficulty with experiencing and expressing deep feelings or emotions, or a variety of avoidance behaviors that support limitations in healthy functioning. Thus, a traumatic past can often be impairing with regard to adult sexual relationships and negatively affect other areas of daily functioning, including activities of daily living. Patients might present with a symptom that appears rather benign (e.g., insomnia), when indeed this is an antecedent problem associated with PTSD.

Anxiety

The role of anxiety, in general, is poorly understood as it relates to sexual risk. This may be in part related to divergence among anxiety disorders and how experienced symptoms may interfere with goals that patients have for their own sexual safety. Social anxiety disorder (SAD; as known as social phobia in the fourth edition of the *Diagnostic and Statistical Manual of Mental Disorders*, text revision), which is characterized by fear of rejection and negative characterization and by chronic and insidious avoidance of feared social situations, has been associated with some degree of impairment with regard to sexual risk behaviors (63). Individuals with SAD experience interference with their ability to keep themselves safe. This may be a particular risk factor among gay and bisexual men given the high prevalence of SAD complicated by—and the greater risk for—HIV seroconversion for MSM (63). Some experts suggest, given the relatively low incidence of treatment relative to the prevalence rates for SAD, that a variety of legal and illegal substances are often used as self-medicating agents to address the anxious symptoms associated with the disorder. In addition, patients with undiagnosed SAD may appear to function normally (i.e., the appearance of functioning in the social sphere). However, risky sexual behaviors, particularly those carried out while disinhibited by substances, may warrant further assessment of SAD because the sexual risk-taking may result from the person's inability to advocate for sexual safety (e.g., asking a sexual partner to use a condom).

Advocacy for condom use is problematic across populations and feels impossible to those with SAD, particularly if they are self-medicating through substance use. Screening for SAD is generally brief and can be accomplished with psychometrically validated questionnaires. Physicians may choose to incorporate these types of brief screeners (e.g., Brief Symptom Inventory [64]) into their new patient intake packets, during annual physical examinations, or based on case presentations. In cases where patients present with concerns about SAD specifically, or anxiety in general, and how these may interfere with functioning in any domain of their lives, cognitive behavioral therapy is brief, safe, effective, and empirically supported (65).

Substance Use

The use of drugs and alcohol, given their disinhibiting effects, results in a greater likelihood of risky sexual behavior and a lower likelihood of ensuring that condoms are used during the riskiest sexual acts. Crystal methamphetamine (also known as, "crystal," "Tina," "speed," "ice," "monster," or "crank") has been documented frequently in the literature as a drug of choice among a subgroup of sexual minority men (see Chapter 10). In 1 study that examined a large sample of HIV-infected men, the mental health and substance abuse problems often co-occurred, as did risky sexual behavior putting patients, and their sexual partners, at increased risk for negative health outcomes (66). Recreational drug use, including polysubstance use, results in multiple negative health outcomes, including increased risk for HIV and other STIs, comorbid mental health problems, more rapid progression of HIV (67,68), and increased HIV transmission risk behaviors (53,60,69–73). Thus, substance problems are of great concern for both HIV-infected and HIV-uninfected men. Risk levels vary greatly based upon the drug, or drugs, used, as well as the frequency and amount used, the health status of the patient, and their sexual behavior.

Syndemics

Although many studies have shown interconnections between psychosocial factors and HIV risk among MSM, recent studies have focused on how these diverse psychosocial issues interact to produce elevated HIV risk behavior among MSM, a phenomena known as a syndemic (60,73–79). A syndemic is the aggregation of two or more disorders or diseases in a given population where some level of interaction extends negative health outcomes of any or all of the syndromes included in the syndemic. Some of the disorders that have been briefly reviewed in this chapter (i.e., depression, PTSD, anxiety, social anxiety disorder, alcohol or other drug abuse) are conditions syndemic with HIV and thus should be addressed in order to achieve optimal patient outcomes for both HIV-uninfected as well as HIV-infected individuals.

Addressing Behavioral Health Issues as Part of HIV Prevention

Given the evidence on psychosocial risk factors, it is particularly important for clinicians to assess for mental health conditions and substance use patterns as part of their HIV prevention efforts with sexual and gender minority patients. This approach is important not only for HIV-uninfected patients but also for HIV-infected patients, as mental health and substance use not only interfere with sexual risk but also with engagement in care, engagement in antiretroviral therapy, adherence to medication, and maintaining and sustaining an undetectable HIV viral load. Evidence suggests that men with an undetectable HIV viral load are much less likely to transmit HIV to their sexual partners (80); therefore, full engagement in HIV care becomes of critical importance to stemming the epidemic. A variety of approaches can be deployed to assess for mental health and substance abuse issues, including the use of psychometrically validated instruments (i.e., brief, empirically validated questionnaires) such as the Patient Health Questionnaire-9, that do not take a great deal of time but can allow clinicians to make subsequent judgments about whether individual counseling, and/or pharmacotherapy may be warranted. Often, brief questions can be added to health history forms that can be completed while patients are in the waiting room. Some clinicians may prefer to approach these risks with routine questions during an examination in order to provide immediate intervention and feedback to patients and their families. Both of these approaches—the use of screeners and direct verbal assessment—can also be combined to maximize accurate risk assessment, time resources, and patient outcomes. See Chapters 8, 9, and 10 for more on these issues.

HIV Testing Tools and Programs

Universal Screening Guidelines

According to the CDC, more than 180,000 Americans have HIV but do not know it, and half of new HIV infections are transmitted by people who are unaware of being infected (81). Given these statistics, both the CDC (82) and the U.S. Preventive Services Task Force (USPSTF) (83) recommend that clinicians screen all patients for HIV infection at least once (grade: A recommendation). The CDC suggests universal screening of everyone between the ages of 13 and 64 years, while USPSTF uses the age range 15 to 65 years. Both also recommend screening pregnant women as well as persons at high risk outside the given age range. Testing in a primary care setting should be opt-out, if allowable by state law. In this way, HIV testing becomes normalized and less threatening to the patient, leading to higher uptake.

The CDC further recommends that those who are considered at high risk for HIV, including MSM (and especially those who have had more than 1 sex partner since their last HIV test), should test more frequently. Annual screening may be sufficient, while the highest-risk patients may benefit from HIV and other STI testing every 3 to 6 months (82,84). Regular testing for MSM is a critical part of HIV prevention, given that knowing one's status is the first step to receiving treatment, which should lead to viral suppression and, consequently, lower transmission to others. Ultimately, if the majority of HIV-infected persons are successfully receiving effective antiretrovirals, the burden of community viral load and/or overall prevalence and incidence of HIV should greatly diminish.

Taking a Sexual History

In preventive medicine, it is important to take routine, non-judgmental sexual histories of all patients, including a discussion about sexual behaviors that may put the patient at risk for HIV infection, STIs, and unwanted pregnancy. Asking about sexual behavior, barrier protection use, gender, and number of partners is crucial to determining which STI tests are needed and whether regular HIV tests are warranted. The CDC's Sexually Transmitted Disease Guidelines (www.cdc.gov/std/treatment/) provide recommendations for testing types based on the likely risk factors for special populations, including tailored recommendations for MSM. Engaging in dialog may also help the patient make healthier decisions in the future. It is advisable to use nonclinical language when there are concerns about literacy or language being a barrier to the patient. Although many providers may not be comfortable talking to their patients about sex, if the health professional assures patients that care will be provided in a confidential, nonjudgmental manner, then patients will likely feel comfortable revealing their history.

As discussed earlier, substance use in the context of sexual activity is also important to discuss with patients because of its association with sexual risk behaviors. In addition, injecting substances such as opiates or methamphetamines is associated with an independent HIV risk because of the sharing of nonsterile injection equipment. For transgender patients, it is also important to ask whether they are using injectable silicone and hormones. Therefore, in addition to inquiring about sexual practices, it is important that clinicians ask about active substance use and make treatment referrals as needed. Chapters 8, 10, and 12 provide more information and strategies for taking sexual and substance use histories. Chapters 5 and 7 offer specific recommendations for youth and older adults, respectively.

Advances in HIV Testing Technology

Recent advances in HIV testing technology have increased access to testing while reducing the window period from the time of exposure to the time HIV antibodies and/or the antigen associated with HIV (p24) are detectable. There are U.S. Food and Drug Administration (FDA) approved rapid antibody testing kits available to providers directly from the manufacturers or in some cases through state and local health departments. The unit costs of these kits run from $11.00 per kit to $20.00. All widely available FDA-approved kits are of similar quality; the time to run the tests varies from 10 to 20 minutes. Some kits are approved for the use of oral mucosal transudate as the test sample, although using whole blood from a finger-stick is considered to be more accurate and the possibility of contamination to the sample is significantly reduced.

A limitation to all currently FDA-approved rapid HIV test kits, including those marketed for home use, is the window period from exposure to the formation of detectable antibodies. The average window period for rapid testing ranges from 6 to 12 weeks after a possible exposure. Because missing a new infection is a potentially serious situation, clinicians should explain this limitation of the test to the patient.

Recently, some health departments and commercial laboratories have begun using a "generation 4" HIV test. This test uses a whole blood sample, which is processed in a laboratory. The algorithm for testing the sample looks for p24 antigen to detect early infection at any time greater than 14 days after exposure. In addition, the algorithm will look for antibodies via enzyme-linked immunosorbent assay and Western blot, and if there are anomalies in the results, the sample will be tested with a viral load test, to eliminate the chance of a false-positive or false-negative result.

Home rapid antibody testing kits have the potential to offer those otherwise unwilling or unable to receive an HIV test in clinical or community settings the ability to perform one on themselves. Although the technology is almost identical to tests of the same brand name offered in clinical settings, the tests use the less accurate oral mucosal transudate sampling, and user error is more likely. In addition, self-administered testing does not allow for in-person support from a counselor. For these reasons, these tests are not a perfect replacement for testing done by a professional. Home kits using antigen testing are available through the Internet from foreign markets. Because these are not FDA approved, they cannot be recommended or endorsed. FDA-approved test kits for consumer use and in vitro use by Clinical Laboratory Improvement Amendments waived personnel can be found on the FDA website at www.fda.gov.

Screening for Acute HIV Infection

Individuals who have been exposed to HIV within the past few days may be asymptomatic and could potentially have acute HIV infection. The screening for this does not involve conventional antibody testing but requires the determination of HIV plasma RNA because it takes weeks to months for HIV antibodies to develop. Some individuals with acute retroviral infection may have influenza-like symptoms, and some may have partial manifestations, such as only severe fever or only a rash or a lymphadenopathy; however, a substantial portion of people with acute HIV infection are asymptomatic. If, however, a patient has had recurrent potential exposures to HIV through unprotected sex or sharing of syringes, conventional antibody testing is the appropriate initial screening test. Individuals who test negative can subsequently be referred for behavioral counseling to decrease sexual risk and/or get treatment for substance abuse. For individuals who indicate that they have frequent ongoing risk-taking behaviors, the clinician should also inquire about potential precipitating factors that may be leading to ongoing risk-taking, such as untreated depression, substance use, and/or being in a coercive relationship. Careful probing for any of these issues can lead to clinical actions that can improve the patient's overall health and reduce his or her risk for HIV transmission or acquisition.

Delivering HIV Test Results

Although offering the patient an HIV test should be presented as something normal and routine, the provider should not neglect to provide a high level of support and attention during the process. Because HIV is a life-changing condition for most newly diagnosed patients, care should be taken to offer clear information without being nonchalant or displaying an abundance of emotion; either response is capable of confusing the patient.

When the result is ready, the provider must deliver it with an understanding that the patient may have a strong emotional reaction, regardless of what the result is. Delivering a "nonreactive" or negative result can be a teachable moment for many patients. What is learned in the moment can, however, be inconsistent. Patients may feel great relief and have a sense that they never want to be in their former state of stress. Another possible reaction to a negative test result may be a sense of immunity or resistance to HIV, and the good news may perpetuate a feeling of invincibility. The clinician may need to discuss this concept with the patient to make the most of the catharsis. Additional behavioral risk-reduction counseling, pre-exposure prophylaxis (PrEP, described later in this chapter), and/or mental health and substance use counseling may be recommended for those exhibiting high-risk behaviors.

In delivering a reactive/preliminary positive (rapid testing) or positive result (serum testing), it is important to be clear and calm. The specific language is a stylistic concern; however, most providers will reassure the patient that with proper medication and monitoring, HIV infection can be controlled to the point that it becomes a chronic, manageable disease. Using active listening, and taking as much time to talk as the patient desires, allows patients to begin to process this new factor in their lives. It is of course critical to try to connect the patient to HIV care at the time the result is delivered. Inform the patient that regular blood monitoring and adherence to anti-HIV medications are critical to long-term health.

HIV Counseling, Testing, and Referral

HIV counseling, testing, and referral (CTR) is a model of service designed to increase knowledge of HIV status; encourage and support risk reduction; and support needed referrals for appropriate services, such as medical and social services. CTR can be delivered by clinics, at dedicated sites, or through outreach services. CTR is substantially more comprehensive than basic HIV screening; in terms of cost-to-benefit ratio, CTR is most appropriate for settings where the HIV prevalence is high (>1% of the population). Detailed information on CTR, including training and implementation material, can be found on the CDC's Effective Interventions website at www.effectivein-terventions.org/en/HighImpactPrevention/PublicHealthStrategies/CTR.aspx.

In its most basic form, CTR includes the following elements:

- Pretest counseling
- The administration of a rapid test, or in the case of a serum test, taking a vial of blood
- The presentation of the result (preliminary positive [rapid test], positive [serum test], nonreactive/negative [rapid test], negative [serum test], or indeterminate)
- Post-test counseling
- Referrals/triage

Organizations interested in implementing a CTR program should consider how and by whom it will be delivered. Often, peers who are representative of the priority population (e.g., MSM) are more credible and understand the subtleties of sexual and substance use behaviors and colloquialisms. CTR may be incorporated into a complete physical examination by a primary care provider, a short visit with a medical assistant or other clinical staff member trained in CTR, emergency department personnel, or trained team members in a nonclinical community-based setting. Regardless of setting or provider, CTR should be conducted within the following framework to ensure the best outcomes for the patient and provider:

- CTR services should be low-barrier (e.g., inviting, non-stigmatizing, easy to find, and not cost prohibitive).
- CTR should be voluntary and should be delivered only after informed consent is obtained.
- State law permitting, anonymous CTR should be offered as an alternative to confidential CTR if substantial confidentiality concerns exist.
- The counseling component of CTR should be client-centered and focused on reducing the patient's risk of acquiring or transmitting HIV, without being directive or judgmental.
- Appropriate referrals for medical or psychological evaluation and social support should be made in the CTR session.
- Should the patient receive an HIV diagnosis, CTR should offer referral for, or help with, notifying sexual and needle-sharing partners. This may be done by CTR staff who are trained and certified, or by disease intervention specialists employed by regional health departments.

Potential challenges can arise in addressing integrated CTR in the medical setting, including language barriers, hypervigilant patients ("over testers"), and patients with serious mental health issues. Work flow issues are also challenging. For example, some rapid tests must be timed carefully; there is also a data collection aspect to CTR. With a provider's often harried schedule, it is advisable to have a medical assistant or counselor dedicated to quality assurance. At times, a provider or counselor will have to make a call as to whether a patient is ready for an HIV test. As with all other practices in the medical setting, the provider must consider the possibility of harm. Intoxicated, hysterical, angry, or potentially suicidal individuals should be stabilized before a priority is placed on CTR.

When considering a testing program, it may be appropriate to offer different levels of counseling based on client need and reported risk. At a basic level, a medical assistant trained in CTR may offer the test and brief counseling along with vital signs and other routine practices at the start of a medical appointment. This version of testing has a nominal intervention component. A middle-level CTR session is appropriate for patients with higher needs, such as anxiety, lack of understanding of HIV risk, or self-proclaimed inability to reduce high-risk behavior. These sessions generally consist of a 40- to 60-minute session with a counselor—either after a medical appointment or as a stand-alone CTR service.

As in the past, before the invention of rapid HIV antibody testing technology, a CTR session may involve 2 sessions. Session 1 includes pretest counseling and a blood draw. The serum is then processed in a laboratory. This is followed up by a return appointment after the results are back. In these types of sessions, the counselor may design a risk-reduction plan with the patient during the pretesting phase and touch base for in-person or phone conversations. For those at increased and consistent risk, the provider should consider the use of PrEP, as described later in this chapter.

With the careful use of HIV counseling and testing resources, those at risk can be offered low-barrier services, and, if needed, they can embark on taking lifesaving medications that not only preserve their immune systems but also dramatically reduce their likelihood of spreading HIV. This test-and-treat philosophy is not at the expense of prevention programs, but rather uses cutting-edge technology to uncover and treat HIV infections.

Couples Testing

Couples testing has gained popularity in the United States recently, in part because of growing evidence that many HIV infections happen in the context of a relationship (21). Originally piloted in Africa for use with serodiscordant couples (85,86), couples HIV testing and counseling has been endorsed by the CDC as an effective intervention, after being piloted in several U.S. cities. The intervention supports the testing and counseling of couples for HIV together, at the same time, and has been found to be safe and acceptable for MSM couples (87).

Testing a couple together for HIV requires a skill set that entails empathy, sensitivity, and a concern for possible coercion by one half of the couple. MSM patients interested in finding sites that offer a "testing together" program can visit www.testingtogether.org, which lists sites across the country.

If testing a couple together is not a realistic activity, it may be advisable to raise awareness that a perception of monogamy may not offer adequate protection from HIV.

HIV Prevention Interventions

Common Theoretical Models

Familiarity with the conceptual models that underlie HIV prevention behaviors is important because it allows clinicians and researchers to develop and refine intervention efforts. For each model described below, the major tenets and strengths of each model are reviewed, along with any frequent criticisms or drawbacks in predicting HIV risk behaviors.

The biomedical model focuses on biological factors in attempting to understand a person's medical illness, disorder, or behavior, excluding psychological and social factors as relevant determinants (88,89). In the biomedical model, individuals are seen as passive agents of their health, with little or no personal responsibility for the presence of, or ability to change, the behavior (89). Although patient characteristics such as age and gender may influence the consequences of illness and play a role in HIV risk behaviors, they are not deemed related to the etiology, development, or manifestations of illness or behavior. For example, anal intercourse increases MSM's and transgender women's risk for HIV acquisition and transmission compared with heterosexuals (90–92), so biomedical interventions will focus on ways to alter transmission, including condoms, oral and topical chemoprophylaxis, or decreasing infectiousness through antiretroviral treatment. However, an exclusively biomedical model has been criticized in HIV prevention because it is viewed as overlooking important factors, such as patients' views of risk behaviors, as well as psychosocial and economic factors that contribute to risk (93).

The behavioral learning model emphasizes the role of antecedents (what comes before acting—i.e., thoughts, environmental cues) and consequences (what comes after acting—rewards/punishments) in shaping overt health behaviors. An example of behavioral learning theory is operant conditioning. According to operant conditioning, behaviors are performed in response to stimuli, and the frequency of occurrence of the behavior post stimuli (response) increases if the behaviors are reinforced (94). For example, if a patient finds condom negotiation with a partner to be difficult and experiences anxiety and negative resistance from the sexual partner every time condom negotiation is initiated, he or she may be more likely to engage in unprotected sex.

Behavior change in this model focuses on either gaining control of the stimuli and reinforcers, and reinforcing only desired behaviors, or presenting only the stimuli, which are already linked to desired behaviors. Learning theories emphasize that learning a new pattern of behavior, such as reducing sexual risk, requires modifying many of the small behaviors that compose the overall complex behavior (e.g., buying condoms in advance of sex, skills building to negotiate condom use). Principles of behavior modification suggest that a complex-pattern behavior can be learned by first breaking it down into smaller segments. Incremental increases are then made as the complex pattern of behavior is "shaped" toward the targeted behavioral outcome goal in successive approximations. The drawbacks of the behavioral learning perspective are that there is little attention to cognition or thought as explanations of behavior and that it does not account for the fact that the relevance of rewards may be individualized and may differ depending on time after the stimulus-response chain.

The communication perspective is a client-centered approach that emphasizes the key role played by good provider–patient relationship and clear communication in determining patient health behaviors, including reducing risk for HIV. The most successful approach related to the communication perspective is motivational interviewing, a client-centered, participatory communication technique that elicits behavioral change by helping clients explore and work through ambivalence about changing their behavior (95–97). From the motivational interviewing perspective, the client is the expert in evaluation of his or her own behavior and generates potential solutions to problems; the provider or practitioner uses Rogerian empathetic and reflective listening (based on the work of U.S. psychologist Carl Rogers, 1902–1987, researcher and founder of client-centered humanistic therapy) to focus on ambivalence associated with behavior change, encouraging the client to examine his or her own behavior (98). Some have criticized that the model overlooks attitudes, motivation, skills, and interpersonal factors that may affect the way messages are received and translated into health behaviors.

The cognitive perspective considers the effects of attitudes, beliefs, and expectations of outcomes on engaging in health behaviors (98). Mental processes, including thinking, reasoning, hypothesizing, and expecting, play an integral role in cognitive theories of behavior. In this perspective, behavior is a function of the subjective value of an outcome and of a subjective expectation (98). Cognitive theorists view reinforcement or consequence of behavior as being important in so far as it influences expectations about a situation, but generally do not consider the role of reinforcement in directly influencing behavior (99). Several models that follow this premise include the health belief model, social cognitive theory, the theory of reasoned action, and the protection motivation theory, which are described in more detail below. Several criticisms have been levied against the cognitive perspective. First, it does not take into account the effect of non-voluntary factors; second, it does not address behavioral skills associated with sexual risk behaviors directly; and third, the theory gives a paucity of attention to the origin of beliefs and how these beliefs may affect behavior (93).

The health belief model (HBM) is a value-expectancy theory and assumes that an individual's behavior is guided by expectations of consequences of adopting new practices (98). The model has 4 key concepts (100,101):

1. Susceptibility: Does the person perceive vulnerability to the specific disease?
2. Severity: Does the individual perceive that getting the disease has negative consequences?
3. Benefits minus costs: What are the positive and negative effects of adopting a new practice?
4. Health motive: Does the person have concerns about the consequences of contracting the disease?

In addition, self-efficacy, an individual's belief in his or her capability to perform a behavior, has recently been integrated into HBM. Thus, increased sexual risk-taking or unprotected sex may be explained and addressed by HBM as follows: One's beliefs about the benefits of condoms (protection from HIV infection or STIs) do not outweigh the costs of condom use (pleasure reduction due to reduced sensation and partner-related concerns, such as creation of distrust in a relationship or reduction of spontaneity). HBM interventions would focus on shifting the benefit–cost perception. A criticism of this model is that it lacks clear definitions of components and the relationship between them; thus, the model has been critiqued for inconsistent measurement in both descriptive and intervention research. HBM has been further critiqued for not fully addressing several behavioral determinants, including sociocultural factors, and for assuming that health is a high priority for most individuals (thus, it may not apply to those who do not place as high a value on health).

Social cognitive theory (SCT) is one of the most frequently applied theories of health behavior (102). SCT posits a reciprocal deterministic relationship between the individual, his or her environment, and behavior; all 3 elements dynamically and reciprocally interact with and upon each other to form the basis for behavior, as well as potential interventions to change behaviors (99,103,104). SCT has often been called a bridge between behavioral and cognitive learning theories because it focuses on the interaction between internal factors, such as thinking and symbolic processing (e.g., attention, memory, motivation), and external determinants (e.g., rewards and punishments) in determining behavior.

A central tenet of SCT is the concept of self-efficacy (105). Behaviors are determined by the interaction of outcome expectations (the extent to which people believe their behavior will lead to certain outcomes) and efficacy expectations (the extent to which they believe they can bring about the particular outcome) (105,106). For example, individuals may hold the outcome expectation that if they consistently use condoms, they will significantly reduce risk for becoming HIV-infected; however, they must also hold the efficacy expectation that they are incapable of such consistent behavioral practice. Behavior change would necessitate bringing outcome and efficacy expectations in alignment with one another. SCT emphasizes predictors of health behaviors, such as motivation and self-efficacy, perception of barriers to and benefits of behavior, perception of control over outcome, and personal sources of behavioral control (self-regulation) (99,105).

Another important tenet with respect to behavior and learning is SCT's emphasis that individuals learn from one another via observation, imitation, and modeling; effective models evoke trust, admiration, and respect from the observer, and they represent a level of behavior that observers are able to visualize attaining for themselves. Thus, a change in efficacy expectations through vicarious experience may be effected by encouraging an individual to believe something akin to the following: "If she can do it, so can I." SCT has been critiqued for being too comprehensive in its formulation, making for difficulty in operationalizing and evaluating the theory in its entirety (93). Moreover, some researchers using SCT as a theoretical basis have been criticized for using only 1 or 2 concepts from the theory to explain behavioral outcomes (102).

The theory of reasoned action (TRA) (107) maintains that volition and intention predict behavior. According to TRA, if people evaluate the suggested behavior as positive (attitude) and if they think others want them to perform the behavior (subjective norm), this results in a higher intention (motivation) and they are more likely to perform the behavior. A high correlation of attitudes and subjective norms to behavioral intention and to behavior has been confirmed in many studies (108). However, results of some studies gesture to a limitation of this theory: behavioral intention does not always lead to actual behavior. A counterargument against the strong relationship between behavioral intention and actual behavior led to the evolution of the theory of planned behavior, a model that includes the effect of non-volitional factors on behavior.

The theory of planned behavior (TPB) (109–111) was developed from the theory of reasoned action and is more applicable when the probability of success and actual control over performance of a behavior are suboptimal. In addition to attitudes and subjective norms that comprise the theory of reasoned action, the TPB's key contribution is the concept of perceived behavioral control, defined as an individual's perception of the ease or difficulty of performing the particular behavior (110). How strong an attempt the individual makes to engage in the behavior and how much control that individual has over the behavior (behavioral control) are influential in whether he or she engages in the behavior. Behavioral intention is produced from a combination of attitude toward the behavior, subjective norm, and perceived behavioral control (112). Behavioral control is similar to self-efficacy and depends on the individual's perception of how difficult it is going to be to engage in the behavior. The more favorable a person's attitude is toward behavior and subjective norms, and the greater the perceived behavioral control, the stronger that person's intention will be to perform the behavior in question. Moreover, given a sufficient degree of actual control over the behavior, people will be expected to carry out their intentions when the opportunity arises (112). Thus, an individual with positive attitudes about always using condoms during vaginal or anal intercourse, who perceives social support for these behaviors from key referent others and who has the conviction that he or she can carry out these behaviors effectively, will likely take consistent HIV preventive actions (113). The model emphasizes the roles played by knowledge regarding necessary skills for performing the behavior, environmental factors, and experience with the behavior (114). Critics have argued that these models would benefit from a more clear and explicit definition of behavior control. Others have suggested that adding the role of beliefs and moral and religious norms would help improve predictive ability of the models (115).

The protection motivation model (116,117) describes processes of adaptive and maladaptive coping with a health threat, emphasizing 2 appraisal processes: 1) a process of threat appraisal and 2) a process of coping appraisal, in which the behavioral options to diminish the threat are evaluated. The appraisal of the health threat and the appraisal of the coping responses result in either the intention to perform adaptive responses (protection motivation) or maladaptive responses (responses that place the individual at high risk and lead to negative consequences, such as unsafe sex) (118). Central to the decision-making process is fear, which is thought to increase both the motivation and the likelihood to engage in protective action. Intention to protect oneself depends on perceptions associated with 4 factors: severity (expected harmfulness), probability (or vulnerability that the event will occur), response efficacy, and self-efficacy. The interaction of these 4 components is in turn responsible for arousing fear. Criticisms of this model are that it does not comprehensively identify sociocultural, environmental, and cognitive variables that affect motivation.

The information-motivation-behavioral skills model (IMB) skills model (100) was originally developed as a simple model to address HIV risk behaviors. Three factors constitute important foci for intervention efforts in this model: basic knowledge and information about the medical condition, motivation based on attitudes about and social support for the behavior, and behavioral skills and self-efficacy specific for the behavior. Moreover, 5 skills are identified by the model as necessary for the practice of HIV prevention: self-acceptance of sexuality, acquisition of behaviorally relevant information, negotiation of preventive behavior with partner, performance of public prevention acts (such as condom purchase), and consistent performance of prevention behavior (100). For example, an IMB-based intervention addressing MSM or transgender women's use of female condoms would focus on ensuring that the patient has basic knowledge about how to use a female condom, is motivated to use it, has the technical skills to properly insert it, and possesses the negotiation skills to get her partner to agree to use it. The IMB model also considers economic and environmental factors, such as living conditions and whether the individual has access to good health care.

Moderators of the IMB model, however, include problems such as depression, substance abuse, and other mental health concerns (119).

The transtheoretical model (TTM) (120–122) is a dynamic theory of change based on the assumption that a common set of change processes can be applied across a broad range of health behaviors. TTM conceptualizes behavior change as a process involving a series of 6 distinct stages: precontemplation, contemplation, preparation, action, maintenance, and termination. These stages are transtheoretical and integrate principles of change from across a variety of theories of intervention. In the early stages of change, individuals apply cognitive, affective, and evaluation processes to progress forward; during the later stages, commitments, conditioning, contingencies, environmental controls, and support to move toward maintenance and termination (122). Each stage brings an individual closer to making or sustaining behavioral changes. Unique variables, processes, and benefits versus costs of behavior change define each stage, and interventions based on this model are meant to increase motivation to change and to resolve ambivalence about change. At times individuals may move back to earlier stages (relapse), but movement through the stages recommences the process of change. TTM is one of the most widely cited and used models for interventions regarding health behavior changes. A criticism of TTM is that such distinct stages cannot capture the complexity of human behavior; the stages may be more properly understood as mere points on a larger continuum of the process of change. Motivational interviewing (described above) is a technique that is also consistent with the transtheoretical model.

The relapse prevention model is based on the principles of social learning theory. As described by Marlatt and George (123), the relapse prevention model integrates skills training, cognitive therapy, and lifestyle change. It aims to increase awareness and begin to change habits in an effort to rebalance lifestyle and improve ability to cope with stressors. Principles of relapse prevention include identifying high-risk situations for relapse (e.g., drug/alcohol use during sex) and developing appropriate solutions (e.g., abstaining from or moderating drug/alcohol use during sex). Helping individuals to distinguish between a slip (e.g., an instance of not participating in the planned activity) and a relapse (e.g., an extended period of not participating) is thought to improve adherence in the relapse prevention model.

The health decision model combining the health belief model and individual preferences, defers to patient preferences in making health decisions with respect to weighing the benefits and risks of behaviors (124,125). In addition to the health belief model's variables (perceived severity, susceptibility, evaluation of action, motivations), the health decision model also incorporates social variables (including knowledge, experience, sociodemographic and sociocultural factors, and patient-provider factors) (126), and recognizes that behaviors and health decisions are often made in an interactional context with other people (127). For example, using a condom to prevent HIV requires 2 people to jointly take action and necessitates the consideration of other people's views—either implicitly or explicitly—to successfully negotiate behavior implementation. Importantly, the health decision model also considers the effect of cultural values on behavior; for example, in Latino culture, condoms have many negative associations (e.g., machismo, religious prohibitions, association with sex work) that may interfere with condom use. As with the health belief model, critics have argued that the health decision model envisions health attitudes and behavior change in a static and linear way (i.e., progressing through a series of stages that lead to the outcome of decision to change) and does not allow for the fluidity, dynamism, and flexibility needed to account for or encourage complex behavior change (127).

The AIDS risk reduction model (ARRM) is one of several stages of change models that posit behavior change to be a process in which individuals move from one step to the next as a result of a given stimulus (128). The ARRM combines aspects of the health belief model, the diffusion of innovation theory and social cognitive theory. In the ARRM, an individual must pass through 3 stages: behavior labeling, commitment to change, and taking action. Consequently, interventions using this model focus on conducting an individual risk assessment, influencing the decision to reduce risk through perceptions of enjoyment or self-efficacy, and assisting the individual with support to enact the change (e.g., access to condoms, social support).

Structure of HIV Prevention Interventions

HIV prevention interventions are generally designed as individual level, group-based, community level, or structural interventions. Individual-level interventions seek to modify knowledge, attitudes, beliefs, self-efficacy, and emotional well-being of the individuals participating. This often involves individualized risk reduction counseling or motivational interviewing delivered by a trained counselor, health educator, peer, or other professional.

Group-level interventions are often designed to influence individual risk behavior by altering knowledge, attitudes, beliefs, and self-efficacy in a small group setting, typically with 5 to 10 individuals per group. Group-based interventions for HIV prevention mainly focus on the development of skills through live demonstrations, role plays, or practice. Examples include teaching skills on learning how to use a condom correctly, how to implement personal decisions to reduce sexual risk, and how to negotiate safer sex/condom use with one's sexual partners.

Community-level interventions seek to motivate and reinforce behavior change in individuals who do not participate directly in the intervention by promoting norms that support safer sex, which is typically accomplished through popular opinion leaders, community mobilization, or social/sexual networks. This type of intervention may have several components, requiring complex coordination and several years or longer to implement.

Finally, structural interventions reduce an individual's risk by changing the current conditions in which people can implement safer behaviors. For example, some sexual and gender minority populations engage in transactional sex as a means of survival. A structural intervention approach could make microfinance loans available for vulnerable and disenfranchised populations that would otherwise turn to sex work. This may affect their need to engage in transactional sex, which may reduce their susceptibility to HIV. Structural approaches include social, economic, and political interventions that can improve HIV risk outcomes by increasing the willingness and ability of individuals to protect themselves.

Systematic reviews and meta-analyses have shown that individual-, group-, and community-level HIV behavioral interventions for adult MSM have resulted in significant reductions in self-reported sexual risk behaviors (129–132). One review of interventions by Herbst and colleagues found that the reduction in odds of unprotected anal intercourse among MSM ranged from 27% to 43%. The authors also found that group- and community-level HIV behavioral interventions for adult MSM were cost-effective (129).

High-Impact Behavioral Interventions

The field of HIV prevention has been expanding over the past decade with the testing of several HIV prevention efficacy trial interventions with a variety of at-risk groups. High Impact HIV/AIDS Prevention Project (HIP) is the CDC's approach to reducing HIV infections in the United States. HIP includes scientifically proven cost-effective, targeted, and scalable interventions for maximum effect on the HIV epidemic. The strategies have been proven effective through research studies that showed positive behavioral (e.g., use of condoms; reduction in number of partners) and/or health outcomes (e.g., reduction in the number of new STIs). This project is formerly known as the DEBI (Diffusion of Effective Behavioral Interventions) and began in 1999 when the CDC published a Compendium of HIV Prevention Interventions with Evidence of Effectiveness to respond to prevention service providers who requested evidence-based interventions that work. The CDC's Compendium now includes more than 74 HIV risk reduction evidence-based behavioral interventions and 8 HIV medication adherence evidence-based behavioral interventions for a variety of at-risk groups. Further description of these interventions can be found at www.effectiveinterventions.org.

Biomedical-based HIV Prevention Interventions

Biomedical HIV interventions center on the concepts that 1) administering antiretroviral medications to persons who are HIV-uninfected but at high risk for becoming infected can protect them from HIV acquisition, and 2) initiation of antiretroviral medications by individuals who are living with HIV infection can reduce their infectiousness to others. These interventions are often referred to as post- and pre-exposure prophylaxis (PEP and PrEP) and as "treatment as prevention," respectively, and are described below.

Chemoprophylaxis (PEP and PrEP)
Early animal studies suggested that chemoprophylaxis is most effective when provided to the animal before an exposure, and dosing immediately after exposure is also important (133). In 1997, a retrospective case-control study conducted by the CDC found that health care workers who took zidovudine (in an era where combination antiretroviral therapy was not yet developed) after a needlestick exposure from an HIV-infected patient were one fifth as likely to become infected than health care workers with similar exposures who did not use antiretrovirals (134). Subsequent observational studies suggested that PEP could also be beneficial for protection after sexual exposure to HIV (135–138); however, definitive randomized controlled trials were never performed because of the relative inefficiency of HIV transmission (i.e., less than 1 per 100 exposures) and the notion that PEP was primarily intended for one-off exposures, not repeated patterns of behavior. Nonetheless, antiretroviral PEP can be used with patients after they have experienced a high-risk sexual, injection drug use, or other nonoccupational exposure. The CDC issued recommendations on non-occupational PEP administration in 2005 (139).

Certain individuals are recurrently exposed to HIV because of lack of desire to use condoms (e.g., to enhance pleasure, or to conceive, for some heterosexuals). Animal data and human pharmacology suggest that certain antiretrovirals might be particularly beneficial for chemoprophylaxis because of achieving high-levels in genital tract secretions (140). The drugs that appear to meet these criteria tended to be reverse transcriptase inhibitors, particularly tenofovir and emtricitabine. Tenofovir by itself or in combination with emtricitabine has been the focus of most of the recent studies of chemoprophylaxis. The first trial to demonstrate the efficacy of PrEP was the iPrEx Study, which randomly assigned 2499 MSM and transgender women from 6 countries in 4 continents to receive oral tenofovir FTC or a placebo pill. iPrEx participants who received the active medication were 44% less likely to become HIV infected (141). There was a high correlation between medication adherence and drug efficacy (142). Among individuals who had detectable tenofovir in their blood, the protection level was well over 90%. Two subsequent studies of heterosexuals in Africa found levels of efficacy exceeding 60% in all the intervention groups (143,144).

The CAPRISA 004 Study, which looked at the efficacy of a topical microbicide gel containing 1% tenofovir, found that South African women in KwaZulu-Natal province were 39% less likely to become HIV infected when they applied the gel pericoitally compared with those applying a placebo gel (145). However, this study was not validated by the VOICE trial, which recruited women from similar populations and asked them to apply a daily vaginal tenofovir gel. It was clear that the major difference between the 2 gel trials was medication adherence (i.e., not using use the gel daily as recommended) (146). Despite these disappointing trial results, the other successful oral and topical PrEP trial results and the high correlation between drug detection and efficacy suggest that proof of concept for chemoprophylaxis exists. New studies are underway to see whether a topical tenofovir gel can protect MSM who are rectally exposed to HIV, with recent studies suggesting that the gel is safe; there are also studies of non–tenofovir-based oral regimens (147). Earlier-phase studies of injectable medications, which do not have to rely on daily adherence, are also underway (www.avac.org), as are studies of different dosing regimens using tenofovir.

Because of the positive results from the first oral PrEP studies, the FDA approved the use of the fixed combination pill containing tenofovir and emtricitabine for chemoprophylaxis against HIV. The guidance suggests that individuals who will benefit from PrEP need to be willing to engage in care (because screening for renal function and hepatitis B status as well as other STIs is an important part of clinical care before initiating PrEP) and willing and able to adhere to the medication regimen. The CDC has issued interim guidance for PrEP use in MSM, injection drug users, and heterosexuals, which can be found at www.cdc.gov/hiv/prevention/research/prep.

To improve understanding of the real-world implementation of PrEP, multiple demonstration projects are underway in the United States and in international settings to obtain more long-term data. Although the clinical trials did not suggest increased-risk compensation, serious clinical toxicities, or antiretroviral drug resistance among those who became infected, these trials were done in very controlled settings. The demonstration projects will be able to ascertain whether longer-term problems may eventuate and whether the initial efficacy findings in the successful clinical trials can be sustained over longer periods of time. One clinical finding in the iPrEx Study does deserve further monitoring: there was a small but statistically significant decrease in bone density in the lumbar spine, but not in the hip, in the participants randomly assigned to the active medication. This was not associated with fractures or other clinical manifestations; however, given that the follow-up time in iPrEx was 72 weeks, this warrants further observation (141).

Although PrEP for HIV prevention is still relatively new, initial data support that excellent adherence to the daily medication regimen greatly reduces risk for seroconversion among the HIV uninfected. That said, mental health and substance use problems still vex researchers and clinicians alike in so far as these problems are thought to directly interfere with medication adherence patterns (54).

Treatment as Prevention

Both observational and prospective randomized multinational studies have demonstrated that treating HIV-infected individuals with antiretroviral therapy can reduce the likelihood that they will transmit HIV to their sexual partners (80). This phenomenon is known as "treatment as prevention." The rationale for treatment as prevention began with early studies evaluating the effect of HIV on plasma viremia. These studies found that in most individuals, decay kinetics were similar in semen and cervicovaginal secretions, suggesting decreased infectiousness in people receiving treatment. Observational studies tended to corroborate this finding (148). Moreover, in the era before combination antiretroviral therapy, a study of discordant couples in Africa found that plasma viremia was the strongest predictor of HIV transmission (43).

HPTN 052 was a randomized controlled trial of 1763 HIV serodiscordant couples with the infected partner having a CD4 count between 350 and 550 cells/mm^3. The infected partners agreed to be randomly assigned to starting antiretroviral therapy immediately or waiting until their CD4 count started declining. The study was stopped prematurely because of the profound positive effect of initiation of antiretroviral therapy on HIV transmission. Out of 28 cases, only 1 was in a couple where the infected partner was receiving antiretroviral therapy; furthermore, in that case, the individual had begun therapy less than 80 days before his partner became infected (149). Because it is well documented that it may take several months before HIV replication is sufficiently suppressed in the plasma to have undetectable levels, these data suggest that treatment as prevention is highly effective but that individuals who are infected may not become significantly less infectious before several months elapse. The data from HPTN 052 have been supported by several ecological studies, including 1 of a primarily MSM epidemic in San Francisco (150) and one of a primarily injecting drug-use epidemic in Vancouver (151,152).

Despite these optimistic findings, treatment as prevention on its own is not a perfect solution to ending the spread of HIV. For example, in several European countries, despite widespread access to antiretroviral therapy and routine health care, decreases in incident infections have not been manifest (153,154). These findings suggest that it is not enough to expand access to antiretroviral therapy for HIV-infected individuals. More focus needs to be on initiating treatment at earlier stages of infection, expanding HIV testing so that all individuals who are infected are aware of their infection, optimizing access to treatment, and supporting medication adherence on an ongoing basis. The United States has a long way to go to make a significant decrease in new infections. Of the more than 1.1 million people living with HIV, approximately 20% are unaware of their infection; among those aware they are infected, many have not accessed care and treatment, or are not being stably maintained in care (155). Thus, the rate of virologic suppression in the United States is still under 30% at the present time. The Department of Health and Human Services recently expanded the guidelines of when to initiate antiretroviral therapy to being permissive to all individuals who are HIV-infected with one of the major goals being the decrease of new HIV infections (156).

Circumcision

As noted earlier, the male foreskin contains many cells that have enhanced susceptibility to becoming HIV-infected. Multiple epidemiologic studies have suggested that for every unprotected sex act, either heterosexual or homosexual, uncircumcised men have a greater risk for becoming HIV infected (43,157,158). Three well-controlled clinical trials conducted in different parts of sub-Saharan Africa all found a net benefit of approximately 50% to 60% in decreasing HIV incidence in men who were offered adult circumcision compared with randomly assigned controls (159–162). The circumcision benefit has been maintained over time in several follow-up studies. It is important to note that male circumcision does not protect female partners or receptive male partners from HIV acquisition. Moreover, for MSM who engage in receptive anal intercourse as well as insertive anal intercourse, there does not appear to be a substantial benefit from circumcision (163). Thus, circumcision provides a benefit only to individuals who are exclusively or primarily insertive.

Combination Biomedical and Behavioral Prevention

Although biomedical interventions are promising, they have been studied as part of a prevention package, in conjunction with behavioral counseling, treatment of sexually transmitted co-infections, and promotion and provision of condoms. This underscores the reality that biomedical and behavioral strategies are most likely to be effective when implemented together as part of a combination approach to HIV prevention. Behavioral health issues are particularly important when considering the use of antiretrovirals for primary or secondary HIV prevention because optimal medication use requires sufficient engagement with the health care system to be tested so that serostatus can be determined, adherence can be optimized, and risk compensation (i.e., engaging in increased unprotected sex) can be minimized. For some individuals, ongoing sexual risk taking may be associated with depression and other affective disorders, and/or significant substance use problems (as described above). Screening for concomitant mental health concerns is a necessary step before treatment or prophylaxis is initiated, since untreated mental health issues can impede antiretroviral adherence, decrease engagement in care, and/or increase sexual risk taking.

Useful HIV Prevention Resources

The field of HIV prevention research has been expanding over the past few years, especially in the areas of treatment as prevention, chemoprophylaxis, and adult male circumcision. With the proliferation of electronic media in the current era, providers and patients may continue to have new questions and seek information on new data. It is impossible for busy primary care clinicians to be aware of all new facts at all times, but the internet provides easy access to a variety of ongoing resources on HIV prevention. Table 13-1 lists several useful resources for clinicians, researchers, and policymakers interested in keeping up to date on current HIV prevention tools, trainings, interventions, and research.

Table 13–1   Resources for Keeping Up to Date on Current HIV Prevention Tools, Trainings, Interventions, and Research

www.thefenwayinstitute.org: The website of The Fenway Institute contains several sections that have updates on new research, particularly PrEP. Fenway Health was one of the first sites in the United States to study PrEP, as well as treatment as prevention. There is also a link to the National Center for LGBT Health Education which provides a range of clinical training programs and materials on HIV prevention.

www.avac.org: The website of the AIDS Vaccine Advocacy Coalition provides up-to-date information about the latest clinical trials of HIV-preventive vaccines, chemoprophylaxis, and treatment as prevention. The site is easily navigable and provides hyperlinks to other resources and new clinical trials and research.

www.rectalmicrobicides.org: The website of the International Rectal Microbicide Advocates (IRMA) contains a substantial amount of new information about prevention technologies, including a focus on studies of rectal microbicides (experimental medications applied directly to the rectal mucosa to prevent HIV). The potential benefits of rectal microbicides over oral medication are that they may be taken right at the time of intercourse and may have less systemic absorption.

www.hivinsite.org: This website sponsored by the University of California in San Francisco (UCSF) provides a compendium of information related to HIV transmission, prevention, and aspects of care. It posts lectures given by UCSF faculty and hyperlinks to many articles from the literature on HIV/AIDS.

www.cdc.gov/hiv: The official website for the CDC has a landing area for HIV/AIDS, including the latest statistics for different jurisdictions in the United States regarding HIV prevalence, incidence, and the success of different prevention interventions.

www.unaids.org and www.who.int: These 2 websites are from United Nations agencies and provide global statistics on the current spread of HIV, rates of access to antiretroviral therapy, and other demographic data regarding the spread of HIV throughout the world. They provide data on the diffusion of new trends in technologies in the populations across the world.

www.adolescentaids.org/healthcare/acts.html: ACTS (Advise, Consent, Test, Support) is an online toolkit for delivering routine HIV testing and counseling in clinical and community-based settings.

www.nccc.ucsf.edu: The Clinician Consultation Center, based at UCSF, offers clinical resources for clinicians serving HIV-infected patients and at-risk patients. Resources include training materials as well as guidance on PEP, PrEP, HIV testing, and HIV management.

www.aidsetc.org: The AIDS Education and Training Center (AETC) National Resource Center offers a central repository of HIV/AIDS prevention and care clinical trainings and materials.

CDC = Centers for Disease Control and Prevention; PEP = postexposure prophylaxis; PrEP = pre-exposure prophylaxis.

Summary Points

- Given that there are 50,000 new HIV infections in the United States each year, the development of effective HIV prevention strategies remains a priority.

- Those at highest risk for HIV infection in the United States are MSM and transgender women, particularly those who are young and black. Latinos are also at elevated risk.
- Behavioral health issues can interact with sexual risk behaviors to produce greater risk for HIV infection and transmission; it is particularly important for clinicians to assess for mental health conditions and substance use patterns, and to treat or make appropriate referrals, as part of their HIV prevention efforts with LGBT patients.
- Recent advances in HIV testing include the CDC's and USPSTF's recommendations for universal screening, the greater availability of rapid antibody testing kits, methods for early detection of HIV, and the option for couples to test together.
- HIV prevention interventions at the individual, group, community, and structural levels can be effective in reducing sexual risk behaviors among MSM. Many conceptual models can help inform the development of effective behavioral interventions.
- Biomedical interventions, including PEP, PrEP, and treatment as prevention, represent a new frontier in HIV prevention but are most likely to be effective when implemented in combination with behavioral strategies.
- The United States has a long way to go in preventing new HIV infections. Providers can make a difference by offering universal HIV testing to all patients; providing routine HIV and STI testing and behavioral counseling to higher-risk patients; and ensuring that infected patients are linked to, and stably maintained in, HIV care.

References

1. **amfAR-AIDS.** Statistics: Worldwide. November 2012. Available at: www.amfar.org/worldwide-aids-stats/.
2. **Centers for Disease Control and Prevention.** Estimated HIV incidence in the United States, 2007–2010. HIV Surveillance Supplemental Report. December 2012. Available at: www.cdc.gov/hiv/pdf/statistics_hssr_vol_17_no_4.pdf.
3. **UNAIDS.** Report on the global HIV/AIDS epidemic 2010 Geneva: UNAIDS; 2010. Available at: http://issuu.com/unaids/docs/unaids_globalreport_2010/9?e=2251159/2047939.
4. **Mayer KH, Wheeler DP, Bekker LG, et al.** Overcoming biological, behavioral, and structural vulnerabilities: new directions in research to decrease HIV transmission in men who have sex with men. J Acquir Immune Defic Syndr. 2013;63 Suppl 2:S161-7.
5. **Centers for Disease Control and Prevention.** HIV among gay, bisexual, and other men who have sex with men. Last updated September 2013. Available at: www.cdc.gov/hiv/risk/gender/msm/facts/index.html.
6. **Mayer KH.** Sexually transmitted diseases in men who have sex with men. Clin Infect Dis. 2011;53 Suppl 3:79-83.
7. **Nussbaum MC.** From Disgust to Humanity: Sexual Orientation and Constitutional Law. Inalienable Rights Series. Oxford, New York: Oxford University Press; 2010.
8. **Delonga K, Torres HL, Kamen C, et al.** Loneliness, internalized homophobia, and compulsive internet use: factors associated with sexual risk behavior among a sample of

adolescent males seeking services at a community LGBT Center. Sex Addict Compuls. 2011;18: 61-74.

9. **Pettifor A, Bekker LG, Hosek S, et al.** Preventing HIV among young people: research priorities for the future. J Acquir Immune Defic Syndr. 2013;63 Suppl 2:S155-60.

10. **Horn SS, Kosciw JG, Russell ST.** Special issue introduction: new research on lesbian, gay, bisexual, and transgender youth: studying lives in context. J Youth Adolesc. 2009;38:863-6.

11. **Centers for Disease Control and Prevention.** HIV among African American gay and bisexual men. February 2014. Available at: www.cdc.gov/hiv/pdf/risk_HIV_among_Black_AA_Gay.pdf.

12. **Millett GA, Flores SA, Peterson JL, Bakeman R.** Explaining disparities in HIV infection among black and white men who have sex with men: a meta-analysis of HIV risk behaviors. AIDS. 2007;21:2083-91.

13. **Reed E, Santana MC, Bowleg L, et al.** Experiences of racial discrimination and relation to sexual risk for HIV among a sample of urban black and African American men. J Urban Health. 2013;90:314-22.

14. **Aidala A, Cross JE, Stall R, et al.** Housing status and HIV risk behaviors: implications for prevention and policy. AIDS Behav. 2005;9:251-65.

15. **Centers for Disease Control and Prevention.** HIV Among Hispanics/Latinos in the United States and dependent areas. November 2013. Available at: www.cdc.gov/hiv/pdf/risk_latino.pdf.

16. **Pouget ER, Friedman SR, Cleland CM, Tempalski B, Cooper HL.** Estimates of the population prevalence of injection drug users among Hispanic residents of large US metropolitan areas. J Urban Health. 2012;89:527-64.

17. **Centers for Disease Control and Prevention.** HIV Surveillance Report, 2008. June 2010. Available at: www.cdc.gov/hiv/pdf/statistics_2008_HIV_Surveillance_Report_vol_20.pdf.

18. **Centers for Disease Control and Prevention.** HIV/AIDS Surveillance Supplemental Report: Cases of HIV infection and AIDS in the United States, by race/ethnicity, 1998-2002. Available at: www.cdc.gov/hiv/surveillance/resources/reports/2004supp_vol10no1/pdf/HIVAIDS_SSR_Vol10_No1.pdf.

19. **Darrow WW, Montanea JE, Gladwin H.** AIDS-related stigma among Black and Hispanic young adults. AIDS Behav. 2009;13:1178-88.

20. **Duran D, Usman HR, Beltrami J, et al.** HIV counseling and testing among Hispanics at CDC-funded sites in the United States, 2007. Am J Public Health. 2010;100 Suppl 1:S152-8.

21. **Sullivan PS, Salazar L, Buchbinder S, Sanchez TH.** Estimating the proportion of HIV transmissions from main sex partners among men who have sex with men in five US cities. AIDS. 2009;23:1153-62.

22. **Williamson LM, Dodds JP, Mercey DE, Hart GJ, Johnson AM.** Sexual risk behaviour and knowledge of HIV status among community samples of gay men in the UK. AIDS. 2008;22:1063-70.

23. **Sandfort TG, Nel J, Rich E, Reddy V, Yi H.** HIV testing and self-reported HIV status in South African men who have sex with men: results from a community-based survey. Sex Transm Infect. 2008;84:425-9.

24. **Lyles CM, Kay LS, Crepaz N, et al.** Best-evidence interventions: findings from a systematic review of HIV behavioral interventions for US populations at high risk, 2000-2004. Am J Public Health. 2007;97:133-43.

25. **Sullivan PS, Zapata A, Benbow N.** New U.S. HIV incidence numbers: heeding their message. Focus. 2008;23:5-7.

26. **Centers for Disease Control and Prevention.** HIV prevalence, unrecognized infection, and HIV testing among men who have sex with men-Five US cities, June 2004-April 2005. MMWR Morb Mortal Wkly Rep. 2005;54:597-601.

27. **Centers for Disease Control and Prevention.** HIV among transgender people. April 2013. Available at: www.cdc.gov/hiv/risk/transgender/index.html.

28. **Baral SD, Poteat T, Strömdahl S, et al.** Worldwide burden of HIV in transgender women: a systematic review and meta-analysis. Lancet Infect Dis. 2013;13:214-22.

29. **Herbst JH, Jacobs ED, Finlayson TJ, et al.** Estimating HIV prevalence and risk behaviors of transgender persons in the United States: a systematic review. AIDS Behav. 2008;12: 1-17.

30. **Garofalo R, Osmer E, Sullivan C, Doll M, Harper G.** Environmental, psychosocial, and individual correlates of HIV risk in ethnic minority male-to-female transgender youth. J HIV/AIDS Prevent Children Youth. 2007;7:89-104.

31. **Nemoto T, Operario D, Keatley J, Nguyen H, Sugano E.** Promoting health for transgender women: Transgender Resources and Neighborhood Space (TRANS) program in San Francisco. Am J Public Health. 2005;95:382-84.

32. **Garofalo R, Deleon J, Osmer E, et al.** Overlooked, misunderstood and at-risk: exploring the lives and HIV risk of ethnic minority male-to-female transgender youth. J Adolesc Health. 2006;38:230-6.

33. **Grossman AH, D'Augelli AR.** Transgender youth: invisible and vulnerable. J Homosex. 2006;51:111-28.

34. **Koken JA, Bimbi DS, Parsons JT.** Experiences of familial acceptance-rejection among transwomen of color. J Fam Psychol. 2009;23:853-60.

35. **Pardo ST, Schantz K.** Growing Up Transgender: Safety and Resilience. ACT for (trans) Youth, Part 2. Ithaca, NY: ACT for Youth Center of Excellence, Cornell University; 2008.

36. **Pardo S. Growing Up Transgender: Research and Theory.** ACT for (trans) Youth, Part 2. Ithaca, NY: ACT for Youth Center of Excellence, Cornell University; 2008.

37. **Lombardi EL, Wilchins RA, Priesing D, Malouf D.** Gender violence: transgender experiences with violence and discrimination. J Homosex. 2001;42:89-101.

38. **Wilson EC, Garofalo R, Harris DR, Belzer M.** Sexual risk taking among transgender male-to-female youths with different partner types. Am J Public Health. 2010;100:1500-5.

39. **Kosenko KA.** Contextual influences on sexual risk-taking in the transgender community. J Sex Res. 2011;48:285-96.

40. **Stieglitz KA.** Development, risk, and resilience of transgender youth. J Assoc Nurses AIDS Care. 2010;21:192-206.

41. **Mayer KH, Venkatesh KK.** Interactions of HIV, other sexually transmitted diseases, and genital tract inflammation facilitating local pathogen transmission and acquisition. Am J Reprod Immunol. 2011;65:308-16.

42. **Sterling TR, Vlahov D, Astemborski J, et al.** Initial plasma HIV-1 RNA levels and progression to AIDS in women and men. N Engl J Med. 2001;344:720-5.

43. **Quinn TC, Wawer MJ, Sewankambo N, et al.** Viral load and heterosexual transmission of human immunodeficiency virus type 1. Rakai Project Study Group. N Engl J Med. 2000;342: 921-9.

44. **Politch JA, Mayer KH, Welles SL, et al.** Highly active antiretroviral therapy does not completely suppress HIV in semen of sexually active HIV-infected men who have sex with men. AIDS. 2012;26:1535-43.

45. **Heffron R, Donnell D, Rees H, et al.** Use of hormonal contraceptives and risk of HIV-1 transmission: a prospective cohort study. Lancet Infect Dis. 2012;12:19-26.

46. **Baggaley RF, White RG, Boily MC.** Infectiousness of HIV-infected homosexual men in the era of highly active antiretroviral therapy. AIDS. 2010;24:2418-20.

47. **Baggaley RF, White RG, Boily MC.** HIV transmission risk through anal intercourse: systematic review, meta-analysis and implications for HIV prevention. Int J Epidemiol. 2010;39: 1048-63.

48. **Millett GA, Peterson JL, Flores SA, et al.** Comparisons of disparities and risks of HIV infection in black and other men who have sex with men in Canada, UK, and USA: a meta-analysis. Lancet. 2012;380:341-8.

49. **Mayer KH, Bekker LG, Stall R, et al.** Comprehensive clinical care for men who have sex with men: an integrated approach. Lancet. 2012;380:378-87.

50. **Bing EG, Burnam MA, Longshore D, et al.** Psychiatric disorders and drug use among human immunodeficiency virus-infected adults in the United States. Arch Gen Psychiatry. 2001;58: 721-728.

51. **Asch SM, Kilbourne AM, Gifford AL, et al.** HCSUS Consortium. Under-diagnosis of depression in HIV: who are we missing? J Gen Intern Med. 2003;18:450-460.

52. **Israelski DM, Prentiss DE, Lubega S, et al.** Psychiatric co-morbidity in vulnerable populations receiving primary care for HIV/AIDS. AIDS Care. 2007;19:220-225.

53. **Koblin BA, Chesney MA, Husnik MJ, et al.** High-risk behaviors among men who have sex with men in 6 US cities: baseline data from the EXPLORE Study. Am J Public Health. 2003; 93:926-32.

54. **O'Cleirigh C, Newcomb ME, Mayer KH, et al.** Moderate levels of depression predict sexual transmission risk in HIV-infected MSM: a longitudinal analysis of data from six sites involved in a "prevention for positives" study. AIDS Behav. 2013;17:1764-9.

55. **Kalichman SC, Kelly JA, Johnson JR, Bulto M.** Factors associated with risk for HIV infection among chronic mentally ill adults. Am J Psychiatry. 1994;151:221-27.

56. **Carey MP, Carey KB, Maisto SA, et al.** HIV risk behavior among psychiatric outpatients: association with psychiatric disorder, substance use disorder, and gender. J Nervous Mental Dis. 2004;192:289.

57. **Carey MP, Carey KB, Kalichman SC.** Risk for human immunodeficiency virus (HIV) infection among persons with severe mental illnesses. Clin Psychol Rev. 1997;17:271-91.

58. **Meade CS, Graff FS, Griffin ML, Weiss RD.** HIV risk behavior among patients with co-occurring bipolar and substance use disorders: associations with mania and drug abuse. Drug Alcohol Depend. 2008;92:296-300.

59. **O'Cleirigh C, Safren SA, Mayer KH.** The pervasive effects of childhood sexual abuse: challenges for improving HIV prevention and treatment interventions. J Acquir Immune Defic Syndr. 2012;59:331-4.

60. **Stall R, Mills TC, Williamson J, et al.** Association of co-occurring psychosocial health problems and increased vulnerability to HIV/AIDS among urban men who have sex with men. Am J Public Health. 2003;93:939-42.

61. **Arreola SG, Neilands TB, Pollack LM, et al.** Higher prevalence of childhood sexual abuse among Latino men who have sex with men than non-Latino men who have sex with men: data from the Urban Men's Health Study. Child Abuse Negl. 2005;29:285-90.

62. **O'Cleirigh C, Traeger L, Mayer KH, et al.** Anxiety specific pathways to HIV sexual transmission risk behavior among young gay and bisexual men. J Gay Lesbian Ment Health. 2013;17: 314-26.

63. **Hart T, Heimberg R.** Social anxiety as a risk factor for unprotected intercourse among gay and bisexual male youth. AIDS Behavior. 2005;9:505-12.

64. **Derogatis LR, Spencer P.** Brief Symptom Inventory: BSI. Upper Saddle River, NJ: Pearson; 1993.

65. **Gordon D, Wong J, Heimberg RG.** Cognitive-behavioral therapy for social anxiety disorder: the state of the science. In Weeks JW, ed. The Wiley Blackwell Handbook of Social Anxiety Disorder. Hoboken, NJ: John Wiley & Sons; 2014.

66. **Skeer MR, Mimiaga MJ, Mayer KH, et al.** Patterns of substance use among a large urban cohort of HIV-infected men who have sex with men in primary care. AIDS Behav. 2012;16: 676-89.

67. **Fong IW, Read S, Wainberg MA, et al.** Alcoholism and rapid progression to AIDS after seroconversion. Clin Infect Dis. 1994;19:337-8.

68. **Wang JY, Liang B, Watson RR.** Alcohol consumption alters cytokine release during murine AIDS. Alcohol. 1997;14:155-9.

69. **Morin SF, Steward WT, Charlebois ED, et al.** Predicting HIV transmission risk among HIV-infected men who have sex with men: findings from the healthy living project. J Acquir Immune Defic Syndr. 2005;40:226-35.

70. **Vaudrey J, Raymond HF, Chen S, et al.** Indicators of use of methamphetamine and other substances among men who have sex with men, San Francisco, 2003-2006. Drug Alcohol Depend. 2007;90:97-100.

71. **Chesney MA, Koblin BA, Barresi PJ, et al.** An individually tailored intervention for HIV prevention: baseline data from the EXPLORE Study. Am J Public Health. 2003;93:933-8.

72. **Mimiaga MJ, Fair AD, Mayer KH, et al.** Experiences and sexual behaviors of HIV-infected MSM who acquired HIV in the context of crystal methamphetamine use. AIDS Educ Prev. 2008;20:30-41.

73. **Stall R, Paul JP, Greenwood G, et al.** Alcohol use, drug use and alcohol-related problems among men who have sex with men: the Urban Men's Health Study. Addiction. 2001;96:1589-601.

74. **Safren SA, Reisner SL, Herrick A, Mimiaga MJ, Stall RD.** Mental health and HIV risk in men who have sex with men. J Acquir Immune Defic Syndr. 2010;55 Suppl 2: S74-7.

75. **Safren SA, Blashill AJ, O'Cleirigh CM.** Promoting the sexual health of MSM in the context of comorbid mental health problems. AIDS Behav. 2011;15 Suppl 1: S30-4.

76. **Singer M.** Introduction to Syndemics: A Critical Systems Approach to Public and Community Health. San Francisco, CA: Jossey-Bass; 2009.

77. **Hirshfield S, Remien RH, Humberstone M, Walavalkar I, Chiasson MA.** Substance use and high-risk sex among men who have sex with men: a national online study in the USA. AIDS Care. 2004;16:1036-47.

78. **Mustanski B, Garofalo R, Herrick A, Donenberg G.** Psychosocial health problems increase risk for HIV among urban young men who have sex with men: preliminary evidence of a syndemic in need of attention. Ann Behav Med. 2007;34:37-45.

79. **Mimiaga MJ, Noonan E, Donnell D, et al.** Childhood sexual abuse is highly associated with HIV risk-taking behavior and infection among MSM in the EXPLORE study. J Acquir Immune Defic Syndr. 2009;51:340-8.

80. **Cohen MS, Chen YQ, McCauley M, et al.** Prevention of HIV-1 infection with early antiretroviral therapy. N Engl J Med. 2011;365:493-505.

81. **Centers for Disease Control and Prevention.** Challenges in HIV prevention. December 2013. Available at: www.cdc.gov/nchhstp/newsroom/docs/HIVFactSheets/Challenges-508.pdf

82. **Centers for Disease Control and Prevention.** Revised recommendations for HIV testing of adults, adolescents, and pregnant women in health care settings. MMWR Recomm Rep. 2006;55(RR14):1-17.

83. **U.S. Preventive Services Task Force.** Screening for HIV. Available at: www.uspreventiveservicestaskforce.org/Page/Topic/recommendation-summary/human-immunodeficiency-virus-hiv-infection-screening

84. **Centers for Disease Control and Prevention.** Sexually transmitted diseasese treatment guidelines, 2010. MMWR Recomm Rep. 2010;59(RR12):1-110.

85. **Allen S, Tice J, Van de Perre P, et al.** Effect of serotesting with counselling on condom use and seroconversion among HIV discordant couples in Africa. BMJ. 1992;304:1605-9.

86. **Painter TM.** Voluntary counseling and testing for couples: a high-leverage intervention for HIV/AIDS prevention in sub-Saharan Africa. Soc Sci Med. 2001;53:1397-411.

87. **Sullivan PS, White D, Rosenberg ES, et al.** Safety and acceptability of couples HIV testing and counseling for US Men who have sex with men: a randomized prevention study. J Int Assoc Provid AIDS Care. 2014;13:135-44.

88. **Porter R.** The Greatest Benefit to Mankind: A Medical History of Humanity from Antiquity to the Present. London: HarperCollins; 1997.

89. **Wade DT, Halligan PW.** Do biomedical models of illness make for good healthcare systems? BMJ. 2004;329:1398-401.

90. **Shattock RJ, Moore JP.** Inhibiting sexual transmission of HIV-1 infection. Nat Rev Microbiol. 2003;1:25-34.

91. **Roehr B, Gross M, Mayer K.** Creating a research and development agenda for microbicides that protect against HIV infection. amfAR AIDS Research. 2001;6(8).

92. **amfAR-AIDS.** Issue Brief: HIV prevention for men who have sex with men. AmfAR AIDS Research. 2006. Available at: www.amfar.org/uploadedFiles/In_the_Community/Publications/HIV%20Prevention%20for%20MSM.pdf

93. **Munro S, Lewin S, Swart T, Volmink J.** A review of health behaviour theories: how useful are these for developing interventions to promote long-term medication adherence for TB and HIV/AIDS? BMC Public Health. 2007;7:104-04.

94. **Skinner BF.** The Behavior of Organisms: An Experimental Analysis. The Century Psychology Series. New York, London: D. Appleton-Century Company, Inc.; 1938.

95. **Miller WR, Rollnick S.** Motivational Interviewing: Preparing People to Change Addictive Behavior. New York: Guilford Press;1991.

96. **Emmons KM, Rollnick S.** Motivational interviewing in health care settings. Opportunities and limitations. Am J Prev Med. 2001;20:68-74.

97. **Lewis MA, DeVellis BM, Sleath B.** Social influence and interpersonal communication in health behavior. In: Glanz K, Rimer BK, Lewis FM, eds. Health Behavior and Health Education: Theory, Research, and Practice. San Francisco: John Wiley & Sons; 2002:240-64.

98. **Janz NK, Champion VL, Strecher VJ.** The Health Belief Model. In: Glanz K, Rimer BK, Lewis FM, eds. Health Behavior and Health Education: Theory, Research, and Practice. San Francisco: John Wiley & Sons; 2002:45-56.

99. **Bandura A.** Social Learning Theory. Englewood Cliffs, NJ: Prentice Hall; 1977.

100. **Fisher JD, Fisher WA.** Changing AIDS-risk behavior. Psychol Bull. 1992;111:455-74.

101. **Romer D, Hornik R.** HIV education for youth: the importance of social consensus in behaviour change. AIDS Care. 1992;4:285-303.

102. **Baranowski T, Perry CL, Parcel GS.** How individuals, environments, and health behavior interact: social cognitive theory. In: Glanz K, Rimer BK, Lewis FM, eds. Health Behavior and Health Education: Theory, Research, and Practice. San Francisco: John Wiley & Sons; 2002.

103. **Bandura A.** Social Foundations of Thought and Action: A Social Cognitive Theory. Prentice-Hall Series in Social Learning Theory. Englewood Cliffs, NJ: Prentice-Hall; 1986.

104. **Bandura A.** Social cognitive theory: an agentic perspective. Annu Rev Psychol. 2001;52: 1-26.

105. **Bandura A.** Self-efficacy: toward a unifying theory of behavioral change. Psychol Rev. 1977; 84:191-215.

106. **Bandura A.** Self-Efficacy: The Exercise of Control. New York: W.H. Freeman; 1997.

107. **Ajzen I, Fishbein M.** Understanding Attitudes and Predicting Social Behavior. Upper Saddle River, NJ: Prentice-Hall; 1980.

108. **Sheppard BH, Hartwick J, Warshaw PR.** The theory of reasoned action: a meta-analysis of past research with recommendations for modifications and future research. J Consumer Res. 1988;15:325-43.

109. **Ajzen I.** From intentions to actions: a theory of planned behavior. In: Kuhl J, Beckmann J, eds. Action-Control: From Cognition to Behavior. Heidelberg: Springer; 1985:11-39.

110. **Ajzen I.** Attitudes, traits, and actions: dispositional prediction of behavior in personality and social psychology. In: Berkowitz L, ed. Advances in Experimental Social Psychology. New York: Academic Press; 1987:1-63.

111. **Ajzen I.** The theory of planned behavior. Org Behav Human Dec Process. 1991;50:179-211.

112. **Ajzen I.** Residual effects of past on later behavior: habituation and reasoned action perspectives. Personal Soc Psychol Rev. 2002;6:107-22.

113. **Fisher WA.** A theory-based framework for intervention and evaluation in STD/HIV prevention. Can J Human Sexual. 1997;6:105-11.

114. **Ajzen I, Madden TJ.** Prediction of goal-directed behavior: attitudes, intentions, and perceived behavioral control. J Exp Soc Psychol. 1986;22:453-74.

115. **Godin G, Kok G.** The theory of planned behavior: a review of its applications to health-related behaviors. Am J Health Promot. 1996;11:87-98.

116. **Rogers RW.** A protection motivation theory of fear appeals and attitude change. J Psychol. 1975;91:93.

117. **Rogers RW.** Cognitive and physiological processes in fear appeals and attitude change: a revised theory of protection motivation. In: Cacioppo J, Pety R, eds. Social Psychophysiology. New York: Guilford Press; 1983:153-76.

118. **Boer H, Seydel E.** Protection motivation theory. In: Conner M, Norman P, eds. Predicting Health Behaviour. Berkshire, United Kingdom:Open University Press;2005:95-120.

119. **Starace F, Massa A, Amico KR, Fisher JD.** Adherence to antiretroviral therapy: an empirical test of the information-motivation-behavioral skills model. Health Psychol. 2006;25:153-62.

120. **Prochaska JO, Redding CA, Harlow LL, Rossi JS, Velicer WF.** The transtheoretical model of change and HIV prevention: a review. Health Educ Q. 1994;21:471-86.

121. **Prochaska JO, Velicer WF.** The transtheoretical model of health behavior change. Am J Health Promot. 1997;12:38-48.

122. **Prochaska JO, Redding CA, Evers KE.** The transtheoretical model and stages of change. In: Glanz K, Rimer BK, Lewis FM, eds. Health Behavior and Health Education: Theory, Research, and Practice. San Francisco: John Wiley & Sons; 2002:99-120.

123. **Marlatt GA, George WH.** Relapse prevention: introduction and overview of the model. Br J Addict. 1984;79:261-73.

124. **McNeil BJ, Keller E, Adelstein SJ.** Primer on certain elements of medical decision making. N Engl J Med. 1975;293:211-5.

125. **Weinstein MC.** Clinical Decision Analysis. Philadelphia: Saunders; 1980.

126. **Eraker SA, Becker MH, Strecher VJ, Kirscht JP.** Smoking behavior, cessation techniques, and the health decision model. Am J Med. 1985;78:817-25.

127. **Fan H, Conner RF, Villarreal LP.** AIDS: Science and Society. Boston, MA: Jones and Bartlett Publishers; 2004.

128. **Catania JA, Kegeles SM, Coates TJ.** Towards an understanding of risk behavior: an AIDS risk reduction model (ARRM). Health Educ Q. 1990;17:53-72.

129. **Herbst JH, Beeker C, Mathew A, et al.** The effectiveness of individual-, group-, and community-level HIV behavioral risk-reduction interventions for adult men who have sex with men: a systematic review. Am J Prev Med. 2007;32(4 Suppl):38-67.

130. **Herbst JH, Sherba RT, Crepaz N, et al.** A meta-analytic review of HIV behavioral interventions for reducing sexual risk behavior of men who have sex with men. J Acquir Immune Defic Syndr. 2005;39:228-41.

131. **Johnson WD, Holtgrave DR, McClellan WM, et al.** HIV intervention research for men who have sex with men: a 7-year update. AIDS Educ Prev. 2005;17:568-89.

132. **Herbst JH, Kay LS, Passin WF, et al; HIV/AIDS Prevention Research Synthesis (PRS) Team.** A systematic review and meta-analysis of behavioral interventions to reduce HIV risk behaviors of Hispanics in the United States and Puerto Rico. AIDS Behav. 2007;11:25-47.

133. **Tsai C-C, Follis KE, Sabo A, et al.** Prevention of SIV infection in macaques by (R)-9-(2-phosphonylmethoxypropyl) adenine. Science. 1995;270:1197-9.

134. **Cardo DM, Culver DH, Ciesielski CA, et al.** A case-control study of HIV seroconversion in health care workers after percutaneous exposure. Centers for Disease Control and Prevention Needlestick Surveillance Group. N Engl J Med. 1997;337:1485-90.

135. **Mayer KH, Merchant C.** Nonoccupational HIV postexposure prophylaxis. JAMA. 2005;294:1615-6.

136. **Shoptaw S, Rotheram-Fuller E, Landovitz RJ, et al.** Non-occupational post exposure prophylaxis as a biobehavioral HIV-prevention intervention. AIDS Care. 2008;20:376-81.

137. **Schechter M, do Lago RF, Mendelsohn AB, et al; Praca Onze Study Team.** Behavioral impact, acceptability, and HIV incidence among homosexual men with access to postexposure chemoprophylaxis for HIV. J Acquir Immune Defic Syndr. 2004;35:519-25.

138. **Roland ME, Neilands TB, Krone MR, et al.** Seroconversion following nonoccupational postexposure prophylaxis against HIV. Clin Infect Dis. 2005;41:1507-13.

139. **Centers for Disease Control and Prevention.** Antiretroviral post exposure prophylaxis after sexual, injection-drug use, or other nonoccupational exposure to HIV in the United States: recommendations from the U.S. Department of Health and Human Services. MMWR Recomm Rep. 2005 ;54(RR02):1-20.

140. **Kashuba AD, Dyer JR, Kramer LM, et al.** Antiretroviral-drug concentrations in semen: implications for sexual transmission of human immunodeficiency virus type 1. Antimicrob Agents Chemother. 1999;43:1817-26.

141. **Grant RM, Lama JR, Anderson PL, et al.** Preexposure chemoprophylaxis for HIV prevention in men who have sex with men. N Engl J Med. 2010;363:2587-99.

142. **Anderson PL, Glidden DV, Liu A, et al.** Emtricitabine-tenofovir concentrations and preexposure prophylaxis efficacy in men who have sex with men. Sci Transl Med. 2012;4:151ra25.

143. **Thigpen MC, Kebaabetswe PM, Paxton LA, et al.** Antiretroviral preexposure prophylaxis for heterosexual HIV transmission in Botswana. N Engl J Med. 2012;367:423-34.

144. **Baeten JM, Donnell D, Ndase P, et al.** Antiretroviral prophylaxis for HIV prevention in heterosexual men and women. N Engl J Med. 2012;367:399-410.

145. **Abdool-Karim Q, Abouzahr C, Dehne K, et al.** HIV and maternal mortality: turning the tide. Lancet. 2010;375:1948-9.

146. **Microbicide Trials Network.** MTN-003-VOICE. Available at: www.mtnstopshiv.org/news/studies/mtn003.

147. **McGowan I, Hoesley C, Cranston RD, et al.** A phase 1 randomized, double blind, placebo controlled rectal safety and acceptability study of tenofovir 1% gel (MTN-007). PLoS One. 2013;8:e60147.

148. **World Health Organization.** Programmatic Update: Antiretroviral Treatment as Prevention (TASP) of HIV and TB. June 2012. Available at: http://whqlibdoc.who.int/hq/2012/WHO_HIV_2012.12_eng.pdf.

149. **Cohen MS, Chen YQ, McCauley M, et al.** Prevention of HIV-1 infection with early antiretroviral therapy. N Engl J Med. 2011;365:493-505.

150. **Das M, Chu PL, Santos GM, et al.** Decreases in community viral load are accompanied by reductions in new HIV infections in San Francisco. PLoS One. 2010;5:e11068.

151. **Montaner JS, Lima VD, Barrios R, et al.** Association of highly active antiretroviral therapy coverage, population viral load, and yearly new HIV diagnoses in British Columbia, Canada: a population-based study. Lancet. 2010;376:532-9.

152. **Montaner JS.** Treatment as prevention: toward an AIDS-free generation. Top Antivir Med. 2013;21:110-4.

153. **Audelin AM, Cowan SA, Obel N, et al.** Phylogenetics of the Danish HIV epidemic: the role of very late presenters in sustaining the epidemic. J Acquir Immune Defic Syndr. 2013;62:102-8.

154. **Birrell PJ, Gill ON, Delpech VC, et al.** HIV incidence in men who have sex with men in England and Wales 2001-10: a nationwide population study. Lancet Infect Dis. 2013;13:313-8.

155. **Hall H, Frazier EL, Rhodes P, et al.** Differences in human immunodeficiency virus care and treatment among subpopulations in the United States. JAMA Intern Med. 2013;173:1337-44.

156. **AIDSinfo.** Panel on Antiretroviral Guidelines for Adults and Adolescents. Guidelines for the use of antiretroviral agents in HIV-1-infected adults and adolescents. Department of Health and Human Services. Available at: http://aidsinfo.nih.gov/contentfiles/lvguidelines/AdultandAdolescentGL.pdf.

157. **Quinn TC.** Circumcision and HIV transmission. Curr Opin Infect Dis. 2007;20:33-8.

158. **Quinn TC.** Circumcision and HIV transmission: the cutting edge [Abstract 120]. Denver, CO: Presented at the Conference on Retroviruses and Opportunistic Infections (CROI); 2006.

159. **Bailey RC, Moses S, Parker CB, et al.** Male circumcision for HIV prevention in young men in Kisumu, Kenya: a randomised controlled trial. Lancet. 2007;369:643-56.

160. **Tobian AA, Kong X, Wawer MJ, et al.** Circumcision of HIV-infected men and transmission of human papillomavirus to female partners: analyses of data from a randomised trial in Rakai, Uganda. Lancet Infect Dis. 2011;11:604-12.

161. **Auvert B, Taljaard D, Rech D, et al.** Association of the ANRS-12126 male circumcision project with HIV levels among men in a South African township: evaluation of effectiveness using cross-sectional surveys. PLoS Med. 2013;10:e1001509.

162. **Gray GE, Allen M, Moodie Z, et al.** Safety and efficacy of the HVTN 503/Phambili study of a clade-B-based HIV-1 vaccine in South Africa: a double-blind, randomised, placebo-controlled test-of-concept phase 2b study. Lancet Infect Dis. 2011;11:507-15.

163. **Goodreau SM, Carnegie NB, Vittinghoff E, et al.** What drives the US and Peruvian HIV epidemics in men who have sex with men (MSM)? PLoS One. 2012;7:e50522.

Chapter 14

Community, Structural, and Policy Approaches to Improve HIV Prevention and Related Health Concerns Among Racial/Ethnic Minority Gay, Bisexual, and Other Men Who Have Sex With Men

PATRICK A. WILSON, PhD
JILL PACE, MPH
MELISSA BOONE BROWN, MPhil
KALVIN LEVEILLE, BS

Introduction

Black and Latino gay, bisexual, and other men who have sex with men (MSM) in the United States experience grave disparities in HIV/AIDS. The goal of this chapter is to provide an overview of community-level, structural, and policy interventions that have great potential to reduce new HIV infections and improve health outcomes among racial/ethnic minority MSM in the United States. In providing this overview, combination prevention/treatment intervention strategies, which integrate interventions at multiple levels, will be emphasized as having the most potential in reducing HIV and other health disparities affecting MSM of color. For a general review of HIV epidemiology and prevention strategies, see Chapter 13.

Historical Trends in HIV/AIDS Among MSM of Color

Since the early days of HIV/AIDS in the United States, black and Latino MSM have been disproportionately affected by the epidemic. Early studies in the United States reported higher HIV/AIDS prevalence and incidence rates for black MSM compared with white MSM, despite comparable risk factors (1,2). This trend continued into the 1990s, with additional studies showing higher rates of HIV/AIDS for black and Latino MSM compared with white MSM (3,4). Between 2001 and 2006, there was a 12.4% increase in HIV diagnosis among all black MSM and a 93.1% increase among black MSM age 13 to 24 years (5). During the same time, HIV/AIDS diagnoses increased by 10.3% among all Latino MSM and by 45.8% among young Latino MSM (age 13 to 24 years) (6). This trend is most recently supported by data from the Centers for Disease Control and Prevention (CDC), which shows that from 2006 to 2009, HIV incidence among people age 13 to 29 years increased 21%, driven largely by a 34% increase in young MSM (7). Among these young MSM, there was a 48% increase among young black MSM. In fact, in 2009, young black MSM accounted for 61% of all new infections (7). In contrast, data show that HIV/AIDS rates in most other high-risk populations are remaining steady or decreasing.

Many hypotheses have been suggested to explain this disparate effect of HIV/AIDS on MSM of color. Researchers have parsed out those hypotheses with evidential support versus those that are not supported by the literature. Hypotheses generally not supported by evidence in the research literature include that black MSM are more likely than other MSM to engage in high-risk sexual behavior and are more likely than other MSM to abuse substances, especially injection drugs, that increase their risk for HIV infection (8). Conversely, hypotheses that are supported by the literature include the following: 1) MSM of color are more likely than other MSM to contract sexually transmitted infections (STIs) that facilitate the acquisition and transmission of HIV; 2) while they are just as likely as other MSM to ever test for HIV, black MSM test less frequently and test positive later in their HIV infection, and thus they may unknowingly expose sexual partners to HIV; and 3) the sexual networks of MSM of color, and notably black MSM, place them at greater risk for HIV infection than the sexual networks of other MSM (8-10). Studies that focus primarily on Latino MSM populations illustrate the diversity of the Latino populations and how variables such as place of birth, socioeconomic status, and substance use affect risk behavior and HIV infection within Latino MSM populations (11-13). More recently conducted work points to access to and engagement in care, antiretroviral (ART) and other treatment access, and adherence to medication as important factors to consider in explaining HIV disparities between racial/ethnic minority MSM and nonminority MSM (10,14-17).

Behavioral Interventions Targeting MSM of Color

Of the more than 30 behavioral interventions listed as effective behavioral interventions for HIV prevention by the CDC, only 4 are tailored specifically to MSM populations. Of these 4, only 2 are geared specifically toward MSM of color, namely black MSM. Below is a description of these 4 MSM-focused interventions, as well as their published results.

1. *D-up: Defend Yourself!* is a community-level intervention for black MSM. It is designed to change social norms and perceptions regarding condom use and uses principles of popular opinion leader theory (18). The efficacy trial of this intervention was implemented in 3 North Carolina counties. During the 12-month trial, 4 community surveys were conducted to test the effects of *d-Up!* in reducing sexual risk behavior. Data showed that in the year after the intervention's implementation, unprotected insertive anal sex decreased by 35.2% and unprotected receptive anal sex decreased by 44.1%. In addition, the number of black MSM reporting always using condoms increased by 23.0% for insertive anal sex and 30.3% for receptive anal sex. The average number of partners for unprotected receptive anal sex decreased by 40.5% (19). With evidence of the efficacy of *d-Up!* in reducing HIV risk for black MSM, the intervention has been taken up and implemented by several HIV/AIDS community-based organizations in cities across the United States.

2. *Many Men, Many Voices (3MV)* is a 7-session, group-level intervention for black MSM. The intervention addresses cultural, social, and religious norms; interactions between HIV and other STIs; sexual relationship dynamics; and the social and psychological influences that racism and homophobia have on HIV risk behaviors. Results from the *3MV* efficacy trial in 2009 showed that 3MV participants reported significantly greater reductions in unprotected anal intercourse with male partners, consistent condom use during receptive anal intercourse with male partners, and significantly greater reductions in the number of male sex partners and greater increases in HIV testing (20). *3MV* is perhaps the most widely disseminated group-level intervention implemented by community-based organizations aiming to reduce HIV among black MSM in diverse communities (20).

3. *Mpowerment* is a community-level intervention for young gay and bisexual men. The Mpowerment project mobilizes young gay/bisexual men to shape a healthy community for themselves, building positive social connections and supporting safer sex. One large-scale trial to test *Mpowerment* for efficacy found that after participation in the *Mpowerment* intervention, the proportion of young men engaging in unprotected anal intercourse decreased from 41% to 30% and the proportion of men engaging in unprotected anal intercourse with non–primary partners decreased from 20.2% to 11%. This research shows that HIV prevention activities can be highly effective when embedded in social activities and community life (21). *Mpowerment* has since been culturally adapted for use specifically with black MSM (22) and continues to be implemented in cities in the United States, notably Detroit and Dallas.

4. *Personal Cognitive Counseling (PCC)* is an individual-level, single-session counseling intervention designed to reduce unprotected anal intercourse among MSM who are repeat testers for HIV. PCC focuses on the person's self-justifications (thoughts, attitudes, and beliefs) he uses when deciding whether to engage in high-risk sexual behavior. PCC has been widely disseminated for use in community-based organizations and health care settings in which MSM test for HIV (23).

Biomedical Interventions

In addition to behavioral interventions, advances in biomedical research have provided additional HIV prevention tools with potential in reducing new HIV infections among MSM. Recently, several research trials have been conducted to look at key clinical and biomedical interventions, such as pre-exposure prophylaxis (PrEP). The Chemoprophylaxis for HIV Prevention in Men Who Have Sex with Men study found that daily use of the drug tenofovir/emtricitabine (i.e., PrEP) was an effective intervention to prevent HIV infection in MSM and transgender women and highlighted the importance of adherence to medication in effective prevention (24). Study subjects who received PrEP had a 44% reduced odds of seroconverting during the study follow-up period. However, those subjects with a detectable drug level in their blood had a 92% relative reduction in HIV risk. Although this research trial focused specifically on MSM and transgender women, the study population was not representative of the HIV epidemic in the United States; only 10% of study participants came from U.S. sites (i.e., San Francisco and Boston). Likewise, few of the participants were from racial/ethnic minority communities in the United States (e.g., only 8.5% of participants were black); however, studies exploring the feasibility and acceptability of PrEP among MSM of color are underway.

Another large-scale study conducted by the HIV Prevention Trials Network (i.e., HPTN 052) looked at the effectiveness of using ART for preventing sexual transmission of HIV in serodiscordant couples. This prevention strategy, known widely as "treatment as prevention," reduced HIV transmission to the HIV-uninfected partner by 96.0% (25). While the study population in HPTN 052 was serodiscordant heterosexual couples, the results of this study have spurred further examination of treatment as prevention in other populations, including MSM, and greater efforts from public health departments to ensure HIV-positive individuals are engaged in care and adherent to ART.

An additional HPTN study, called Broadening the Reach of Testing, Health Education, Resources and Services for Black Men Who Have Sex with Men (i.e., the BROTHERS study, HPTN 061) is a recently conducted trial focusing specifically on black MSM living in the United States. This study used peer health navigators to increase access to and uptake of HIV prevention and treatment services among black MSM. The trial showed that the rate of new HIV infection among black MSM was 2.8% per year, nearly 50% higher than rates among white MSM in the United States (26). The BROTHERS study demonstrated that the overall infection rate among black MSM in the sample (n = 2418) was similar to that in countries in sub-Saharan Africa with generalized epidemics. Correlates of infection included being younger than age 30 years and having had unprotected receptive anal intercourse with an HIV-positive or unknown-status partner (26). The scientists who conducted the BROTHERS study concluded that the trial clearly showed a need for tailored and culturally appropriate HIV prevention strategies incorporating behavioral, social, and biomedical strategies in order to decrease rates among black MSM (26).

Community Mobilization and MSM of Color

Community mobilization has been instrumental in increasing rates of condom use and curbing the HIV epidemic among gay men and other MSM in the United States (27,28). However, these mobilization efforts, for the most part, have not included large numbers of racial/ethnic minority MSM. This is largely due to early perceptions that HIV and AIDS were diseases of white gay men, community-level stigma surrounding homosexuality and AIDS, and programs of social exclusion (29–32). Even as the color of U.S. epidemic has become more and more "black and brown," mobilization of racial/ethnic minority MSM around HIV/AIDS has largely sputtered, although there have been calls for heightened community response (33,34).

While more intensive mobilization efforts are needed to curb the epidemic among racial/ethnic minority MSM, some national and community-level initiatives have focused on reducing the impact of HIV on this population. These efforts have largely focused on increasing HIV testing among MSM of color and reducing stigma related to homosexuality and HIV/AIDS through the implementation of wide-reaching local and national social marketing campaigns. These campaigns provide a foundation that can be built upon and referenced as greater efforts are made to increase mobilization efforts and implement community-level responses to HIV and related health issues affecting racial/ethnic minority MSM. They are explained in more detail below.

Community Mobilization Around HIV Testing

Given the importance of HIV testing as a way to identify undiagnosed HIV-positive individuals, link them to care, and prevent the transmission of HIV to uninfected individuals, a vast number of HIV/AIDS social marketing campaigns have focused on increasing routine HIV testing in high-risk populations. At the national level, the CDC launched a multiyear initiative called Act Against AIDS (AAA), which aims to raise awareness about HIV/AIDS and increase HIV testing and prevention behaviors, including condom use. The AAA campaign seeks to reduce the prevalence and incidence of HIV in the communities hardest hit by the epidemic—blacks, Hispanics/Latinos, and gay men—through the use of prevention messaging via public service advertisements, media placements, Internet advertising, and billboard advertising. AAA also involves the implementation of and consultation from a leadership initiative composed of civic, business, and education organizations within black and Latino communities across the United States. The goal of the leadership initiative is to help galvanize communities to respond and mobilize around HIV by disseminating testing and prevention messages through social and business organizations that are not necessarily focused on public health.

A component of AAA that specifically targets black MSM is the campaign "Testing Makes Us Stronger." This social marketing campaign has appeared in advertisements in national publications and websites, as well as local transit, print, and online media in select U.S. cities experiencing high levels of HIV infection among black MSM (e.g., Atlanta, Baltimore, Houston, New York, Oakland, and Washington, DC). It focuses specifically on increasing routine HIV testing among black MSM. Although the efficacy of wide-scale social marketing campaigns in increasing HIV testing and mobilizing racial/ethnic minority populations has yet to be documented, these efforts represent first steps at the national level to mobilize communities around HIV. An example of a print advertisement used in the "Testing Makes Us Stronger" campaign can be found in Figure 14-1 (panel A).

Another component of AAA called "REASONS/RAZONES" focuses broadly on Latino populations, and specifically Latino MSM. It launched in 2013 in Los Angeles and Miami, 2 cities with large HIV epidemics among Latinos. The campaign uses images of family, friends, and partners as reasons to test for HIV and emphasizes a strong sense of self and interconnectedness in an effort to mobilize Latino MSM to engage in routine HIV testing. An example print ad used in the "REASONS/RAZONES" campaign appears in Figure 14-1 (panel B). Both "Testing Makes Us Stronger" and "REASONS/RAZONES" highlight approaches that CDC has taken to engage in culturally tailored messaging that speaks to experiences of racial and ethnic minority MSM in the United States, while appreciating the diversity and heterogeneity that exist in these populations. It is notable that these campaigns feature openly gay men, often engaging in emotional expressions with their partner, as shown in Figure 14-1. Racial and ethnic minority MSM who are open about their sexuality and self-label as homosexual or gay are the most vulnerable to HIV infection (17) and thus are the targets of these 2 AAA campaigns.

At the local level, several communities experiencing high HIV prevalence have implemented local campaigns that aim to mobilize the community to engage in HIV testing. For example, in New York City, which experiences some of the highest rates of HIV among racial/ethnic minority MSM in the nation, the local health department implemented the "Bronx Knows" campaign (35–37). Epidemiologic data in New York City showed extremely high rates of undiagnosed HIV infection in the Bronx, particularly in the

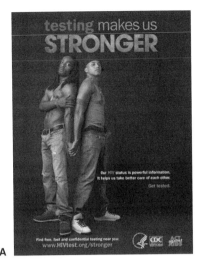

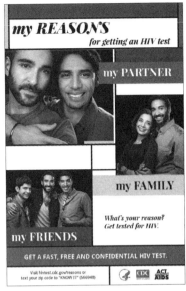

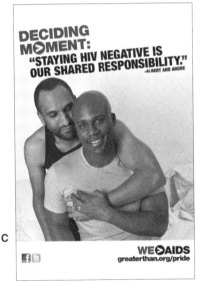

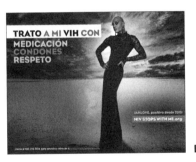

Figure 14-1 Examples of community mobilization campaigns targeted toward racial/ethnic minority gay, bisexual, and other men who have sex with men in the United States. **A.** Centers for Disease Control and Prevention (CDC) Act Against AIDS campaign: "Testing Makes Us Stronger." **B.** CDC Act Against AIDS campaign: "REASONS/RAZONES." **C.** "Greater Than AIDS" campaign. **D.** "HIV Stops With Me" campaign.

areas where populations of color reside. In response, the "Bronx Knows" campaign was initiated on National HIV Testing Day in 2008 in an effort to conduct 250,000 HIV tests in 1 year. The "Bronx Knows" campaign was New York City's first borough-specific HIV testing initiative and one of the largest local mobilization campaigns implemented in the United States; through the campaign, more than 600,000 tests were conducted, thousands of new infections were identified, and undiagnosed individuals were linked to care (38). It has since been replicated in other boroughs of New York City.

Community Mobilization Around Stigma Reduction

Stigma surrounding HIV/AIDS and homosexuality has had profound negative effects on responses to HIV at the national, state, and local levels (34). While efforts have been made to reduce stigma surrounding HIV, and mainstream lesbian, gay, bisexual and transgender (LGBT) communities have been galvanized around national and state laws surrounding gay marriage, the effectiveness of these campaigns and efforts to mobilize the community have been unclear with regard to reducing HIV/AIDS stigma and improving HIV-related outcomes at the population level (29,39).

One recently and widely implemented national campaign aimed at reducing stigma around HIV/AIDS within black, Latino, and other communities is the "Greater Than AIDS" campaign. Developed by the Black AIDS Institute and implemented, in part, by the Kaiser Family Foundation, "Greater Than AIDS" focuses on emphasizing hope, unity, and personal empowerment as a way to confront stigma and reduce the spread of HIV in communities of color. Like other mass communication campaigns, "Greater Than AIDS" uses advertisements located in transit venues, community print media, and online. The campaign also involves personal testimonies and celebrity spokespersons in an attempt to normalize HIV and promote uptake of treatment in communities that continue to stigmatize the disease and people living with HIV and AIDS. There is a focus on identifying inspirational and motivating stories targeting racial/ethnic minority gay, bisexual, and other MSM. Although efficacy of the campaign in reducing stigma and improving HIV-related outcomes in communities of color is unknown, the campaign has been deemed widely successful from acceptability and dissemination standpoints. A print ad example from the "Greater Than AIDS" campaign appears in Figure 14-1 (panel C).

There are also examples of locally initiated campaigns that aim to reduce HIV/AIDS stigma and homophobia. For example, in 2007 the "HIV Stops With Me" campaign was implemented in New York City with the aim of reducing HIV-related stigma by featuring HIV-positive persons, many highly visible and well-known community leaders, talking about issues related to living with HIV. "HIV Stops With Me" has since been implemented in several U.S. cities and states, including Buffalo, New York; Los Angeles; Maryland; and Virginia. The campaign is one of the most well-evaluated stigma-reduction campaigns implemented on a national scale, with several process evaluations that have been conducted or are underway, according to the campaign's website, www.hivstopswithme.org. Also worth noting, the "HIV Stops With Me" campaign has been nominated for best advertising campaign by the Gay and Lesbian Alliance Against Defamation (GLAAD) and has won awards for its web outpost, which includes media and other interactive features. An example ad from New York City featuring Jahlove, a well-known activist and entertainer in the local Latino gay community, is included in Figure 14-1 (panel D).

Barriers to Community Mobilization

Of all the barriers that thwart community mobilization within racial/ethnic minority communities and among MSM of color, stigma may be the most important. Stigma related to race/ethnicity (i.e., racial discrimination, prejudice, and stereotyping), homosexuality (i.e., homophobia, sexual stigma), and HIV/AIDS (i.e., AIDS stigma) all affect the lack of community-level interventions and mobilization efforts targeting racial/ethnic minority MSM. For example, racial and ethnic minority gay men often experience high levels of racism within the gay community (40–43). These stigma experiences, which can be considered to be experienced at interpersonal and community/institutional levels, may lead MSM of color to distance themselves from the mainstream gay community and the issues it supports, such as marriage equality.

Racial/ethnic minority MSM also experience stigma within their families and social networks, neighborhoods, jobs, health care institutions, and other institutional settings (e.g., churches, prisons, and detention facilities) that impedes mobilization. Stigma creates situations in which these men feel they have to hide their sexual identity and, if they are HIV-positive, their HIV status (44,45). The lack of self-identification with gay/bisexual and HIV-positive communities translates into a lack of the ability to create visibility around HIV and other health problems affecting MSM of color.

Community-level and institutional stigma around homosexuality and HIV may be internalized among many racial/ethnic minority MSM, and thereby influences men's perceptions regarding same-sex sexual behaviors and HIV. This internalized stigma is tied to an inability to talk about sexuality within many racial/ethnic minority communities and hinders community-level responses to HIV among MSM of color. Community-level homophobia diminishes open, meaningful dialogues about homosexuality and sexual behaviors in which gay men engage—instead of talking about sexuality in an open and healthy manner, discussions within many racial/ethnic minority communities are more focused on MSM as engaging in deviant behaviors that propagate HIV within the community (46). This type of discourse pathologizes MSM of color, increases fear and fatalism among MSM, and impedes mobilization (47,48).

Finally, understanding priorities and unmet needs among MSM of color may also help to explain the lack of mobilization and community-level efforts around HIV. Racial/ethnic minority MSM experience greater rates of homelessness, joblessness, incarcerations, abuse experiences, and other traumatic life events compared with white MSM (17,49,50). Without having basic needs met, it is highly unlikely that MSM of color will mobilize around issues that may be perceived to be low priority or not relevant to their lives.

Approaches to Facilitate Community Mobilization

To facilitate community mobilization, even greater efforts need to be made to reduce stigma around HIV, as well as levels of homophobia, in racial/ethnic minority communities across the United States. Existing antistigma campaigns need to be further implemented and evaluated, and new campaigns that are culturally tailored and take advantage of existing technologies (such as social media) need to be developed and tested.

Additionally, greater alliances among public health departments, community-based organizations, and private-sector companies need to be developed. These alliances can help to create norm changes within and across community and institutional settings. Programs such as the CDC's Act Against AIDS Leadership Initiative need to be replicated on the state and local levels. These alliances should make their missions, at least in part, to reduce stigma around HIV and homosexuality.

Finally, more HIV-positive black and Latino MSM need to be empowered to publicly disclose their HIV status. Attempts to normalize HIV, promote community perceptions of HIV as a manageable disease, and highlight the presence of HIV-positive MSM of color in all parts of the community, from churches to corporate offices, will help reduce stigma and negative perceptions around HIV.

Structural Interventions and MSM of Color

In the past, most HIV prevention interventions for MSM have focused on changing individual-level behaviors, knowledge, or attitudes, such as teaching participants how to use a condom correctly or teaching about HIV transmission routes (51). Few interventions, however, have focused on removing structural barriers to HIV prevention in MSM. There is some evidence that individual-level behavioral interventions can benefit from attention to structural-level factors that shape individual behavior, such as poverty, access to care, and policy (52). However, structural factors are often difficult to define and target for public health interventions. Structural factors are typically challenging to change and require long-term solutions; this often makes researchers and community organizers skip them in favor of behavioral interventions, which can be implemented in shorter periods of time and have more immediate outcomes (51).

Structural factors that affect HIV risk and prevention have been defined as "physical, social, cultural, organizational, community, economic, legal, or policy aspects of the environment that impede or facilitate persons' efforts to avoid HIV infection" (53). Tawil and colleagues distinguish between prevention approaches with a goal of changing individual-level behavior and those approaches that "enable change to occur" by focusing on environmental and social determinants that facilitate behavior change (54). Structural interventions, therefore, do not aim to change HIV risk behavior directly but work to make conditions amenable for reducing risky behavior and enacting protective behaviors. Structural interventions address 3 types of contextual factors: 1) increasing availability of tools and settings that aid individuals in preventing health problems, 2) increasing social acceptability of protective health behaviors and decreasing social acceptability of risky behaviors, and 3) manipulating power and policies to promote accessibility of resources integral to preventing health problems (55).

Structural factors fall into 2 categories: factors that have been shown to shape risk behavior and environmental mediators that act as protective factors and increase people's resilience to HIV infection (56). Thus, structural factors are elements that are likely outside of individuals' awareness and have the potential to influence the vulnerability of any given group (56). Concrete examples include social factors, such as stigma and gender inequality; legal factors, such as laws that criminalize MSM and limit their ability to seek prevention services; cultural factors, such as religious beliefs; and economic factors, such as poverty.

Structural Factors That Influence HIV Prevention in MSM of Color

Several structural factors prevent MSM of color from reducing HIV risk behavior. Many of these factors are compounded in MSM of color because of the intersection of their marginalized racial identity with their marginalized sexual orientation or behavior. For HIV-positive racial/ethnic minority MSM, this compounding is even greater because of HIV/AIDS stigma.

Access to Health Care

As noted previously, access to health care and treatment is regarded as a major structural barrier to HIV prevention, care, and treatment. The widely presented treatment cascade and continuum of care research clearly delineates gaps between HIV testing, linking to and engaging in care, and adherence to ART medications. These gaps are only enhanced for MSM of color. Millett and colleagues describe evidence showing that from the start, black MSM are more likely than white MSM to be unaware of their serostatus, thus not even entering the treatment continuum of care (8). Low-income MSM of color may be unable to afford health care services, often because they are uninsured or underinsured (10). In a study of black MSM in Massachusetts, being publically insured by Medicaid plus reporting difficulty accessing health care was a strong correlate of poor mental health outcomes, namely severe depression (57). Men most in need of long-term health insurance may be the least likely to get it, as the health insurance structure in the United States has historically permitted insurers to deny insurance to people with HIV or to charge extraordinarily high premiums if they are accepted. Policy interventions such as the Affordable Care Act help to create systemic and structural changes that have the potential to facilitate access to care among MSM of color.

A lack of access to insurance may send many MSM to community health clinics and other health centers where they can receive free or reduced-cost health care. However, community clinics may have less experienced medical providers and may have staff who lack cultural sensitivity toward MSM and other LGBT people (34). Medical providers who work with MSM of color may know less about HIV prevention and care of HIV-positive individuals because of their inexperience (58,59). In addition, many community health clinics suffer from huge turnover because staff may leave for lower-load, higher-pay positions (34). This leads to a lack of continuity in care for precisely the population that needs it the most.

Additional barriers to accessing care for MSM of color include the location of health care providers, stigma associated with receiving care, and the patient-provider relationship. Black and Latino people in HIV care reported traveling longer and waiting longer for care compared with their white counterparts (60). Many community clinics that provide HIV prevention or treatment may also be housed in LGBT centers or marketed as safe spaces for LGBT people, which may alienate MSM who do not identify as gay or bisexual. In addition, many MSM of color may be unable to identify compassionate or tolerant medical providers with whom they feel comfortable disclosing their identity or behavior. Stein and Bonuck found that nearly one fifth of lesbians and gay men reported delaying or avoiding seeking health care because of fears that providers would not accept their sexual orientation (61).

In addition, being black has been associated with lower retention in medical care of various types, including HIV treatment (16,62,63). Results with Latinos have been mixed, with some studies finding that they delay care and others finding that they access care more quickly than their white counterparts (16,62–64). MSM of color, particularly black MSM, may have lower adherence to medical regimens because of medical mistrust brought on by a cultural history of mistreatment by the medical system and possible individual perceived discrimination. In a study of black, mostly gay and bisexual men in Los Angeles, belief in treatment-related HIV conspiracies was associated with nonadherence to ART (65). However, very few studies have specifically addressed engagement in care of MSM of color; this is an area of research that requires further exploration.

Immigration and Migration

Immigration and migration are also structural factors that affect HIV risk prevention and treatment among MSM of color. Historically, immigrants have used less health care overall than native-born residents (66–68). Because of welfare reform in the mid-1990s, even legal immigrants are unable to access Medicaid until after they have resided in the United States for 5 years. This leaves poor immigrants vulnerable to a lack of health insurance, especially because they are less likely to be insured through employers (69). Undocumented immigrants are especially vulnerable, being much less likely to be insured and more often employed in job sectors that are outside of the legal employment structure for little pay (68,70,71). Undocumented immigrants have also been more likely to delay or avoid access to care because of a fear of "the system" and the risk of being deported to their home countries (67). Many immigrants also have to rely on English-speaking family members to translate during communications with health care providers; this may add the complication of HIV disclosure and stigma management—many of these immigrants may not want family members or friends to know about their sexual identity or HIV status, but also may be unaware or unable to avail themselves of the services of medical translators. MSM of color who are immigrants and also identify as gay or bisexual may feel that they must identify with, and become involved with, sexual minority communities in order to access HIV prevention and treatment care. This may not appeal to these groups because of deep-seated stigma in their home countries or cultural enclaves and their desire to avoid disclosure to family members.

Incarceration and Criminal Justice

Incarceration and criminal justice policy are also structural factors that affect vulnerability to poor health outcomes among MSM of color. Black men represent not only the largest proportion of all incarcerated men but also the largest proportion of HIV-infected men in federal and state prisons in the United States (72). The HIV infection rate is 5 times higher in prisons than in the general population (72). Despite these staggering numbers, there have been few studies of incarcerated MSM, which report incongruent results (8). One study found no racial differences in reported incarceration history among MSM (73). Another other found young black MSM were more likely to report a history of incarceration (74). The previously mentioned BROTH-ERS Study (i.e., HPTN 061) showed an extremely high level of engagement in the criminal justice system among black MSM, with an estimated incarceration rate of 35% in the sample (75).

Because black MSM are more likely than other MSM to be incarcerated and because of the high rates of HIV infection while incarcerated, structural interventions in correctional facilities have the potential for a strong effect on reducing HIV infection among incarcerated populations. Proposed structural interventions include implementing testing, treatment, and prevention programs; providing linkage to care and support services for prisoners after their release; and broader distribution of condoms within correctional facilities (76,77).

Poverty and Homelessness

Poverty and homelessness are overarching structural factors that affect not only HIV prevention and care among MSM of color but also interact with other structural factors that have been mentioned previously. In a 2010 CDC study, HIV prevalence in the United States was significantly correlated with having an income at or below the poverty threshold, being unemployed or disabled, and experiencing homelessness within the past year (78). In addition, the HIV prevalence rate in urban poor areas of the United States was similar to rates found in low-income countries with generalized HIV epidemics (78). In a study of homeless people in San Francisco, MSM not only were more likely to have HIV but were twice as likely compared with others to be lifetime injection drug users (79). Reflecting the national epidemic, rates of HIV among homeless black MSM were significantly higher than homeless white MSM (79). These results were also seen in studies in other urban U.S. cities (80,81).

Barriers to Creating, Implementing, and Scaling Up Structural Interventions

Structural interventions for prevention and treatment of HIV are difficult to design, implement, and evaluate. The very structural issues that these interventions hope to address often re-emerge as barriers to initially designing and implementing such an intervention. For example, successfully implementing a structural intervention that focuses on access to care and treatment depends largely on the availability of culturally competent health care, the capacity of trained health care providers, and stable supply chains for antiretroviral medication (82). In addition, some structural interventions that have been implemented in the past can themselves be seen as barriers to the ultimate goal of primary prevention of HIV. Structural interventions in the United States that may be barriers to prevention include laws against nondisclosure, travel bans on HIV-infected foreign nationals, name-based HIV reporting, and partner notification (83).

Even for structural interventions that are proven effective, the ability to scale up and implement such interventions largely depends on the characteristics of the intervention. Among the characteristics of successful structural interventions are simple and adaptive design and implementation, wide acceptance, strong leadership and governance, active engagement of key stakeholders, and an acceptable economic cost (83). Creating, implementing, and scaling up a structural intervention specifically for MSM of color add layers of additional barriers. For MSM of color, particularly black MSM, who account for such a large percentage of all new HIV infections in the United States, socio-structural factors such as poverty, incarceration, unemployment, and discrimination are key targets of structural interventions to prevent HIV; yet these are the same factors that build barriers to creating and implementing structural interventions (84).

There is a well-documented association between socio-structural factors that disproportionately affect MSM of color and an increased risk for HIV; however, there is a dearth of research and interventions that address these factors specifically for MSM of color. To successfully implement structural interventions, researchers, clinicians, and policymakers need to work collectively to address these barriers and ensure that structural interventions are developed and scaled up in diverse settings and communities.

Approaches to Take in Structural Interventions

There are many ways that structural interventions can influence barriers to care and treatment for MSM of color. These include expanding HIV testing venues and providing linkage to care support at the time of testing; working to decrease stigma of HIV/AIDS prevention, care, and treatment; revising health insurance policies to ease restrictions on vulnerable populations; and working with HIV care providers to increase culturally sensitive care and to strengthen patient–provider relationships. Likewise, efforts to increase the number of clinicians, researchers, and public health practitioners who are MSM of color comprise a form of structural intervention that can facilitate improvements in health outcomes among MSM of color (50).

Implementing structural interventions with the potential to address these extremely large and all-encompassing issues can seem daunting. However, spurred by community mobilization and local and national policy, structural interventions can be developed and implemented, particularly given current changes in health care access and LGBT rights. On a community level, structural interventions can include providing secure housing for MSM of color, particularly young MSM who may be living outside of family care and are at high-risk for HIV infection; increasing access to education and employment programs; and policies that ensure marriage equality and same-sex couple rights. On a national policy level, programs that help to relieve socioeconomic stressors and provide living wages, stable employment, and/or access to affordable housing among historically marginalized populations, which include MSM of color, can facilitate wide-scale change.

National Policy Interventions and MSM of Color

National policy interventions not only affect health and access to health services among MSM of color; they affect health among all U.S. citizens.

Broad-scale reforms that have the capacity to reshape the landscape of health care are difficult to achieve for the same reasons that structural interventions can be difficult to implement. They require input and buy-in from multiple stakeholders and are often very slow to be developed and implemented. However, several recent policy interventions have had direct effects on racial/ethnic minority MSM in the United States. They include the National HIV/AIDS Strategy (NHAS), the CDC's revised HIV/AIDS funding plan for health departments, and the Affordable Care Act (ACA).

In the summer of 2010, the White House released the NHAS. NHAS represents the first comprehensive coordinated HIV/AIDS plan in the United States, with specific and measurable targets to be achieved in the short term. NHAS emphasizes a need for greater efforts to prevent and treat HIV among MSM of color, namely black gay men. For example, it notes (85):

> What is sometimes less recognized is the extent to which the HIV epidemic among African Americans remains concentrated among Black gay men, who comprise the single largest group of African Americans living with HIV. Fighting HIV among African Americans is not mutually exclusive with fighting HIV among gay and bisexual men. Efforts to reduce HIV among Blacks must confront the epidemic among Black gay and bisexual men as forcefully as existing efforts to confront the epidemic among other groups.

The need for community-level responses is noted in NHAS, as is the need for more resources targeted to reducing vulnerability to HIV among MSM of color, in order to successfully curb the epidemic in the United States. In addressing this enhanced vulnerability to HIV among MSM of color, it is important to take a holistic approach that aims to treat and intervene upon multiple problems and issues affecting MSM of color. For example, the NHAS (85) states:

> HIV is often only one of many conditions that plague communities at greater risk for HIV infection. In many cases, it is not possible to effectively address HIV transmission or care without also addressing sexually transmitted diseases, substance use, poverty, homelessness and other issues . . . Because of these many co-occurring issues, it is important to employ a holistic approach to HIV prevention and care that extends beyond risk behaviors of the individual and address not only mental health, but contextual factors such as sexual and drug use networks, joblessness or homelessness and others that increase risk for infection or suboptimal access or response to care.

In response to the NHAS, the CDC made significant changes to its plan for providing funding to state and local health departments for HIV programs and services (i.e., CDC FOA PS12-1201). The new plan provides funds to many U.S. health departments in three categories: basic HIV prevention programs, expanded HIV testing initiatives, and demonstration projects to implement highly innovative prevention strategies. A key component of this change is a focus on high-impact prevention, encouraging health departments to implement programs and other scalable interventions that have demonstrated the potential to reduce new HIV infections in the right populations in order to yield a greater impact on the HIV epidemic (86). The release of the NHAS and changes to the way health departments are funded for HIV prevention represent a unique opportunity for public health leaders, HIV/AIDS and sexual health practitioners, and community stakeholders to reassess and evaluate public health efforts to reduce HIV infection. Notably, efforts to prevent and treat HIV/STIs among MSM of color must be critically evaluated and new programs that aim to improve prevention efforts directed toward this population should be implemented.

Another wide-scale policy that has the potential to effect significant change to improve health among MSM of color is the ACA. The ACA integrates specific programs that increase health care availability for people living with HIV/AIDS and lower-income individuals, 2 populations that MSM of color are more likely to belong to than non-MSM and white MSM. One key example is that the ACA limits the ability of insurance companies to deny coverage to individuals because of their HIV status. Provisions within the ACA also increase access to antiretroviral medications among low-income HIV-positive MSM, and improve the availability of prevention tools, such as condoms and PrEP. The ACA also provides opportunities to implement programs that encourage cultural sensitivity and that train providers on the unique needs of MSM of color. These types of efforts will be critical as the ACA is rolled out in states across the country. Details on the ACA and its potential effects on MSM of color are described in Figure 14-2.

Leveraging Policy Interventions to Reduce HIV/AIDS Vulnerabilities and Improve Health Outcomes Among MSM of Color

NHAS, the CDC funding plan, and the ACA each provide opportunities for clinicians, researchers, and public health practitioners to improve health outcomes among racial/ethnic minority MSM. For example, targeted HIV testing initiatives should be coupled with greater efforts to increase racial/ethnic minority MSM's level of motivation to be linked to HIV care once they are diagnosed with HIV infection, and to enhance their ability to stay engaged in care over time. In addition, HIV testing and treatment clinics should integrate mental health counseling both at the time of diagnosis and in the months following, as newly diagnosed HIV-positive MSM of color are linked to care and begin to make decisions with their health providers about their course of treatment. Similarly, mental health treatment should be accessible to HIV-positive MSM of color who are actively engaged in care

Community Mobilization	Structural	Policy
NYC Council Faith-based HIV/AIDS Initiative	**Housing Programs for LGBTQ Youth**	**The Affordable Care Act**
• In 2003 the National Black Leadership Commission on AIDS (NBLACA) launched the *NYC Council Faith-based HIV/AIDS Initiative.* This innovative project focuses on building the capacity of clergy and faith-based communities to implement HIV/AIDS and STI screening and testing, prevention, treatment, and care programs in NYC. • The program focuses on congregations in black communities in NYC, and aims to improve HIV prevention efforts targeting gay men/MSM. • As a result of the *NYC Council Faith-based HIV/AIDS Initiative,* thousands of racial/ethnic minority men and women in NYC have been tested and screened for HIV and other STIs, received sexual health education and safer sex materials, and have been referred to HIV treatment and care. • The initiative was recently expanded to include ecumenical communities and civic groups across the U.S. NBLCA affiliates in Atlanta, Baltimore, Detroit, Tampa, and Washington, D.C. have conducted community town halls and policy workshops to promote community dialogue and action to identify solutions to the HIV/AIDS epidemic affecting the black community. • As a part of the initiative, The National Black Clergy for the Elimination of HIV/AIDS Act of 2009 was developed. The act is a comprehensive proposal for fighting HIV/AIDS in the black community, and includes far-reaching steps improve HIV outcomes and health among MSM.	• Two successful housing programs for LGBTQ youth are YouthCare's ISIS House and the Ali Forney Center. • Based in Seattle, Washington, YouthCare builds confidence and self-sufficiency for homeless youth by providing a continuum of care that includes outreach, basic services, emergency shelter, housing, counseling, education, and employment training. • In 1998, YouthCare opened ISIS House, the first transitional living program in Washington State to focus on the unique needs of homeless LGBTQ youth. • In New York City, the Ali Forney Center (AFC) was started in 2002 in response to the lack of a safe shelter space for LGBTQ youth. • ACF is the largest and most comprehensive program in the nation dedicated to meeting the needs of homeless LGBTQ youth. • AFC sees over 1,000 homeless LGBTQ youth each year. In addition to hot meals, shower facilities, and clothing, AFC also provides youth with on-site medical and mental health services, HIV and STI testing and treatment, substance abuse support, career and educational counseling and life skills mentoring.	• The Affordable Care Act (ACA) includes many new benefits for LGBT people in the United States. • ACA expands coverage options available to all Americans, including those without access to coverage through a domestic partner or employer, and those with pre-existing health conditions. • ACA offers new patient protections to help end discrimination that LGBT individuals have experienced in the health care system. These protections include prohibiting insurance companies from refusing coverage because of a pre-existing condition and ensuring that companies can no longer turn someone away because of his or her sexual orientation. • ACA also aims to improve access to preventative care and to fight health disparities. Moreover, ACA is aligned with the National HIV/AIDS Strategy to improve HIV/AIDS prevention and treatment. • The National Alliance of State and Territorial AIDS Directors (NASTAD) has outlined three steps to ensure that ACA is addressing the specific health care needs of MSM and that MSM are aware of the potential new benefits to their health care. • These three steps include 1) ensuring that community organizations focused on MSM are part of ACA outreach and enrollment programs; 2) developing tailored messages on what ACA means for MSM; and 3) continuing to address stigma in health care settings.

Figure 14-2 Case studies focusing on community mobilization, structural, and national policy interventions affecting racial/ethnic mionority gay, bisexual, and other men who have sex with men. LGBTQ = lesbian, gay, bisexual, transgender, queer; MSM = men who have sex with men; STI = sexually transmitted infection.

and may need resources to stay engaged, even during times when they experience high levels of stigma within their communities and personal difficulties maintaining their treatment regimen.

A critical action step that should be taken while the ACA is being implemented is improving provider education and competence in providing culturally appropriate and holistic HIV care to MSM of color. As biomedical and behavioral health interventions, including HIV prevention programs and adherence interventions, become more routinely implemented in medical settings and/or medical care homes, it is important that those working within these settings are well equipped to deliver HIV prevention services to black, Latino, and Asian/Pacific Islander MSM. Currently, most medical providers do not receive training on the unique health concerns and issues affecting racial/ethnic minorities and LGBT individuals. Medical schools and continuing education programs rarely include courses on LGBT and minority health. This oversight has meant that providers working with patients that are racial/ethnic minority MSM have to learn about these populations on the job, if they learn about them at all. Greater efforts must be made to change the way health care providers are educated and to make training on racial/ethnic minority and LGBT health a mandatory component of medical education.

Lastly, stigma around HIV and sexuality serves as a barrier for MSM of color to equip themselves with knowledge about STIs and available treatments and feel empowered to have honest and open discussions with their health care providers about their sexual behaviors. Tools need to be developed for patients and providers that can facilitate these actions and reduce the stigma around testing for STIs and protecting one's sexual health. Multi-pronged approaches, including social marketing campaigns that demystify sexual health and in-person trainings for providers and practitioners that improve knowledge of and comfort with gay men's sexual health concerns, are imperative.

Combination Prevention: The Best Hope for HIV/AIDS Prevention Among MSM of Color

There are a growing number of proven approaches to reduce the risk for HIV infection. These proven approaches include behavioral, biomedical, community-level, and structural programs. Regardless of the potential effectiveness of these programs, each still experience gaps in efficacy that can likely be answered by combining programs. For example, HIV testing is an important tool in HIV prevention. Coupling HIV testing with programs emphasizing linkage and engagement in care makes testing a formidable tool in the prevention of HIV transmission. We know from recent studies that treating people living with HIV early in their infection greatly reduces the risk for transmitting the virus to others. However, we also know major challenges to successfully implementing this intervention include adherence to medication and access to care. These challenges can be met by combining treatment as prevention with medication adherence interventions, as well by focusing efforts on structural and national policy issues surrounding access to care. Related to treatment as prevention, PrEP has proven to be a new prevention intervention that lowers the chances of HIV transmission to HIV-uninfected people. This biomedical intervention must be combined with behavioral interventions focused on medication adherence, risk-reduction behaviors, and access to care in order to maximize effectiveness.

In 2009, the U.S. President's Emergency Plan for AIDS Relief (PEPFAR) initiative identified combination prevention as its foremost approach to HIV prevention, stating that successful prevention programs must include a combination of biomedical, behavioral, and structural interventions that are routed in evidence. In their 2010 publication "Combination HIV Prevention: Tailoring and Coordinating Biomedical, Behavioural and Structural Strategies to Reduce New HIV Infections" UNAIDS (87) defined *combination prevention* as:

> ...rights-based, evidence-informed, and community-owned programmes that use a mix of biomedical, behavioural, and structural interventions, prioritized to meet the current HIV prevention needs of particular individuals and communities, so as to have the greatest sustained impact on reducing new infections. Well-designed combination prevention programmes are carefully tailored to national and local needs and conditions; focus resources on the mix of programmatic and policy actions required to address both immediate risks and underlying vulnerability; and they are thoughtfully planned and managed to operate synergistically and consistently on multiple levels (e.g. individual, relationship, community, society) and over an adequate period of time. They mobilize community, private sector, government and global resources in a collective undertaking; require and benefit from enhanced partnership and coordination; and they incorporate mechanisms for learning, capacity building and flexibility to permit continual improvement and adaptation to the changing environment.

Planning, implementing, and monitoring combination prevention programs depend largely on the interdisciplinary coordination and cooperation of many key players in the HIV prevention field.

Recommendations for Future Combination Prevention Interventions for MSM of Color

In response to the growing rates of HIV infection among MSM, PEPFAR released guidance on implementing combination prevention programs for MSM (88). PEPFAR identified the core elements of a comprehensive package of HIV-prevention services for MSM as community-based outreach; distribution of condoms and lubricants; HIV counseling and testing; programs related to linkage to care and treatment; targeted information, education, and communication; and STI prevention, screening, and treatment. Central to these core elements is that all HIV prevention programs for MSM should be based on equity, nondiscrimination, and voluntariness and be sensitive to the stigma and discrimination experienced by MSM worldwide.

Prevention programs for MSM should be rooted in the community and should attempt to build the capacity of community organizations, particularly MSM-specific organizations, to lead and implement the intervention among their peers. It is essential that participants in these programs feel confident that their privacy is protected at all times and that staff are trained to provide high-quality services that are nondiscriminatory, confidential, and responsive to the needs of the population. Also important for future combination prevention programs is the need to integrate services for HIV prevention and treatment. This will increase access to HIV testing and prevention programs, provide natural links to care and treatment, and streamline the delivery of MSM-focused services. The future of combination prevention programs should also capitalize on new technologies involving mobile phones and applications and should consider the rapidly changing evidence from new and ongoing research trials (88).

Conclusion

Since the beginning of HIV/AIDS in the United States, black and Latino MSM have been disproportionately affected by the epidemic. While many effective

---

Table 14–1   HIV Prevention Approaches for MSM of Color: Clinical Implications and Resources

- New biomedical interventions, such as PrEP, can prevent HIV infection in MSM. PrEP can be prescribed to MSM in primary care settings. For current information and guidelines, visit www.cdc.gov/hiv/prevention/research/prep and www.iprexole.com.

- Patients at risk for HIV may be referred to effective behavioral interventions in their communities. Visit www.effectiveinterventions.org to find behavioral interventions for MSM and MSM of color.

- Health care institutions can reduce barriers to access by making their facilities welcoming, inclusive, and respectful of sexual, gender, and racial/ethnic minorities. See Appendix A for strategies and visit www.lgbthealtheducation.org for resources.

- Health care providers can help curb the HIV epidemic by implementing routine HIV testing for all populations and by encouraging racial/ethnic minorities to get tested for HIV and other STIs. Recommendations for routine testing can be found at www.uspreventiveservicestaskforce.org/Page/Topic/recommendation-summary/human-immunodeficiency-virus-hiv-infection-screening or www.cdc.gov/hiv/guidelines/index.html.

- Providers should also develop systems and programs that link and engage HIV-infected people into treatment and care. An example program, Anti-Retroviral Treatment and Access to Services (ARTAS), can be found at www.effectiveinterventions.org.

- Medical providers and students should access more training and education on the unique health concerns of MSM of color. For training resources, visit www.lgbthealtheducation.org.

MSM = men who have sex with me; PrEP = pre-exposure prophylaxis; STI = sexually transmitted infection.

behavioral and biomedical interventions have been identified for HIV prevention, very few focus on MSM of color. Community mobilization efforts have at once proven effective for HIV prevention and highlighted the need for more campaigns focused on MSM of color. In addition to community-level interventions, structural and policy interventions have potential to reduce new HIV infections and improve health outcomes among racial/ethnic minority MSM in the United States. Combination prevention/treatment intervention strategies, which integrate interventions at multiple levels, have the greatest ability to reduce HIV and other health disparities impacting MSM of color. Additional clinical resources on preventing HIV in racial/ethnic minority MSM are listed in Table 14-1.

Summary Points

- MSM of color, particularly black MSM and young MSM are among the highest risk populations for HIV infection in the United States. Evidence-based explanations for this disparity point to a need for greater efforts to improve and enhance culturally-tailored HIV prevention, linkage to care, and treatment programs.
- The CDC disseminates information on four evidence-based effective behavioral interventions specifically for MSM and two interventions tailored for MSM of color. These can be found at www.effectiveinter ventions.org.
- There is a great need for tailored and culturally appropriate HIV prevention strategies incorporating behavioral, social, and biomedical strategies in order to lower rates among MSM of color.
- Advances in biomedical research have provided additional HIV prevention tools with potential in reducing new HIV infections among MSM; these include PrEP and "treatment as prevention." Internalized and institutional stigma around race, homosexuality, and HIV have impeded the implementation of interventions and mobilization efforts among MSM of color.
- Community mobilization efforts for MSM of color have largely been focused on increasing HIV testing and/or reducing stigma related to homosexuality and HIV/AIDS through the implementation of local and national social marketing campaigns, such as the CDC's Act Against AIDS campaign, "Greater Than AIDS," and "HIV Stops with Me."
- Structural factors can be defined broadly as the "physical, social, cultural, organizational, community, economic, legal, or policy aspects of the environment that impede or facilitate persons' efforts to avoid HIV infection." These factors are compounded for MSM of color, who are marginalized not only because of their race/ethnicity but also due to their sexual orientation.

- For MSM of color, important structural factors that need to be addressed in interventions and health programs include access to care and treatment, immigration and migration, incarceration and re-entry, poverty, and homelessness.
- Successful structural interventions often have simple designs, are cost-effective, are facilitated by community mobilization efforts, and require wide acceptance from leadership, governance and community stakeholders.
- The NHAS, the CDC's revised HIV/AIDS funding plan for health departments, and the Affordable Care Act are 3 policy interventions that affect health and access to health care programs among MSM of color.
- NHAS supports targeted approaches to improve health and well-being among MSM of color, notably black MSM. Holistic interventions that address multiple factors enhancing vulnerability to poor health among MSM of color are needed.
- Combination prevention, which mixes biomedical, behavioral, and structural interventions, is the best hope for HIV prevention among MSM of color in the United States.

References

1. **Grant RM, Wiley JA, Winkelstein W.** Infectivity of the human immunodeficiency virus: estimates from a prospective study of homosexual men. J Infect Dis. 1987;156:189-93.
2. **Winkelstein W, Lyman DM, Padian N, et al.** Sexual practices and risk of infection by the human immunodeficiency virus. The San Francisco Men's Health Study. JAMA. 1987;257: 321-25.
3. **Easterbrook PJ, Chmiel JS, Hoover DR, et al.** Racial and ethnic differences in human immunodeficiency virus type 1 (HIV-1) seroprevalence among homosexual and bisexual men. The Multicenter AIDS Cohort Study. Am J Epidemiol. 1993;138:415-29.
4. **Ruiz J, Facer M, Sun RK.** Risk factors for human immunodeficiency virus infection and unprotected anal intercourse among young men who have sex with men. Sex Transm Dis. 1998;25:100-7.
5. **Mitsch A, Hu X, Harrison KM, Durant T.** Trends in HIV/AIDS diagnoses among men who have sex with men—33 States, 2001-2006 . MMWR Morb Mortal Wkly Rep. 2008;57:681-6.
6. **Phillips G, Wohl A, Xavier J, et al.** Epidemiologic data on young men of color who have sex with men. AIDS Patient Care STDS. 2011;25:S1-8.
7. **Prejean J, Song R, Hernandez A, et al.** Estimated HIV incidence in the United States, 2006-2009. PLoS One. 2011;6:e17502.
8. **Millett GA, Peterson JL, Wolitski RJ, Stall R.** Greater risk for HIV infection of black men who have sex with men: a critical literature review. Am J Public Health. 2006;96:1007-19.
9. **Marks G, Millett GA, Bingham T, et al.** Understanding differences in HIV sexual transmission among Latino and black men who have sex with men: the Brothers y Hermanos Study. AIDS Behav. 2009;13:682-90.
10. **Oster AM, Wiegand RE, Sionean C, et al.** Understanding disparities in HIV infection between black and white MSM in the United States. AIDS. 2011;25:1103-12.
11. **Diaz RM, Ayala G, Bein E, et al.** The impact of homophobia, poverty, and racism on the mental health of gay and bisexual Latino men: findings from 3 US cities. Am J Public Health. 2001;91:927-32.

12. **Stall R, Paul JP, Greenwood G, et al.** Alcohol use, drug use and alcohol-related problems among men who have sex with men: the Urban Men's Health Study. Addiction. 2001;96: 1589-601.

13. **Ramirez-Valles J, Garcia D, Campbell RT, et al.** HIV infection, sexual risk behavior, and substance use among Latino gay and bisexual men and transgender persons. Am J Public Health. 2008;98:1036-42.

14. **Losina E, Schackman BR, Sadownik SN, et al.** Racial and sex disparities in life expectancy losses among HIV-infected persons in the united states: impact of risk behavior, late initiation, and early discontinuation of antiretroviral therapy. Clin Infect Dis. 2009;49: 1570-8.

15. **Moore RD.** Epidemiology of HIV infection in the United States: implications for linkage to care. Clin Infect Dis. 2011;52:S208-13.

16. **Christopoulos KA, Das M, Colfax GN.** Linkage and retention in HIV care among men who have sex with men in the United States. Clin Infect Dis. 2011;52:S214-22.

17. **Millett GA, Jeffries WL, Peterson JL, et al.** Common roots: a contextual review of HIV epidemics in black men who have sex with men across the African diaspora. Lancet. 2012; 380:411-23.

18. **Kelly JA, St Lawrence JS, Stevenson LY, et al.** Community AIDS/HIV risk reduction: the effects of endorsements by popular people in three cities. Am J Public Health. 1992;82: 1483-89.

19. **Jones KT, Gray P, Whiteside YO, et al.** Evaluation of an HIV prevention intervention adapted for Black men who have sex with men. Am J Public Health. 2008;98:1043-50.

20. **Wilton L, Herbst JH, Coury-Doniger P, et al.** Efficacy of an HIV/STI prevention intervention for black men who have sex with men: findings from the Many Men, Many Voices (3MV) project. AIDS Behav. 2009;13:532-44.

21. **Kegeles SM, Hays RB, Coates TJ.** The Mpowerment Project: a community-level HIV prevention intervention for young gay men. Am J Public Health. 1996;86:1129-36.

22. **Miller RL, Forney JC, Hubbard P, Camacho LM.** Reinventing Mpowerment for black men: long-term community implementation of an evidence-based program. Am J Community Psychol. 2012;49:199-214.

23. **Dilley JW, Schwarcz S, Murphy J, et al.** Efficacy of personalized cognitive counseling in men of color who have sex with men: secondary data analysis from a controlled intervention trial. AIDS Behav. 2011;15:970-5.

24. **Grant RM, Javier RL, Anderson PL, et al.** Preexposure chemoprophylaxis for HIV prevention in men who have sex with men. N Engl J Med. 2010;363:2587-99.

25. **Cohen MS, McCauley M, Gamble TR.** HIV treatment as prevention and HPTN 052. Curr Opin HIV AIDS. 2012;7:99-105.

26. **Koblin BA, Mayer KH, Eshleman SH, et al.** Correlates of HIV acquisition in a cohort of Black men who have sex with men in the United States: HIV prevention trials network (HPTN) 061. PLoS One. 2013;8:e70413.

27. **Escoffier J.** The invention of safer sex: vernacular knowledge, gay politics and HIV prevention. Sexuality. Berk J Sociol. 1998-99;43:1-30.

28. **Shilts R.** And the Band Played On: Politics, People, and the AIDS Epidemic. New York: Martin's Press; 2007.

29. **Mahajan AP, Sayles JN, Patel VA, et al.** Stigma in the HIV/AIDS epidemic: a review of the literature and recommendations for the way forward. AIDS. 2008;22:S7.

30. **Parker R.** Sexuality, culture, and power in HIV/AIDS research. Annu Rev Anthropol. 2001; 163-79.

31. **Parker R, Aggleton P.** HIV and AIDS-related stigma and discrimination: a conceptual framework and implications for action. Soc Sci Med. 2003;57:13-24.

32. **Quimby E, Friedman SR.** Dynamics of Black mobilization against AIDS in New York City. Soc Prob. 1989;36:403-15.

33. **Jaffe HW, Valdiserri RO, De Cock KM.** The reemerging HIV/AIDS epidemic in men who have sex with men. JAMA. 2007;298:2412-14.

34. **Wilson PA, Moore TE.** Public health responses to the HIV epidemic among Black men who have sex with men: a qualitative study of US health departments and communities. Am J Public Health. 2009;99:1013-22.

35. **Centers for Disease Control and Prevention (CDC).** HIV surveillance—United States, 1981-2008. MMWR Morb Mortal Wkly Rep. 2011;60:689-93.

36. **HIV Epidemiology and Field Services Program, New York City Department of Health and Mental Hygiene.** New York City HIV/AIDS annual surveillance statistics 2010. Updated 2012. Available at: www.nyc.gov/html/doh/downloads/pdf/ah/surveillance2010-tables-all.pdf.

37. **Department of Health and Mental Hygiene.** Unprotected anal intercourse among young men who have sex with men (MSM) in New York City. Epi Data Brief. 2012;13. Available at: www.nyc.gov/html/doh/downloads/pdf/epi/databrief13.pdf.

38. **Myers JE, Braunstein SL, Shepard CW, et al.** Assessing the impact of a community-wide HIV testing scale-up initiative in a major urban epidemic. J Acquir Immune Defic Syndr. 2012; 61:23-31.

39. **Bertrand JT, O'Reilly K, Denison J, et al.** Systematic review of the effectiveness of mass communication programs to change HIV/AIDS-related behaviors in developing countries. Health Educ Res. 2006;21:567-97.

40. **Díaz RM.** Latino gay men and the psychocultural barriers to AIDS prevention. In: Levine MP, Nardi PM, Gagnon JH, eds. In Changing Times: Gay Men and Lesbians Encounter HIV/AIDS. Chicago: University of Chicago Press; 1997:221-44.

41. **Stokes JP, Vanable PA, McKirnan DJ.** Ethnic differences in sexual behavior, condom use, and psychosocial variables among Black and White men who have sex with men. J Sex Res. 1996;33:373-81.

42. **Wilson PA, Valera P, Ventuneac A, et al.** Race-based sexual stereotyping and sexual partnering among men who use the Internet to identify other men for bareback sex. J Sex Res. 2009; 46:1-15.

43. **Wilson PA, Yoshikawa H.** Experiences of and responses to social discrimination among Asian and Pacific Islander gay men: their relationship to HIV risk. AIDS Educat Prev. 2004; 16:68-83.

44. **Mamary E, Mccright J, Roe K.** Our lives: an examination of sexual health issues using photovoice by non-gay identified African American men who have sex with men. Culture Health Sexual. 2007;9:359-70.

45. **Lichtenstein B.** Secret encounters: black men, bisexuality, and AIDS in Alabama. Med Anthropol Q. 2000;14:374-93.

46. **Fullilove MT, Fullilove RE.** Stigma as an obstacle to AIDS action. Am Behav Sci. 1999;42: 1117-29.

47. **Harawa NT, Williams JK, Ramamurthi HC, Bingham TA.** Perceptions towards condom use, sexual activity, and HIV disclosure among HIV-positive African American men who have sex with men: implications for heterosexual transmission. J Urban Health. 2006;83: 682-94.

48. **Wilson PA, Wittlin NM, Muñoz-Laboy M, Parker R.** Ideologies of Black churches in New York City and the public health crisis of HIV among Black men who have sex with men. Global Public Health. 2011;6:S227-242.

49. **Dyer TP, Shoptaw S, Guadamuz TE.** Application of syndemic theory to black men who have sex with men in the Multicenter AIDS Cohort Study. J Urban Health. 2012;89:697-708.

50. **Wilson PA, Nanin J, Amesty S, et al.** Using syndemic theory to understand vulnerability to HIV infection among black and Latino men in New York City. J Urban Health. 2014 Aug 26. [Epub ahead of print].

51. **Gupta GR, Parkhurst JO, Ogden JA, et al.** Structural approaches to HIV prevention. Lancet. 2008;372:764-75.

52. **Coates TJ, Richter L, Caceres C.** Behavioural strategies to reduce HIV transmission: how to make them work better. Lancet. 2008;372:669-84.

53. **Sumartojo E.** Structural factors in HIV prevention: concepts, examples, and implications for research. AIDS. 2000;14:S3-10.

54. **Tawil O, Verster A, O'Reilly KR.** Enabling approaches for HIV/AIDS prevention: can we modify the environment and minimize the risk? AIDS. 1995;12:1299-1306.

55. **Blankenship KM, Bray SJ, Merson MH.** Structural interventions in public health. AIDS. 2000;14:S11-21.

56. **Parkhurst JO.** HIV prevention, structural change and social values: the need for an explicit normative approach. J Int AIDS Soc. 2012;15:1-10.

57. **Resiner SL, Mimiaga MJ, Skeer M, et al.** Clinically significant depressive symptoms as a risk factor for HIV infection among black MSM in Massachusetts. AIDS Behav. 2009;13:798-810.

58. **Malebranche DJ, Peterson JL, Fullilove RE, Stackhouse RW.** Race and sexual identity: perceptions about medical culture and healthcare among Black men who have sex with men. J Natl Med Assoc. 2004;96:97-107.

59. **Millett GA, Ding H, Marks G, et al.** Mistaken assumptions and missed opportunities: correlates of undiagnosed HIV infection among black and Latino men who have sex with men. J Acquir Immun Defic Syndr. 2011;58:64-71.

60. **Korthuis PT, Saha S, Fleishman JA, et al.** Impact of patient race on patient experiences of access and communication in HIV care. J Gen Intern Med. 2008;23:2046-52.

61. **Stein GL, Bonuch KA.** Attitudes on end-of-life care and advance care planning in the lesbian and gay community. J Palliat Med. 2001;4:163-90.

62. **Hightow-Weidman LB, Jones K, Wohl AR, et al.** Early linkage and retention in care: findings from the outreach, linkage, and retention in care initiative among young men of color who have sex with men. AIDS Patient Care STDS. 2011;25:S31-8.

63. **Hall HI, Gray KM, Tang T, et al.** Retention in care of adults and adolescents living with HIV in 13 U.S. areas. J Acquir Immune Defic Syndr. 2012;60:77-82.

64. **Magnus M, Jones K, Phillips G, et al.** Characteristics associated with retention among African American and Latino adolescent HIV-positive men: results from the outreach, care, and prevention to engage HIV-seropositive young MSM of color special project of national significance initiative. J Acquir Immune Defic Syndr. 2010;53:529-36.

65. **Bogart LM, Wagner G, Galvan FH, Banks D.** Conspiracy beliefs about HIV are related to antiretroviral treatment nonadherence among African American men with HIV. J Acquir Immune Defic Syndr. 2010;53:648-55.

66. **Leclere FB, Jensen L, Biddlecom AE.** Health care utilization, family context, and adaptation among immigrants to the United States. J Health Soc Behav. 1994;35:370-84.

67. **Berk ML, Schur CL, Chavez LR, Frankel M.** Health care use among undocumented Latino immigrants. Health Aff (Millwood). 2000;19:51-64.

68. **Ortega AN, Fang H, Perez VH, et al.** Health care access, use of services, and experiences among undocumented Mexicans and other Latinos. Arch Intern Med. 2007;167:2354-60.

69. **Ku L, Matani S.** Left out: immigrants' access to health care and insurance. Health Aff (Millwood). 2001;20:247-56.

70. **Kullgren JT.** Restrictions on undocumented immigrants' access to health services: the public health implications of welfare reform. Am J Public Health. 2003;93:1630-33.

71. **Nandi A, Galea S, Lopez G, et al.** Access to and use of health services among undocumented Mexican immigrants in a US urban area. Am J Public Health. 2008;98:2011-20.

72. **Dwyer M, Fish DG, Gallucci A, Walker SJ.** HIV care in correctional settings. HRSA. 2014. Available at: http://hab.hrsa.gov/deliverhivaidscare/2014guide.pdf.

73. **Bingham TA, Harawa NT, Johnson DF, et al.** The effect of partner characteristics on HIV infection among African American men who have sex with men in the Young Men's Survey, Los Angeles, 1999-2000. AIDS Educ Prev. 2003;15:39-52.

74. **MacKellar DA, Valleroy LA, Secura GM, et al.** Repeat HIV testing, risk behaviors, and HIV seroconversion among young men who have sex with men: a call to monitor and improve the practice of prevention. J Acquir Immune Defic Syndr. 2002;29:76-85.

75. **Brewer RA, Magnus M, Kuo I, Wang L, Liu TY, Mayer KH.** Exploring the relationship between incarceration and HIV among Black men who have sex with men in the United States. J Acquir Immune Defic Syndr. 2014;65:218-25.

76. **May JP, Williams EL Jr.** Acceptability of condom availability in a U.S. jail. AIDS Educ Prev. 2002;14:85-91.

77. **Centers for Disease Control and Prevention.** HIV in correctional settings. Sept 13, 2013. Available at: www.cdc.gov/hiv/risk/other/correctional.html.

78. **Denning P, DiNenno E.** Communities in crisis: is there a generalized HIV epidemic in impoverished urban areas of the United States? XVIII International AIDS Conference. Vienna, July 18-23, 2010. Abstract WEPDD101. Available at http://hivandhepatitis.com/2010_conference/AIDS2010/docs/0723e_2010.html

79. **Robertson MJ, Clark RA, Charlebois ED, et al.** HIV seroprevalence among homeless and marginally housed adults in San Francisco. Am J Public Health. 2004;94:1207-17.

80. **Stall R, Mills TC, Williamson J, et al.** Association of co-occurring psychosocial health problems and increased vulnerability to HIV/AIDS among urban men who have sex with men. Am J Public Health. 2003;93:939-42.

81. **Hixson BA, Omer SB, del Rio C, Frew PM.** Spatial clustering of HIV prevalence in Atlanta, Georgia and population characteristics associated with case concentrations. J Urban Health. 2011;88:129-41.

82. **Sullivan PS, Carballo-Diéguez A, Coates T, et al.** Successes and challenges of HIV prevention in men who have sex with men. Lancet. 2012;380:388-99.

83. **Shriver MD, Everett C, Morin SF.** Structural interventions to encourage primary HIV prevention among people living with HIV. AIDS. 2000;14 Suppl 1:S57-62.

84. **Bowleg L, Teti M, Malebranche DJ, Tschann JM.** "It's an Uphill Battle Everyday": intersectionality, low-income black heterosexual men, and implications for HIV prevention research and interventions. Psychol Men Masc. 2013;14:25-34.

85. **National HIV/AIDS strategy for the United States.** Available at: www.whitehouse.gov/sites/default/files/uploads/NHAS.pdf.

86. **Centers for Disease Control and Prevention.** HIV prevention in the United States: expanding the impact. December 10, 2013. Available at: www.cdc.gov/nchhstp/newsroom/hivfactsheets/future/high-impact-prevention.htm.

87. **UNAIDS.** Combination HIV prevention: tailoring and coordinating biomedical, behavioural and structural strategies to reduce new HIV infections. 2010. Available at: www.unaids.org/en/media/unaids/contentassets/documents/unaidspublication/2010/JC2007_Combination_Prevention_paper_en.pdf.

88. The United States' President's Emergency Plan for AIDS Relief. Technical guidance on combination HIV prevention. May 2011. Available at: www.pepfar.gov/documents/organization/164010.pdf.

Chapter 15

Self-Discovery: A Toolbox to Help Clinicians Communicate With Clarity, Curiosity, Creativity, and Compassion

JENNIFER POTTER, MD

Importance of Connection, Affirmation, and Support

Social support and interpersonal connection promote healing and the ability to thrive in the face of adversity, while social isolation and loneliness exacerbate illness and increase overall mortality (1). Although social support includes several elements, studies have shown that the relational aspect is of preeminent importance (1). This translates into the clinical realm, in which higher-quality clinician–patient communication and relationships have been shown to be key factors associated with improved patient engagement, satisfaction, and adherence to care (2). The quality of relationships between health care team members in the work setting also facilitates recruitment and retention of clinicians and other staff members, prevents burnout, and fosters ongoing growth and renewal (3). Thus, cultivation of sustained connections over time is essential for our own well-being as well as that of our patients.

As discussed extensively in other chapters, a history of exclusion, perceived social isolation, and experience of overt interpersonal trauma predisposes some lesbian, gay, bisexual, transgender, and queer/questioning (LGBTQ) people to social withdrawal and lack of engagement—including difficulty engaging in relationships with health care providers—and to reliance on a wide variety of maladaptive coping behaviors that may pose a substantial threat to their health. Therefore, a primary objective for clinicians in working with LGBTQ patients is the establishment of solid, trusting relationships, which provide the foundation on which connection to a broader social context can be encouraged and more adaptive and healthier attitudes and behaviors can be nurtured and strengthened over time. The overall goal, variously referred to as "starting where the patient is," developing "unconditional positive regard," or providing "validation" or "affirmation," is to accept each patient's unique identity and individuality; to allow patients to safely share their feelings and thoughts; to demonstrate respect for their perception of things in the moment; and to help patients feel heard, acknowledged, and understood.

About This Chapter

As LGBTQ people and issues have become more mainstream in U.S. society, greater familiarity has led to a less prejudicial atmosphere, where people are more accepting and less afraid of diverse sexual and gender identities and relationships. Parallel changes have occurred in clinical and research environments, as evidenced by system-wide efforts to 1) establish clinical guidelines and training materials for LGBTQ care (4–9); 2) develop educational competencies to guide training for medical students (10); 3) create a repository of relevant curricular materials to be used in teaching (11); and 4) set an expanded research agenda (12). These efforts to make needed changes at the macro level are discussed in detail elsewhere in this book (see Chapter 1).

Systems-wide changes have profound importance in establishing a standard-of-care benchmark—that is, societal expectations regarding how a clinician should act when caring for LGBTQ patients. However, setting expectations and providing a script may not adequately address the internal doubts, fears, and reluctance many clinicians experience when they contemplate asking patients questions about sexual orientation and gender identity for the first time, nor the personal tools they need to cope most effectively with all of the emotional reactions that can arise during interactions with individual patients. Recognition of and attention to these factors are critical if we are to succeed in being fully present and able to work most effectively with LGBTQ patients.

As humans, we normally have a wide variety of emotional reactions when we encounter patients whose life stories are unfamiliar or seem strange. Many of these reactions, especially those that are particularly extreme, such as shock, disbelief, horror, disgust, fear, paralysis, pity, anger, fascination, or intrigue, can be harmful to patients if we allow these reactions to dictate our words or actions. We may also have additional, judgmental reactions about even having these feelings at all and may be disinclined to discuss them with peers out of fear that we might be perceived to be narrow-minded, lacking in compassion, or overtly prejudiced. If, however, we are able to acknowledge—and, indeed, welcome—all of our internal reactions, becoming curious about them, and seeking to learn what they can tell us about both ourselves and our patients, we will often find that they can be very informative, and ultimately help us transform our interactions into ever more sensitive and compassionate interchanges.

The intent of this chapter is give you a set of tools (summarized in bullet points at the end of this chapter) you can use to perform this kind of internal inquiry. Because this is a text about LGBTQ issues, the cases that will be discussed are LGBTQ-focused; however, you will likely find these techniques universally helpful in working with many different kinds of patients who may provoke similar kinds of reactions—that is, if you use these tools, you will become a better caregiver for *all* of your patients.

Addressing Feelings and Thoughts That Can Interfere With Engagement

A variety of common feelings and thoughts may distract or otherwise prevent clinicians from engaging effectively with LGBTQ patients. Otherwise known as "showstoppers," these feelings and thoughts must be identified and addressed promptly so we can move forward, practice asking new questions, gain new knowledge, and continually develop our skills as clinicians. Table 15-1 lists common showstopper feelings and thoughts with which you may identify, as well as a variety of "antidote" thoughts that may help you stay on track. As with other aspects of self-discovery discussed in this chapter, through the process of self-inquiry you will realize the "antidotes" that are most effective for you to overcome your own personal "showstoppers" efficiently.

At one extreme lies the belief that one is already so familiar with the lifestyles and needs of LGBTQ people that there is nothing to be gained by performing any self-inquiry or pursuing additional learning. In reality, it is well to remember that no one can ever truly become an LGBTQ "expert"—or, for that matter, any other type of "expert"—as each patient is an individual with unique needs, desires, and goals. Acting on the basis of an expert view may alienate LGBTQ patients because it involves making assumptions that may not represent each patient's actual experience. It therefore behooves even the most experienced clinicians, including those who identify as LGBTQ themselves, to regularly engage in self-reflection to identify the presence of potentially interfering biases and assumptions in the course of interacting with every patient.

At the other extreme lies the conviction, often culturally or religiously based, that it is fundamentally wrong to be LGBTQ, or that behaviors LGBTQ people engage in are perverted or sick. If acted upon unilaterally, these biased views can lead to avoidance and outright rejection of LGBTQ patients. Fortunately, we are not uni-dimensional creatures: Whenever we identify a part of ourselves that holds an extreme belief, we should remember that it represents only one part of ourselves. With a little internal investigation we will inevitably be able to identify other feelings or thoughts, some of which will be less extreme and can facilitate acceptance and engagement.

Most of the feelings or thoughts in the left column of Table 15-1 arise from a clinician's desire to avoid experiencing discomfort, embarrassment, or awkwardness during medical encounters related to navigating previously unfamiliar and uncharted waters; beginning to explore traditionally secret

Table 15–1   Antidotes to "Showstopper" Feelings and Thoughts

Feelings and Thoughts That Can Interfere With Engagement	Helpful "Antidote" Thoughts That Can Keep You on Track
I don't need to learn anything more about LGBTQ people because I'm already an expert.	It is impossible to ever become a true "expert." We are all learning, all the time. Maintaining an explicit "co-expert" status with patients levels the playing field and empowers them to engage productively in their own care.
I'm afraid I'll say the wrong thing or offend someone.	It takes courage to be imperfect. It is inevitable that I will make mistakes. The appropriate response is to apologize by acknowledging the mistake, understanding the experience of the mistake, and learning not to make the same mistake twice.
I feel too uncomfortable and embarrassed to talk about issues relating to sexuality/gender.	It is normal to feel uncomfortable when trying something new. It may help diffuse the discomfort to "name it" (see text). With practice, I will gain greater comfort over time.
I can't possibly ask all the questions in the chapter on taking a history—there will never be time!	Rome was not built in a day. It is sufficient to start the conversation at the first encounter and continue the dialogue over time.
I'm afraid to ask screening questions because I won't know what to say next.	It is okay not to know and to seek consultation from colleagues. When in doubt, a good next step is to ask: "Tell me more."
I'm afraid to ascertain all of the person's health needs because they'll be overwhelming and I won't be able to help.	It will never be possible to meet all of a patient's needs—we are not redeemers. I need to trust that each patient has internal resources and sources of resilience. My job is to partner with the patients to strengthen their coping skills over time. Sometimes it takes a village . . .
I just can't relate to LGBTQ people; their experience is utterly foreign and unfathomable to me.	It is normal to feel off-balance in the face of the unknown. I need to hang in there and develop greater familiarity so that people who are different from me no longer feel so strange . . . I recognize that I am feeling uncomfortable. If I understand why I'm feeling this way, I can learn how to overcome it.
I think LGBTQ people are sick.	People come from different backgrounds that may not always resemble or mesh with my own.
I think the behaviors LGBTQ people engage in are wrong.	I can value LGBTQ people as human beings even if I dislike or disapprove of their actions or behaviors.

or forbidden topics (e.g., sexuality); or potentially releasing the lid of a Pandora's box. It is important to address these anxieties so they do not result in paralysis. The bottom line is that it is normal to feel uncomfortable when trying something new, okay to admit when you do not know, and always a good idea to ask for help when you feel you are out of your depth.

In some situations it can be helpful to name one's discomfort in the presence of the patient. For example, when becoming embarrassed while discussing an element of the sexual history, you might say something like: "You may notice that I am blushing, which reflects how common it is to feel embarrassed while discussing a topic that our society considers to be taboo. I'm glad we're doing it anyway, since sexuality is a very important aspect of your health." This kind of statement demonstrates your willingness to "go there" with the patients even though it can be embarrassing and invites patients to explore an area about which they themselves may also feel anxious.

One final point deserves emphasis. Confronting a new and unfamiliar situation should not be viewed as a solely uncomfortable experience—it can often be stimulating and exhilarating as well. The process of exploration and practice can be fun, presenting an opportunity to be gentle with yourself when you make an assumption, misunderstand, or otherwise blunder; to share your experiences with colleagues; and to appreciate the educational value of both your successes and your mistakes.

Ascertaining and Acknowledging Biases and Assumptions

Studies show that it is a widespread reaction to resist the idea that one is biased: for example, "I'm not homophobic . . . I'm a member of the LGBTQ community myself!" Or, alternatively, "I'm totally open to LGBTQ issues . . . some of my best friends are gay." Similarly, given changing mores, it may not be immediately obvious that bias continues to exist in society: "I don't really see what the big deal is . . . LGBTQ people seem to have it much easier these days, and I don't really think discrimination is much of a problem anymore." If you find yourself having a similar reaction, you may want to take a quick self-assessment test to increase your awareness and acceptance of your own biases and assumptions and the persistence of societal stigma toward LGBTQ people (see Table 15-2, Table 15-3, and Table 15-4).

Table 15-2 presents two tests to elicit awareness of *internal* bias. The Implicit Association Test (available at: https://implicit.harvard.edu) examines how words describing sexual orientation (e.g., *gay, straight*) and positive versus negative concepts (e.g., *joyful, beautiful, marvelous, wonderful, pleasure, glorious, lovely,* and *superb* on the one hand and *agony, terrible, horrible, humiliate, nasty, painful, awful,* and *tragic* on the other hand) are paired in people's minds. Analysis of tens of thousands of these tests has

Table 15–2   Self-Assessment Tests to Demonstrate the Presence of Internal Bias

- **Sexuality Implicit Association Test (IAT)**
  Please go to the Sexuality IAT at: https://implicit.harvard.edu.

- **Clarifying Beliefs Scale**
  Please read each of the following statements and rate your level of agreement based on the scale.
    5: Strongly agree
    4: Somewhat agree
    3: Indifferent
    2: Somewhat disagree
    1: Strongly disagree

—I refrain from making homophobic remarks or jokes about LGBTQ people.

—I always confront homophobic remarks and jokes made by others.

—I believe that homophobic harassment and violence are serious issues and it is important to seriously sanction perpetrators.

—I believe that LGBTQ people are equally entitled to all of the same rights and privileges as everyone else.

—I believe that LGBTQ people are capable of the same normal, healthy relationships as everyone else.

—I do not worry about what kind of effect an LGBTQ individual might have on my children or any other children.

—I use language and examples that are inclusive of LGBTQ individuals and their experiences.

—I am comfortable publicly expressing my affection for friends of the same gender.

—I am knowledgeable about the histories, cultures, psychosocial development, and needs of LGBTQ people.

—I value the contributions that "out" [students] [faculty] [colleagues] [staff] make to the culture and climate of my [school] [workplace].

—I do not make judgments about people based on what I perceive their sexual orientation to be.

—I respect the confidentiality of LGBTQ people by not gossiping about their sexual orientation or gender identity.

—I actively advocate for, financially support, and/or participate in LGBTQ organizations.

—I have questioned/thought about/seriously considered my own sexuality.

—I have questioned/thought about/seriously considered my gender identity.

—I am comfortable with being assumed to be LGBTQ. (If you identify as LGB, answer whether you would feel comfortable being assumed to be transgender).

—I am comfortable around people who dress, act, or present themselves in ways that are not traditionally associated with their assumed biological sex.

—I am comfortable seeing open expressions of affection between people of the same gender.

—It does not bother me if I cannot identify the gender of a person just by looking at that person.

—I believe that homophobia and transphobia affect all people, regardless of their sexuality or gender.

Clarifying Beliefs Scale adapted from the California State University, Chico Safe Zone Program Resource Guide. Available at: http://www.csuchico.edu/diversity/documents/safe-zone-resources.pdf

Table 15–3   Self-Assessment Test to Demonstrate the Effect
of External Bias (Heterosexual Privilege)

On a daily basis, as a straight person . . .

—I am not identified/defined by my sexual orientation.

—People don't ask when I first realized I was heterosexual.

—I can go for months without being called straight.

—Nobody calls me straight as an insult.

—People can use terms that describe my sexual orientation and mean positive things (e.g., "straight as an arrow," "standing up straight" or "straightened out") instead of demeaning terms (e.g., "ewww, that's gay" or being "queer").

—I am never asked to speak for everyone who is heterosexual.

—If I pick up a magazine, watch TV, or play music, I can be certain my sexual orientation will be represented.

—I can easily find a religious community that will not exclude me for being heterosexual.

—I can count on finding a therapist or health provider willing and able to talk about my sexuality.

—I am guaranteed to find sex education literature for couples with my sexual orientation.

—People do not assume I am experienced in sex (or that I even have it) merely because I am heterosexual.

—If I talk about my partner, I am not viewed as pushing my sexual orientation onto others.

—I can hold hands or kiss in public with my significant other and not have people double-take or stare.

—I do not have to fear that if my family or friends find out about my sexual orientation there will be economic, emotional, physical or psychological consequences.

—Because of my sexual orientation, I do not need to worry that people will harass or assault me.

—I can be open about my sexual orientation without worrying about how it will affect my job.

Adapted from: Unpacking the invisible knapsack II: Sexual orientation. Available at: www.cs.earlham.edu/~hyrax/personal/files/student_res/straightprivilege.htm

shown that 81% of heterosexuals demonstrate implicit biases for straight people over gay men and lesbians (13). Interestingly, the Implicit Association Test shows that minorities often internalize the same biases as majority groups: For example, 38% of gay men and lesbians taking this test demonstrated a bias for straight people over homosexuals (13).

Table 15-2 also offers a brief questionnaire that will give you a sense of your degree of familiarity, comfort, and support for LGBTQ people. Other scales that measure internal bias towards LGBTQ people include those developed by Riddle (14) and by Wright, Adams, and Bernat (15).

In addition, 2 tests are helpful in demonstrating ongoing existence of external bias and may foster greater compassion for what it feels like to live

Table 15–4   Self-Assessment Test to Demonstrate the Effect
of External Bias (Cisgender Privilege)

On a daily basis, as a person who is not transgender . . .

—I do not have to choose between either invisibility ("passing") or being consistently "othered" and/or tokenized based on my gender.

—My validity as a man/woman/human is not based upon how much surgery I've had or how well I "pass" as a nontransgender person.

—I don't have to hear "so have you had THE surgery?" or "oh, so you're REALLY a [incorrect sex or gender]?" each time I come out.

—Strangers do not ask me what my "real name" [birth name] is and then assume they have a right to call me by that name.

—People do not disrespect me by using incorrect pronouns.

—I am not excluded from events that either explicitly or de facto admit only men-born-men or women-born-women (e.g., when establishing candidacy for participation in competitive sports).

—Strangers don't assume they can ask me what my genitals look like and how I have sex.

—When becoming intimate with someone, I do not have to worry that they won't be able to deal with my parts or that having sex with me will cause them to question their own sexual orientation.

—People assume that because I'm cisgender, I must do sex work.

—I do not have to worry about whether I will be able to find a bathroom to use or whether I will be safe changing in a locker room.

—When I express my gender identity, I don't have to worry that I will be considered mentally ill.

—I am not required to undergo extensive psychological evaluation in order to receive basic medical care.

—My health insurance provider does not specifically exclude me from receiving benefits or treatments available to others because of my gender.

—If I end up in the emergency room, I do not have to worry that my gender will keep me from receiving appropriate treatment or that my medical issues will be seen as a result of my gender.

—I don't have to worry about losing my housing or job because of my gender.

Adapted from: Gender privilege. University of Texas Gender and Sexuality Center. Available at: www.utexas. edu/diversity/ddce/gsc/downloads/resources/Gender_Privilege.pdf

in a society that stigmatizes LGBTQ identities and lifestyles. Both tests are derived from the work of Peggy McIntosh, who demonstrated the power, in confronting racism, of looking at the degree to which being white confers advantage in society (16). Table 15-3 and Table 15-4 present revised lists of questions developed by university students working on diversity initiatives; answering these questions will help to elucidate the privilege inherent in being heterosexual/straight (17) or nontransgender (also known as cisgender) (18).

If you are surprised by your results or reactions to any of these self-assessment tests, you are not alone. It is a common reaction to feel guilt, shame, or other emotions when confronted with one's own privilege. Rather than allowing these emotions to overwhelm or hinder further reflection and action, you should remember they are usually a testament to cherished principles of justice and equality that conflict with the biases and assumptions that may result from the pervasive effects of socialization in an imperfect and unequal society. The key is to use this realization as a wake-up call to remain continuously alert for any thoughts, feelings, and behaviors that might signal the presence of a subtle bias that could be communicated to and be hurtful to an LGBTQ patient, and to consciously identify and challenge all of your assumptions.

Questioning and Challenging Biases and Assumptions

As any person who has ever tried to change any aspect of themselves can attest, it does little good to attempt to merely censor unwanted thoughts or feelings (and associated behaviors) because we develop and hold on to our beliefs for good reasons. With a little investigation (discussed more below), it becomes clear that even attitudes and beliefs that are biased, judgmental, unfair, and potentially harmful to others initially developed with a protective intent in mind. Therefore, when we attempt to summarily banish any of our beliefs without understanding the reasons we developed them in the first place, we often find that they become even more tenacious and entrenched than before (e.g., we dig in our heels and cling to the status quo when our stability and sense of safety are shaken).

It is important to note that the same belief systems can exist across all sexual and gender identities. For example, consider the example of a lesbian or gay person who has difficulty understanding the concept of bisexuality. This person then meets a bisexual person at a community support group and feels threatened by the presence of a person "not like me." In response, this person ignores the bisexual support group member, and thereby perpetuates bisexual stigma and lack of trust within the LGBTQ community. Fortunately, it is possible to change our belief systems. Forward motion can be accomplished if we 1) acknowledge and "own" our current attitudes; 2) come to understand and appreciate why they developed in the first place and how well they serve us now; 3) examine the costs of holding on to them and how they may limit us or harm others; and 4) consider the potential benefits of changing perspective. Useful questions to ask include the following:

- How do my current beliefs serve me?
- What might I lose if I change my beliefs?
- What are the costs of maintaining my current perspective?
- How might it benefit me to change?

Language that expresses readiness for change exists on a spectrum from "I may never be able to (believe/act any differently) . . ." to "I should . . ." to "I am willing to . . ." to "I am completely ready to . . ." to "I am currently (believing/acting in a different way)." It is important to remember that change of any kind requires significant time and conscious effort. It is always possible to nudge oneself along from one point on this spectrum to the next by making a deliberate choice to do so, no matter how immutable one's starting position may at first seem.

Let's take a closer look at how we develop our belief systems and why we sometimes cling to these beliefs even when ample evidence shows they are no longer effective or are actually harmful to ourselves or to others. At an instinctual level, our survival as human beings depends on our ability to rapidly assess the environment for potential danger, to make reasonably accurate predictions about the level of threat (if any), and to act accordingly to achieve or maintain our safety. Throughout our lives we continually encounter unfamiliar people, places, and things—all potential threats to our well-being—and we have to make split-second fight-or-flight decisions in order to remain safe. Because time is of the essence, we have developed cognitive strategies (short cuts) that rely on superficial characteristics and associations to these characteristics to rapidly form initial impressions to guide our behavior.

In social encounters, we start putting each other into boxes the minute we see each other, based initially on purely visual characteristics, such as age, gender, skin color, height, weight, clothing, mannerisms, and overall demeanor. If we have the opportunity to talk with one another, we continue this categorization by asking targeted questions: "Where are you from? What do you do? What are your interests? Do you have children?" Many of these categories are socially constructed and perpetuated by an unequal social order. Thus, we do not have to resist only a random set of categories when we try to overcome this sorting process; we must resist norms and injustices pervading and continually reinforced by our society—a more formidable task. It may be helpful to remember that what we really seek are answers to basic questions: "Am I going to be able to relate to this person? What do we have in common? Is this person a potential friend or might this person hurt me?"

A similar questioning and sorting process occurs in the clinical arena. Patients continually size us up in order to assess: "Will this provider see me as I really am? Will the provider respect me without judgment? Will the provider treat my body with care? Is this a person with whom I can expose my vulnerabilities and nakedness?" These questions are particularly common among LGBTQ patients, whose prior negative experiences with the medical profession often color expectations of future encounters. As clinicians, we also continually size up our patients: When meeting any individual for the first time, we need to remember that sexual orientation and gender identity are often invisible—that is, it is generally not possible to make accurate predictions that a person is LGBTQ based on superficial visual characteristics. Therefore we should not assume a patient is straight or nontransgender, as this may lead LGBTQ patients to feel unseen and invalidated.

Once an LGBTQ patient self-identifies, our human tendency to categorize can pose additional hazards. The fact that patients self-identify as LGBTQ tells us little about what the sexual or gender minority term they choose to identify with actually means to them. Sexual and gender minority identities cannot be pigeonholed into discrete categories. For example, the attractions of many people who identify as gay may encompass people of the opposite sex, and therefore fall on a spectrum that is actually grey. In addition, the fact that patients self-identify as LGBTQ tells us nothing about their other identities, beliefs, and behaviors. If we want and/or need to know about any of these details, we have to ask. Many people have multiple identities, some of which may be more important to their sense of self and more important to safeguard than their LGBTQ identity. Focusing unduly on sexual or gender minority identity may therefore be irrelevant, or may undermine efforts people make to express to you who they really are in their entirety.

Clinicians have a particular tendency to associate certain risk behaviors (e.g., unsafe sexual behavior) with certain LGBTQ subgroups (e.g., men who have sex with men) but not others (e.g., lesbians) as a result of social stereotyping. It is vital to resist this temptation so we do not form rapid, unfounded judgments that may affect how we interact or communicate with a patient, potentially causing us to offend (e.g., assume a gay man has multiple partners when he is in a monogamous relationship) or miss a key piece of the history (e.g., assume discussion of contraception with a lesbian is unnecessary, only to discover that she has occasional unprotected vaginal sex with men).

How we use results of LGBTQ health research to inform our practice also requires careful consideration. While such research is invaluable in providing needed information about the prevalence of risk factors, related illnesses, and outcomes of treatment in various LGBTQ population subgroups, we need to remember not to overgeneralize findings from one sexual minority study cohort to all patients who share certain characteristics with that cohort. The scientific method itself, which emphasizes the importance of order, making a definitive diagnosis, and setting forth confidently on a course of action, can contribute to leading us astray because human beings do not fit into neat, tidy packages that are easily classified. For example, some sexual and gender minority people reject identity labels such as L, G, B, T, and Q outright, feeling that who they are transcends any existing definition and that any possible description will be by nature overly constraining.

Humans tend to become especially uncomfortable in the face of ambiguity. Thus, we may feel quite unsettled sitting with patients who are questioning their sexual orientation or gender. We may find ourselves struggling more with the concept of bisexuality than either heterosexuality or homosexuality. And we may feel entirely at sea when we first start working with patients on the transgender spectrum, especially with those who do not identify as exclusively male or female, or with those starting to transition, when their physical characteristics may not yet match their gender identity.

We are at greatest risk of rejecting patients—whether overtly or more subtly by communicating disinterest or disengagement by our demeanor—when we perceive them as "other"; that is, we find nothing in their experience we can relate to, and their lives seem unfathomable and utterly foreign. This type of reaction, which can be summed up as "I don't understand what's going on here, so I'd better keep my distance" arises most often in relationship to transgender patients because most of us cannot relate to the experience of being born in the wrong body. The challenge is to remain open-hearted despite feeling off-balance, reminding ourselves that although some of our patients have vastly different life experiences from our own and may view the world through a different lens, there is still one huge area of commonality—we are all human, and therefore share a universal need for acceptance and connection.

Paradoxically, it is only when we stop trying to categorize, control, and predict that we find ourselves able to be truly open, compassionate, and ready to meet our patients where they are. This allows us to be open to any possibility with every patient, ensures that we are careful to ask comprehensive questions in every interview, and enables us to obtain a complete and accurate history. Identifying assumptions and choosing to set them aside require deliberate and continual vigilance, since assumptions arise from the unconscious and we tend to act from them before we are even aware of their presence.

Clinicians may find it useful to take a mental time-out before each new interaction in order to make a conscious commitment to leave assumptions at the door. Upon entering the room, you should repeatedly self-question throughout the encounter by asking:

- Am I making any assumptions?
- What are those assumptions?
- In what way are my assumptions preventing me from being fully present and open to any possibility with this patient?
- How can I set my assumptions aside so I can get to know this person as this person is?

Table 8-2 in Chapter 8 lists assumptions clinicians frequently make about LGBTQ patients. Readers with little experience working with sexual and gender minority patients may find it helpful to study this list to be aware of mistakes they may make, and to inform their best effort to avoid making the same mistakes repeatedly.

Welcoming Internal Reactions and Using Them to Maintain Connection With the Patient

All clinician–patient interactions include 3 sets of dialogue: the nonverbal and verbal interaction going on in the room between the clinician and the patient; the internal dialogue going on within the patient (who experiences thoughts about and emotional reactions toward the clinician); and the internal dialogue going on within the clinician (who experiences thoughts about and emotional responses toward the patient). Freud termed the patient's reactions *transference* and the clinician's reactions *countertransference*. In psychoanalytic circles, countertransference is understood to represent blind spots and self-protective aspects of the clinician that can get in the way of productive engagement with the patient. However, these reactions can also be used beneficially if the clinician is able to identify and understand them, and learns how to use them productively to help understand and form a therapeutic connection with the patient. This portion of the chapter uses case examples to illustrate the enormous clinical value inherent in welcoming and addressing all of the internal reactions that surface for us during interactions with patients and presents a method (see Table 15-5) to teach you how to do this routinely.

Case 1: Reactions Toward a Patient Who Is Questioning His Sexual Orientation

A 40-year-old man you have known for some time returns for an episodic visit with a chief complaint of anxiety. He says he has been happily married for 7 years and loves his wife and 4-year-old daughter. He has a community of close friends and family and a solid job in which he was just promoted. He and his wife share many interests and until recently were actively talking about having a second child. Despite all of these positive things, he has been feeling very anxious and confused. For the past month, he has been unable to stop thinking and fantasizing about a male coworker who is an out gay man. Nothing like this has ever happened to him before, and he doesn't know what to make of it.

He has many questions: "What does this mean? Am I gay? How am I ever going to talk about this with my wife? Should I even tell her about it? Do I stand to lose everything we have built together? What will happen if I let this man know I am attracted to him? Will he reject me? What if he is attracted to me too? Are we going to act on our feelings? What would it be like to be with another man? What on earth am I going to do?"

Sitting with this patient might be expected to trigger a variety of possible internal reactions in a clinician. Many of us might feel overwhelmed: "Oh no! I feel totally out of my league. I've never encountered a situation like this

Table 15-5   Suggested Framework for Welcoming and Addressing Internal Reactions

• Perform a quick internal scan to identify any internal reactions that have been triggered by sitting with the patient. For example, ask yourself: "What am I thinking and feeling?"

• Find out if there is any sense of urgency attached to your thoughts and feelings. For example, ask yourself: "Am I at risk of speaking or acting impulsively on the basis of these thoughts/feelings?"

• Push the "pause button" before responding. This pause will help prevent you from speaking or acting impulsively on the basis of an unbalanced, polarized, or reactive standpoint.

• Become curious about the source and purpose of each of your reactions. For example, ask yourself: "Where did these thoughts/feelings come from? What is their function? Is there anything my reactions can tell me about the patient's experience?"

• Validate and appreciate what your thoughts/feelings are doing for you (e.g., serving a protective function, mirroring the thoughts/feelings of the patient). Most internal reactions make sense once we understand where they're coming from.

• See if there is anything else you need to do in order to 1) take care of yourself and 2) set your thoughts/feelings aside in order to be maximally helpful to (e.g., present with) the patient.

• It is often sufficient to take a moment to re-center yourself (e.g., breathe, remind yourself it is not your job to come up with the solution), letting the stirred up parts of yourself know you will get back to them later.

• If necessary (e.g., if being asked to prescribe medications that are unfamiliar), let the patient know that you need to learn more, and schedule a mutually agreeable time in the near future to continue the conversation after you have had a chance to do some research and/or obtain consultation from a colleague.

• You will know you are on safe ground to continue your interaction with the patient when you feel clear, calm, and connected and can approach yourself and the patient with curiosity and compassion. In general, "C" words indicate groundedness and safety. Other "C" words to keep in mind include courage, creativity, confidence, and collaboration.

• If you are repeatedly stirred up by the same reactions, to the extent that they consistently interfere with working productively with patients, you may want to seek personal help (e.g., counseling).

before. I have no idea what to say or do. There's no way I'm going to be able to help this person. I think I'd better figure out who I can refer him to and get him out of here as soon as possible." If we inadvertently or overtly communicate these feelings to the patient (e.g., by disengaging emotionally) or act out on the basis of these feelings (e.g., by precipitously ending the encounter), we risk contributing to the patient's confusion, shame, isolation, and sense of panic. However, if we take a moment to validate our internal reactions and ask what we need in order to steady ourselves and be present for the patient, the outcome will likely be very different. Positive clinician reactions can have enormous therapeutic benefit. Since self-acceptance (19) and an internal sense of control (20) mitigate the psychological distress that arises from discrimination and victimization, an accepting interaction that supports patient autonomy may instill resilience among members of the LGBTQ community.

As we discussed before, it makes all the sense in the world to feel uncomfortable and unsure in the face of the unfamiliar. The protective urge to create distance and escape from an uncomfortable situation is also understandable. Simply validating these feelings/urges may be sufficient to restore a sense of calm; if not, taking a few centering breaths is often an effective way to restore balance. It can also be very useful to ask what our reactions might suggest about the patient's internal experience. For example, when we find ourselves feeling extreme emotions in the presence of a patient—such as feeling overwhelmed, confused, or panicked as in this example—chances are that we are picking up on the very feelings with which the patient is also grappling. Using this insight, it is then easy to formulate an initial compassionate response, such as, "It must be hard to sit with all of these conflicting and confusing feelings. I'm glad you shared them with me. I'll support you regardless of what you decide is best for you."

It is difficult for many clinicians to sit with a patient's ambivalence. Depending on one's personal experiences, view of the world, and ability to tolerate uncertainty, this discomfort may tempt a clinician to influence patients in one direction of their ambivalence or the other. One polarized response may involve placing undue value on maintaining the status quo (e.g., "He has a nice relationship with his wife and a young child—why does he want to rock the boat? I can't believe he'd consider throwing it all away. This is an impending disaster"). An opposite but still polarized response would be to place excessive value on exploration (e.g., "We only have one life to live. It would be sad to pass up an opportunity to find true passion and fulfillment"). Note that values-laden responses such as some of these will detract from the patient's internal locus of control and autonomy and may therefore be detrimental to the patient.

Another set of reactions stems from clinicians' feelings and attitudes about sexual orientation in particular and may be heavily influenced by any unresolved feelings about their own sexual orientation and/or behavior. A heterosexually biased viewpoint might include the thought, "Why would he give up a socially acceptable heterosexual marriage for a lifestyle that can bring isolation and shame?" A homosexually biased viewpoint might include thoughts such as "He must be gay. I know how to help—I can refer him to a great coming-out group for gay men." It is crucially important for clinicians to refrain from expressing an opinion in one direction or the other because patients need to go through their own unique process in order to arrive at a solution that feels right to them. It is also critical that clinicians avoid framing a sexual orientation dilemma in binary terms, since this neglects the real possibility that the patient may ultimately come to embrace a bisexual, queer, or other identity. What is really needed—for both the clinician and the patient—is to accept that this is one of those situations where "don't just do something, sit there" is the wisest strategy. Clinicians can carefully explain that questioning will be a process that takes some time to sort out, commit to working with patients over time, and help find other supports and resources as needed.

Case 2: Reactions Toward a Gay Man Presenting With Anal Discomfort

A 55-year-old, self-identified gay man presents for follow-up of an anal fissure. Although he holds a steady job, he is fairly isolated, and his major form of connection is frequent anonymous sex. He is a "bottom" and does not always use condoms. He comes to the clinic frequently for sexually transmitted infection (STI) testing: To date, he has been treated for gonorrhea twice but has thus far remained HIV negative. Despite having been advised to abstain from anal sex to permit healing, he had an anal encounter a few days ago, and is now experiencing more pain than before. He says he "just wasn't able to hold back any longer and had to get out there again."

This case might be expected to produce a variety of reactions. Some are related to the experience of sitting with a patient who engages repeatedly in a behavior that results in self-injury, and generally reflect a clinician's sense of hopelessness/powerlessness or dismay, frustration, and/or anger. Examples include: "He'll never heal if he keeps re-injuring himself. He keeps putting himself and his sexual partners at risk. He has no motivation to change. I'm wasting my time. I'm sick of seeing this guy." Others are related to the clinician's attitudes about sexuality in general and/or anal sex in particular. These reactions might include disgust/revulsion: "Ugh, how pathetic, wanting sex this much is not okay. This guy is disgusting/revolting/unacceptable. Anal sex is dirty and gross. I can't believe I'm going to have to examine this guy's anus again." There might also be shame: "Who am I to try to counsel this guy when I myself have desires or fantasies or engage in behaviors that others may find disgusting or unacceptable." It is also important for clinicians to acknowledge feelings of curiosity/titillation, such as: "I wonder what it feels like to have anal sex? I wonder what chat rooms and cruising areas are like. Maybe I'll go online and check it out." It is important to point out that none of these reactions are unique to working with gay male patients. Rather, they may come up when working with any patient who engages in sexual behaviors about which there are cultural taboos (e.g., a heterosexual woman who enjoys anal sex) or any patients who engage in behaviors that have unfavorable health/life consequences (e.g., patients of any sexual orientation/gender identity who compulsively overeat and are obese, or patients with diabetes who are repeatedly nonadherent to treatment recommendations).

The urge associated with many of these reactions is to distance yourself from the patient rather than sit with your feelings and stay in the work. If acted on in case 2, the urge to create distance might take the form of doing a perfunctory exam/STI testing and sending the patient on his way, or lecturing him in a judgmental and dismissive manner. A more helpful strategy would be to follow the suggested frame for welcoming and addressing internal reactions as outlined in Table 15-5. It is often helpful to remind oneself that the aspect of the patient that is provoking a negative reaction is only one part of the patient, who invariably, just like the clinician, has a variety of other parts that hold other (e.g., more easily accepted) feelings, thoughts, and urges. In addition, as we saw in case 1, a clinicians' reactions often mirror how patients feel about themselves. For example, the patient described in case 2 likely also has parts that hold frustration, hopelessness, self-judgment/recrimination, and shame. Realizing that the presenting part of the patient is not the only part of the patient creates a sense of hope. Recognizing patients' levels of "stuckness" and despair about their own predicaments, even when the patients overtly express only denial and disinterest in change, can be instrumental in moving clinicians from a place of wanting to give up to a place of feeling compassion and curiosity. In situations like case 2, it is very easy to fall into enacting a polarization where clinicians stand at one extreme of the dichotomy (e.g., "You should/must stop [the behavior in question] . . .") and patients have their heels dug in at the other extreme (e.g. "I can't/won't stop [the behavior in question] . . ."). The temptation to do this stems in part from a clinician's desire to solve the dilemma; after all, the wish to help patients is a prime motivator for why we choose to become clinicians in the first place. However, it is impossible for us to fix situations for our patients, no matter how much they and we may sometimes wish we could do so. What is needed is for us to recognize our own limitations and to trust in the internal resources of our patients. Only then can we let go of our investment in specific outcomes, becoming curious and compassionate, and partnering with our patients to explore all of the facets of their dilemmas.

An overriding principle in working with patients who repeatedly engage in behaviors that have harmful consequences (as in this patient's continual reopening of an anal fissure by engaging in compulsive sexual activity) is to remember that acceptance of where the patient is does not mean denying or ignoring our feelings about or condoning the behavior. Rather, it means developing curiosity about the functions of the behavior and collaborating creatively to brainstorm potential solutions. Frequently, a harm reduction approach works best. This starts by accepting and validating where the patient is coming from: "I'm getting that you're frustrated and probably scared that the fissure is taking so long to heal." It then moves to a statement of fact: "Your body is telling you that it needs more time to recover" and an attempt to engage the patient in arriving at a workable approach: "Let's think together about what might seem doable. What feels like the next right step?"

When working with patients who are struggling with a compulsive or addictive behavior, you should remember that finally admitting powerlessness over the behavior (whether it involves food, alcohol, drugs, sex, or anything else) typically represents a critical turning point for the patient. This is the cornerstone of 12-step self-help fellowships such as Alcoholics Anonymous (www.aa.org) and Overeater's Anonymous (www.oa.org). For a clinician, recognition of one's own powerlessness to change the behaviors of a patient is also pivotal because it returns responsibility to the patient, where it rightly belongs, and facilitates the development of a true collaboration in which both parties bring unique expertise and creativity to the table.

It can be truly terrifying to work with patients whose self-destructive behaviors may ultimately be life threatening or fatal. While the impulse to create distance from patients in order to escape this fear (e.g., by telling patients you will not be able to continue the work if they continue to engage in the behavior) is understandable, it is liable to backfire because it enacts a polarization as already described above. For clinicians to stay engaged in the work, 2 things are crucial: 1) to be very clear with patients under what circumstances you will need to intervene to assure their safety (e.g., by hospitalizing them) and 2) to obtain consultation and support from colleagues because the feelings that arise when working with patients who harm themselves are too difficult to carry alone.

Case 3: Reactions Toward a Lesbian Couple Requesting Help With Insemination

A 32-year-old lesbian presents with her partner to discuss conception. A male friend has agreed to be the sperm donor and to participate in raising a child. The couple has decided that your patient will be the one to attempt conception. They now ask you to 1) recommend tests the donor should undergo to rule out communicable and genetic diseases and 2) teach them how to perform home inseminations.

As with the previous cases, case 3 may provoke a variety of reactions. One possibility is judgment: "This is wrong. I don't want any part of it." Another possibility is uneasiness or fear regarding the potential impact on the child and each adult in the situation, as well as the possibility of the clinician's own liability. Examples include: "I don't know if this is really a good idea. What would it be like for a child to grow up in an unconventional family? What role will this man have in the child's life? Is this a gay or heterosexual man? Does the man's sexual orientation even matter? What will happen if/when he gets involved in an intimate relationship? What standing will my patient's partner have in this situation? It's hard enough raising a child with 2 parents; how will it work if there are 3? What if my patient contracts some hitherto unsuspected disease from the donor? What is my responsibility here? Do I have any right to even be asking any of these questions or exploring any of these issues with this couple? Will I have any liability if I choose to get involved?" Finally, one can imagine that many clinicians will have a part that feels enthusiastic about the couple's requests ("Let's go for it! Of course I want to help!")

Acting on any of these reactions impulsively might result in alienating the patient on the one hand (in the case of a judgmental reaction) and failing to help her think through possible logistical and legal complexities (in the case of an overly enthusiastic reaction). The challenge here is to be able to provide anticipatory guidance and education while realizing that you cannot know what is best for the patient and refraining from imposing your own wants or beliefs. The LGBTQ patient who has questions about conception and parenting presents a unique scenario in the sense that questions of this sort may provoke an urge in some clinicians to give personal or culturally biased advice in a manner that arises less frequently in interacting with heterosexual patients or couples. This is a situation in which any sense of urgency to provide advice or attachment to a particular outcome signals the clinician's reactivity, and it is best to push the pause button and to proceed as outlined in Table 15-5.

Some clinicians with experience (or after referring to Chapter 6 in this book to learn what guidance is appropriate) will feel calm, clear, and comfortable carrying out testing of the patient (and possibly also the donor, if requested). Other clinicians will feel comfortable teaching the couple how to perform home inseminations and may perhaps even be motivated to offer or learn to perform intrauterine inseminations in their own offices. However, it is always an option for clinicians who lack the requisite experience or do not feel comfortable providing guidance themselves to refer LGBTQ prospective parents to a clinic that offers comprehensive support and services (resources can be found at www.theafa.org/family-building/lgbt-family-building).

Case 4: Reactions Toward a Transgender Man Who Presents With Vaginal Bleeding

A 45-year-old individual who self-identifies as a transgender man and requests to go by the pronoun "he" presents for evaluation of abnormal vaginal bleeding. According to the chart, his legal name is "Susan," but he uses the first name "Sandy." During the history, you learn that he has been taking testosterone prescribed by an endocrinologist and had no menstrual periods from the beginning of treatment until 1 year ago, when he started to experience intermittent, heavy vaginal bleeding. He has avoided primary care and pelvic examinations/Papanicolaou tests for the past 10 years because of reluctance to expose his natal female genitalia and previous negative clinical experiences during which he felt he was on display. He is now "dragged in" by his cisgender female partner, who is concerned that the bleeding may represent something serious.

This case may evoke several reactions. Many clinicians may feel confused by the different names, lack of concordance between the patient's gender and presence of natal sex organs, and difficulty understanding transgender experience: "How do I wrap my brain around this. He has a beard, but also a uterus and vagina? I just don't get it—he's still with the same female partner as before his hormonal transition . . . what was wrong with living life as a lesbian?" Curiosity is natural: "I wonder what all of this has been like for the partner? What will his body look like?" Many clinicians will also feel anxious, hyperaware of their choice of language during the encounter, and concerned about what may come up for them and the patient during the exam: "This whole interaction feels really awkward. What if I use the wrong pronoun? I'd better be really careful so I don't cause offense. How will I feel doing a pelvic exam on a person who looks like a man? How can I help make him feel more comfortable with an exam that has clearly been traumatic in the past?" Other reactions may also arise, including worry/concern ("Why did he wait so long to seek help? What if he now has uterine or cervical cancer?"). Judgmental and dismissive reactions on the part of the clinician may also occur in response to transgender patients but are not considered further here because reactions of this type were already discussed in previous cases.

Confusion is common, as we live in a society in which one of the earliest ways we categorize people is according to their perceived gender. For example, think about the first question that is typically asked about a new baby: "Is it a girl or a boy?" Simply recognizing that it makes sense to feel confusion and anxiety when encountering a transgender or gender-nonconforming patient for the first time can help reduce a clinician's anxiety considerably. It may also be helpful to remember that the degree to which the clinician feels anxious or worried serves as a useful barometer for the level of anxiety and worry the patient, too, is likely experiencing. Sometimes is it useful to name these feelings: "I can imagine that you must be feeling quite anxious and worried about the bleeding you've been having." You can then validate the patient's decision to seek help ("I'm so glad you came in today to get this evaluated") and the clinician's intention to see the evaluation through to conclusion ("Let's talk about what might be going on and what needs to be done to determine the cause of the bleeding. Once we know the cause, we can figure out how to treat you appropriately").

When you knowingly encounter transgender or gender-nonconforming patients for the first time, you have several opportunities to optimize the likelihood of a successful interaction: 1) Be honest with the patients about your lack of experience while at the same time expressing your desire to work with them and a willingness to learn; 2) explicitly ask the patients to let you know immediately if anything you do or fail to do makes them feel uncomfortable; 3) avoid being overly curious (e.g., voyeuristic) by asking questions about their life story that are not pertinent to their medical care (e.g., previous name); 4) apologize promptly when you make a mistake; and 5) discuss various options to make the exam as safe and non-traumatic as possible (see Chapters 8, 17, and 18). Most patients are willing to forgive well-meaning clinicians who make unintentional insensitive remarks, and apologies can be very powerful, providing corrective/reparative experiences for patients who have previously been treated with preponderant disrespect.

Transgender issues are still enough of a societal hot button topic that clinicians caring for transgender and/or gender-nonconforming patients also need to be on the lookout for judgmental reactions and insensitive comments that are voiced by other members of the health care team. If these biased reactions are not addressed appropriately, they may threaten the tentative trust a clinician has started to build with such patients. Examples of common reactions, and suggestions regarding appropriate responses, are considered in the following section.

Case 5: What to Do When an Extreme Reaction Will Not Budge

A clinician who was raised to believe that LGBTQ people are immoral is unable to dispel this thought despite following suggestions similar to those in this chapter, including consultation with a colleague. While he feels able to provide competent care under emergency circumstances, he is aware that his lack of tolerance is preventing him from establishing a warm working relationship with a transgender patient who recently joined his practice and from providing an optimal level of support and guidance.

The situation described in this case is likely to be rare if clinicians follow the suggestions outlined in this chapter. Nonetheless, there may be situations in which clinicians are unwilling to engage in self-inquiry or find themselves unable to change their perspectives toward and ways of interacting with LGBTQ patients despite their best efforts to do so. When this is the case, the overriding principle is the clinician's duty to do no harm, and the best thing to do is to be fully honest both with oneself and the patient and to make a referral to a clinician who will be able to treat the patient with respect and compassion.

When referring an LGBTQ patient to another clinician, you should do so in a manner that communicates caring and respect, rather than disdain and dismissal. Consider the responses of 2 different clinicians to a transgender man's request for a refill of his testosterone prescription after relocating to a new city. Both clinicians were surprised by the request. Clinician A said, in an indignant and disdainful tone, "I can't believe you are asking this of me! Why can't you find some other doctor to do it? I have to deal with all types of people in this profession, and when I don't understand them, I always refer." These responses communicated a derogatory attitude (who wants to be seen as a "type of people"?) and a desire to have nothing further to do with the patient. Clinician B, on the other hand, said, in a thoughtful tone, "I have never knowingly worked with anyone who is transgender before. I'm interested in learning more and figuring out how to help you. I'm sorry that I don't yet know how to prescribe the hormones, but I'm glad you came to see me so I can help you find a provider with this expertise." By offering an apology, the clinician and affirmed the patient's choice to seek care and acknowledged that this may have been a struggle. Inclusion of the word *knowingly* was also affirming, as it demonstrated acceptance of the fact that transgender people exist and may often be invisible, as well as a willingness to embrace that aspect of the patient's identity. Similarly, use of the word *yet* indicated the clinician's intention to learn more and an investment in the care and concerns of the patient. Finally, providing a referral to an educated provider who would be able to help with hormone treatment conveyed a willingness to advocate on behalf of the patient and engendered trust that the clinician would do no harm.

Responding Productively When You See Other People Reacting in a Biased or Insensitive Manner

As we have seen, the process of continually examining and addressing biases and assumptions about people with sexual orientations and gender identities that differ from our own can be challenging, but is also rewarding and necessary if we are to succeed in providing complete and equal care to LGBTQ patients. However, it remains true that many clinicians, trainees, and other personnel working in health care environments have little experience working with LGBTQ patients and may not understand the value of or feel committed to this process. Conscious clinicians can serve as role models and have a responsibility to respond productively when they witness others reacting toward LGBTQ patients in an insensitive manner.

Insensitivity can be expressed intentionally or unintentionally, and may include demeaning comments or jokes about sexual orientation and gender identity and/or derogatory physical gestures (e.g., rolling the eyes or flicking a limp wrist). Real-life examples that have been overheard in the health care setting include: "Who gave my patient such a 'homosexual' dose of diuretic?" (attending physician on an inpatient service). "They should charge homosexuals more for health insurance than they charge the rest of us" (one office staff member to another). "I don't care what they say . . . I think it's just weird for 2 gay men to have a baby" (one office staff member to another). "A lot of people identify as bisexual before they come out as lesbian or gay" (trainee to patient questioning sexual orientation). "Look at that dude in a dress! Is that person a he, a she, or an it?" (one office staff member to another). "You make a beautiful woman—you must have been a handsome man. What did you look like before? Have you had the entire surgery?" (clinician comments to various patients). "Welcome back to being a woman!" (clinician remark after having performed a Papanicolaou test on a transgender man). "She only wants to be a man because she was sexually abused" (preceptor to trainee). While these comments range from some that are overtly unacceptable to others that more subtly lack understanding, all are potentially hurtful. Injury can be avoided and all patients treated with dignity and respect in a health care environment that encourages caregivers to openly examine their biases and to choose their words carefully before speaking.

Table 15–6   Suggested Frame for Constructively Addressing Insensitive Remarks/Jokes

• Notice concrete events you think imply or express insensitivity/bias.

• Push the "pause button" before responding in order to:

• Perform an emotional check-in. Do you have the clarity to respond effectively on the spot, or do you need to take a time-out before proceeding?

• Evaluate the risk of responding. Is it safe to proceed immediately, or do you need to seek assistance or support (as may be the case if the person who made the remark/joke is your supervisor/boss) before you intervene?

• Consider whether this is a "teachable moment." When an insensitive remark or joke is made in front of bystanders, consider the merits of a public (educates others, makes a broader statement) versus a private (less likely to cause embarrassment/humiliation) response.

• When it feels safe and the timing and context are appropriate, reach out to the person who made the insensitive/biased remark or joke.

• Start with a statement, a question, or a statement-question pair (see below). Use "I," not "you," statements in a nonconfrontational and nonjudgmental tone. The goals are to let the offender know how you feel about what was said and to express curiosity about their beliefs, not to criticize or focus on what they did "wrong."

• Listen respectfully to the person's responses, then ask additional clarifying questions and/or provide factual information that contradicts stereotypes and alternate language that is not derogatory.

• Continue the dialogue over time. Sometimes people need to hear more than once that their remarks or jokes are not acceptable.

• Be firm and set limits when necessary. None of us has the right to dictate another person's beliefs/sense of humor; however, we do have the right to request that insensitive remarks or jokes not be used in our own or our patients' presence.

Adapted with permission from the work of Diane Goodman (Goodman D. Promoting Diversity and Social Justice: Educating People from Privileged Groups. New York: Routledge; 2011).

It is not always easy to respond productively when colleagues express negative attitudes about LGBTQ patients or when a coworker makes a homo-, bi- or trans-phobic remark or joke. This is especially true when there is a power dynamic in play, as when a trainee hears an attending physician make the disparaging comment. However, silence is the voice of complicity, and if we don't speak up when we feel we should do so, we are likely to experience a sense of personal disappointment and guilt. Clinicians can serve as invaluable role models by treating all patients with respect and being clear with others that, while they have a right to their own beliefs and opinions, anti-LGBTQ remarks or jokes cannot be tolerated in the health care environment. The goal is not to start an argument or generate hostility but rather to build bridges across differences and to increase understanding.

Project Implicit (21), the Anti-Defamation League (22), Diane Goodman (23), and others have developed guidelines that can be used to address insensitive remarks or jokes. Tables 15-6 and 15-7 and 15-8 present an

Table 15-7   Sample Statements and Questions for Constructively Addressing Insensitive Remarks/Jokes

Sample Statements

Use "I" versus "you" statements:

I feel differently.

I don't believe that's true.

My experience has been different, and rather than letting that statement stand, I'd like to share my perspective.

I'm concerned that making generalizations like that can be hurtful.

It seems to me that we might be treating patient A differently than other patients because of their LGBTQ identity.

Express your feelings:

I'm uncomfortable when I hear you talk about a person (or specific group) in that way. I'd like you to stop.

Separate intent from impact:

I'm sure you didn't intentionally mean to be hurtful, but when you use that term . . .

I know you were just trying to be funny, but I found that joke offensive because . . .

I'm sure you can find jokes that don't put down other people.

Appeal to values and principles:

I've always thought of you as a fair-minded person, so it surprises me when I hear you say something like that.

I know you want to have a respectful and inclusive work environment; those kinds of statements just aren't consistent with that.

Consider what's in it for them:

I know you didn't support him being hired, but our trainees have been asking for more diversity in our staff and for more people who share their experiences. I think he will be an important addition and will enhance our department and enrollments.

She will really help us work with some of our patients. She understands LGBTQ culture and can help reduce the distrust.

Talk about how you used to feel, think, or say similar things but have changed:

I used to make assumptions like that too, but then I learned that they are untrue generalizations or stereotypes, so now I try to catch myself.

I used to use those terms, but then I heard they can be offensive because . . .

Better language I've learned is . . .

I used to laugh or tell jokes like that, but then I realized how hurtful they are to people. I don't do it anymore and I'd like you to stop too.

Focus on fairness/kindness and ensuring dignity and respect:

I believe in treating every patient the way I want to be treated myself.

All of our patients deserve to be treated fairly and with respect.

Remind people of their obligation and liability:

In this workplace, our rules of conduct obligate us to speak respectfully of LGBTQ people.

That behavior could be considered discriminatory against LGBTQ people and we have a policy against discriminating on the basis of [sexual orientation] [gender identity].

Table 15-7   Sample Statements and Questions for Constructively Addressing Insensitive Remarks/Jokes (*Continued*)

Sample Questions

Repeat back what was said to ensure you are hearing the person correctly and to help them hear the bias and stereotyping in their remarks:

What I hear you saying is that all gay men practice unsafe sex. Am I hearing you correctly?

It seems that you're describing all bisexual people as unstable or undecided. Am I hearing you correctly?

Ask clarifying questions to determine why these persons hold these views to provide you with more information so you can address misconceptions and to help them realize how what they are saying is unfounded or does not make a lot of sense:

I'm wondering . . . how did you develop that belief?

How many people have you treated who are LGBTQ?

Do you know what research shows about the adjustment of children who have gay parents?

Play dumb to force people to think more about their remarks/jokes:

I'm sorry; what's so funny?

I'm sorry, but I'm not sure I know what you meant by "bull dyke." Can you explain that term?

I notice you used the pronoun "she" when you were talking about Jimmy during rounds. I'm curious . . . how did you decide to do that?

I'm not sure what his [sexual orientation] [gender identity] had to do with the story . . . did I miss something?

Encourage empathy:

I know you meant it as a joke, but how would you feel if someone said something like that about your spouse/girlfriend/sister/daughter?

I know you hate it when people make jokes that are anti-[religious group] [racial group] [other group with which the person identifies]. It's not OK to make jokes about other minority groups either.

Tie tolerance to the bottom line:

Is "faggot" really a word we should be throwing around? We don't know who's gay and who's straight, who has gay relatives and who doesn't. I think that comment could really upset some people and distract them from their work.

Adapted with permission from the work of Diane Goodman (Goodman D. Promoting Diversity and Social Justice: Educating People from Privileged Groups. New York: Routledge; 2011).

adapted framework based largely on Dr. Goodman's work. It starts by noticing or recognizing when a colleague or coworker makes an insensitive joke or remark, and involves expressing curiosity about the source of the person's beliefs and providing factual information that challenges those perspectives. It is based on an assumption of good will (giving the person the benefit of the doubt) and a desire to maintain a connection with (as opposed to potentially alienating) the person who made the remark or joke. Most people who make insensitive comments do so out of ignorance. Similarly, most people do not tell jokes to purposefully hurt or embarrass others, and will stop if they realize this is the effect of their attempt at humor. Finally, people tend to listen better and to be more open when they know that they matter to the person who is speaking up or intervening.

In addition to addressing bias on a personal level, as outlined in Table 15-6 and Table 15-7, clinicians can play a leadership role in raising institutional awareness by ensuring that LGBTQ issues and topics are regularly included in formal training seminars, curricula, programming, and professional development workshops, whenever appropriate. A variety of training and educational resources are available at www.lgbthealtheducation.org.

Cultivating, Enriching, and Maintaining Sustained Connections With Ourselves and Others

In behavioral health disciplines, inclusion of supervision sessions, in which not only beginning trainees but also seasoned practitioners have an opportunity for regular reflection and self-inquiry, is considered to be an integral aspect of clinical practice. Surprisingly, few such opportunities exist in medical and surgical disciplines. A sizable literature addresses the problem of clinician burnout, which results from excessive workload, loss of autonomy, administrative burdens, litigation threats, a reduction in personal meaning due to less time spent with patients and colleagues, and difficulties integrating/balancing personal and professional life. It can manifest as numbness, disconnection, and heightened reactivity, and clinicians who suffer burnout are more prone to errors, less empathetic, and more likely to treat patients like diagnoses or objects. Solutions are desperately needed to build resiliency and restore inspiration, creativity, balance, and a sense of joy in our calling (3). While not directly related to care of LGBTQ patients specifically, this topic is so important to the maintenance of a clinician's clarity, curiosity, creativity, and compassion that it is included as an integral part of this chapter.

Table 15-8 presents several strategies clinicians can use to reduce stress and promote connection with all aspects of themselves—not just their clinical practitioner/academician/researcher personas—and with all of the other important people in their lives, including friends, family, and colleagues. Doing no harm begins with oneself, as expressed by the oft-quoted phrase: "Physician, heal thyself."

Summary Points on How to Form Creative and Compassionate Partnerships With LGBTQ Patients

- Make this an explicit goal for yourself.
- Be willing to step outside your comfort zone to stretch your experience and grow.

Table 15–8   Strategies to Promote Inspiration, Creativity, Connection, and Renewal

At work:

* Regularly set aside a "check-out" time in which to breathe and "check in" with yourself to see what your needs are in the moment.
* Make time in your schedule periodically to have coffee with a colleague.
* Find mentors with whom you can talk about personal reactions that come up in the context of your work.
* Start a group activity with colleagues that will foster support and connection:
  * Convert peer review sessions (which can at times feel punitive) into case discussions where participants feel comfortable sharing their questions and doubts.
  * Consider starting a writing group in which participants reflect on their clinical practice and have an opportunity to share their writing with other members of the group.
* Consider starting a regular rounds (such as the Schwartz Center Rounds; please see www.theschwartzcenter.org/supporting-caregivers/schwartz-center-rounds), during which clinicians and other members of the care team have an opportunity to talk about the joys and challenges of being caregivers.
* Set limits (boundaries) that will support work-life balance (e.g., don't be afraid to advocate for a flexible-hours, part-time, or job-sharing arrangement).
  * Try to maintain your sense of humor.

Outside work:

* Take care of your body: obtain adequate sleep, nutrition, and regular exercise.
* Engage in specific stress-reduction techniques, such as meditation or yoga.
* Commit to a spiritual practice, if this is meaningful to you.
* Make time in your schedule to spend with friends and family members.
* Pursue hobbies, travel, and other non–work-related activities you enjoy.
* Consider working with a psychotherapist or life coach.

---

* Be open-minded to the possibility that every new patient may have any gender identity or sexual orientation, or engage in any sexual behavior; avoid making assumptions based on stereotypes or generalizing from your own experience.
* Seek training experiences in venues that cater to large numbers of LGBTQ individuals so you will have many opportunities to practice, but remain mindful that you may encounter an LGBTQ person anywhere, when you least expect it.
* Go through the motions even if you don't feel ready ("fake it till you make it"; act "as if"). Start by asking open-ended or specific questions suggested in clinical guidelines and Chapter 8 in this book, even if it feels uncomfortable at first.
* Routinely perform a quick internal scan, looking for and acknowledging any emotional reactions that arise in response to being in an

unfamiliar situation or meeting a person whose life story and circumstances you have not encountered before.

- Be kind to yourself. Refrain from self-recrimination if you identify a reaction that seems excessive, extreme, or otherwise unacceptable at first glance. Generally, the more intense the reaction, the greater the underlying sense of threat to the status quo and the more urgently your attention and care are needed. It is also helpful to keep in mind that we all have many different, seemingly contradictory reactions at any time, and any one reaction is just that—it represents just one part of you and not all of you.

- At the same time that you are self-scanning and carrying out your internal inquiry, be careful to maintain safety for the patient by making a conscious commitment to refrain from speaking or acting impulsively from the perspective of any extreme reaction.

- Ask each reaction to reveal itself more to you: Where is it coming from? What is its intention? Generally even our most extreme reactions make sense when we take the time and make the effort to understand them better.

- Validate the intention of each reaction if it makes sense to you, and ask if anything further is needed in order for you to proceed in your encounter with the patient. Often simple acknowledgment will be enough for a reaction to relax back and feel less urgent.

- You will know you are on safe ground to continue your interaction with the patient when you feel clear, calm, and connected, and can approach yourself and the patient with curiosity, creativity, and compassion. In general, "C" words are highly indicative of groundedness and safety. Other C words to keep in mind include courage, confidence, and collaboration.

- If you continue to feel highly reactive and detect an urge to speak or act from the perspective of any of your reactions, excuse yourself from the clinical encounter to give yourself an opportunity to "unblend" from the extreme viewpoint, and obtain consultation to help you understand why the patient is provoking such a strong response. Chances are that if you are feeling this way, your mentor or peer has been there too at some point and may be able to help.

- If and when consultation is not successful, it is always acceptable—and indeed the responsible thing to do—to refer the patient to another provider who will be able to maintain a constructive approach.

- Even when you are on track and have the best intentions, you will still occasionally make mistakes that may hurt or otherwise offend a patient. When this happens, acknowledge the mistake, apologize to the patient, and set an intention to learn from the experience so it is not repeated in the future.

- It is okay—even desirable—not to be an expert. Be honest when you don't know something and offer to try to find out. Resist the impulse to pretend you know more than you know; this might result in providing harmful misinformation. In essence, none of us is ever truly expert, as learning is a continual process, and all cultures are fluid and ever changing.

- Ask for feedback—from mentors, peers, and especially from patients. Consider talking about the clinician–patient relationship as a partnership up front and asking patients to let you know when and if something isn't working for them. Inviting people who have been neglected and marginalized to join in arriving at a solution sends a powerful message and can be very healing.

- Whether you are or will be in a formal teaching role, the culture of health care training ("watch one, do one, teach one") and the team structure of health care delivery mean that you will frequently find yourself in a teaching role of sorts toward other members of the care team (e.g., as a role model or mentor). Remember that your behavior sets an example for others and take care to always act in a responsible and respectful manner.

- Speak up when you witness others making insensitive remarks or jokes about or displaying reactive behaviors toward LGBTQ patients. Silence implies indifference to or even approval of what was said, and lack of action condones unacceptable behaviors.

- Don't go it alone. Be in it with others. Share the discomforts (a little sense of humor can go a long way) and celebrate the successes. We all need support. We can all learn from one another.

Acknowledgments

I would like to thank Richard C. Schwartz, who developed the Internal Family Systems model (24) on which much of this chapter is based, as well as Ida Bernstein, Kristen Eckstrand, and Ruben Hopwood for their helpful suggestions on the manuscript.

References

1. **Steptoe A, Shankar A, Demakakos P, Wardle J**. Social isolation, loneliness, and all-cause mortality in older men and women. Proc Natl Acad Sci U S A. 2013;110:5797-801.
2. **Flickinger TE, Saha S, Moore RD, Beach MC**. Higher quality communication and relationships are associated with improved patient engagement in HIV care. J Acquir Immune Defic Syndr. 2013;63:362-6.
3. **Swetz KM, Harrington SE, Matsuyama RK, Shanafelt TD, Lyckholm LJ**. Strategies for avoiding burnout in hospice medicine and palliative care: peer advice from physicians on achieving longevity and fulfillment. J Palliative Med 2009;12:773-7.
4. **GLMA**. Guidelines for Care of Lesbian, Gay, Bisexual, and Transgender Patients. 2006. Available at: www.glma.org.
5. **Coleman E, Bockting W, Botzer M, et al**. Standards of care for the health of transsexual, transgender, and gender nonconforming people, 7th version. World Professional Association for Transgender Health; 2013. Available at: www.wpath.org.

6. **Center of Excellence for Transgender Health.** Primary care protocol for transgender patient care. 2011. Available at: http://transhealth.ucsf.edu/trans?page=protocol-00-00.

7. **The National LGBT Health Education Center.** Available at: www.lgbthealtheducation.org.

8. **The Joint Commission.** Advancing effective communication, cultural competence, and patient- and family-centered care for the lesbian, gay, bisexual, and transgender (LGBT) community: a field guide. 2011. Available at: www.jointcommission.org/lgbt/.

9. **Hollenbach AD, Eckstrand KL, Dreger A, eds.** Implementing Curricular and Institutional Climate Changes to Improve Health Care for Individuals Who Are LGBT, Gender Noncon-forming, or Born With DSD: A Resource for Medical Educators. Association of American Medical Colleges. November 2014. Available at: www.aamc.org/lgbtdsd.

10. **MedEdPORTAL.** Lesbian, Gay, Bisexual, Transgender and/or Differences of Sex Development-affected Patient Care Project. Available at: https://www.mededportal.org/icollaborative/about/initiatives/lgbt/.

11. **MedEdPORTAL.** Lesbian, Gay, Bisexual, Transgender and/or Differences of Sex Develop-ment-affected Patient Care Project: a call for submissions for innovative and effective prac-tices and competency-based teaching & assessment resources for the undergraduate medical education curriculum. Available at: https://www.mededportal.org/icollaborative/about/initiatives/lgbt/.

12. **Institute of Medicine.** The Health of Lesbian, Gay, Bisexual, and Transgender People: Build-ing a Foundation for Better Understanding. Washington, DC: The National Academies Press; 2011.

13. **Jost JT, Banaji MR, Nosek BA.** A decade of system justification theory: accumulated evidence of conscious and unconscious bolstering of the status quo. Polit Psychol 2004;25:881-919.

14. **Riddle D.** The Riddle Scale. Alone No More: Developing a School Support System for Gay, Lesbian and Bisexual Youth. St. Paul: Minnesota State Department; 1994.

15. **Wright LW, Adams HE, Bernat J.** Development and validation of the homophobia scale. J Psychopathol Behav Assess 1999;21:337-47.

16. **McIntosh P.** White privilege and male privilege: a personal account of coming to see corre-spondences through work in women's studies. Working paper #189. Wellesley, MA: Wellesley College Center of Research on Women; 1988.

17. **Unpacking the invisible knapsack.** II. Sexual orientation. www.cs.earlham.edu/˜hyrax/personal/files/student_res/straightprivilege.htm

18. **Gender privilege.** University of Texas Gender and Sexuality Center. Available at: www.utexas.edu/diversity/ddce/gsc/downloads/resources/Gender_Privilege.pdf.

19. **Woodford MR, Kulick A, Sinco BR, Hong JS.** Contemporary heterosexism on campus and psychological distress among LGBQ students: the mediating role of self-acceptance. Am J Orthopsychiatry. 2014 Aug 11. [Epub ahead of print]

20. **Carter L, Mollen D, Smith NG.** Locus of control, minority stress, and psychological distress among lesbian, gay, and bisexual individuals. J Couns Psychol. 2014;61:169-75.

21. **Project Implicit.** Available at: https://implicit.harvard.edu/implicit/demo/selectatest.html.

22. **Anti-Defamation League.** Education & outreach. Available at: www.adl.org/education.

23. **Diane J. Goodman, EdD.** Available at: www.dianegoodman.com.

24. **Schwartz RC.** Introduction to the Internal Family Systems Model. Oak Park, IL: Trailheads Publications; 2001.

Gender Identity and Health

Chapter 16

Gender Nonconformity and Gender Discordance in Childhood and Adolescence: Developmental Considerations and the Clinical Approach

SCOTT LEIBOWITZ, MD
STEWART ADELSON, MD
CYNTHIA TELINGATOR, MD

Introduction

In recent years there has been growing social awareness, as reflected in media and popular culture, that some children and adolescents' gender identity or gender-related behavior varies substantially from population averages and societal norms. Health care providers are increasingly being asked to play a key role in supporting the unique physical and mental health care needs of these youth and to do so at earlier ages (1,2). Guidelines and standards shaped by scientific study and social advocacy have begun to emerge to guide clinical practice, although there remains a pressing need for further research to fully inform policies and best practices in this area (3–5).

Clinicians caring for these children and adolescents may encounter various challenges. For example, when the possibility of social gender transition, cross-sex hormonal therapy, and/or gender affirmation surgery are raised by youths and/or their parents, the informed consent procedures that apply in patient-initiated gender transition by adults must be adapted to the developmental and medico-legal status of minors. Complicating this type of decision-making is the fact that youths' gender-related developmental outcome is not always clear, and that their developmental stage may not allow them to understand or verbalize their gender-related experiences in adult terms.

Furthermore, current best practice models of care for these youths sometimes presume the availability of a multidisciplinary team that includes mental health specialists working in collaboration with primary care providers over a sustained period. However, in some communities, that may not be a readily available option. Many communities lack ideal resources or present unique challenges related to local social and cultural factors. Nonetheless, providers in these communities do find themselves caring for gender-variant children and adolescents who desire support and/or medical intervention.

The goal of this chapter, therefore, is to provide clinicians a framework for understanding and addressing many of the concerns and issues raised by children, adolescents, and their parents around gender-variant behaviors and identities. To that end, the chapter will 1) describe basic concepts related to gender-variant children and adolescents; 2) explain what is currently known about the gender and sexual identity outcomes of these youths; 3) provide an approach within a developmental framework for the assessment and clinical care of these youths; 4) explain how to apply best practices in a variety of clinical settings, with an emphasis on guiding the primary care provider to promote healthy outcomes; and 5) help promote an awareness of the limits of current knowledge and the need for further research to guide best clinical practice.

Definitions and Concepts

It is important for clinicians working with children and adolescents to understand several terms and concepts related to gender role behavior and gender identity development. Children and adolescents may present with a variety of gender-variant behaviors and feelings. These variations may be mild or marked; transient and limited to childhood or persistent through adolescence into adulthood; and related to a developing gay, lesbian, or bisexual sexual orientation, transgender identity, neither, or both (6). The definitions below reflect current terminology in the medical and mental health literature.

Gender Role Behavior and Gender Nonconformity

The American Academy of Child & Adolescent Psychiatry's Practice Parameter on Gay, Lesbian, or Bisexual Sexual Orientation, Gender Nonconformity, and Gender Discordance in Children and Adolescents (AACAP LGBT Practice Parameter) defines *gender role behavior* as "personal and social attributes that are recognized as masculine or feminine. This can relate to a youth's activities, interests, use of symbols, styles, or other personal and social attributes that are recognized as masculine or feminine," and is connected to how one portrays one's subjective sense of gender in such areas as dress, speech, and/or mannerisms, which is often defined as *gender expression* (4). *Gender role norms* refer to societal expectations of various aspects of gender that are conventionally identified as masculine or feminine. How one's expression of gender is perceived by others depends on the cultural context. Certain aspects of gender role behavior emerge as early as age 2 years, when male and female toddlers begin to display culturally defined gender-specific preferences in toys (e.g., dolls for girls and trucks for boys). As children develop, gender-specific preferences also show up in interests, hobbies and pastimes, clothing styles, and other personal attributes, as well as in means of expressing emotions.

Gender nonconformity refers to variation from developmental norms in gender role behavior. In males, examples of gender nonconforming behaviors might include an aversion to rough-and-tumble play or a predilection for conventionally feminine clothing, toys, games, and other pastimes. In females, gender nonconformity might include an aversion to wearing stereotypical feminine clothing, interest in rough-and-tumble play, or a preference for toys and games that are typically preferred by boys. In many cultures, gender nonconformity in childhood is a common developmental precursor to same-sex sexual orientation, especially in males, and may be a main reason why many gay men and lesbian women report having felt different from their peers as children.

Gender Identity and Gender Discordance

Gender identity is a concept distinct from gender role behavior. The AACAP LGBT Practice Parameter defines gender identity as "an individual's personal sense of self as male or female. For most, it develops by age three, is concordant with a person's sex and gender, and remains stable over the lifetime. For a small number of individuals it can change later in life" (4).

Gender discordance describes a disjunction between gender identity and the sex that a person was assigned at birth (also known as *natal sex*). Unlike gender nonconformity, which involves behavior and expression, gender discordance relates to identity. Gender discordance is a basic aspect of being transgender: that is, a transgender person is someone whose gender identity varies from their natal sex and/or assigned gender. Some transgender people have a gender identity that is the opposite of their natal sex (e.g., a natal female whose gender identity is male), and some have a gender identity that is not exclusively male or female.

Gender Dysphoria

Gender dysphoria refers to the distress, or affective disturbance, that individuals may experience when their gender identity does not match their physical anatomy (i.e., feelings of distress related to gender discordance). Gender dysphoria is the new diagnostic term used in the fifth edition of the American Psychiatric Association's *Diagnostic and Statistical Manual of Mental Disorders* (*DSM-5*) for children, adolescents, and adults experiencing this type of distress (7). It replaces "gender identity disorder (GID)," which many felt stigmatized transgender people by labeling them as "disordered." These changes to the DSM were made at a time when the biological, social, and other influences on gender development remain unclear. Policy implications continue to be debated by professionals, advocates, and society at large. Some have called for removing gender dysphoria from the DSM altogether, but the APA has kept it in as a way to continue to facilitate access to individualized health care treatments that alleviate distress and allow people to feel comfortable with their own body, identity, and expressions. Because gender dysphoria typically diminishes or disappears after appropriate treatments are given, the DSM-5 also includes a post-transition specifier to continue to allow access to appropriate maintenance treatments, such as cross-sex hormones. Gender discordance in children and youth is often, but not always, accompanied by gender dysphoria. The extent of dysphoria may be very much influenced by current cultural norms that view gender as binary (male or female) and as always concurrent with birth sex, in addition to the distress created by a discrepancy between physical sex and gender identity. As cultural norms shift more toward acceptance of nonbinary views of gender, and if stigma against transgender identities decreases, experiences of dysphoria may greatly diminish.

Comparison of Gender Nonconformity and Gender Discordance

Gender nonconformity and gender discordance are fundamentally different in phenomenology, influences, and developmental course, although these phenomena can occur together or overlap in an individual. Gender-discordant youth feel their gender is the opposite of, or otherwise different from, their natal sex, and they typically feel comforted when perceived by others in that way. In contrast, youth who are gender nonconforming but not gender discordant might be distressed by the perception that they are a gender that differs from the one they were assigned at birth; for them, despite gender-nonconforming behavior, there is no discordance between gender identity and natal sex. While many youths display gender nonconformity without experiencing gender discordance, youths with gender discordance frequently display extreme gender nonconformity. To illustrate the differences between gender-nonconforming youths with and without gender discordance at different life stages, and to begin to present some of the challenging health care needs for these youths, we offer the following vignettes:

Vignette: Gender Nonconformity Without
Gender Discordance in a Prepubertal Child
Tommy, an 8-year-old natal boy, dislikes rough-and-tumble sports that other boys relish, enjoys toys and games such as playing with dolls and occasional dress-up (in some boys, this might involve wearing an occasional costume; for others, this might include occasional cross-gender dressing). He prefers the companionship of female playmates

who tend to play more gently. This leads to some teasing by peers, as well as parental anxiety and disapproval. Although Tommy sometimes seems sad, self-conscious, and embarrassed about not being like the other boys, he has never expressed a desire to be perceived of as a girl, and in fact gets upset when other boys tease him for being "like a girl."

This case illustrates a child whose gender role behavior does not conform to cultural norms in favored games and playmate preference (gender nonconformity). It is a common pattern in boys who may grow up to be gay, although it does not always precede homosexuality. While Tommy likes to do things that many girls often like to do, there is no evidence that this boy thinks of himself as or wants to be a girl (i.e., no evidence of gender discordance).

Vignette: Gender Nonconformity With Gender Discordance in a Prepubertal Child

Brianna, an 8-year-old natal girl, has displayed a preference for toy trucks, action hero figures, and various sports ever since she could verbalize her wishes. From a young age, she threw tantrums when asked to wear a dress or a skirt. More recently, she quit playing softball with the "girl team" and asked her parents if she can play baseball on the "boy team" instead. Her mother explains that Brianna has asked to use the boys' bathroom at school because she prefers the urinal, and her mother suspects Brianna is standing to urinate over the toilet because she has found urine on the floor next to the toilet several times. On a few occasions, Brianna has said to her mom, "I wish I was a boy." Brianna has asked to be called "Brian," and her mother wonders whether she should go ahead and do so in order to avoid upsetting her child and causing tantrums.

This vignette illustrates a prepubertal child who displays both variation from expected gender roles, such as preferred games and pastimes (gender nonconformity), and also behavior, feelings, and verbalizations indicating a wish to be, or comfort in being perceived as, belonging to the gender opposite to that assigned at birth (gender discordance). This child may continue to experience gender discordance as she ages, but it is also possible that her feelings of gender discordance will fade by puberty.

Unfortunately, it is sometimes clinically challenging when working with younger children to determine unequivocally whether they are gender nonconforming, gender discordant, or both. Many children do not yet have the cognitive development, maturity, or coping skills necessary to clearly experience, organize, and express their gender experiences. This can be especially true for children who are experiencing shame, guilt, anxiety, or social or family pressure to conform to prevailing norms. Because of these factors, some children who are gender discordant but unable to say so may express gender discordance through extreme and persistent gender nonconformity.

The understanding of these issues, for both the child and the clinician, may evolve as the child develops cognitively, emotionally, and physically. This child's current expressed wish to "be a boy" raises a typical clinical challenge in knowing how to best respond. There are potential risks and benefits to different approaches, as will be discussed later in the chapter.

Vignette: Gender Nonconformity and Discordance in a Pubertal Youth

Aiden, a 12-year-old natal male, presents with a lifelong history of cross-gender behaviors and has asked to be referred to as Allison on many occasions. He has only female friends and has enjoyed wearing princess dresses ever since he was a young child. He would throw temper tantrums when taken for haircuts. As a result, his parents relented and allowed him to grow his hair out. They report that he would refuse to play sports and would become angry when grouped together with boys in academic and social settings. In the past 2 months, his parents note that Aiden has become extremely sad and withdrawn. They also observe that he appears uncomfortable about his developing secondary sexual characteristics; for example, since showing signs of puberty he tucks his penis between his legs so it is not noticeable when wearing bathing suits.

This youth displays persistently pronounced gender-nonconforming behaviors that suggest gender discordance, with a possible diagnosis of gender dysphoria at the beginning stages of puberty. Although this child is older, he still may not have the cognitive development skills to clearly express his gender experience. Adolescents are generally more capable than children of abstract thinking and self-reflection, but they may also have challenges in organizing and expressing gender-related concerns, especially if family non-acceptance, peer harassment, or other forms of stigma are present. For some youths, it will not be possible to clarify their gender status; these youths need more time before their gender development and needs become clear. Interventions for youths this age might include pubertal suppression therapy that delays the onset of physical changes associated with puberty in order to allow more time for identity development; more on this type of intervention will be discussed later in this chapter.

Vignette: Gender Nonconformity Without Gender Discordance in Adolescence

Maggie, a 15-year-old adolescent female, enjoys physical play and sports and prefers the companionship of male peers. She feels she shares more interests with male peers than female peers, and she feels physically and emotionally uncomfortable in dresses, skirts, and other clothing that may be perceived as "feminine." She has a short haircut and eschews the make-up that other female classmates wear. She is ostracized by many peers and is not invited to be a part of the popular cliques that exist in the high school, and she has experienced tension with her parents over her choices of clothing, hairstyle, and grooming. She nevertheless has an unequivocal sense of herself as being a girl. She feels very warmly toward female friends and is confused about whether she is attracted to them sexually, wondering if she might be bisexual or lesbian. Because of feelings of isolation and shame, she experiences bouts of depression, and recently has implied she has occasional suicidal thoughts.

This teenage girl has persistent gender nonconformity in play, style of dress and grooming, and peer affiliation, but no signs of gender discordance or dysphoria. This pattern is seen in some, although by no means all, females growing up lesbian or bisexual; it is also seen in some young women who grow up to be heterosexual adults. This case also points to the possible mental health impact of gender nonconformity in teenagers, including a greater likelihood of depression, anxiety, substance use, self-injurious behavior, and suicidal thought or behavior.

As can be inferred from these 4 vignettes, the health care and support needs of gender-nonconforming children and adolescents without gender discordance are quite different from youth with gender discordance. It is vitally important for clinicians to understand this difference in order to know when different types of support are needed, as well as when certain mental health and medical interventions should be considered. The details of how to clinically approach these differing needs will be explored in detail later in this chapter.

Other Terms to Know

Gender variance is a term that has been used to refer broadly to the entire spectrum of variation from population norms in both gender role behavior and gender identity, subsuming gender nonconformity and gender discordance with or without gender dysphoria. Another broader term that can be used to refer to youth who are gender variant is *gender minority youth*. This term differs from *sexual minority youth*, which refers to those who identify as having same-sex attractions, arousal patterns, same-sex sexual behaviors, or identities along the spectrum of sexuality. Today's youth have used other terms in colloquial language. *Pansexual* often refers to having a sexual identity that includes attractions to members of any gender, not strictly those along the male-female binary. *Genderqueer* is a term of gender identity used to identify those who blur or bend the gender binary, identify outside of the gender binary (i.e., neither male nor female, agender) and/or identify as both male and female. *Cisgender*, an antonym for *transgender*, refers to individuals whose gender identity is concordant with their natal sex (i.e., anyone who is not transgender).

Historical Context

Contextualizing the scientific understanding, theoretical conceptualizations, and clinical matters pertaining to gender and sexuality within a historical framework is important. Changing social and medical attitudes and increased awareness and appreciation of the complexity of being human have led to revisions of the *DSM*, including the removal of "homosexuality" in the 1970s and the inclusion of categories of "gender identity disorder" (GID) in the *DSM-III* in 1980 (8,9). Historically, the constructs of gender identity and sexual orientation were conflated as one phenomenon, which restricted research and clinical efforts and prevented practitioners from identifying both the overlapping and divergent health needs. The diagnosis of homosexuality in the original *DSM*, consistent with the thinking at the time, broadly included individuals whose gender identity did not conform to societal norms. Many have argued that the inclusion of these phenomena as diagnoses within the *DSM* perpetuated societal stigmatization of people whose expression of gender role or sexual behavior deviated from the majority (10). The removal of homosexuality from the *DSM* and the inclusion of GID in subsequent DSM versions reflected an evolved understanding that gender identity and sexual orientation are distinct phenomena, yet led many to question why transgenderism continued to constitute pathology when homosexuality no longer did.

In 2013, GID was replaced in the *DSM-5* with the less pathologizing "gender dysphoria," described above. The intent of these changes was to recognize the distress that can accompany gender discordance and need for interventions to alleviate that distress through strategies that may include sex reassignment, without pathologizing the individual's transgender identity itself. The changes were also intended to depathologize the experience by removing the word "disorder" and adding a "post-transition" specifier that implies gender transition to be a valid intervention for individuals experiencing gender dysphoria.

Despite these changes, bias against lesbian, gay, bisexual, and transgender (LGBT) individuals has persisted in society and within health care (3,5). As described in other chapters of this textbook (see especially Chapter 5), the scientific medical and mental health literature has established associations with poor health outcomes for LGBT youth that included higher rates of suicidal ideations, parasuicidal behaviors, and suicide attempts, health risk behaviors (substance abuse, high-risk sexual behavior leading to higher risk for sexually transmitted infections), and mental health disorders (affective and anxiety disorders) (3). These poor health outcomes do not necessarily reflect inherent pathology. Rather, the literature has established that the increased prevalence of mental health and substance use disorders is largely or entirely mediated by social or environmental stress (often referred to as "minority stress") created by marginalization, victimization, and isolation within society (11,12). Professional organizations are prioritizing the understanding of LGBT populations to determine appropriate health interventions and research initiatives. For example, the Institute of Medicine published a report of LBGT health disparities research (3), and AACAP published practice guidelines for clinicians to reference in the clinical management of issues pertaining to sexuality and gender (4).

Developmental Outcomes for Gender-Variant Youth

Research on Sexual Orientation Outcomes

A limited but growing number of research studies have looked at the sexual orientation and gender identity outcomes of gender-nonconforming youths, including those with and those without gender discordance. Several research studies have found that gender-nonconforming behavior in childhood is significantly correlated with a homosexual sexual orientation in adulthood for both females and, especially, males. For example, retrospective studies in a diversity of cultures (13–15) have found that gay men and lesbian women in adulthood recall more gender-nonconforming behaviors and/or cross-gender identities in childhood compared with heterosexual men and women. Several prospective studies have found that males who display cross-gender behaviors in childhood have more than a 60% likelihood of becoming bisexual or homosexual in late adolescence or young adulthood (13). Prospective studies of children with definitive or likely gender discordance who were referred to specialty clinics and followed into adolescence also found high rates (24% to 82%) of bisexual or homosexual developmental outcomes (16–19). Despite these strong findings, gender nonconformity and discordance in childhood were not absolutely correlated with homosexuality in any of these studies: that is, not all gender-nonconforming or -discordant children became gay or bisexual and not all gay or bisexual adults were gender nonconforming in childhood.

Research on Gender Discordance Outcomes

Prospective studies of children referred to specialty clinics have also looked to see how often gender discordance persisted into adolescence, and what characteristics predicted this outcome. These studies found that the percentage of children who continued to experience gender discordance (or possible gender discordance) in adolescence ranged from 1.5% to 37% (16–20). The variability in ranges may reflect differences in the cohorts studied. The study finding the lowest rate of persistent gender discordance possibly included extremely gender-nonconforming, but not clearly gender-discordant, children among the participants, while studies finding greater rates of persistence included only clearly gender-discordant children by *DSM-IV* GID criteria. These findings suggest that "most children with gender dysphoria will not remain gender dysphoric after puberty" (16) in clinically referred samples.

Two of these prospective studies (both from Amsterdam, the Netherlands) suggest that many factors predicted the persistence of these feelings into adolescence (16,20). The most significant predictive factor was intensity of childhood gender discordance. Other predictive factors included cognitive and/or affective cross-gender identification, age at presentation with gender dysphoria (particularly for natal girls), and having made a social role transition (particularly for natal boys). In addition, gender-discordant natal girls presenting to a gender identity specialty clinic were more likely to continue to experience gender discordance in adolescence (50%) than were natal boys (29%) (20).

A qualitative retrospective study on the experiences of adolescents whose gender discordance persisted compared with those whose discordance did not persist indicated differences in the motivations of their early childhood cross-gender identifications (21). While they all reported a desire to be the other gender in childhood, those whose discordance subsided seemed to have been motivated more by a desire to have the opportunity to live in their preferred gender role; in contrast, those adolescents whose gender discordance persisted experienced a cognitive and affective cross-gender identification (i.e., the thought and feeling that their true gender did not match their natal sex) when they were younger. This study, which included 25 adolescents, determined that the period between 10 and 13 years of age was crucial in consolidating their identities. The anticipated actual feminization or masculinization of their bodies, changes in their social environment (including the perception of increased social distance between males and females), and first experiences of sexual attractions to others occurred during this period. During this time, youth whose cross-gender identifications diminished began developing more typically cisgender interests and behaviors, although gender-nonconforming behaviors also persisted. Many of those who came to identify as cisgender in adolescence occupied what might be an intermediate point in a nonbinary gender identity spectrum. For others, cross-gender identification greatly increased in intensity and consolidated a transgender identity. Many developed attractions to others of their natal sex, although because of their cross-gender identifications, none considered themselves to be gay or lesbian.

The data from most of these (more recent) studies were obtained from clinically referred samples, and therefore the results cannot be generalized to the entire population. Further research is needed to confirm the developmental relationship between prepubertal gender discordance and later transgender or cisgender identity, and/or homosexuality and bisexuality. Finally, although gender discordance in prepubertal children may or may not persist with pubertal advancement, at least one study has shown that when gender discordance presents in adolescence, it tends to persist and lead to an enduring transgender identity (22).

In conclusion, on the basis of research studies alone, it is not possible to definitively predict the future sexual orientation or gender identity for a particular prepubertal child who presents as gender nonconforming or gender discordant. Therefore, clinicians should bear in mind the complex range of outcomes for gender-discordant youths and provide care that supports flexible, adaptive coping and a satisfactory outcome of gender and sexual development that is not needlessly constrained by rigid, unrealistic categories or expectations.

Mental Health Risks in Gender-Variant Youths

Risks Related to Gender Nonconformity

The literature on mental health risks in LGBT children and adolescents has found that being perceived as LGBT, including being gender nonconforming, is associated with increased risk for victimization, including bullying, school and peer nonacceptance, and family rejection, which are in turn associated with negative psychosocial adjustment later in life (12,23,24). LGBT adults recall increased prevalence of childhood sexual abuse and physical and psychological abuse as youths by caregivers. This has been correlated to the development of post-traumatic stress later in life (25,26). In addition to these overt risk factors, gender-nonconforming children routinely encounter negative attitudes ("microaggressions") that cause distress, including feelings of shame and low self-esteem. For example, childhood gender nonconformity is associated with higher risk for depression later in life, which is mediated by exposure to victimization and bullying both inside and outside the home (27). Poor self-esteem in gay adults is associated with having experienced rejecting attitudes and behaviors directed towards their gender nonconformity in childhood and is not inherently connected to the identity itself (28).

Early detection of and intervention for these risk factors are an important strategy to prevent harmful outcomes. Pediatric health care providers are in a unique position to detect signs of physical, sexual, and emotional abuse in children; problematic interactions between children and caregivers; and stigmatizing experiences that include microaggressions in the social environment. For these reasons, clinicians must remain particularly vigilant for suspected abuse when a gender-nonconforming child presents for treatment.

Adolescents also experience substantial mental health risks associated with gender nonconformity. One study of gender-nonconforming adolescents indicated that abuse (both psychological and physical) is significantly associated with the development of major depression and suicidality (29). A history of family rejection during youth significantly predicts increased risk for several adverse health outcomes, including suicide attempts, depression, illegal drug use, and unprotected sex in gay, lesbian, and bisexual young adults, when compared with sexual minority peers whose families were more accepting (12). Other studies demonstrate that gender nonconformity and being LGBT or being perceived as such are associated with victimization and negative psychosocial adjustment in adolescence (30–33). Some adverse effects of gender nonconformity may be entirely due to the social reaction to it; one study found that school victimization of gender-nonconforming LGBT adolescents fully mediated outcomes of life satisfaction and depression in young adulthood (24). The effects of stigma against gender nonconformity during an important developmental period may have significantly harmful effects on establishment of an individual's positive self-image.

Risks Related to Gender Discordance

Gender discordance may be associated with additional mental and behavioral health risks for children and adolescents. Wallien and colleagues investigated the prevalence of comorbid psychiatric disorders in children with *DSM-IV* GID and found that 52% of those children had 1 or more mental health diagnoses in addition to GID (34). They also found that behavioral problems in these youths are associated with increased risk for social ostracism. Research evidence and clinical experience suggest that the following factors may be associated with poorer outcomes in these children: 1) lack of supportive caretakers; 2) differing levels of support in caretakers (particularly in custody situations); 3) higher degrees of victimization, marginalization, bullying, and/or microaggressions from peers and community members; 4) unhealthy communication patterns among family members; 5) limited coping mechanisms in the child; and/or 6) the presence of a significant psychiatric comorbidity (such as anxiety, depression, and/or peer relation and behavior problems).

Of the first 97 patients presenting with gender discordance to a medical clinic that specializes in cross-sex hormonal therapy, 43% presented with a psychiatric illness and 20% had a history of self-mutilation (35). Another study of 55 gender-discordant youth indicated that the following factors are significantly associated with making a suicide attempt: suicidal ideation related to transgender identity, experiences of past parental verbal and physical abuse, and low body esteem (particularly with respect to weight satisfaction and perceptions of how others perceive the youths' bodies) (36). For adolescents, research evidence and clinical experience suggest that the following risk factors may be associated with poorer outcomes for gender-discordant adolescents: 1) experience of school victimization; 2) experiences of family rejection; 3) presence of comorbid psychopathology, including substance abuse; 4) body dissatisfaction; and 5) experiences of verbal or physical abuse.

Providing Care and Support for Gender-Variant Children and Adolescents in Primary Care Settings

Issues related to gender variance in childhood and adolescence may present in a variety of ways in different clinical settings. Primary care clinicians may be the first to be made aware of a problem such as bullying or anxiety about school in a gender-variant youth. In other situations, a child's behavior distresses parents enough to seek consultation from a mental health professional. While some parents may seek professional consultation for significant issues, such as depression, bullying, or high-risk behavior, others may seek consultation for guidance in addressing their child or adolescent's gender nonconformity. Negative attitudes about homosexuality or being transgender may influence parental or other family members' concerns about the child/adolescent. Conversely, a parent or guardian may avoid seeking professional help out of fear that the provider will confirm (or deny) a particular approach or outcome. A patient or parent's feelings of helplessness, hopelessness, or stigma about seeking mental health care may be barriers to accessing specialized care. Therefore, the pediatrician, family physician, or allied health provider may be the most acceptable source of care for these youths and families. The remainder of this chapter will focus on ways in which a primary care provider can support the healthy development of gender-variant children and adolescents, including creating inclusive environments for care; fostering relationships with parents and schools; partnering with mental health providers, endocrinologists, and other specialists in gender issues; assessing for gender dysphoria; and providing clinical management and treatment for gender dysphoria.

Creating a Welcoming Office

Creating an office environment that offers a sense of safety for gender-variant children and adolescents, as well as for LGB youths and their families, is extremely important. Other chapters in this book (see Chapters 8, 17, and Appendix A) provide suggestions for creating inclusive clinical environments for LGBT people. Ways to enhance the comfort of patients can include posting clear signage indicating that patients are welcome to use bathrooms of their affirmed gender identity, and/or offering gender-neutral bathrooms (this may be especially important for individuals who do not affirm a binary gender identity); training all staff to not make assumptions regarding gender, name, or pronoun use; creating a system where staff members are alerted in medical records when they should use the preferred gender-affirming name and pronouns of gender-discordant patients; and creating a narrative section in the documentation that specifies "Name and Pronoun Use," which allows the practitioner to justify the use of the most appropriate name and pronoun when the gender marker and legal name differ from the patient's desires. The same might be done with a prescription where the legal name and birth sex are listed or computer generated. A provider might consider working with the pharmacist to determine the possibility of using the preferred name choice that reflects a gender-discordant patient's affirmed gender on the medication bottle. Such gestures can apply to other forms of written communication, such as patient instruction forms and appointment reminder cards.

Such efforts to validate and affirm a gender-discordant patient's gender identity can increase the potential for treatment adherence and a positive therapeutic alliance. At the same time, providers and staff should be careful not to assume that all gender-nonconforming youths are discordant; hesitation in recognizing natal gender could be very upsetting to a youth who is gender nonconforming but not gender discordant (including many cisgender youth growing up gay or lesbian). For this reason, it is very important for clinicians and staff to understand the difference between gender-nonconforming youths with and without gender discordance, to know various strategies for making each welcome (including knowing when and when not to affirm natal gender), and to use clinical judgment and tact when uncertain.

A Multidisciplinary Team Approach

Because of the complexity of caring for gender-discordant and/or gender-nonconforming youth experiencing clinically significant mental health issues, it is recommended that a primary care clinician work as part of a multidisciplinary team familiar with gender issues in youths that includes a psychiatrist or other mental health professional and, in the case of gender discordance in an adolescent, an endocrinologist. The multidisciplinary perspective that characterizes an integrated team approach is frequently desirable to help weigh treatment options, obtain appropriate consent, guide treatment, and achieve optimal long-term outcomes. For gender dysphoric youth, this recommendation is consistent with the World Professional Association for Transgender Health Standards of Care for the Health of Transsexual, Transgender, and Gender-Nonconforming People (WPATH SOC-7) (5). According to the SOC-7, the role of a mental health professional in caring for gender-dysphoric youths can include assessing gender dysphoria in children and adolescents; counseling and psychotherapy to help explore gender identity, alleviate distress, and ameliorate psychosocial difficulties; providing care for any coexisting mental health problems; referring adolescents for additional physical interventions, such as endocrinological treatment for gender dysphoria; engaging in education and community advocacy on behalf of gender dysphoric children, adolescents, and their families; and offering referral for peer support.

In this model, mental health providers do not play a "gatekeeping" role for care. They are explicitly enjoined not to be dismissive or rejecting of variant gender identities and not to make efforts to alter them. Offering mental health care is especially important for gender-dysphoric children and adolescents undergoing social transition (including starting to live in the opposite or some alternative gender role), who may benefit from additional support in coping with stresses of disclosure, potential victimization, and rejection within the community and family (5). In addition, some gender-discordant or -nonconforming youth without dysphoria may benefit from mental health care if they need help with identity exploration, coping with stigma and its effects, or problems related to adjustment in school or at home. For youths with significant psychiatric symptoms, such as depression, anxiety, substance abuse, or a history of suicidal behavior, clinically appropriate efforts must be made to obtain a psychiatric assessment. Conversely, for well-adjusted gender-nonconforming youths with supportive, well-functioning families, ongoing mental health treatment may not be necessary.

Identifying a mental health provider who specializes in gender issues is not always easy, and a team approach is not always feasible. However, developing a network of licensed mental health clinicians with training in pediatric mental health consistent with leading professional organizations' guidelines on gender and sexual orientation issues is useful. These organizations, such as the American Gay and Lesbian Psychiatric Association, AACAP, WPATH, or the Lesbian and Gay Child and Adolescent Psychiatric Association, as listed in Table 16-1, may help in locating a local specialist. When making a referral, primary care clinicians will want to convey the reasons for the referral to ensure effective collaboration, and to make clear

---

Table 16-1   Resources for Accessing Pediatric Gender and Mental Health Specialists

Professional organizations

American Academy of Child & Adolescent Psychiatry (AACAP): www.aacap.org

Association of Gay and Lesbian Psychiatrists (AGLP): www.aglp.org

Gay and Lesbian Medical Association (GLMA): www.glma.org

Lesbian and Gay Child and Adolescent Psychiatric Association (LAGCAPA): www.lagcapa.org

World Professional Association for Transgender Health (WPATH): www.wpath.org

Multidisciplinary child and adolescent gender clinics in the United States (partial listing)

Ann & Robert H. Lurie Children's Hospital of Chicago: Gender & Sex Development Program: www.luriechildrens.org/en-us/care-services/specialties-services/gender-program/Pages/index.aspx

Boston Children's Hospital Gender Management Service (GeMS): www.childrenshospital.org/centers-and-services/disorders-of-sexual-development-dsd-and-gender-management-service-program/disorders-of-sexual-development-program

Children's Hospital Los Angeles: Center for Transyouth Health and Development: www.chla.org/transyouth

Children's National Medical Center in Washington, DC: Gender and Sexuality Development Program: www.childrensnational.org/departments/gender-and-sexuality-development-program

Ackerman Institute for the Family: Gender and Family Project: www.ackerman.org/#/posts/view/142-the-gender-and-family-project

NYU Child Study Center: Gender and Sexuality Service: www.aboutourkids.org/families/care_at_the_csc/gender_sexuality_service

UCSF Benioff Children's Hospital: Child and Adolescent Gender Center Clinic: www.ucsfbenioffchildrens.org/clinics/child_and_adolescent_gender_center

that the aim is to provide support, without inappropriately implying mental illness or inducing shame.

When specialists are not locally available, clinicians may be able to receive consultation by phone or email with a mental health professional identified through the organizations listed in Table 16-1. In addition, resources such as listservers and websites are increasingly being used to aid providers in underserved areas or those with limited availability to specialists. At the same time, patient needs must be adapted realistically to the local community. According to WPATH SOC-7, "health professionals must be sensitive to [cultural] differences and adapt the *SOC* according to local realities" (5).

Finally, some pediatricians, family practitioners, and adolescent medicine health specialists may have competence in dealing with gender variance in childhood and adolescent gender variance, behavioral health and developmental psychopathology and may be able to independently provide evaluation and care to gender-variant youth when specialists are not available.

Supporting Parents and Other Family Members

Primary care clinicians can provide ongoing support to families of gender-variant children and adolescents that will enhance the likelihood of positive outcomes. Parents and caregivers may express concern about a gender-variant child ranging from questions about how to best support their child to expressions of distress. Understanding parental assumptions and attitudes about gender variance, who in the family is concerned about what, and what sources of support are available to the family is crucial (37). Doing so requires trust and may take time.

A primary parental concern, particularly for those with younger prepubertal children, often revolves around developmental outcomes; that is, they want to know whether their child will grow up to be transgender, gay, straight, et cetera. Clinicians should educate parents about the limitations in predicting these outcomes and help parents tolerate any unavoidable ambiguity about the future, stressing that the goal is to ensure their children always feel safe and supported. Parents may also question whether acceptance of their child's gender-variant behaviors will increase the likelihood of a gender or sexual orientation outcome they fear. Some may ask whether discouraging gender-variant behaviors is desirable. Others, seeking to support their child, may want to implement a social gender transition. Appropriately guiding parents involves helping them understand the difference between gender nonconformity and discordance, and stressing the importance of acceptance, support, and healthy family relationships.

As a primary care provider develops a relationship with a family over time, it may become apparent that different family members react in different ways to their gender-variant child or adolescent. Sometimes, observing child/adolescent–parent interactions will give valuable information about how a family member reacts to their youth's gender-based behaviors.

If the clinician has a strong rapport with that family member, it may be helpful to set aside some time to meet with that individual to explore the concerns and provide education about gender nonconformity being a normal variant of human behavior. Families may experience relief in dealing with these issues if they detect that their clinician is comfortable addressing questions and concerns that may arise for the child, siblings, parents, and other family members. Sometimes, a family therapy referral may help address interpersonal challenges, or an individual mental health referral may be useful for a family member (e.g., a sibling, grandparent, or father) who is particularly struggling with their family member's gender-nonconforming behaviors and/or identifications. It may also help to encourage parents and other family members to seek out local resources, such as support groups. National organizations that provide support and resources relevant to gender nonconforming children and their families include Parents, Friends, & Families of Lesbians and Gays (www.pflag.org) and TransActive (www.transactiveonline.org). The literature has noted the value of connecting parents with other parents of gender nonconforming children in helping promote tolerance and support (38,39). Finally, if any form of emotional, sexual, or physical abuse by a family member is detected, the clinicians should follow appropriate protocols in response. This will help ensure the safety and well-being of all members of the family.

Working With Schools and Community Groups

When caring for gender-variant children and adolescents, the clinician should consider consulting with the child's school, especially if the child or parent reports bullying and victimization occurring in the school setting. The AACAP Practice Parameter recommends that a clinician should "seek information about the sexual beliefs, attitudes and experiences of these social systems, and whether they are supportive or hostile in the patient's perception and in reality" (4). A helpful resource in working with schools is the Gay, Lesbian, & Straight Education Network (www.glsen.org). If the child is already seeing a mental health professional, it would be critical to engage early in a collaborative discussion regarding the best manner to involve the child's school in minimizing bullying and victimization while promoting support and tolerance. All health care providers should recognize when it is necessary to advocate for an adolescent experiencing school victimization, parental rejection, and/or discrimination in the community, and should be familiar with pertinent abuse reporting requirements.

Promoting Self-Esteem and Coping Skills

All providers who work with gender-variant children and adolescents should aim to promote healthy self-esteem and coping skills, which are critical to resilience. Addressing any discomfort about being "different" from what others expect may be very helpful. Examples include helping a child appropriately cope with any victimization in school and any unavoidable threatening situations, minimize exaggerated reactions to perceived harms, and get help when needed. Supportive adults can foster and enhance development of these social skills. For example, a gender-nonconforming boy who may be repeatedly picked last for sports teams and lacks positive coping strategies may feel isolated and victimized. The same would be true for a teenage girl who has an aversion to or disinterest in wearing make-up, painting her nails, or going shopping for more feminine clothing, leaving her feeling isolated and alone. With adult support, these youths may be able to develop strategies to pursue desired interests and friendships. The clinician can help in part by discussing with parents how their child can safely and flexibly cope with invalidating experiences (such as bullying), while providing validating experiences within the home, family, and community whenever possible.

Clinical Care for Gender-Variant Children

Promoting healthy psychosocial adjustment for gender-variant children and adolescents is the pediatrician or family physician's primary goal in caring for these youth. However, many of the clinical strategies for achieving this goal differ depending on whether a child is prepubertal or adolescent. Therefore, clinical care for gender-variant children is discussed here first, followed by a discussion of adolescent care needs.

The major aims for the clinical care of gender-variant children within a pediatric setting, which may take time over many appointments, are to 1) identify children with gender-nonconforming behavior or gender discordance, even when not a chief complaint of the patient or family; 2) consider whether the child meets criteria for *DSM-5* diagnosis of gender dysphoria; 3) assess the effect of gender-related issues on psychological functioning, such as feelings of low self-esteem, guilt, anxiety, other problems in mood, behavior, or parent–child interactions; 4) understand the meaning of any gender nonconformity or discordance within the child's social and cultural environment; 5) evaluate supportive or rejecting attitudes and behavior of the parent/guardian related to any gender variance, and how these change over time; 6) assess the need for referral for consultation and/or ongoing treatment with a mental health professional comfortable in assisting families with these issues; and 7) assess the degree of pubertal advancement in a latency-age child who is approaching puberty to assist in correlating any changes (emergence, intensification, or desistance) in gender dysphoria with the presence of secondary sexual characteristics.

Assessing Gender Dysphoria in Children
When presented with a child who shows signs of gender dysphoria, clinicians can use the *DSM-5* diagnostic criteria for gender dysphoria as part of

a parent and/or child interview. Compared with the *DSM-IV* criteria for gender identity disorder of childhood, the new criteria capture both cognitive (e.g., identification as the opposite gender) and affective (e.g., a preference for, or comfort manifesting behavior typical of, the opposite gender) domains (7,40). To meet the criteria, children must exhibit a marked incongruence between their experienced/expressed gender and assigned gender. This must be manifested for at least 6 months' duration by criterion A: 1) a strong desire to be of the other gender or an insistence that one is the other gender. In addition, the child must exhibit 5 of the following 7 additional indicators for at least 6 months: 2) in natal boys, a strong preference for wearing female attire, or in natal girls, a strong preference for wearing only typical masculine clothing and aversion to wearing typical feminine clothing; 3) a strong preference for cross-gender roles in make-believe or fantasy play; 4) a strong preference for the toys, games, or activities stereotypically used or engaged in by the other gender; 5) a strong preference for playmates of the nonassigned gender; 6) in natal boys, a strong rejection of typically masculine toys, games, and activities (including an avoidance of rough-and-tumble play), or in natal girls, a strong rejection of typically feminine toys, games, and activities; 7) a strong dislike of one's sexual anatomy; and 8) a strong desire for the primary and/or secondary sex characteristics that match one's experienced gender. To meet the *DSM-5* criteria for gender dysphoria, the child must also display criterion B: clinically significant distress or impairment in social, school, or other important areas of functioning.

The *DSM-5* diagnosis of gender dysphoria in children requires verbalization of cross-gender wishes or identification as a cardinal feature. Assessing whether a child meets these criteria may be clinically challenging in children who have difficulty verbalizing their feelings and for whom extreme gender-nonconforming behavior may be the primary manifestation of their gender dysphoria. The AACAP Practice Parameter includes information that can assist clinicians in diagnosis. This includes both clinical descriptions and guidelines and also information about rating scales, such as the Gender Identity Interview for Children and the Gender Identity Questionnaire for Children, which is a parent questionnaire (41–43).

Clinical Management of Gender Dysphoria in Childhood

For children who meet the *DSM-5* criteria for gender dysphoria, additional clinical management and support beyond what is presented above may be needed. While more research is required to guide best evidence-based clinical practices (4), many different treatment approaches have been proposed in recent years (44). These include 1) supporting any natural subsiding of cross-gender feelings (e.g., attempting to support naturally burgeoning comfort in expressing behaviors and identifications consistent with natal sex) through multimodal approaches including group therapy and parental guidance; 2) helping children attain flexible concepts of gender not dependent on conventional preconceptions, and redirecting the child to neutral expressions of gender while enhancing flexibility to safely adapt to avoid harassment; and 3) helping parents support youth with persistent cross-gender identifications and, when appropriate, facilitating a cross-gender social transition by changing their child's name and using opposite pronouns in some or all situations. Each of these general approaches has potential risks and benefits that must be addressed as ethical issues in treatment (37,45).

Selecting an appropriate clinical approach can be challenging because of the difficulty in distinguishing children who will continue to experience gender dysphoria from those in whom gender dysphoria will naturally subside by adolescence.

Risks and Benefits of Social Transition in Gender-Dysphoric Children

One might reasonably argue that a child with gender dysphoria, which might or might not persist into adolescence, would benefit from a partial or complete social transition to the opposite gender in order to alleviate the dysphoria as soon as possible. However, in light of the natural course of gender dysphoria in children and the high rates of subsiding of dysphoria by adolescence, a social gender transition might carry several risks: 1) Consolidating a cross-gender identity that might otherwise have subsided, thereby actually prolonging the child's experience of dysphoria beyond puberty; 2) causing a child to feel pressured to live in a cross-gender role past puberty when gender dysphoria has subsided; and/or 3) causing distress by creating a situation in which the child must undergo a later, second social gender transition back to the gender role of their natal sex. Despite these risks, prepubertal social gender transition has occurred with successful outcomes in some cases (5).

One important potential benefit of prepubertal social gender transition is the possibility that psychosocial functioning will improve if the child's gender identity is affirmed by others; however, informed consent from the parents/guardians and developmentally appropriate assent from the child includes consideration of the current lack of information regarding indications for and outcomes of this option, and the possible need for a second gender transition back to the natal gender if the child's gender dysphoria lessens with pubertal advancement. As a practical matter, the provider might consider making sure the patient and family know that many, if not most, gender-dysphoric children continue to explore their gender identity for a while, frequently not making a final decision until adolescence or young adulthood. Educating the families that the changes puberty will eventually bring on will also be valuable in helping their child explore their gender identity as they get older is important. Clinicians might recommend that patients and families consider a gradual and exploratory change, first starting in the home setting or on family vacations, and then progressing to other settings, in order not to lock a child into a premature decision.

Whatever the risks and benefits for an individual child, in general, data from Amsterdam's specialty gender identity clinic suggests that in the last decade there has been a fourfold increase in the number of children who present at the initial visit having already undergone a full social cross-gender transition (45). The article reports that before 2000, only 2 prepubertal boys out of 112 children (1.7%) referred to the gender identity clinic had initially presented with having completely transitioned to the female role. Between 2005 and 2009, however, 16 of 180 children (10 boys and 6 girls; about 9%) presented having completely made a social transition to the opposite gender at the time of the initial visit. These data may indicate that parents are increasingly implementing gender transition before seeking guidance from gender identity specialists. Primary care clinicians therefore may play an increasingly important role in helping to guide such decisions. For this reason, when presented with a child with gender dysphoria, it is important for primary care clinicians to discuss with patients and their families the potential benefits and risks of cross-gender social transition.

To help patients and families with these decisions, consultation with a mental health specialist with competence in pediatric gender identity issues is advisable if possible. Families navigating the complexities of childhood gender transition may benefit from knowledge and experience that mental health professionals have around these very complicated issues. A collaborative approach between the primary care clinician and mental health professional is ideal. As noted earlier, finding a local specialist may be challenging; professional organizations, such as the ones in Table 16-1, should be able to offer assistance in locating a nearby specialist, or in identifying someone who can offer consultation as needed.

In light of the need for further research evidence to guide best practices for gender-dysphoric children, it is necessary to adapt currently accepted practices to the unique clinical needs of each child as development unfolds, taking into account the risks and benefits of the options in ongoing treatment planning. To date, no large-scale prospective study has followed gender-nonconforming and/or dysphoric children in community primary care settings into adolescence in order to help establish primary care guidelines.

Clinical Care for Gender-Variant Adolescents

Adolescence is characterized by physical, cognitive, and emotional changes. Puberty is a physical maturation process demarcated by the 5 Tanner stages. It includes the development of masculine (e.g., deeper voice, body and facial hair) and feminine (e.g., breast development, change in fat distribution) secondary sexual characteristics. It also includes brain development and associated processes, both cognitively (normally including progression from concrete thought processes to abstract reasoning) and emotionally (including increased sexual and aggressive feelings, susceptibility to adult forms of mood disorders, and normally the establishment of affective regulation). The response of gender-nonconforming or -discordant youths to the physical changes of puberty can provide critical diagnostic clues about the emergence or intensification of gender dysphoria. Determining whether medical hormonal interventions might be useful in alleviating any gender dysphoria is an important strategy during puberty and adolescence (46).

The primary care clinician's role in promoting healthy outcomes for gender-nonconforming and/or -discordant adolescents is important and includes the following: 1) recognize the difference between gender role behavior and gender identity, and the unique clinical needs of youth who are gender nonconforming, gender discordant, and gender dysphoric (this includes recognizing that an adolescent need not express gender-nonconforming behaviors to internally experience gender discordance); 2) obtain a psychosexual history without assuming a developmental outcome; 3) create a safe office environment where youths can discuss their gender development and sexuality confidentially within the parameters of mandated disclosure policies; 4) conduct a physical examination in a sensitive manner that recognizes the potential distress that some gender-dysphoric adolescents may have with unwanted aspects of their physical anatomy (see Chapters 8 and 18 for recommendations); 5) appropriately collaborate with mental health providers for adolescents with gender dysphoria, including those who seek hormonal or surgical intervention for gender reassignment as part of gender affirmation; 6) appropriately screen for mental health and psychosocial problems, such as depression, anxiety, self-endangering behaviors, school victimization, bullying, or family rejection and refer for appropriate mental health treatment or psychosocial support; 7) recognize the different hormonal interventions that exist for the treatment of gender dysphoria, their indications across specific stages of puberty, and the associated risks and benefits; and 8) intervene appropriately in the event that verbal, physical, or sexual abuse or other clinically important psychosocial problems are detected.

Assessment of Gender Dysphoria in Adolescents
As discussed earlier, recognizing whether an adolescent experiences gender dysphoria is important not only for the patient–provider relationship but also for meeting the unique health needs of these youths, who may desire a clinical intervention for gender affirmation. In assessing for evidence of gender dysphoria, a provider should approach the assessment in a developmentally appropriate and nonjudgmental manner that makes no assumptions about gender or sexual identities or outcomes, as depicted in Figure 16-1. Observing the parent–adolescent interaction, including the name and pronoun that the parent uses when referring to the son or daughter, helps to

Open-ended interaction questions

"Do you have a preferred name that you would like me to refer to you as?"
"Do you have a preference for pronouns that I should use?"

Screening questions to assess for gender dysphoria

"Have you ever thought about living life in the opposite or some other gender?"
"Do you feel you are a different gender from the way others have thought of you since you were born?"
"Are there any aspects of your body that bring you displeasure or that you wished you did not have?"
"Have you thought about your body having certain characteristics or features of another gender?"

Specific questions to understand the gender dysphoria

"Which aspects of your body bring you displeasure the most? The least?"
"Of the body features that bring you the most displeasure, are any of them more distressing to you over the others?"

Figure 16-1 Clarifying questions for possible gender discordance in adolescents. These questions are best asked when alone with the adolescent.

determine how to conduct the interview, including whether to speak with the adolescent privately in the beginning. If gender discordance is suspected (e.g., if an adolescent presents in a gender-ambiguous manner or it is not clear whether they are gender nonconforming, discordant, or both), the provider may want to privately ask an open-ended question about the adolescent's name preference, such as "How would you like me to refer to you?" This might lead to questions about pronoun preference and any specific situations where the adolescent prefers reverting back to assigned name and natal sex pronouns (e.g., when his/her parents are in the room). The provider should also assess whether the patient *currently* identifies in a particular way, without suggesting that the patient should have identity fully sorted out or implying that this identification should or should not change over time.

When initial screening indicates it is clinically appropriate, the clinician should assess for the presence of gender dysphoria in a manner that does not presume a transgender identity or desire for steps toward gender reassignment. An example of a clarifying question is: "Do you feel you are a different gender from the way others have thought of you since you were born?" Other questions can be found in Figure 16-1. If any of these questions yield affirmative answers, further assessment would include the degree to which the adolescent experiences them. An example of one question might be: "Of the body features that bring you the most displeasure, are any of them more distressing to you over the others?"

The AACAP LGBT Practice Parameter includes additional information on the clinical assessment of gender dysphoria in adolescents. This includes information about rating scales, such as the Gender Identity/Gender Dysphoria Questionnaire for Adolescents and Adults (47). For sexually active adolescents, sexual behavior screening questions often yield important information pertaining to the adolescent's ability to derive pleasure from their genitals, a useful aspect of the history when considering medical hormonal interventions that have the potential to irreversibly disrupt sexual functioning of natal genitals (5).

A more detailed interview would be necessary to diagnose gender dysphoria according to *DSM-5* criteria (7). A diagnosis of gender dysphoria in adolescents and adults requires that an individual have certain symptoms (A and B criteria). To meet criterion A, an adolescent must display a "marked incongruence between one's experienced/expressed gender, of at least 6 months' duration, as manifested by at least 2 of the following 6 indicators: 1) a marked incongruence between one's experienced/expressed gender and primary and/or secondary sex characteristics (or anticipated characteristics for a young adolescent); 2) a strong desire to be rid of one's primary and/or secondary sex characteristics because of the marked incongruence between one's experienced/expressed gender (or a desire to prevent the development of the anticipated sex characteristics in a young adolescent); 3) a strong desire for the primary and/or secondary sex characteristics of the other gender; 4) a strong desire to be the other gender or some alternative gender different from one's assigned gender; 5) a strong desire to be treated as the other gender or some alternative gender different from one's assigned gender, and/or 6) a strong conviction that one has the typical feelings and reactions of the other gender or some alternative gender. Criterion B specifies that the condition is associated with clinically significant distress or impairment in social, occupational, or other important areas of functioning.

Two specifiers may be used if warranted: presence of a disorder of sex development and/or an indication of post-transition. The post-transition specifier can refer to adolescents who have transitioned full-time to living in the desired gender (with or without legal recognition of the gender change) and have started or prepared to start at least one cross-sex medical/surgical procedure. It does not include those adolescents who are on pubertal suppression solely. Because gender dysphoria can present in childhood or adolescence, an adolescent does not have to have met the criteria for the childhood subtype of gender dysphoria in order to meet criteria in adolescence. In addition, since because gender dysphoria may or may not persist, children with gender dysphoria may not continue to meet criteria for it in adolescence.

In addition to ordinary clinical interviews, specialized psychometric measures are sometimes used to help develop a more comprehensive understanding of the adolescent and help clarify a diagnosis of gender dysphoria (1,48). Such measures may also help in understanding the interactions between any gender identity issues and other psychiatric areas of functioning, and are therefore especially helpful with adolescents who present with significant psychiatric comorbid conditions, such as autism spectrum disorder, which the literature has shown to be correlated with gender dysphoria in clinically referred samples (49). The use of such specialized measures may be beyond the scope of practice of a pediatric setting and would typically be completed by a mental health professional. It is especially recommended that pediatricians work in collaboration with mental health specialists in such complex cases.

Medical and Other Interventions for Gender-Dysphoric Youth

For gender-dysphoric adolescents, providers can consider offering endocrine and nonmedical interventions to help relieve the dysphoria and provide affirmation. Choice of intervention depends on the adolescent's physical and emotional maturity, defined by Tanner staging and psychosocial functioning. Consultation with a mental health professional can help with choosing the most appropriate interventions. Similar to the approach with children, obtaining informed consent from parents or other legal guardians of minor patients, as well as developmentally appropriate assent from minors, by discussing the known risks and benefits of possible interventions is crucial. Several multidisciplinary gender specialty clinics exist, both in the United States and abroad, and each of their clinical protocols has been described in the literature (1,48,50–52). Different models of transgender health care pertinent to youth have been described. These have been generally categorized as standard of care models (5) and informed consent models (53,54).

Non-endocrine Interventions

Non-endocrine intervention options to alleviate gender dysphoria summarized in the WPATH SOC-7 (5) include 1) in-person and online support groups or community organizations that provide social support and advocacy; 2) in-person and online resources for friends and families; 3) voice and communication therapy to help the individual develop both verbal and nonverbal communication skills that facilitate comfort with their gender identity; 4) hair removal through electrolysis, laser treatment, or waxing; 5) breast binding or padding, genital tucking or penile prostheses, or padding of the hips or buttocks; and 6) changes in name and gender markers on identity documents. When hormonal options are not available (lack of access to care or insurance coverage) or are not indicated at that point in time (e.g., too much psychiatric instability to obtain informed consent/ assent), then these non-endocrine interventions can precede hormonal intervention. However, these interventions can also be used in conjunction with hormonal intervention when those options are indicated.

The mental health goals of SOC-7 outlined above are especially important for gender-dysphoric adolescents undergoing social transition (including starting to live in the opposite or some alternative gender role), who may benefit from support in coping with stresses of disclosure, potential victimization, and rejection within the community and family. Providers can help adolescents who are considering various gender identities, including nonbinary ones, and who may undergo social transition, to carefully consider the risks and benefits of various strategies for achieving their goals.

When endocrine treatment intervention is a consideration, the choice of intervention depends largely on stage of pubertal advancement. For younger gender-dysphoric adolescents (Tanner stages 2 and 3), gonadotropin-releasing hormone agonists (GnRH agonists) have been used to achieve reversible pubertal suppression and can be considered (55). Cross-sex hormone treatment (estrogen for natal males and testosterone for natal females), which promotes partially irreversible secondary sexual characteristics, can be considered in older adolescents (Tanner stages 4 and 5) if their maturity is sufficient to allow them to participate in providing appropriate assent or informed consent along with any relevant legal guardians. It is important for clinicians to bear in mind the current limits of knowledge from existing research when weighing the risks and benefits of these options, which may include unknown risks or irreversible effects. In multidisciplinary teams, it is important that providers and consultants from all disciplines, including pediatrics, endocrinology, and mental health, collaborate in developing an appropriate treatment plan. This requires that all providers be familiar with the risks and benefits of proposed treatment and nontreatment options, as well as any clinically relevant mental health issues, in determining endocrine treatment recommendations and their timing.

Familiarity with all locally relevant medicolegal issues, such as consent to medical care for minors and child protection laws, is part of competent care for all youths, including those who are gender variant. Supportive family involvement is almost always desirable if possible. However, in certain situations an adolescent may be entitled to make independent treatment decisions based on local health regulations, such as when the adolescent is an emancipated minor, mature minor, or of similar legal status. Clinicians should seek legal consultation to clarify any uncertainties about medical consent.

Pubertal Suppression with GnRH Analogues

The Endocrine Society's 2009 guidelines describe pubertal suppression for adolescents in Tanner stage 2 or 3 following appropriate mental health assessments (56). The rationale for GnRH analogue treatment in younger gender-dysphoric adolescents is to reversibly prevent the development of unwanted secondary sexual characteristics, which are irreversible and may be highly distressing to the adolescent. In doing so, one may relieve the immediate distress and allow for deferral of decisions about interventions that are irreversible (such as cross-sex hormone treatment or surgery) until maturity allows the youth to provide informed consent. Additionally, one hypothetical advantage to using pubertal suppression in these youth is that the patient will ultimately develop an outward appearance that more closely resembles the affirmed gender, which is associated with better psychological adjustment later in life (57). This intervention may reduce the degree of invasive surgeries required by adolescents and adults to achieve an appearance that resembles their affirmed gender, avoiding not only the medical risks but also financials barrier to surgery, which may be very expensive and not covered by insurance.

Results of studies of pubertal suppression with GnRH analogues published by the Amsterdam Gender Dysphoria Clinic in 2006 and follow-up studies document a psychosocial benefit of this intervention (55,58–60). A prospective study that followed adolescents who had received GnRH analogue treatment to 1 year after subsequent sexual reassignment surgery and/or cross-sex hormone treatment found that none of 27 young adult participants (11 female-to-male and 16 male-to-female) regretted the irreversible interventions (cross-sex hormone therapy or surgeries) (61). Further research is needed on pubertal suppression to fully assess its short- and long-term psychological and physical benefits and risks for gender-dysphoric patients.

WPATH guidelines specify the following minimum criteria for GnRH treatment: 1) The adolescent has demonstrated a long-lasting and intense pattern of gender nonconformity or dysphoria; 2) gender dysphoria emerged or worsened with the onset of puberty; 3) any coexisting psychological, medical, or social problems that could interfere with treatment have been addressed; and 4) the adolescent or parents/caretakers have given informed consent (depending on the age of medical consent) while supporting the adolescent throughout the treatment. When considering an individual's eligibility for pubertal suppression, a multidisciplinary team that includes a mental health professional and endocrinologist is ideal and recommended by the WPATH standards of care. The mental health professional can help explore issues around gender identity before and during treatment and help provide any necessary follow-up. Ideally, an endocrinologist would help monitor physical development and manage treatment risks, such as low bone mineral density and decreased growth.

The novelty and relative lack of evidence of outcome research for GnRH analogue treatment of adolescent gender dysphoria raise important ethical and practical clinical issues that clinicians must weigh on an individual basis (62). Further outcomes research is needed on pubertal suppression for pediatric gender dysphoria to inform best clinical practice related to such things as the selection criteria for pubertal suppression, optimal timing of endocrine interventions, and information about long-term risks, if any, of treatment. Providers should be familiar with these issues and prepared to discuss them with patients and parents, who may educate themselves as well through resources including blogs, online support groups, and community networks. A review by Kreukels and Cohen-Kettenis in 2011 summarizes many of these dilemmas (55). One hypothetical concern about the use of GnRH analogues relates to the fact that growth and development of the central nervous system in childhood and adolescence depend on the brain's natural exposure to sex hormones, such as testosterone and estrogen, produced and metabolized both outside and within the central nervous system. Sex hormones are trophic on development in puberty, and their blockade might theoretically adversely affect neuropsychiatric development; this is an area that requires further research. A recent study on bone development in gender-dysphoric adolescents who received pubertal suppression and subsequent cross-sex hormone treatment is reassuring with respect to bone mineral density results (63). This area requires further research for confirmation in the peer-reviewed literature. The potential risks and benefits of currently available treatments, including those known and not yet known for future surgical options (such as vaginoplasty and metoidioplasty) and physical and mental health, must be weighed against the benefits and risks of not treating gender dysphoria, including the risk that progression of secondary sexual characteristics might lead to harmful psychiatric outcomes, both immediately and in the long term.

Increasing use of pubertal suppression in clinical practice, as well as media coverage and increasing public awareness of this option, may lead some families to seek pubertal suppression in youth whom they incorrectly assume to be gender dysphoric. When gender discordance is suspected, dysphoria related to the initial development of secondary sexual characteristics may actually help confirm the diagnosis of gender dysphoria. In addition to unnecessary treatment, risks of premature use of pubertal suppression may include preventing natal males from having an opportunity to bank sperm for future reproductive efforts. Other ethical concerns include possible unintended social consequences of the widespread use of pubertal suppression, such as the possibility that an unquestioned clinical goal of aligning a patient's physical sex and appearance with gender identity might inadvertently reinforce stigma against individuals whose gender identity is actually nonbinary (64). Medical paradigms that undertake treatment based on overly rigid and binary conceptions of gender might also inadvertently exacerbate stigma against gender-nonconforming individuals, including many who are gay, lesbian, or bisexual (65).

Despite these potential risks, existing evidence supports the conclusion that pubertal suppression of gender-dysphoric adolescents is an important innovative treatment option that may improve quality of life, which warrants further research. Details of its dosing and administration can be found in the WPATH SOC-7 (5). Unfortunately, the intervention has very limited insurance coverage and is quite costly, making it accessible to only a small percentage of the population, adding to the significant health disparity that already exists for these youths (66). The SOC-7 includes reversible interventions for pubertal suppression in younger gender-dysphoric adolescents that may be less cost prohibitive than GnRH analogues. For adolescents with male genitalia, they include progestins or spironolactone, which have contra-androgenic activity. For adolescents with female genitalia, they include continuous oral contraceptives with a progestin that blocks menses. Primary care clinicians may want to consider these options, including possible consultation with or referral to specialists in fields such as endocrinology, obstetrics and gynecology, or adolescent medicine, who are familiar with these interventions in adolescents (5).

The authors of the WPATH SOC-7 make this important observation: "Neither puberty suppression nor allowing puberty to occur is a neutral act . . . the long-term effects can only be determined when the earliest-treated patients reach the appropriate age"; at the same time, "refusing timely medical interventions for adolescents might prolong gender dysphoria . . . withholding puberty-suppression and subsequent feminizing or masculinizing hormone therapy is not a neutral option for adolescents" (5). Clinicians must therefore weigh the benefits and risks—both known and hypothetical—of all options, recognizing that non-treatment may carry significant risks, and obtain appropriate informed consent and assent from youth and their guardians in forming an individualized treatment plan.

Cross-sex Hormone Treatment

In gender dysphoric adolescents, the initiation of cross-sex hormone therapy (estrogen for natal males and testosterone for natal females) around the age of 16 is sometimes considered to promote the development of secondary sexual characteristics of the affirmed gender. Informed consent and assent require detailed discussion and understanding of the fact that the physical changes they induce are partially irreversible. These include irreversible effects on the reproductive system, among others, and discussion of the preservation of gametes when applicable. Providers across disciplines should familiarize themselves with the expected changes that come with exogenous cross-sex hormone administration. Details of dosing, administration, and the timeline of these expected changes can be found in the WPATH SOC-7 (5). The Endocrine Society guidelines have hormone regimens adapted specifically for adolescents (56). It may be clinically appropriate to consider use of cross-sex hormonal treatment in youths who previously received pubertal suppression treatment. For example it may be in the best interest of a youth to proceed with cross-sex pubertal development contemporaneously with the youth's peers. For younger adolescents in situations where the benefits far outweigh risks, cross-sex hormone therapies may be considered medically necessary, especially if prognostic signs of persistent cross-gender identity are present. When making such complex decisions, discussion among a multidisciplinary team of specialists, the youth, and the family may help weigh the risks and benefits for each adolescent. Providers who are considering interventions for a patient should become familiar with the WPATH SOC-7's "eligibility and readiness criteria" for adolescents seeking hormonal intervention (5).

General principles of mental health treatment with adolescents seeking hormonal intervention include exploration of the following: 1) degree of distress that specific aspects of anatomical incongruence bring to the adolescent; 2) understanding of the effects of hormonal interventions and how those effects correlate with the alleviation of distress; 3) thorough exploration of the potential risks and benefits of various hormonal interventions; 4) degree of psychosocial support from families or others; and 5) psychiatric comorbid conditions, including their potential effect on mature consent and participation in treatment. The presence of a psychiatric condition is not necessarily a contraindication to proceeding with medical interventions for gender reassignment; indeed, certain psychiatric conditions may be ameliorated by them.

Surgical Options

Several surgical techniques have been developed to help transgender adults transition to the sex that is consistent with their gender identity. Such options include mastectomy, metoidioplasty, phalloplasty, and vaginoplasty. These techniques, while potentially quite beneficial when appropriately used, have limitations and associated risks. Some adolescents have unreasonable expectations about the outcomes of these surgical procedures. For adolescents who are considering surgery in the future, discussion should therefore carefully explore the risks and benefits. Providers should not assume that all adolescent patients desire to pursue surgical interventions.

Surgical options and standards for their use are described in Chapter 18 and in the WPATH SOC-7 (5). In general, deferral of such techniques until adulthood may be preferable for many reasons. First, their irreversibility makes it important that they be undertaken when it is clear and unequivocal that the individual has a persistent transgender identity and can provide mature consent for them. These may not be clear until adulthood, which is one rationale for the use of pubertal blockade with GnRH. Second, especially in the case of genital reconstruction, the technical feasibility and long-term success of surgery may depend on adequate tissue growth of secondary sexual characteristics. Whether and how GnRH analogues affect the feasibility of these surgical techniques later on remains to be studied.

These general considerations notwithstanding, appropriate care is based on a thoughtful assessment of the needs of the individual, taking into account the psychosocial aspects of care, ideally involving important sources of support, such as family, and always proceeding with informed consent of whoever is legally responsible for the youth as well as the youth's own assent. As with other aspects of medical intervention, the age of legal consent for surgery varies by state, and these elements of care are usually best conceived as a process that is undertaken in the context of a long-term, supportive, and affirming health care relationship in which trust and effective communication are established, patient concerns addressed, options clarified, adaptive coping supported, and goals established and achieved. This approach, which helps assure the appropriateness of surgical interventions and supports the likelihood of their eventual success and acceptability to the patient, illustrates the usefulness of multidisciplinary care that includes a mental health and wellness perspective as one aspect of care—not to function as a gatekeeper to surgical interventions, but as a facilitator of beneficial planning when they are appropriate.

Case: Gender Dysphoria in Adolescence

The following case has been developed to illustrate various potential issues that can present in the clinical care of an adolescent with gender dysphoria. The case does not represent all gender-dysphoric adolescents, nor does it intend to associate gender dysphoria with challenging psychosocial situations, extreme risk-taking behaviors, and access to care issues. Rather, multiple complex issues are presented here in order to demonstrate how different circumstances can influence decisions for care and treatment.

> Julia is a 15-year-old natal male with strong and persistent cross-gender feelings who presents to a pediatrician in a rural health clinic. Her birth name was Oscar, but she has been asking others to refer to her as Julia and to use female pronouns when speaking about her. Julia is seeking assistance in gender transition, and is accompanied by a caseworker at a group home for runaway youth where Julia lives. There is no mental health clinician in the clinic, and none in the community with specific expertise in gender issues in youth. Julia has had a lifelong preference of stereotypical feminine interests, which led to extreme harassment and bullying by peers in school, and several arguments with her family, including corporal punishment. In a particularly severe argument 6 months ago, her father punched her, causing a lip laceration. Julia subsequently ran away and was homeless for several weeks, including a period of prostitution, until an arrest led to social service intervention. Julia was then placed in temporary foster care. Because of ongoing paternal threats,

Julia's court-appointed legal guardian has petitioned for status as an emancipated minor; for the time being, Julia remains in foster care as a ward of the state.

Julia reports feeling depressed ever since the development of facial hair and a deepening voice and, in the last 6 months, severely depressed mood on a daily basis with frequent hopelessness. Julia has long hair and painted nails and makes an effort to have a higher-pitched voice. She wishes to be placed in a female group home and for the past 6 months has been shaving her legs and wearing exclusively female-typical clothing. The caseworker reports that in speaking with other transgender youth, Julia learned that some blood pressure medicines can help grow breasts; she has been trading sex for such pills from men on the street. On physical exam, she has numerous self-induced cutting injuries at various stages of healing, with some appearing recently inflicted. A suicide screen yields passive suicidal thought (wish to be not alive). Although she denies immediate intentions or plans to kill herself, Julia says that estrogen treatment will be the only way she can proceed in life, and would like to start the hormone therapy as soon as possible.

This case illustrates several complex gender-related issues in an adolescent. In addition to gender dysphoria, this youth is experiencing several psychosocial problems, including abuse, running away, homelessness, depression, self-injurious behavior, and a history of prostitution, with possible exposure to HIV and other health risks. It is difficult to know to what degree this adolescent's intense distress results from the discrepancy between her gender identity and body, as opposed to other factors, such as the social environment's reaction to her or pre-existing depression or other psychiatric illness. The clinician must weigh these various possible causes of distress in choosing a treatment plan. Although the patient's sole priority is hormonal intervention, the clinician must independently evaluate to what degree and how the broader contextual psychosocial problems should be addressed first. In addition, the clinician must make a judgment about whether the hormonal intervention this patient requests is in her best interest; to what degree the psychiatric symptoms would need to be stable before proceeding with hormone therapy, if indicated; how giving or withholding hormone therapy might affect psychiatric symptoms and/or risk behaviors; and how to obtain informed consent for treatment.

Because of the limitations of a rural setting, the clinician must make these important judgments without ready access to the subspecialty consultation that would help with the complex endocrine issues and potential morbidity and mortality associated with the psychiatric and behavioral issues. Financial resources are lacking for travel to a city where clinical resources are available for consultation and follow-up. Despite these obstacles to care, this patient needs help. To bridge these service gaps, the provider must consider several issues: when it is helpful or necessary to seek consultation from colleagues with specialization in transgender health in fields such as endocrinology and psychiatry; how to do so; how to manage the case if these are not obtainable; and how and whether to involve the family and other systems in the youth's care when there are social challenges.

Each patient's health needs must be evaluated in the psychosocial context in order to formulate appropriate treatment recommendations. Doing so requires understanding various gender-related clinical phenomena in children and adolescents, their developmental course, current standards of best practice in the field, and limitations of the evidence base. Bearing these issues in mind, standard practices of informed consent, weighing the risks and benefits of options, can help guide treatment. Keeping a long-term perspective in the context of a treatment relationship with a clinician can help patients, families, and other legal guardians to give appropriate informed assent and consent for treatment decisions, taking into consideration overall health and psychosocial well-being.

Conclusion

Within the historical context of shifting social and medical paradigms, health care providers are approaching the spectrum of gender variance from new perspectives. Some gender and sexual variance that historically was seen as pathologic is now viewed as normal variation in human behavior; further changes will undoubtedly occur. Children, adolescents, and their families are presenting in greater numbers and at younger ages with these issues, providing new opportunities for a variety of clinical disciplines to help them. The primary care physician is uniquely exposed to children and adolescents of parents who might not seek help from mental health professionals when it might be clinically helpful or indicated. The task of that physician is complex and has many layers, which include helping families support and accept their child or adolescent; understanding basic aspects of psychosexual development; distinguishing sexual orientation, gender nonconformity, discordance, and dysphoria from one another; recognizing when distinguishing between these phenomena is difficult; determining when a mental health referral or interdisciplinary team is warranted; learning how to consult with a mental health gender specialist when one is not readily accessible in their area; and intervening when the child or adolescent is exposed to harm. Medical fields related to gender have evolved relatively quickly within the past few decades. As more gender specialty clinics establish services across the world, newer research will likely clarify some of the unanswered questions, guide the clinical approach in a more systematic way, and help bridge the gaps where consensus among the experts has not yet been reached.

Summary Points

- Health care providers are increasingly being asked to play a key role in supporting the unique physical and mental health care needs of children and adolescents who display variation from population averages in gender role behavior and gender identity.
- Gender nonconformity refers to variation from developmental norms in gender role behavior, such as an aversion to rough-and-tumble play or team sports in males or an aversion to wearing stereotypical feminine clothing in females.
- Gender discordance describes incongruence between gender identity and the sex that a person was assigned at birth.
- Gender nonconformity and gender discordance are distinct phenomena; however, they can occur in the same individual and have significant developmental relationships to one another.
- Many, but not all, gender-nonconforming children (with and without gender discordance) grow up to be cisgender (nontransgender) with a gay, bisexual, or lesbian sexual orientation.
- Gender discordance in a child can cause clinically significant distress. Distress related to gender discordance and marked gender nonconformity are diagnostic features of the *DSM-5* diagnosis "gender dysphoria."
- Gender dysphoria can present before or after puberty. When it presents in childhood, it subsides in a majority of cases; when it presents in adolescence, it often persists (as in adulthood).
- Clinicians should inform parents and other caregivers of the various possible developmental outcomes for these children, as well as the limitations in predicting these outcomes, and help them to tolerate ambiguity about the future. The focus should be on ensuring that their children feel safe and supported.
- In addition to routine pediatric health care, gender-nonconforming and gender-discordant youth sometimes need additional psychosocial and mental health support and, in the case of gender dysphoria, possibly current and future endocrinological and surgical interventions.
- Care for gender-nonconforming and gender-dysphoric youth may also include interventions within the family or community for support, education, advocacy, and referral.
- Reasonable efforts to include appropriate mental health services provided by clinicians with competency in pediatric mental health and gender and sexual development are part of the standard care for gender-dysphoric and -nonconforming youth.
- Treatment for gender dysphoria includes nonmedical interventions, such as support groups, breast binding, and name and other social gender changes, as well as endocrine treatments, such as pubertal suppression and cross-sex hormonal treatment. Interventions may have risks and benefits.

- It is important to obtain informed consent (including consent from any legal guardians) as well as developmentally appropriate assent based on consideration of the risks and benefits, both known and hypothetical, of treatment and nontreatment options.
- Although clinical practice guidelines and parameters in this field of medicine exist, there remains a pressing need for further research to fully inform best practices. Clinicians must therefore flexibly adapt the current guidelines to the needs of each individual patient and community.

References

1. De Vries AL, Cohen-Kettenis PT. Clinical management of gender dysphoria in children and adolescents: the Dutch approach. J Homosex. 2012;59:301-320.
2. Wood H, Sasaki S, Bradley SJ, et al. Patterns of referral to a gender identity service for children and adolescents (1976–2011): age, sex ratio, and sexual orientation. J Sex Marital Ther. 2013;39:1-6.
3. Institute of Medicine. The Health of Lesbian, Gay, Bisexual, and Transgender People: Building a Foundation for Better Understanding. Washington, DC: The National Academies Press; 2011.
4. Adelson S, Walter H, Bukstein O, et al. Practice parameter on gay, lesbian or bisexual sexual orientation, gender-nonconformity, and gender discordance in children and adolescents. J Am Acad Child Adolesc Psychiatry. 2012;51:957-74.
5. Coleman E, Bockting W, Botzer M, et al. Standards of care for the health of a transsexual, transgender and gender non-conforming people, version 7. Int J Transgender. 2011;13: 165-232.
6. Adelson SL. Development of AACAP practice parameters for gender nonconformity and gender discordance in children and adolescents. Child Adolesc Psychiatr Clin North Am. 2011;20:651-63.
7. American Psychiatric Association. Diagnostic and Statistical Manual of Mental Disorders. 5th ed. Arlington, VA: American Psychiatric Publishing; 2013.
8. American Psychiatric Association. Diagnostic and Statistical Manual of Mental Disorders. 2nd ed. Washington, DC: American Psychiatric Association Press; 1968.
9. American Psychiatric Association. Diagnostic and Statistical Manual of Mental Disorders. 3rd ed. Washington, DC: American Psychiatric Association Press; 1980.
10. Drescher J. Queer diagnoses: parallels and contrasts in the history of homosexuality, gender variance, and the diagnostic and statistical manual. Arch Sex Behav. 2010;39:427-60.
11. Meyer IH. Prejudice, social stress, and mental health in lesbian, gay, and bisexual populations: conceptual issues and research evidence. Psychol Bull. 2003;129:674-97.
12. Ryan C, Huebner D, Diaz RM, Sanchez J. Family rejection as a predictor of negative health outcomes in white and Latino lesbian, gay, and bisexual young adults. Pediatrics. 2009;123: 346-52.
13. Bailey JM, Zucker KJ. Childhood sex-typed behavior and sexual orientation: a conceptual analysis and quantitative review. Dev Psychol. 1995;31:43-55.
14. Whitam FL. The prehomosexual male child in three societies: the United States, Guatemala, Brazil. Arch Sex Behav. 1980;9:87-99.
15. Whitam FL, Mathy RM. Childhood cross-gender behavior of homosexual females in Brazil, Peru, the Philippines, and the United States. Arch Sex Behav. 1991;20:151-70.
16. Wallien MSC, Cohen-Kettenis PT. Psychosexual outcome of gender-dysphoric children. J Am Acad Child Adolesc Psychiatr. 2008;47:1413-23.

17. **Zucker KJ, Bradley SJ.** Gender Identity Disorder and Psychosexual Problems in Children and Adolescents. New York: Guilford Press; 1995.

18. **Green R.** The "Sissy-Boy Syndrome" and the Development of Homosexuality. New Haven: Yale University Press; 1987.

19. **Drummond KD, Bradley SJ, Peterson-Badali M, Zucker KJ.** A follow-up study of girls with gender identity disorder. Dev Psychol. 2008;44:34-45.

20. **Steensma TD, McGuire JK, Kreukels BP, Beekman AJ, Cohen-Kettenis PT.** Factors associated with desistence and persistence of childhood gender dysphoria: a quantitative follow-up study. J Am Acad Child Adolesc Psychiatry. 2013;52:582-90.

21. **Steensma TD, Biemond R, de Boer F, Cohen-Kettenis P.** Desisting and persisting gender dysphoria after childhood: a qualitative follow-up study. Clin Child Psychol Psychiatry. 2011; 16:499-516.

22. **Smith YL, van Goozen SH, Cohen-Kettenis PT.** Adolescents with gender identity disorder who were accepted or rejected for sex reassignment surgery: a prospective follow-up study. J Am Acad Child Adolesc Psychiatry. 2001;40:472-81.

23. **Birkett M, Espelage DL, Koenig B.** LGB and questioning students in schools: the moderating effects of homophobic bullying and school climate on negative outcomes. J Youth Adolesc. 2009;38:989-1000.

24. **Toomey R, Ryan C, Diaz R, Card NA, Russell ST.** Gender nonconforming lesbian, gay, bisexual, and transgender youth: school victimization and young adult psychosocial adjustment. Dev Psychol. 2010;46:1580-89.

25. **Roberts AL, Rosario M, Corliss HL, Koenen KC, Austin SB.** Childhood gender nonconformity: a risk indicator for childhood abuse and posttraumatic stress in youth. Pediatrics. 2012;129:410-7.

26. **Roberts AL, Rosario M, Corliss HL, Koenen KC, Austin SB.** Elevated risk of posttraumatic stress in sexual minority youths: mediation by childhood abuse and gender nonconformity. Am J Public Health. 2012;102:1587-93.

27. **Roberts AL, Rosario M, Slopen N, et al.** Childhood gender nonconformity, bullying victimization and depressive symptoms across adolescence and early adulthood: an 11 year longitudinal study. J Am Acad Child Adolesc Psychiatry. 2013;52:143-52.

28. **Friedman RC, Downey JI.** Sexual Orientation and Psychoanalysis: Sexual Science and Clinical Practice. New York: Columbia University Press; 2002.

29. **Nuttbrock L, Hwahng S, Bockting W, et al.** Psychiatric impact of gender-related abuse across the life course of male-to-female transgender persons. J Sex Res. 2010;47:12-23.

30. **Kosciw JG, Diaz EM, Greytak EA.** The 2007 National School Climate Survey: The Experiences of Lesbian, Gay, Bisexual and Transgender Youth in Our Nation's Schools. New York: Gay, Lesbian, and Straight Education Network; 2008.

31. **O'Shaughnessy M, Russell S, Heck K, Calhoun C, Laub C.** Safe Place to Learn: Consequences of Harassment Based on Actual or Perceived Sexual Orientation and Gender Non-conformity and Steps for Making Schools Safer. San Francisco, CA: California Safe Schools Coalition; 2004.

32. **D'Augelli AR, Grossman AH, Starks MT.** Childhood gender atypicality, victimization, and PTSD among lesbian, gay, and bisexual youth. J Interpers Violence. 2006;21:1462-82.

33. **Pilkington NW, D'Augelli AR.** Victimization of lesbian, gay, and bisexual youth in community settings. J Commun Psychol. 1995;23:34-56.

34. **Wallien MS, Swaab H, Cohen-Kettenis PT.** Psychiatric comorbidity among children with gender identity disorder. J Am Acad Child Adolesc Psychiatry. 2007;46:1307-14.

35. **Spack NP, Laura Edwards-Leeper, HA Feldman, et al.** Children and adolescents with gender identity disorder referred to a pediatric medical center. Pediatrics. 2012;129:418-25.

36. **Grossman AH, D'Augelli AR.** Transgender youth and life-threatening behaviors. Suicide Life Threat Behav. 2007;37:527-37.

37. **Pleak RR.** Ethical issues in diagnosing and treating gender-dysphoric children and adolescents. In: Rottnek M, ed. Sissies and Tomboys: Gender Nonconformity and Homosexual Childhood. New York: New York University Press; 1999:34-51.

38. **Menvielle EJ, Tuerk C.** A support group for parents of gender-nonconforming boys. J Am Acad Child Adolesc Psychiatry. 2002;41:1010-3.

39. **Menvielle EJ, Rodnan LA.** A therapeutic group for parents of transgender adolescents. Child Adolesc Psychiatr Clin N Am. 2011;20:733-44.

40. **American Psychiatric Association.** Diagnostic and Statistical Manual of Mental Disorders. 4th ed. Washington, DC: American Psychiatric Association Press; 1994.

41. **Zucker KJ, Bradley SJ, Sullivan CB, Kuksis M, Birkenfeld-Adams A, Mitchell JN.** A gender identity interview for children. J Pers Assess. 1993;61:443-56.

42. **Wallien MS, Quilty LC, Steensma TD, et al.** Cross-national replication of the gender identity interview for children. J Person Assess. 2009;91:545-52.

43. **Johnson LL, Bradley SJ, Birkenfeld-Adams AS, et al.** A parent- report gender identity questionnaire for children. Arch Sex Behav. 2004;33:105-16.

44. **Zucker KJ.** On the "natural history" of gender identity disorder in children. J Am Acad Child Adolesc Psychiatry. 2008;47:1361-3.

45. **Steensma TD, Cohen-Kettenis PT.** Gender transitioning before puberty? Arch Sex Behav. 2011;40:649-50.

46. **Leibowitz SF, Telingator C.** Assessing gender identity concerns in children and adolescents: evaluation, treatments, and outcomes. Curr Psychiatry Rep. 2012;14:111-20.

47. **Singh D, Deogracias JJ, Johnson LL, et al.** The Gender Identity/Gender Dysphoria Questionnaire for Adolescents and Adults: further validity evidence. J Sex Res. 2010;47:49-58.

48. **Edwards-Leeper L, Spack NP.** Psychological evaluation and medical treatment of transgender youth in an interdisciplinary "Gender Management Service" (GeMS) in a major pediatric center. J Homosex. 2012;59:321-36.

49. **de Vries ALC, Noens ILJ, Cohen-Kettenis PT, et al.** Autism spectrum disorders in gender dysphoric children and adolescents. J Autism Dev Disord. 2010;40:930-6.

50. **Zucker KJ, Wood H, Singh D, Bradley SJ.** A developmental, biopsychosocial model for the treatment of children with gender identity disorder. J Homosex. 2012;59:369-97.

51. **Menvielle E.** A comprehensive program for children with gender variant behaviors and gender identity disorders. J Homosex. 2012;59:357-68.

52. **Ehrensaft D.** From gender identity disorder to gender identity creativity: true gender self child therapy. J Homosex. 2012;59:337-56.

53. **Callen Lorde Community Health Center.** Transgender health program protocols. 2012. Available at: http://callen-lorde.org/our-services/sexual-health-clinic/transgender-health-services/

54. **Tom Waddell Health Center.** Protocols for hormonal reassignment of gender. 2006. Available at: www.sfdph.org/dph/comupg/oservices/medSvs/hlthCtrs/TransGendprotocols122006.pdf.

55. **Kreukels BP, Cohen-Kettenis PT.** Puberty suppression in gender identity disorder: the Amsterdam experience. Nat Rev Endocrinol. 2011;7:466-72.

56. **Hembree W, Cohen-Kettenis PT, Delemarre-van de Waal HA, et al.** Endocrine treatment of transsexual persons: an Endocrine Society clinical practice guideline. J Clin Endocrinol Metab. 2009;94:3132-54.

57. **Lawrence AA.** Factors associated with satisfaction or regret following male-to-female sex reassignment surgery. Arch Sex Behav. 2003;32:299-315.

58. **de Vries AL, Steensma TD, Doreleijers TA, Cohen-Kettenis PT.** Puberty suppression in adolescents with gender identity disorder: a prospective follow-up study. J Sex Med. 2011;8:2276-83

59. **Delemarre-van de Waal HA, Cohen-Kettenis PT.** Clinical management of gender identity disorder in adolescents: a protocol on psychological and paediatric endocrinology aspects. Eur J Endocrinology. 2006;155:S1131-7.

60. **Cohen-Kettenis PT, Delemarre-van de Waal HA, Gooren LJ.** The treatment of adolescent transsexuals: changing insights. J Sex Med. 2008;5:1892-7.

61. **de Vries ALC, Steensma T, Wagenaar TAH, et al.** Puberty suppression followed by cross-sex hormones and gender reassignment surgery: a prospective follow-up of gender dysphoric adolescents into adults. Gender dysphoria in adolescents; mental health and treatment evaluation [Thesis]. Amsterdam, the Netherlands: VU University Medical Center; 2010.

62. **Stein E.** Commentary on the treatment of gender variant and gender dysphoric children and adolescents: common themes and ethical reflections. J Homosex. 2012;59:480-500.
63. **Delemarre-van de Waal HA.** Medical intervention in transgender adolescents appears to be safe and effective. Presented at the Endocrine Society 95th Annual Meeting, San Francisco, 2013. Available at: www.sciencecodex.com/medical_intervention_in_transgender_adolescents_appears_to_be_safe_and_effective-114120
64. **Sadjadi S.** The endocrinologist's office-puberty suppression: saving children from a natural disaster? J Med Human. 201334:255-60.
65. **Schwartz D.** Listening to children imagining gender: observing the inflation of an idea. J Homosex. 2012;59:460-79.
66. **Leibowitz S, Spack NP.** The development of a gender identity psychosocial clinic: treatment issues, logistical considerations, interdisciplinary cooperation, and future initiatives. Child Adolesc Psychiatr Clin North Am. 2011;20:701-724.

Chapter 17

Creating a Foundation for Improving Trans Health: Understanding Trans Identities and Health Care Needs

JOANNE G. KEATLEY, MSW
MADELINE B. DEUTSCH, MD
JAE M. SEVELIUS, PhD
LUIS GUTIERREZ-MOCK, MA, MPH

Introduction

In discussions of lesbian, gay, bisexual, and transgender (LGBT) populations, transgender (trans) people are often included with the assumption that the reader understands the differences inherent to this population when compared to LGB-identified individuals. This leads to many inaccurate beliefs and complications, particularly when it comes to matters concerning health and well-being. The common practice of including trans people with LGB people also leads to the misunderstanding that all trans people identify as lesbian, gay, or bisexual and engage in same-sex behaviors, when in fact trans people represent the full range of sexual identities and behaviors. This practice has led to the relative invisibility of the population and has accentuated a lack of understanding of the overall health care needs of trans people. In addition, there has been limited research on trans health issues, and few medical schools provide their students with a curriculum that covers what is known about trans health (1,2). As a result, health care providers have come to depend on anecdotal, at times inconsistent, information to make treatment decisions. Despite these limitations, health care providers are in a unique position to make a positive impact on trans people's lives. When given accurate information and training, they become empowered and able to provide culturally appropriate care and treatment. This chapter was developed to educate health care providers about basic concepts related to trans people in order to help them optimize care for their patients. To this end, the chapter aims to clarify distinctions and acknowledge diversity among trans people, define terms and issues frequently associated with certain trans identities, detail processes of gender identity formation, and lay out strategies for providing affirming care to trans people.

The Transgender Population: Health Disparities and Population Size

The profound health disparities experienced by trans people in the United States have been well documented (2–4). In the 2011 report "Injustice at Every Turn: A Report of the National Transgender Discrimination Survey," 50% of the 6450 trans respondents reported that their medical providers were not adequately prepared to respond to their specific health care needs (4). Nineteen percent of the respondents reported being refused medical care, and 28% reported postponing medical treatment because of discrimination in health care. As a result of high levels of discrimination and social and economic marginalization, transgender people experience higher rates of substance use, violence and harassment, and suicide attempts (41% reported attempting suicide) compared with the general population (2,4).

Nationally, the disparities are startling, but they are even more striking given that, to date, we have not done an adequate job of documenting, tracking, or measuring the population itself and the range of health issues that affect them (2). In 2011, 30 years into the HIV epidemic, the Centers for Disease Control and Prevention (CDC) added a gender identity variable as an optional field in the electronic HIV/AIDS Reporting System. The U.S. Census does not ask questions related to one's gender identity, and to date no national population-based studies on gender identity have been conducted in the United States.

Because of the lack of consistent data collection methods, as well as the diversity and in many cases hidden nature of trans communities, it is not possible to accurately estimate the size of the trans population. Nonetheless, we can estimate a range by looking at studies that collect data from existing pathology-based sources, such as *Diagnostic and Statistical Manual of Mental Disorders* (*DSM*) codes, or by using limited data from studies on the rates of suicidality, tobacco use, and HIV among trans populations. In addition, emergency departments and state departments of health sometimes collect gender identity information. From all of these sources, the limited understanding of the trans population size in the United States indicates that an estimated range of 0.1% to 0.5% of the population present with a form of gender identity, expression, or presentation that could be included in the trans spectrum (5–8).

A recent well-conducted landline phone survey of 28,662 residents of Massachusetts between ages 18 and 64 years found trans rates at the high end of this range (7). On this survey, respondents were asked the following question: "Some people describe themselves as transgender when they experience a different gender identity from the birth sex. For example, a person born into the male body, but who feels female or lives as a woman. Do you consider yourself to be transgender?"

Additional information was provided to respondents who did not understand the question. A total of 131 respondents (0.5%; 95% confidence interval, 0.3% to 0.6%) responded "yes" to this question. This study's methods serve well as a template for additional studies of the prevalence of transgender identities. With the rising visibility of gender diversity among younger generations, the study might even have found a higher prevalence if it had used a mobile phone survey, as younger generations are less likely to have a landline telephone. The potential impact of 0.5% of a randomly selected U.S. population identifying as trans on such factors as insurance coverage, research funding, and public health programming is profound; trans people are no longer a rare exception but are in fact becoming recognized as a substantial portion of the general population and as such a natural component of the human experience.

Trans Terminology

Like many minority communities, the trans community is not a homogenous group but rather represents a diversity of identities that cut across ethnic, linguistic, national, socioeconomic, and generational lines (9,10). Attempting to define the trans community through a single or small number of identities would be akin to describing the community of Beatles fans; there may be little in common between 2 members of the community beyond their musical tastes. Instead, taking a broader view of both the community and defining terminology will not only help to understand the community but also enhance patient–provider interactions through improved understanding and fluency.

Terminology used in describing trans people is as diverse as the community itself. The term *transsexual* was first used by Mangus Hirschfeld in 1923 to describe a patient who underwent an early genital reassignment procedure (11). Table 17-1 defines *transsexual* and other common terms. For the purposes of this discussion, the term *trans* (the abbreviation of *transgender*) will be used for convenience to describe the overarching community of those whose gender identity differs from the sex that they were assigned at birth; *trans* will also include other gender-nonconforming people who may or may not identify as transgender or trans, but whose gender expression may vary from the stereotypical expression of someone assigned male or female at birth. For example, a butch woman or effeminate man are examples of gender-nonconforming people who may still experience discrimination and face barriers and social determinants of health similar to those encountered by trans-identified persons.

Table 17–1   Definitions of Terms Related to Transgender Health and Identities*

Term	Definition
Sex	Refers to a combination of biological markers (chromosomes and hormones) and anatomic characteristics (reproductive organs and genitalia). In the United States, all people are assigned 1 of 2 dichotomous sexes at birth or shortly after birth: male or female.
Gender	Refers to the rules and norms that a society assigns to varying degrees of maleness and femaleness. Gender in the United States is usually expressed as a binary construct: you are either a man or a woman. However, many people believe the gender binary to be overly simplistic and harmful to those whose gender identity and/or expression falls outside this simple dichotomy (such as those who identify as genderqueer, discussed below).
Gender identity	A person's internal sense of their[†] own gender. All people have a gender identity; however, transgender people feel their gender identity does not reflect the sex they were assigned at birth.
Gender expression	How one externally manifests their gender identity through behavior, mannerisms, speech patterns, dress, and hairstyles. Gender expression falls along a spectrum and may not directly correlate with gender identity.
Gender nonconforming	Refers to people whose gender expression differs from their gender identity based on a given society's norms for males and females: e.g., a woman who dresses primarily in what is considered male style clothing or a young boy who prefers stereotypically "feminine" toys, such as dolls, and rejects stereotypically "masculine" games, such as rough-and-tumble games.
Transgender	Refers to a person whose gender identity does not correspond to their sex assigned at birth. *Transgender* (or the shortened version, *trans*) may be used to refer to an individual person's gender identity and is sometimes used as an umbrella term for all people who do not conform to traditional gender norms.
Cisgender/ Non-trans	Refers to a person who is not transgender; a person whose gender identity corresponds with their sex assigned at birth. The terms *cisgender* and *non-trans/non-transgender* may be used interchangeably.
Genderqueer	A person who blurs or bends the gender binary, identifies outside of the gender binary (i.e., neither male nor female gender) and/or identifies as both male and female. Similar terms include *gender variant* and *gender fluid.*
Trans man (sometimes referred to as FTM)	A person who was assigned female sex at birth and who now identifies as male. Some trans people use the term *FTM* (female-to-male) to refer to the same concept.
Trans woman (sometimes referred to as MTF)	A person who was assigned male sex at birth and who now identifies as female. Some trans people use the term *MTF* (male-to-female) to refer to the same concept.

(continued)

Table 17-1   Definitions of Terms Related to Transgender Health and Identities* *(Continued)*

Term	Definition
Transsexual	Historically been used as a medical term to refer to individuals seeking medical or surgical intervention to affirm their gender; also a term used by some people to describe their gender identity. People who identify as transsexual will likely have received some gender-affirming procedures; however, not all transsexual identified people take cross-sex hormones or have had any gender-confirming surgeries. Unlike *transgender*, *transsexual* is not an umbrella term and should be used only if an individual self-identifies as a transsexual person.
Transition	Generally refers to the period that a person "transitions" from one gender to another. This may include some or all of the following: coming out to oneself and accepting oneself as a different gender; coming out to friends/family/coworkers; changing legal documents to reflect a different gender (e.g., birth certificate, driver license, social security); changing name, dress, and voice; undergoing cross-sex hormone therapy and/or other gender-affirming procedures.
Gender-affirming procedures	Surgical or other medical procedures that are used to help to affirm an individual's gender identity, including but not limited to cross-sex hormone therapy, vaginoplasty, phalloplasty, metoidioplasty, facial feminization surgery, chest reconstruction surgery (mastectomy), breast augmentation, and soft tissue filler injections. Gender-affirming surgical procedures may also be referred to as gender-confirming surgeries, sex reassignment surgeries, reassignment surgeries, and "sex change" surgeries.
Cross-sex hormone therapy	Cross-sex hormones (estrogens in people assigned a male sex at birth and androgens in people assigned a female sex at birth) are used to induce or maintain the physical and psychological characteristics of the sex that matches a person's gender identity. Not all trans people want to take cross-sex hormones.

*Terminology is always evolving and can vary in different cultures. In addition to the terms defined here, there are many other words that people use to describe themselves and their experiences.

†The gender-neutral pronoun *their* is used here in place of *his/her* in order to be inclusive of nonbinary gender identities.

Identity Processes and Gender Affirmation

As our understandings of trans people and their experiences have evolved over the years, we have come to recognize that there is no singular trans identity. A great deal of work remains to be done in terms of conceptualizing a trajectory of trans identity development and understanding what constitutes healthy resolution of the process of trans identity development. Below is a summary of some of the academic literature to date on gender identity development and processes. See also Chapter 4 for further discussion of this topic.

Stage Models of Identity Development

Borrowing from research on gay and lesbian identity development, stage models have been proposed for conceptualizing trans identity development (12). Most of these models assume a trajectory that includes a "coming out" process that is similar to the gay and lesbian experience, where one's "true identity" is sensed internally early in life, is initially hidden, and is then revealed to others as the person achieves a higher degree of self-acceptance (13). In these stage models, coming out is often closely preceded or followed by the exploration and possible pursuit of medical transition, which is then followed by identity resolution and possibly even invisibility as a trans person once transition is complete. Many of these models include the caveat that some people may not experience these stages of identity development in a linear fashion and may cycle back through earlier stages at various points in one's lifetime. In addition, not all trans people experience identity resolution and integration (13).

For example, Bockting's (14) model of the stages of trans coming out process draws from Erikson's (15) ideas about how identity development is influenced by social interactions and interpersonal relationships. The stages he proposes include pre–coming out, coming out, exploration, intimacy, and identity integration. Recently, Morgan and Stevens (12) proposed a similar stage model where one's internally felt sense of being trans is experienced as "mind-body dissonance" followed by the negotiation and management of identity, and ultimately the process of transitioning.

These stage models are useful in guiding health professionals in their work with trans people, but there is much work still to be done. As our cultural understanding and acceptance of trans people increase, more young people are growing up in families that are supportive and seek appropriate care for their children early on in their development. These children may have very different developmental trajectories due to changes in both the social and medical environment, where, for example, some have access to puberty-suppressing medication and thus never have to endure an adolescence that is incongruent with their identity (for more on this topic, see Chapter 16).

In addition, we still have much to learn about differences in trans identities and their development by race/ethnicity, culture, region, age, etc. In light of a wide variety in cultural notions about gender and gender diversity, trans people's experiences and identities are significantly shaped by their cultural environment. This includes generational differences in identity and expression among trans people within the same Western culture.

Identity Processes and the Role of Gender Affirmation

While many stage theories propose similar trajectories that culminate in a resolved, integrated trans identity, more attention has recently been given

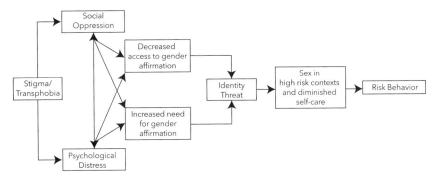

Figure 17-1 Model of gender affirmation.

to the fact that identity management is life-long and ever evolving. Trans peoples' identities may shift over time and may range from integrating a trans identity into a gender presentation that is consistent with the sex assigned at birth, to gender presentations that do not conform to the male-female binary, to full social and medical transition from the sex assigned at birth to an opposite binary sex and gender presentation.

Gender affirmation refers to an interpersonal, interactive process whereby a person receives social recognition and support for gender identity and expression (14,16,17). While a number of investigators have observed an intense need for (and often lack of access to) gender affirmation among trans individuals, its relationship to health has rarely been directly investigated (16,17). Recently, the Center of Excellence for Transgender Health proposed a Model of Gender Affirmation (18) to provide a trans-specific framework for research and intervention development focused on risk-taking and self-care behaviors among trans women. The Model of Gender Affirmation (see Figure 17-1) posits that in the context of transphobia, a high need for gender affirmation among trans people coupled with low access to gender affirmation procedures, results in an unmet need for gender affirmation, which constitutes identity threat (18,19). Trans people may attempt to reduce identity threat (or meet their needs for gender affirmation) by seeking affirmation in contexts that can pose health risks and subsequently undervalue important health seeking behaviors (18,20). Interventions that emphasize self-care motivated by empowerment, gender pride, and understanding gender-based power inequalities, may be successful in building sexual negotiation skills and inspiring healthy behaviors that are supported by a sense of self-worth.

Gender Identity and the Process of Transition/Affirmation

The process by which trans people undergo a social and/or medical transition is often called *transition* or *gender identity affirmation* (the term *affirmation*, sometimes written as *confirmation*, is used to acknowledge that outward changes are simply affirming a person's inner gender identity). This may involve a combination of medical and surgical processes, legal document changes, and social change, which is often the most difficult component and involves coming out to friends and family and reorienting oneself to moving through the world in a different gender (in some cases with needed psychotherapeutic support).

For successful gender affirmation processes to occur, the World Professional Association for Transgender Health (WPATH), which publishes the Standards for the Care of Transsexual, Transgender, and Gender Nonconforming Persons (SOC), used to recommend a triadic pathway involving psychotherapy followed by hormone replacement and then surgery (21). The current seventh version of the SOC recognizes that the components of transition are individualized; not all people need all components, and the order in which they occur must be flexible and individualized (22).

Gender Identity and Sexual Orientation

It can be difficult for some to separate the concepts of sexual orientation and gender identity. Both represent distinctive spectra that on some levels are related, but not intimately linked. Trans women are not gay men who were so gay and effeminate that they became women, and trans men are not butch lesbians who were so butch that they became men. As with the general population, trans people have a range of sexual orientations; trans men and women may be attracted to men, attracted to women, attracted to both, or attracted to neither. As with sexual orientation, it is always best to allow trans persons to define their own sexual identity and terminology; however, in general the terminology should reflect the affirmed gender (i.e., a trans woman who is attracted to other women is a lesbian, and a trans man attracted to other men is a gay man). As with people who are non-transgender, these sexual identities may also have deep meaning in political and social contexts; trans lesbians may have an intense connection to the larger lesbian community, and trans gay men may feel strongly about gay male identity and culture (reminding us that trans people have more aspects to their individual identities than simply being trans) (23,24).

Regarding sexual behavior, trans people exhibit a range of sexual practices; some but not all trans people are opposed to using their natal genitals in a sexual manner. Some trans women may use their penis for penetrative sex, and some trans men may engage in vaginal receptive sex (25,26). Because cross-sex hormone therapy is not reliable contraception, such practices without adequate barriers may place trans people at risk for pregnancy or impregnating someone else, in addition to the risk for acquiring a sexually transmitted infection, including HIV infection (27).

Customs and terminology become even more varied when looking at cultures outside of the European–North American context. The lines between sexual orientation and gender identity may be less well defined, or the concepts and terminology related to gender identity may be completely different or even lacking. For example, in Latin America some trans women retain a connection to their male identity and use the term *gay* to describe themselves (28); some cultures in Southeast Asia and the Indian subcontinent recognize a third gender that is neither male nor female and in general comprises people on the trans spectrum (29). There is great variation even within the United States. African-, Asian- and Latin-American subcultures can differ widely from European-American paradigms. A detailed discussion of these cultural intersections is beyond the scope of this text; however, suffice it to say that an open mind should be kept around trans identity, culture, and terminology.

Gender Identity: A Diagnosis?

Given the wide range of identities, sexual orientations, and gender expressions encountered among trans people, the existence of a single diagnosis (or small set of diagnoses) related to "being trans" may at first glance appear counterintuitive, or in the very least difficult to clearly define. The trans community remains divided on the debate over whether trans people should be given a mental health diagnosis—and with good reason. On the one hand, maintaining a diagnosis for what many feel is within the normal range of human expression may bring an undue degree of pathologization; on the other hand, the existence of a diagnosis allows for access to treatments that may otherwise be unavailable (or in the very least not covered by insurance) were an official diagnosis not to exist.

Both the *DSM* (published by the American Psychiatric Association [APA]) and the *International Classification of Diseases* (*ICD*, published by the World Health Organization [WHO]) contain gender-identity related diagnostic categories, although terminology differs between the two, and there is debate over which diagnoses to use and for what purposes (30). Both are meant to be used by a range of clinicians and researchers and are tools for collecting epidemiologic statistics (31,32), although the *DSM* is considered the "standard classification of mental disorders used by mental health professionals in the United States" (31), whereas the *ICD* is considered "the standard diagnostic tool for epidemiology, health management, and clinical purposes" (32).

DSM Diagnoses

The most recent revision to the *DSM* (*DSM-5*) was launched at the May 2013 annual conference of the APA in San Francisco, California, and contains numerous updates with respect to gender identity (33). The previous version, *DSM-IV-TR*, used the diagnosis of "gender identity disorder" (GID) with specifiers "in adults/adolescents" (302.85) or "in children" (302.6); additional specifiers were used for sexual orientation (attracted to men, women, both, or neither), and "GID not otherwise specified" (NOS) was included for those with concurrent intersex conditions or otherwise not specified (34). In addition, a separate diagnosis of "transvestic fetishism" (TF; 302.3) existed only for heterosexual males with sexual arousal, behaviors, or urges upon cross-dressing behavior. Both were listed in the "Sexual and Gender Identity Disorders" chapter, while GID was listed in its own "Gender Identity Disorders" section. TF was contained within the "Paraphilias" section housed between "Sexual Sadism" and "Voyeurism."

Indeed, while both GID and TF contained "distress" criteria (i.e., the behaviors or conditions had to cause emotional distress or interfere with daily living in order to lead to a diagnosis), the general sentiment among many community activists was that both of these diagnoses were pathologizing, especially TF's placement among paraphilias such as frotteurism and pedophilia. Several years of debate and academic discussions leading up to the revision included requests for commentary from the APA as well as input from WPATH and countless professionals and members of the community (35). Finally, for the *DSM-5*, the diagnosis of GID was eliminated and a new diagnosis "gender dysphoria" was included in its place. The *DSM-5* criteria for gender dysphoria in adolescents and adults (33) are as follows:

A. Marked incongruence between one's experienced and expressed gender, of at least 6 months' duration; as manifested by at least 2 of the following:

1. Incongruence between one's expressed gender and primary and/or secondary sex characteristics
2. Strong desire to be rid of one's primary and/or secondary sex characteristics
3. Strong desire for the primary and/or secondary sex characteristics of the other gender
4. Strong desire to be of the other gender, or of some alternative gender that differs from assigned gender
5. Strong desire to be treated as the other gender, or as someone of an alternative gender that differs from assigned gender
6. Strong conviction that one has the typical feelings and reactions of the other gender, or as someone of an alternative gender that differs from assigned gender

B. Condition is associated with clinically significant distress or impairment in social, occupational, or other important areas of functioning.

The *DSM-5* criteria contain several important updates of note: 1) the recognition that gender dysphoria is a multicategorical concept rather than a dichotomy, eliminating the strict view of a gender binary (as opposed to more of a spectrum of gender), and 2) removal of the sexual orientation specifiers. A post-transition specifier has been added to recognize the ongoing need for a diagnostic category to allow continued access to services for those who no longer suffer distress due to their gender identity. Childhood criteria have been tightened somewhat, now requiring a strong desire to be of the other gender. Transvestism remains and has in fact been renamed "transvestic disorder" with additional autogynephilic and autoandrophilic specifiers—both of which signify a largely unproven theory that transvestism is rooted in a sexual arousal by the thought of becoming a woman (autogynephilia) or a man (autoandrophilia) (36).

ICD Diagnoses

Many in the community have expressed disappointment with the renaming and reclassification in the *DSM*; in fact, many had called for complete removal of gender dysphoria, preferring to rely entirely on the use of codes within the *ICD* (37). On some levels this does make sense; as noted in the *DSM-5*, gender dysphoria is a unique condition in that it is a diagnosis that may be made by mental health professionals but is primarily treated medically and surgically. Nonetheless, there is also debate over how the ICD defines and diagnoses gender identity–related health. The *ICD-10* contains a gender-related diagnosis in section F64, "Gender Identity Disorders," under the Mental and Behavioral Disorders section, "Disorders of Adult Personality and Behavior" subsection, but no strictly medical codes exist. Thus, some medical providers use other codes, such as for "endocrine disorder NOS" (259.9). Furthermore, the United States, as of early 2014, still uses *ICD-9* and is preparing for a changeover to *ICD-10*, while the rest of the world is already using *ICD-10* and is preparing for a changeover to *ICD-11*. Currently, WPATH and other stakeholders (including the Global Action for Trans* Equality) have been reviewing language and drafting recommendations for consideration for the upcoming *ICD-11* revision. While the recommendations have been made, nothing has yet been decided. WPATH published a report in 2013 on their ongoing consensus process regarding the *ICD-11* (38).

The Application of a Gender Identity Diagnosis

Beyond the letter of the actual content in both the ICD and the DSM lies the application of such diagnoses. Like many DSM diagnoses, gender dysphoria is defined as such only if it "causes undue distress." Such a statement may assuage concerns that gender dysphoria is in need of an "exit clause" that would allow someone to no longer carry the diagnosis once they have navigated their transition to a place of comfort and self-satisfaction. A theoretical concern, however, may be that the existence in the *DSM* of such a diagnosis in any capacity results in a situation where diagnoses may be used incorrectly or may further pathologize. France, for example, has formally declassified gender dysphoria as a mental illness (39). In any case, a diagnosis of some kind is likely needed in the long term to allow trans people to continue to access care and receive insurance benefits related to hormonal and other care (40). As such, it would seem appropriate to partner efforts for *DSM* and *ICD* reform with efforts to better educate users on the correct and appropriate application of such diagnoses. Clear recommendations for clinicians in the United States are difficult to make, however. Some believe that compliance with coding guidelines requires all trans-specific care to be coded using one of the *ICD* gender-related categories (e.g., 302.85) effectively for life. In this case, a trans person who is decades past social transition and surgery would still face the use of this diagnosis as there is currently no diagnostic code for the medical care (i.e. hormone maintenance) of transgender people who are post-transition. Others argue that because the *ICD* is incomplete with respect to a "maintenance phase" diagnosis, it is better to instead use codes for such conditions as endocrine disorder NOS (259.9), endocrine disorder not elsewhere classifiable (259.8), or a code for a related condition, such as for gonadal failure or early menopause.

Delivering Trans-Competent Medical Services

Establishing services for trans people can seem like a daunting and intimidating prospect because many health professionals are taught little to nothing about this in school or training (1). Nevertheless, as the needs of trans people become better known, visibility of the community increases, and insurance exclusions from trans care coverage wane, service providers will face an increasing mandate to provide culturally appropriate and evidence-based trans care. To begin, it is important to define several related terms. *Culturally appropriate* refers to services of any type that are provided in a fashion sensitive to the needs and culture of trans people and that provide a welcoming, inclusive, and safe environment. *Trans-inclusive* specifies services that may not be trans-specific but are rendered in a fashion that considers the needs of trans people. *Trans-specific* refers to services that address the unique needs of trans people.

As with the general population, trans people require culturally appropriate routine primary and preventive care (41). Just as a clinic with a large ethnic Chinese population will likely have Chinese art on the wall, a clinic or agency that serves trans people would be well served to have trans-themed art or pamphlets in the waiting area. Gender-neutral bathrooms or a clear policy that allows people to use the bathroom of their choice is essential.

In addition, trans-inclusive services will ensure that the needed steps are taken to provide appropriate care for trans people. Such steps should include

- Amending intake forms, charts, and electronic health record (EHR) systems to allow for the unique needs of trans people (see below for more on this topic; Appendix A provides more recommendations for creating an inclusive clinical environment).

- Equipping the facility with appropriate equipment and supplies, such as smaller vaginal speculums for trans men, having practices in place to allow the processing of cervical Papanicolaou smears in trans men, and ensuring that providers and staff are appropriately trained in the particulars of trans primary health and screening needs.

Trans-specific care is addressed in detail in Chapter 18. Selected additional resources are listed in Table 17-2. In general, trans-specific care refers to a variety of medical and surgical procedures as well as, in many cases, mental health services. Some services are more complex and require extensive training (i.e., surgery), while others involve application of existing primary care skills with slight modifications to current practices

---

Table 17-2   Additional Resources on Transgender Health Care

Updated recommendations from the World Professional Association for Transgender Health Standards of Care (WPATH SOC). Am Fam Physician. 2013;87:89-93.

Review of updates and changes in WPATH SOC version 7 as compared to version 6 relevant to primary care settings.

A long-term follow-up study of mortality in transsexuals receiving treatment with cross-sex hormones. Eur J Endocrinol. 2011;164:635-42.

Long-term follow-up on 966 male-to-female (MTF) and 365 female-to-male (FTM) individuals.

University of California San Francisco Center of Excellence for Transgender Health Primary Care. Protocol for Transgender Care. 2010. Available at www.transhealth.ucsf.edu/protocols

Evidence-based expert consensus opinion on transgender care in resource-limited settings.

Providing care to transgender persons: a clinical approach to primary care hormones and HIV management. J Assoc Nurses AIDS Care. 2010;21:221-9.

Primary and hormonal care HIV and transgender care.

Principles of Transgender Medicine and Surgery. Binghamton, NY: Haworth Press; 2007

Textbook covering a wide range of transgender health subjects, including primary care, hormones, surgery, and mental health.

Endocrine therapy for transgender adults in British Columbia: suggested guidelines. 2006.

Comprehensive set of evidence based endocrine primary care and mental health treatment and training guidelines tailored for the Canadian health system. Currently being revised.

Endocrine treatment of transsexual persons: an Endocrine Society clinical practice guideline. J Clin Endocrinol Metab. 2009;94:3132-54.

Endocrinologist-oriented in-depth review. Contains some outdated recommendations based on sixth version of SOC.

Hormone therapy in adults: suggested revisions to the sixth version of the Standards of Care. Int J Transgender. 2009;11:146-82.

In-depth review of hormonal care.

Table 17-3   Care and Treatment Commonly Sought by Transgender People

---

Medical
  • Cross-sex hormone therapy
  • Preoperative medical evaluations
  • Routine postoperative care and office management of surgical complications
  • Facial hair removal via laser or electrolysis (including prescription of pain
    medication and topical anesthetics)

Surgical: Trans Women/Male-to-Female (MTF)
  • Vaginoplasty
  • Orchiectomy
  • Breast augmentation
  • Facial feminization
  • Adam's apple removal (reduction thyrochondroplasty)
  • Liposuction and body contouring

Surgical: Trans Men/Female-to-Male (FTM)
  • Mastectomy ("top surgery")
  • Hysterectomy with or without oophorectomy
  • Vaginectomy
  • Scrotoplasty
  • Phalloplasty
  • Metoidioplasty (clitoral reconstruction)

Psychotherapeutic
  Transgender persons may require any one or combination of the following:
  • Exploration of gender identity
  • Assistance and support in coming out and transitioning socially
  • Dealing with mood and behavioral conditions that arise from the stresses of living as
    a transgender person (i.e., trauma)
  • Addressing mental health issues that may be unrelated to gender or one's
    transgender experience (i.e., psychiatric disorders)

(i.e., hormone therapy, orchiectomy, or psychotherapeutic support for coming out), and of course not all agencies will offer all such services. Table 17-3 lists care and treatments commonly sought by trans people. Capacity and expertise in these areas can be obtained through the use of resources listed in Table 17-2 as well as attending conferences such as the WPATH Biennial Conference; the biennial National Transgender Health Summit convened by the University of California, San Francisco Center of Excellence for Transgender Health; or the annual Philadelphia Trans-Health Conference. Unfortunately, formal clinical training programs in trans care are limited, albeit developing. Several large LGBT-oriented clinics offer some degree of medical or mental health training opportunities, including Fenway Health in Boston, Callen-Lorde in New York City, Lyon-Martin Health Services in San Francisco, and the Los Angeles Gay & Lesbian Center; in addition, there are initiatives to develop formal training programs at the University of California, San Francisco. Surgical training opportunities in the United States are almost nonexistent, and many United States–based surgeons seek training in Europe.

Using Preferred Names, Pronouns, and Other Terms

A key component of providing trans-affirming health care is to allow patients to identify themselves using their own terminology. Consecutive trans patients may have seemingly opposite approaches to identity and terminology. While asking patients how they would like to be addressed is potentially awkward for clinicians and other staff in health care settings, in fact most trans patients are pleased to be asked, and doing so may enhance overall primary care (42). In particular, clinicians may use common sense judgment when entering the room of a patient whose listed name or sex marker is in obvious discordance with the expressed gender. In other words, upon entering the room of a patient whose name is listed as "John Smith," and whose sex is listed as male, but who is wearing a skirt or women's jewelry, it would be prudent and appropriate for the clinician to ask the patient what name and pronoun are preferred. This inquiry should occur regardless of the clinician's own judgment of how "well" the patient is "passing" or "blending" as their intended gender, or how "far along" the patient seems to be in the transition. It is important that all staff in health care settings learn about possible discordance between names and information on official records and a patient's identity to avoid embarrassment. When mistakes do occur, it is best to apologize. Teaching all staff about these issues is important. Table 17-2 offers resources for training clinicians and other health care staff in these areas.

Gender Marker on Identity Documents

Trans people often seek a legal change of name as well as an amendment of the listed gender marker on legal documents, such as a passport, birth certificate, or driver license. While the name change process in the United States is a fairly straightforward and standardized process involving a court order, the concept of "legal gender" is more complex and is a patchwork of local, state, and federal policies and documents. Having documentation that appropriately reflects one's affirmed gender and a preferred and congruent name is essential for purposes of housing, employment, travel, and other basic needs. Failing to obtain appropriate documentation may put trans people at risk for violence and may press them into an underground economy, with inherent risks for HIV infection and hepatitis (28,43). Historically, many jurisdictions required documentation of transition-related surgery (and in some cases sterilization or specifically genital surgery) to amend document gender markers. In recent years the U.S. State Department (passports), Social Security Administration, and many states (driver license) have introduced processes that allow gender-marker amendment with a physician letter documenting that a patient has undergone "appropriate treatment." Still, other states lag behind on driver licenses and birth certificates, and some states and New York City do not permit changing these documents at all. The problem is compounded for undocumented immigrants or those with visas or who are permanent residents; in these cases neither name nor gender may be amended on these documents before such changes are made in the country of origin, a process that may be prohibitive or even impossible (44).

Documenting Gender Identity in Electronic Health Records

The issues of preferred versus legal name and preferred pronouns versus the gender marker listed on legal documents and insurance plans complicate the use of electronic health records (EHRs) in the care of trans patients. An ideal EHR interface would allow appropriate documentation of a patient's trans status for both medical and population health research purposes but at the same time limit the availability of that information to those settings and personnel for whom knowledge of trans status is required. Such a system would also allow providers as well as allied health and front office workers to be promptly and clearly alerted to a patient's preferred name and pronoun when they differ from those under which the patient is registered in the system. Naturally this is easier said than done and EHR implementation in the United States is still in relatively early stages. In addition to patient concerns about privacy, other challenges include how to standardize gender identity data and where exactly to place them in the EHR. Another challenge has developed largely in response to the meaningful use regulations that require a consolidated data document be sharable among medical providers. The benefit to this requirement is that it provides a relevant summary of care for a provider; the challenge is that it becomes difficult to segment data, particularly when a patient wants to restrict sharing of certain types of data.

Initial recommendations from the WPATH EHR Working Group were published in May 2013, and the Institute of Medicine has held several forums on the topic (45,46). In general, a 2-step method for collection of gender parameters is recommended: 1) querying the patient's gender identity and 2) querying the birth-assigned sex (see Appendix B for sample questions) (47). This process has been in use by the U.S. Centers for Disease Control and Prevention (CDC) enhanced HIV/AIDS Reporting System for some time and has been recommended by the University of California, San Francisco, Center of Excellence for Transgender Health and the National LGBT Health Education Center. However, depending on social, financial, and legal status situation, a patient may have several gender identities that simultaneously need to be accommodated in the EHR: self-identified gender, the gender on health insurance, and the legal gender marker in a given state. (Appendix D provides an example of how to ask about different names and gender markers in an intake form.) The provider may also wish to use a different gender for certain laboratory tests, depending on the patient's hormonal status. Unfortunately, EHRs are not currently designed to record gender fluidity. Providers will need to be transparent with their patients about the limitations of their EHR when appropriate adaptations are not possible. Other considerations for EHRs include allowing for "gender-neutral" history, review of systems, and physical examination sections; this change would permit, for example, the documentation of a vaginal examination on a male patient or a prostatic history or complaint on a female patient. EHRs might also include a list of commonly sought transition-related procedures that may not otherwise be listed.

Conclusion

There is growing awareness of the diversity of transgender identities and health care needs. Health care providers who familiarize themselves with the needs of trans people and offer a gender-affirming environment can make a significant difference in the lives of their patients, many of whom must bear the daily burden of stigma, harassment, and discrimination. Additional resources for health care providers and organizations looking to increase their knowledge and skills can be found through the Center of Excellence for Transgender Health, the National LGBT Health Education Center, and an increasing number of local and national organizations (see Table 17-2 and Appendix C for resources).

Summary Points

- The trans community is not a homogenous group but rather includes diverse identities that cut across ethnic, linguistic, national, socioeconomic, and generational lines, as well as a range of sexual orientations.
- Terms and language used to describe trans individuals and identities similarly vary; it is important for providers to ask patients about their preferred gender terminology and pronouns.
- Many different stage models have been proposed to conceptualize trans identity development, all of which assert the importance of gender affirmation (the interpersonal process whereby a person receives social recognition and support for gender identity).
- Providers should educate themselves about the medical and psychological needs of their trans patients. Trans patients all require the same types of primary care as all people, and many also have unique needs directly related to the transition process.
- The current Standards of Care for the Health of Transsexual, Transgender, and Gender Nonconforming Persons (published by the World Professional Association for Transgender Health) recognizes that the components of transition are individualized; not all people need all components, and the order in which they occur needs to be flexible and individualized.

- The utility and appropriateness of the current diagnoses related to trans identity in the *ICD* and *DSM* are under debate. While pathologization of trans identities is not ideal, many providers find that they must provide a diagnosis in order to continue to provide treatment to their trans patients.
- Efforts are underway to revise electronic health record systems to allow for appropriate documentation of trans patients' preferred name, pronoun, and health history.

References

1. **Obedin-Maliver J, Goldsmith ES, Stewart L, et al.** Lesbian, gay, bisexual, and transgender-related content in undergraduate medical education. JAMA. 2011;306:971-77.
2. **Institute of Medicine.** The Health of Lesbian, Gay, Bisexual, and Transgender People: Building a Foundation for Better Understanding. Washington, DC: The National Academics Press; 2011.
3. **Herbst JH, Jacobs ED, Finlayson TJ, et al.** Estimating HIV prevalence and risk behaviors of transgender persons in the United States: a systematic review. AIDS Behav. 2008;12:1-17.
4. **Grant JM, Mottet LA, Tanis J, et al.** Injustice at Every Turn: A Report of the National Transgender Discrimination Survey. Washington, DC: National Center for Transgender Equality and National Gay and Lesbian Task Force; 2011.
5. **Gates GJ.** How many people are lesbian, gay, bisexual, and transgender? Los Angeles: The Williams Institute.2011. Available at: http://williamsinstitute.law.ucla.edu/wp-content/uploads/Gates-How-Many-People-LGBT-Apr-2011.pdf
6. **Division of HIV and STD Programs, Los Angeles County Department of Public Health, 2013.** Los Angeles County Transgender Population Estimates 2012. Available at: http://ph.lacounty.gov/aids/reports/TransgenderPopulationEstimates2-12-13.pdf.
7. **Conron KJ, Scott G, Stowell GS, Landers SJ.** Transgender health in Massachusetts: Results from a household probability sample of adults. Am J Public Health. 2012;102:118-22.
8. **Bye L, Gruskin E, Greenwood G, et al.** California Lesbians, Gays, Bisexuals, and Transgender (LGBT) Tobacco Use Survey-2004. Sacramento, CA: California Department of Health Services. 2005. Available at: www.cdph.ca.gov/programs/tobacco/Documents/CTCP-LGBTTobaccoStudy.pdf.
9. **Kuper LE, Nussbaum R, Mustanski B.** Exploring the diversity of gender and sexual orientation identities in an online sample of transgender individuals. J Sex Res. 2012;49: 244-54.
10. **Lombardi E.** Varieties of transgender/transsexual lives and their relationship with transphobia. J Homosex. 2009;56:977-92.
11. **Pfaefflin F.** Sex reassignment, Harry Benjamin, and some European roots. Int J Transgenderism. 1997;1.
12. **Morgan SW, Stevens PE.** Transgender Identity Development as Represented by a Group of Transgendered Adults. Issues Mental Health Nurs. 2012;33:301-8.
13. **Lev AI.** Transgender Emergence: Therapeutic Guidelines for Working With Gender-Variant People and Their Families. Binghamton, NY: Haworth Clinical Practice Press; 2004.
14. **Bockting W, Coleman E.** Developmental stages of the transgender coming-out process. In Etter R, Monstrey S, Eyler A, eds. Principles of Transgender Medicine and Surgery. New York: Hawthorne Press; 2007:185-208.
15. **Erikson E.** The problem of ego identity. J Am Psychoanal Assoc. 1956;4:56-121.
16. **Melendez R, Pinto R.** 'It's really a hard life': love, gender and HIV risk among male-to-female transgender persons. Culture Health Sexual. 2007;9:233-45.

17. **Nuttbrock L, Bockting W, Hwahng S, et al.** Gender identity affirmation among male-to-female transgender persons: a life course analysis across types of relationships and cultural/lifestyle factors. Sex Relationship Ther. 2009;24:108-25.

18. **Sevelius J.** Gender affirmation: a framework for conceptualizing risk behavior among transgender women of color. Sex Roles. 2013;68:675-89.

19. **Major B, O'Brien L.** The social psychology of stigma. Annu Rev Psychol. 2005;56:393-421.

20. **Nuttbrock L, Hwahng S, Bockting W, et al.** Lifetime risk factors for HIV/sexually transmitted infections among male-to-female transgender persons. J AIDS. 2009;52:417-21.

21. **Meyer III W, Bockting W, Cohen-Kettenis P, et al.** (2001). The standards of care for gender identity disorders, sixth version. Int J Transgender. 2001;5.

22. **Coleman E, Bockting W, Botzer M, et al.** Standards of care for the health of transsexual, transgender, and gender-nonconforming people, version 7. Int J Transgender. 2012;13:165-232.

23. **Sevelius J.** 'There's no pamphlet for the kind of sex I have': HIV-related risk factors and protective behaviors among transgender men who have sex with nontransgender men. J Assoc Nurses AIDS Care. 2009;20:398-410.

24. **Rowniak S, Chesla C, Rose CD, Holzemer WL.** Transmen: the HIV risk of gay identity. AIDS Educ Prev. 2011;23:508-20.

25. **Meier SC, Pardo ST, Labuski C, Babcock J.** Measures of clinical health among female-to-male transgender persons as a function of sexual orientation. Arch Sex Behav. 2013;42:463-74.

26. **Kenagy GP.** The health and social service needs of transgender people in Philadelphia. Int J Transgender. 2005;8:49-56.

27. **Baral SD, Poteat T, Strömdahl S, et al.** Worldwide burden of HIV in transgender women: a systematic review and meta-analysis. Lancet Infect Dis. 2013;13:214-22.

28. **Silva-Santisteban A, Raymond HF, Salazar X, et al.** Understanding the HIV/AIDS epidemic in transgender women of Lima, Peru: results from a sero-epidemiologic study using respondent driven sampling. AIDS Behav. 2011;16:872-81.

29. **Reisner SL, Lloyd J, Baral SD.** Technical Report: The Global Health Needs of Transgender Populations. USAID's AIDS Support and Technical Assistance Resources, AIDSTAR-Two, Task Order 2. Arlington, VA; 2013

30. **De Cuypere G, Knudson G, Green J.** WPATH Consensus Process Regarding Transgender and Transsexual-Related Diagnoses in ICD-11. World Professional Association for Transgender Health. 2013. Available at: www.wpath.org/uploaded_files/140/files/ICD%20Meeting%20Packet-Report-Final-sm.pdf.

31. **American Psychiatric Association.** Diagnostic and Statistical Manual of Medical Disorders. Arlington, VA: American Psychiatric Association; 2013Available at: www.psychiatry.org/practice/dsm.

32. **World Health Organization.** International Classification of Disease (ICD), version 10. Geneva: World Health Organization; 2013.

33. **American Psychiatric Association.** Diagnostic and Statistical Manual of Mental Disorders, fifth edition. Washington, DC: American Psychiatric Publishing; 2013:451-60.

34. **American Psychiatric Association.** Diagnostic and Statistical Manual of Mental Disorders, fourth edition, text revision. Washington, DC: American Psychiatric Association; 2000.

35. **Zucker KJ.** DSM-5: call for commentaries on gender dysphoria, sexual dysfunctions, and paraphilic disorders. Arch Sex Behav. 2013;42:669-74.

36. **Nuttbrock L, Bockting W, Rosenblum A, et al.** Sexual arousal associated with private as compared to public feminine dressing among male-to-female transgender persons: a further response to Lawrence (2011). Arch Sex Behav. 2011;40:1093-6.

37. **Bouman WP, Bauer GR, Richards C, Coleman E.** World Professional Association for Transgender Health consensus statement on considerations of the role of distress (criterion D) in the DSM diagnosis of gender identity disorder. Int J Transgender. 2010;12:100-6.

38. **De Cuypere G, Knudson G, Green J.** WPATH Consensus Process Regarding Transgender and Transsexual-Related Diagnoses in ICD-11. Minneapolis, MN: World Professional Association of Transgender Health; 2013.

39. La transsexualité ne sera plus classée comme affection psychiatrique. Le Monde.fr. 2009. Available at: www.lemonde.fr/societe/article/2009/05/16/la-transsexualite-ne-sera-plus-classee-comme-affectation-psychiatrique_1193860_3224.html.

40. **Corneil TA, Eisfeld JH, Botzer M.** Proposed changes to diagnoses related to gender identity in the DSM: a world professional association for transgender health consensus paper regarding the potential impact on access to health care for transgender persons. Int J Transgender. 2010;12:107-14.

41. **Deutsch MB, Feldman JL.** Updated recommendations from the world professional association for transgender health standards of care. Am Fam Physician. 2013;87:89-93.

42. **Melendez RM, Pinto RM.** HIV prevention and primary care for transgender women in a community-based clinic. J Assoc Nurses AIDS Care. 2009;20:387-97.

43. **Khan SI, Hussain MI, Parveen S, et al.** Living on the extreme margin: social exclusion of the transgender population (Hijra) in Bangladesh. J Health Popul Nutr. 2009;27:441-51.

44. Advancing Transgender Equality. Policy Brief: Birth Certificate Gender Markers. National Center for Transgender Equality. 2011. Available at: http://transgenderequality.wordpress.com/2011/06/22/policy-brief-birth-certificate-gender-markers/.

45. **Deutsch MB, Green J, Keatley J, et al.** Electronic medical records and the transgender patient: recommendations from the World Professional Association for Transgender Health EMR Working Group. J Am Med Inform Assoc. 2013;20:700-3.

46. **Institute of Medicine.** Collecting Sexual Orientation and Gender Identity Data in Electronic Health Records: Workshop Summary. Washington, DC: The National Academies Press; 2013.

47. **Tate CC, Ledbetter JN, Youssef CP.** A two-question method for assessing gender categories in the social and medical sciences. J Sex Res. 2012;18:1-10.

Chapter 18

Medical and Surgical Management of the Transgender Patient: What the Primary Care Clinician Needs to Know

JAMIE FELDMAN, MD, PhD
KATHERINE SPENCER, PhD

Introduction

Transgender people represent an underserved community in need of sensitive, comprehensive health care. Delivery of quality medical care to this population can be challenging for several reasons. Transgender identity and behavior are often socially stigmatized, leading many individuals to maintain a traditional male or female presentation and public role while keeping their transgender identity and related health concerns concealed. Lack of health insurance, the experience of discrimination in the health care setting, lack of access to medical personnel competent in transgender medicine, and possible discomfort with the body can lead transgender patients to avoid medical care altogether (1–3). Thus, they often lack access to preventive health services and timely treatment of routine health problems.

In addition, most physicians and other health care professionals do not receive training in health issues specific to transgender patients and lack ready access to appropriate information or to a knowledgeable colleague (2). Long-term, prospective studies for most transgender-specific health issues are lacking, resulting in variable preventive care recommendations based primarily on expert opinion (2,4). However, by using an increasing body of peer-reviewed, scientific research on transgender health, along with relevant data from the general population, one can develop an evidence-based approach to preventive care for transgender patients.

This chapter presents a general medical approach to transgender health care for primary care clinicians who seek to increase their skills to provide quality care to this population. The chapter includes recommendations about elements of an appropriate history and how to perform the physical examination. Recommendations for screening and prevention are presented, categorized appropriately for individuals with varying physiologic (hormonal) and anatomic (surgical) presentations. While the nuances of transgender hormone therapy are not discussed in detail here, major published guidelines are briefly reviewed.

General Guidelines

Patients explore issues related to their gender identity and expression best in an environment of trust. Providers should refer to transgender patients by their preferred name and pronouns, reassure them about confidentiality, educate frontline and other clinical staff and colleagues regarding transgender issues, and respect patients' concerns regarding potentially sensitive physical examinations and tests (such as pelvic examinations or mammography). Familiarity with commonly used terms and the diversity of identities within the transgender community is essential (see Chapter 17). While specialists who provide hormonal treatment and surgeries play important roles in preventive care, optimally every transgender person should partner with a primary care provider for overall health care needs (5). Many of these will be active in maintenance, if not initiation, of treatments.

Hormonal and surgical treatment, discussed later in this chapter, can increase the quality of life for transgender individuals who desire to bring their bodies into greater congruence with their gender identity (6,7). Efforts should be made to address health concerns that arise related to hormonal interventions or planned surgeries through behavior change, lifestyle change, or medication. Reduction or discontinuation of hormones, unless desired by the patient, should be a last rather than first resort and not be undertaken lightly because of potentially serious psychological consequences.

The Transgender-Oriented Health History

As with any patient establishing care, providers should perform a comprehensive health history. However, specific areas within the history take on a greater importance for transgender patients because of greater experience of stigma, discrimination, and lower economic status, and desire for or actual use of cross-sex hormones and gender affirmation surgeries. The transgender-oriented history is described in detail in *Transgender Primary Medical Care* (8). In addition, Chapter 8 offers recommendations on taking a general medical history with transgender people, and Chapter 17 details ways to offer transgender-competent health services. Questions should be framed in a sensitive and respectful manner that recognizes the patient's self-identification, including pronoun choice. To clarify for the purposes of this chapter, the term "transgender woman" refers to a person assigned as male at birth who identifies as female/feminine, and "transgender man" refers to a person assigned as female at birth who identifies as male/masculine. The transgender-oriented health history should include the following general elements:

The *general health history* should review current and past medical conditions, including all medications and the most recent physical examination (including Papanicolaou [Pap] smear, testicular, and rectal examinations, where appropriate). A thorough gynecologic and obstetric history is important in transgender men because this population may have an increased incidence of polycystic ovarian syndrome (PCOS) or hyperandrogenicity (9,10).

In the *family history*, particular attention should be paid to any clotting disorders, cardiovascular disease, hypertension, diabetes, and mental illness. Any family history for breast, ovarian, uterine, or prostate cancer should also be noted because these cancers are known to be influenced by exogenous hormones and may require different or more frequent screening if patients are taking feminizing or masculinizing hormones.

A *sexual health* history requires particular sensitivity for transgender patients. Discussion should be initiated gradually, and pacing should depend on patient comfort. A screening sexual history should cover sexual orientation, risk behaviors related to sexually transmitted infections (STIs) (including engaging in sex for money) and unintended pregnancy, and sexual function. If the screening history raises concerns, a more detailed sexual history is warranted. See Chapters 8 and 12 for more detailed recommendations on taking a sexual history.

The *psychosocial history* should include a review of a transgender patient's family, economic, and larger social environments, which can be sources of support or stress. Social isolation, rejection by family or community of origin, harassment, and discrimination can significantly affect a transgender individual's health. As a result of employment discrimination and family abandonment, many transgender people live in poverty in both rural and urban areas, and housing concerns, including homelessness, are not uncommon (1). Psychiatric conditions, including depression, anxiety, chemical dependence, and post-traumatic stress disorder (including a history of history of physical, sexual, or emotional trauma or abuse) should be addressed, either here or in the general health history (11).

History of Feminizing or Masculinizing Interventions

Some transgender individuals use hormonal, surgical, or other interventions to bring their bodies into greater alignment with their gender identity. In establishing care with a transgender patient, a thorough history of these interventions is essential. For other patients, hormonal and surgical concerns are less prominent, and this part of the history is accordingly brief. Questions may include:

1. Has the patient ever taken cross-sex hormones? Are there any complications or concerns regarding past or current hormone use?

Feminizing and masculinizing medications have the potential for numerous drug interactions, and the primary care provider needs to recognize these before prescribing anything new. Medically unsupervised use of hormones is common among transgender patients with limited access to care (12,13). Increasingly, transgender persons are purchasing hormones over the Internet, usually from foreign suppliers and with little to no clinician involvement. The primary care provider should also inquire about "herbal hormones"—phytoestrogens or androgen-like compounds sold as dietary supplements, such as red clover, black cohosh, and dehydroepiandrosterone. Transgender patients with coexisting chronic medical problems will need closer follow-up once they begin hormones.

2. Has the patient undergone any feminizing or masculinizing surgical procedures, including silicone injections? Are there any complications or concerns regarding past surgeries?

Common surgeries for individuals seeking greater gender identity congruence are listed in Table 18-1 and may also include procedures to masculinize or feminize facial and body contours. Complications relating to genital surgery are not infrequent, particularly in patients who underwent surgery many years ago when techniques were less sophisticated and follow-up care less consistent. Surgical interventions will be discussed in more detail later in this chapter.

Some transgender women may have undergone injections of free silicone oil into their hips, buttock, thighs, breasts, lips, or face, often by a layperson using potentially industrial-grade silicone oil with minimal or absent sterile techniques. Risks associated with these procedures include

Table 18-1   Common Gender-Related Surgeries

Masculinizing Surgical Procedures	*Feminizing Surgical Procedures*
Mastectomy and chest reconstruction	Orchiectomy
Hysterectomy	Surgery to elevate voice pitch
Vaginectomy	Penectomy
Metoidioplasty	Vaginoplasty
Phalloplasty	Breast augmentation/augmentation mammoplasty
Urethral lengthening	Facial feminization
Scrotoplasty	Tracheal shave/Adam's apple reduction

local and systemic infection, embolization, painful granuloma formation, and a systemic inflammatory syndrome (13).

3. Does the patient plan to pursue hormone therapy or surgeries in the future? Does the patient seek additional feminizing/masculinizing interventions?

Awareness of future plans is useful in coordinating referrals and planning relating to care for any coexisting medical, social, or psychological concerns. Offline and online peer support resources, groups, or community organizations are often useful for assistance relating to appearance and changes in legal name or sex designation and provide avenues for social support and advocacy. Referrals may be sought for voice therapy, hair removal through laser or electrolysis, or hair transplant (14).

Transgender Physical Examination

Physical examinations should be structured according to the organs present rather than the perceived gender of the patient. For example, transgender men who have had no breast surgery or only breast reduction need routine breast/chest examinations and mammography according to published guidelines for natal females. Those who have had chest reconstruction ("top surgery") usually still have some small amount of residual breast tissue, but mammography is not routinely indicated. In these patients a chest examination is advisable.

The prostate is not removed in vaginoplasty; therefore, prostate examinations should be performed for transgender women. If the uterus and cervix are present in transgender men, pelvic examinations and Pap smears should be done as a part of preventive care, although the onset and frequency of these examinations will vary depending on the age and sexual activity of the patient.

Transgender patients may be uncomfortable with their bodies and find some elements of physical examination traumatic. Unless there is an immediate medical need, sensitive elements of the examination (particularly breast, genital, and rectal examination) should be delayed until strong clinician–patient rapport has developed. Sensitive examinations can be managed in a variety of ways, depending on patient preference; some patients prefer the examination to be done as quickly as possible, while others require a slow pace or even light sedation. It is important to discuss the purpose and specifics of the examination (when, where, and how you will touch the patient) before proceeding: When this is done clearly, most patients will understand. The physical examination provides an important opportunity to educate patients about their bodies and about the need for ongoing health maintenance.

A range of physical development is seen in patients undergoing hormone therapy. Transgender men may have beard growth, clitoromegaly, acne, and androgenic alopecia; those who have bound their breasts for numerous years may have rash or yeast infection of the skin under the breasts. Transgender women may have feminine breast shape and size, often with relatively underdeveloped nipples; breasts may appear fibrocystic if there have been silicone injections. Galactorrhea is sometimes seen in patients with high prolactin levels, especially among those using breast pumps to stimulate development (15). There may be minimal body hair and variable facial hair (depending on length of time on hormones and manual hair removal treatments, such as electrolysis). Testicles may become small and soft; defects or hernias at the external inguinal ring may be present due to the practice of "tucking" the testicles up near (or into) the inguinal canal. In the absence of hormone therapy, findings suggestive of intersex conditions should be further evaluated.

Physical findings in postoperative patients will depend on the types of surgeries that have been done, the quality of the surgical work, the impact of postoperative complications, and any revisions that have been performed after the initial surgery. Transgender men after chest surgery will have scar tissue consistent with the type of procedure and may have large nipples or small grafted nipples. The neophallus created from the release of an augmented clitoris (metoidioplasty procedure) looks like a small penis; a grafted penis constructed by phalloplasty will be adult-sized but more flaccid than in the natal male (erection is obtained through use of an implanted prosthetic device). Transgender women may have undergone breast augmentation with implants. Genital surgery typically involves simultaneous removal of the penis or testicles and creation of a neovagina; some patients may just have the testes removed, prior to or instead of vaginoplasty. There may be varying degrees of labial reconstruction and clitoral hooding, depending on the completion of surgical revisions. The neovagina typically appears less moist than in natal women and may be stenosed internally if the patient does not dilate regularly or is not sexually active.

Laboratory Requisition Forms

Most requisition forms for laboratory tests ask for the sex of the patient to furnish the provider with normal ranges for the results (which are often sex-dependent) and to flag abnormal results. Normal values for transgender persons who are undergoing or have completed gender transition have not been established for any laboratory test, and there is no consensus about how sex should be recorded on laboratory requests for the transgender patient. Clinicians must therefore balance consideration of the following issues in order to designate sex on laboratory orders in an appropriate manner:

1. The stress a patient experiences going into the laboratory with a sex on the form that conflicts with their name/appearance;

2. The need to obtain laboratory tests that are most appropriate to a patient's physiology;
3. The need to minimize laboratory error; and
4. The need to match the gender marker on the patient's insurance identification card.

Gender Identity and Electronic Health Records

Electronic health records (EHRs) present opportunities and challenges in providing health care for transgender patients. In a recent report on the health of LGBT people, the Institute of Medicine recommended that information on patients' sexual orientation and gender identity be collected in EHRs (as are race and ethnicity) because such demographics provide the foundation for understanding any population's status and needs (2). However, the primary concerns of collecting this information remain those of accurately representing the patient's gender identity in the context of the EHR while simultaneously respecting privacy and avoiding complications with coding and insurance coverage (16). For more detailed explanations of these issues, see Chapters 1, 8, and 17.

Evidence-Based Decision-Making in Transgender Care

Currently, few prospective, large-scale studies exist regarding transgender health care. The best available evidence comes from a Dutch historical cohort involving 966 transgender women and 365 transgender men, with hormone use of at least 1 year and median follow-up duration of 18.5 years (17). Morbidity and mortality were compared with age- and gender-specific statistics in the general Dutch population. Because the study did not track a specific cohort over a long period, particularly into the over-65 age range, the long-term health effects of hormone therapy remain uncertain. Smaller-scale studies on specific issues, such as osteoporosis, do exist, along with non–trans-specific evidence (i.e., studies involving men and women who are not transgender). In many areas, case reports or series are the major source of trans-specific data. Case studies suggest that certain conditions occur in the transgender setting; however, further research is needed to determine incidence and clinical significance.

In applying knowledge from the nontransgender setting to transgender patients, clinicians should look for rigorous studies that are highly relevant to the clinical context. For example, a large prospective study involving nontransgender women on postmenopausal hormone therapy may be relevant for transgender women older than age 50 who are taking similar types of hormones. Evidence from nontransgender studies can be directly applied to similar transgender patients who have not had surgical or hormonal interventions (e.g., findings from studies involving nontransgender women apply to transgender men who have not taken testosterone or have not had masculinizing surgery).

Risk assessment and recommendations for preventive care often depend on the patient's hormonal and surgical status and will be discussed according to these categories where applicable. The recommendations below are based on a systematic, evidence-based review of the transgender and appropriate nontransgender literature, supplemented by peer-reviewed expert opinion.

Vaccinations

Recommended vaccinations are the same for transgender and nontransgender patients. While vaccination of all children for hepatitis B is now recommended, many transgender adults are not immune and could benefit from vaccination—particularly persons with more than one sexual partner in the last 6 months, patients with a recent STI, individuals who share needles to inject hormones or other substances, and those traveling to endemic areas.

Cancer Screening: Breast Cancer

Transgender Women Without Hormone Use
There is no evidence of increased risk for cancer compared with natal male patients, in the absence of other known risk factors (e.g., Klinefelter syndrome). Routine screening, in the form of regular breast examinations or mammography, is not indicated.

Transgender Women With Past or Current Hormone Use
Patients who have taken feminizing hormones may be at increased risk for breast cancer compared with natal males but probably have much lower risk than natal females. No evidence supports routine screening mammography for all transgender women receiving hormone therapy (18). The duration of feminizing hormone exposure, family history, body mass index greater than 35 kg/m^2, and use of progestins may further increase breast cancer risk (18). On the basis of current U.S. Preventive Services Task Force (USPSTF) guidelines developed for nontransgender women (19), screening mammography every 1 to 2 years would be advisable for transgender women age 50 years and older with additional risk factors (e.g., estrogen or progestin use for >5 years, positive family history, body mass index >35 kg/m^2). Annual clinical breast examination and periodic self-breast examination are not recommended for cancer screening but may serve an educational purpose. Breast augmentation, which is common among transwomen, does not appear to increase risk for breast cancer, although it may impair the accuracy of screening mammography (20).

Transgender Men Without Chest Surgery, With or Without Testosterone Use

Breast examinations and screening mammography are recommended as for natal females.

Transgender Men, After Chest Surgery, With or Without Testosterone Use

Patients who undergo breast reduction or mastectomy (chest reconstruction) retain some degree of underlying breast tissue for good cosmetic result. Case series of breast cancer among transgender men after chest surgery and on hormones have been published (21). The risk for breast cancer is reduced with chest surgery but appears higher than the risk in natal men, based on breast reduction studies in nontransgender women. Risk is affected by age at chest surgery and the amount of breast tissue removed. Mammography before chest surgery is not recommended unless the patient meets usual natal female recommendations (22). Yearly chest wall screening and axillary examinations, along with education regarding the small but possible risk for breast cancer, are recommended.

Cancer Screening: Cervical Cancer

Transgender Women, Following Vaginoplasty

There is only one published case report of vaginal dysplasia in this population, and disease-oriented evidence suggests that the risk for neoplasia is extremely small (23,24). In addition, the USPSTF recommends against screening nontransgender women after hysterectomy for benign disease (25). Case reports of neovaginal condyloma in transgender patients are noted in the literature (26,27), and physicians may consider screening these patients for vaginal neoplasia, especially if they are immunosuppressed.

Transgender Men, Cervix Intact (Partial Hysterectomy or No Hysterectomy)

Pap smears can be traumatic for transgender men and should be kept to a minimum for those at low risk for human papillomavirus (HPV) transmission (i.e., little sexual activity involving the genitals). Pap smears should follow recommended guidelines for natal females in patients with an intact cervix, and can often be as infrequent as every 3 to 5 years (25). There is no evidence that testosterone increases or reduces the risk for cervical cancer (18). Because testosterone therapy can result in atrophic dysplasia-like changes to the cervical epithelium, the pathologist should be informed of the patient's hormonal status (28). For patients otherwise at low risk for cervical cancer, atypical squamous cells of uncertain significance and low-grade squamous intraepithelial lesion Pap smears are unlikely to represent precancerous lesions, especially in the absence of high-risk strains of HPV (29,30). Any patient with a cervix should have cancer risk surveillance with cytology with or without HPV cotesting as indicated. Total hysterectomy should be considered in the presence of high-grade dysplasia or if the patient is entirely unable to tolerate Pap smear, unless the patient wishes to preserve the option for pregnancy.

Transgender Men After Total Hysterectomy (Cervix Completely Excised)

If there is no history of high-grade cervical dysplasia and/or cervical cancer, no future Pap smears are needed. Patients with a history of high-grade cervical dysplasia or cervical cancer should have regular surveillance as recommended by their gynecologist or oncologist. The timing and nature of this surveillance depend on how far out the patient is from their diagnosis and treatment.

Cancer Screening: Ovarian or Uterine Cancer

Transgender Men Intact Ovaries, and/or Uterus (No Hysterectomy), With or Without History of Hormones

Incidence of hyperandrogenism and PCOS is increased among transgender men even in the absence of testosterone use (9,10,31). PCOS is a hormonal syndrome complex characterized by some or all of the following: failure to ovulate, absent or infrequent menstrual cycles, multiple cysts on the ovaries, hyperandrogenism, hirsutism, acne, hidradenitis suppurativa, acanthosis nigricans, obesity, and glucose intolerance or diabetes. PCOS is associated with infertility as well as increased risk for cardiac disease, high blood pressure, and endometrial cancer (32). Screening at least once by history and physical examination for signs and symptoms of PCOS is therefore reasonable in all transgender men. A positive screen would prompt a diagnostic evaluation and appropriate monitoring for the medical conditions associated with PCOS if indicated.

No long-term studies have assessed the incidence of ovarian cancer among transgender men receiving testosterone. Case reports do exist; the risk for ovarian cancer may also be increased among natal women with PCOS, but the evidence is inconclusive (18). There is no USPSTF-recommended screening test for ovarian cancer for any patient. The risk for ovarian cancer is increased among all nontransgender women as they age, particularly those older than 40 years. Other risk factors include nulliparity, a history of infertility, and family history or genetic mutations associated with ovarian cancer. Providers should consider screening with a history and bimanual pelvic examination every 1 to 3 years for patients at increased risk. Transgender men with suspected genetic mutations should be referred for genetic counseling regarding their prevention options. An oophorectomy may be a reasonable consideration if the patient is older than 40 years of age or cannot tolerate pelvic examinations, if maintenance of fertility is not desired, and if surgery will not impair the patient's health.

The risk for endometrial cancer is increased among all nontransgender women older than age 40 and all women with PCOS, while the evidence regarding the effects of testosterone on the uterine lining in transgender men is mixed (18). Providers should evaluate uterine bleeding with transvaginal ultrasonography, pelvic ultrasonography, or endometrial biopsy if bleeding is prolonged. Because pelvic examinations may be distressing for transgender men, a total hysterectomy should be considered if patients cannot tolerate ongoing pelvic examinations, particularly if fertility is not desired, the patient is older than age 40 years, and surgery will not harm the patient's health.

Cancer Screening: Prostate Cancer

Transgender Women, No Current/Past Hormones, No Surgery

Routine prostate-specific antigen (PSA) screening in any usual-risk population is not supported by evidence (33). The risks and possible benefits of PSA screening should be discussed with all patients, and screening may be considered in high-risk patients (African American, family history of prostate cancer) starting at ages 45 to 50 years. While a digital rectal examination is invasive and uncomfortable, it is often part of the standard screening for colorectal cancer starting at age 50 years and thus is gender-neutral, but as in any practice should be explained to the patient.

Transgender Women, Past or Current Hormones, With or Without Surgery

Feminizing hormone therapy appears to decrease the risk for prostate cancer, but the degree of reduction is unknown. PSA screening is not recommended because PSA levels may be falsely low in an androgen-deficient setting (34), even in the presence of prostate cancer. The prostate is not removed in feminizing genital surgery, and cases of prostate cancer have been reported among patients receiving feminizing therapy, both before and after gender reassignment surgery (18), although these cases began in people who transitioned later in life (after 50 years old). A digital rectal examination, along with education regarding the small but present risk for prostate cancer even after reassignment surgery, is recommended starting at age 50 for usual-risk patients.

Cancer Screening: Other Cancers

Currently, there is no evidence that transgender persons are at increased or decreased risk for other cancers. Screening recommendations for other cancers (including colon cancer, lung cancer, and anal cancer) should be followed as with nontransgender patients.

Cardiovascular Disease

All Transgender Patients

Assessing and treating cardiovascular risk factors is an essential primary care intervention for transgender patients. Regardless of hormone status, the transgender population as a whole has several risk factors for cardiovascular disease; feminizing or masculinizing hormone therapy can further increase cardiovascular risks. Smoking is a concern for both transgender men and transgender women. Transgender women tend to present for transgender care at an older age (35,36) with increased comorbidities of hypertension, diabetes, and hyperlipidemia—cardiovascular risk factors encountered earlier in male bodies (37). Transgender men who present with PCOS are at increased risk for hypertension, insulin resistance, and hyperlipidemia (18). Finally, cardiovascular risk factors are often undiagnosed or undertreated among transgender patients because of their relative lack of primary care. Prompt identification and management of cardiovascular risk factors may decrease the hazards associated with hormone therapy in these patients. As in nontransgender patients, daily aspirin therapy may be considered in patients at risk for coronary artery disease.

Transgender Women Patient, Currently Taking Feminizing Hormones

Retrospective studies of long-term use of feminizing hormones suggest a possible increase in cardiovascular risk over time. Studies have been mixed in terms of detecting any elevations in cardiovascular morbidity or morality, though more recent retrospective data involving a greater proportion of older patients showed excessive mortality and morbidity (17,38,39). Several case reports have described myocardial infarction and ischemic stroke among transgender patients taking estrogen (18). In addition, Gooren and colleagues (40) performed a retrospective chart and literature review of changes in cardiovascular risk factors (such as lipids and insulin sensitivity) among patients receiving feminizing therapy, noting an overall deleterious effect on these variables.

Both the Heart and Estrogen/Progestin Replacement Study (HERS) and Women's Health Initiative (WHI) trials, prospective studies of hormone replacement among postmenopausal women, indicated no benefit and a probable increased risk for cardiovascular events with combined estrogen and progesterone therapy (41,42). The estrogen-only arm of the WHI trial demonstrated an increase in cerebrovascular events but not cardiac events. The HERS and WHI trials were conducted using oral conjugated estrogen; it is unclear whether these effects extend to other oral or transdermal estrogens (which show reduced risk for venous thromboembolic events) (43). In light of these data, transgender women older than age 50 with preexisting coronary artery disease or stroke, or with cardiovascular risk factors, appear to be at an increased risk for future events with estrogen and/or progestin use. The extent of risk, and of resulting morbidity and mortality, is unclear. It may be substantial, as doses used for feminization in transgender women are typically higher than in postmenopausal hormone replacement therapy. It may be possible to reduce risks by using transdermal estradiol, decreasing the estrogen dose, and omitting progestin from the regimen. As with all patients, it is important to be attentive to modifiable risks for cardiovascular disease.

Transgender Men, Currently Taking Testosterone

The effect of testosterone on cardiovascular events among transgender men is unclear. Retrospective studies found no increase in cardiovascular events (17,38,39), although the populations may not have been old enough or followed-up long enough to detect any difference. There are case reports of myocardial infarction among patients receiving testosterone therapy (44,45). Masculinizing hormone therapy increases lipid measures associated with increased cardiovascular risk (4,18), but its effects on other cardiovascular risk factors, such as blood pressure and insulin sensitivity, are inconclusive or minimal in average-risk persons (18). While hyperandrogen states among natal women increase several cardiac risk factors, current evidence of any increase in cardiac morbidity or mortality with PCOS is limited (18). However, supraphysiologic levels (i.e., those sometimes achieved by male athletes using androgen supplementation) also increase cardiac risk, and sometimes result in premature death (46).

Use of physiologic dosing of testosterone should minimize the risk for cardiovascular disease over the lifespan in all patients receiving masculinizing therapy (4). Patients with cardiovascular risk factors or preexisting coronary artery disease should have their risk factors well controlled and be monitored for any signs and symptoms.

Hypertension

All Transgender Patients, Not Currently Taking Hormones

Hypertension screening and treatment should follow Eighth Joint National Committee (JNC 8) guidelines recommended for nontransgender patients (47). Ideally, blood pressure should be well controlled before initiation of feminizing or masculinizing hormone therapy.

Transgender Women Patients, Currently Taking Estrogen

Exogenous estrogen, whether in oral contraceptives, postmenopausal hormone replacement, or feminizing hormone therapy, increases blood pressure (18,39,40). Providers should monitor blood pressure at every visit, with a systolic blood pressure goal of less than 140 mm Hg and a diastolic goal of less than 90 mm Hg. Use of the antiandrogen spironolactone may be considered as part of an antihypertensive regimen in patients desiring feminizing therapy.

Transgender Men Patients, Currently Taking Testosterone

Exogenous testosterone may increase blood pressure in natal males (48–50), especially at supraphysiologic doses (51), while natal females with PCOS are at increased risk for hypertension (18). Among transgender men receiving testosterone therapy, prospective studies have been mixed, with 2 showing no change (52,53) and another demonstrating a significant increase in blood pressure (54). Providers should monitor blood pressure at every visit to evaluate patients who might be prehypertensive, with recommended blood pressures goals of 140 mm Hg systolic or less and 90 mm Hg diastolic or less, especially in patients with PCOS.

Diabetes Mellitus

All Transgender Patients, Not Currently Taking Hormones

Providers should follow diabetes screening and management guidelines as for the nontransgender population. Additionally, providers should consider screening (by patient history) all transgender men for PCOS and screen for diabetes if PCOS is present.

Transgender Women, Currently Taking Estrogen

Patients taking estrogen may be at increased risk for type 2 diabetes, particularly those with a family history of diabetes or other risk factors. There have been case reports of new-onset type 2 diabetes within a year of beginning estrogen (55) and an increase in fasting insulin levels and decrease in insulin sensitivity among patients receiving feminizing therapy (40). Studies of nondiabetic women using exogenous estrogen have shown mixed effects on glucose tolerance (18). Patients receiving feminizing hormones experience a modest weight gain (4 kg) (52,56) and as much as a 21% increase in body fat (52), both of which contribute to diabetes risk (57,58). An annual diabetes screening test (hemoglobin A1c or fasting glucose) is recommended in patients with a family history of diabetes or weight gain greater than 5 kg, and further monitoring for all patients with evidence of impaired glucose tolerance. Diabetes should be managed according to guidelines for nontransgender patients, but insulin-sensitizing agents are recommended if medications are indicated, given the underlying mechanism of insulin resistance associated with hormonal therapy.

Transgender Men, Currently Taking Testosterone

As noted above, individuals with PCOS, which may be increased among transgender men have an increased risk of glucose intolerance. Retrospective studies do not indicate an altered risk for type 2 diabetes among transgender patients receiving testosterone (18). In prospective studies, masculinizing testosterone therapy increases visceral fat and decreases fasting glucose but increases insulin resistance (40,52,59). Providers should consider an annual diabetes screening test (hemoglobin A1c or fasting glucose) in patients with family history of diabetes or weight gain greater than 5 kg. Guidelines for managing diabetes mellitus are the same as for the nontransgender population.

Lipids

In November, 2013, the American College of Cardiology/American Heart Association Task Force on Practice Guidelines published new recommendations for managing lipids as a means of reducing cardiovascular risk. One key element of this guideline includes the recommendation of statin therapy for individuals without clinical atherosclerotic cardiovascular disease or diabetes with low-density lipoprotein (LDL) cholesterol of 70 to 189 mg/dL and estimated 10-year ASCVD risk >7.5%. Unfortunately, the risk calculators used to estimate ASCVD risk in this guideline do not account for transgender individuals on current or past masculinizing or feminizing hormone therapy (64). Until the new guidelines can be appropriately modified for transgender patients, recommendations are based on the previous ATP guidelines (65).

All Transgender Patients
Screening for and treatment of hyperlipidemia should follow guidelines for nontransgender patients. Ideally, lipids should be well controlled before initiation of feminizing or masculinizing hormones. Exercise is recommended in all groups to treat low high-density lipoprotein (HDL) levels.

Transgender Women, Currently Taking Estrogen
Studies in both nontransgender women and transgender women receiving estrogen therapy demonstrate increased HDL and decreased LDL cholesterol (18,40). Oral estrogen therapy, both in postmenopausal women and transgender patients, increases triglycerides and has precipitated pancreatitis in several cases of postmenopausal hormone replacement therapy (60,61). Transdermal estrogen is preferred for patients with hyperlipidemia, particularly hypertriglyceridemia, because it decreases triglycerides and is neutral or beneficial with regard to levels of HDL and LDL (62,63).

An annual fasting lipid profile is thus recommended for transgender women taking estrogen. To incorporate the cardiovascular effects of feminizing hormone therapy into existing evidence-based guidelines, estrogen use can be considered as an additional cardiac risk factor. Target lipid levels for patients on treatment include an LDL level less than 130 mg/dL for low- to moderate-risk patients and less than 100 mg/dL for high-risk patients, consistent with current National Cholesterol Education Program Adult Treatment Panel guidelines (65).

Transgender Men Patients, Currently Taking Testosterone

Studies of testosterone therapy among transgender men patients tend to show a decrease in HDL cholesterol, with no changes or, more commonly, increases in LDL cholesterol (18,66). A meta-analysis concluded that the effects of testosterone enanthate on total cholesterol (HDL and LDL) among hypogonadal natal males showed small but significant decreases in both HDL and LDL (67). Supraphysiologic doses may increase the risk for lipid abnormalities, while transdermal administration appears to be lipid neutral (48) in this setting. Natal women with PCOS are at increased risk for dyslipidemia and other metabolic disturbances, although the effect on the risk for cardiac events is undetermined (18).

An annual fasting lipid profile is recommended for patients receiving testosterone, and supraphysiologic testosterone levels should be avoided, particularly in patients with known hyperlipidemia. Daily topical or weekly intramuscular testosterone regimens are thus preferable to more extended intramuscular regimens. Target lipid levels for patients receiving treatment should follow National Cholesterol Education Program Adult Treatment Panel guidelines, as noted above.

Smoking

All Transgender Patients

The transgender population in the United States experiences a higher prevalence of smoking than the population as a whole. Among a national sample of more than 7000 transgender respondents, 30% reported smoking daily or occasionally, compared with 20.6% of U.S. adults (1). Among the transgender population, there are commonly multiple identified risk factors for smoking, including poverty, stressful living and work environments, and societal marginalization. The trans-specific risks associated with smoking include an increased risk for venous thromboembolic events with estrogen therapy and reassignment surgery, possible increased risk for cardiovascular disease with both feminizing and masculinizing hormone therapy (especially in patients older than age 50), and delayed healing following surgery. Providers should screen all transgender patients for past and present tobacco use.

Although little is known about cessation patterns in the transgender population, inclusion of smoking cessation as part of comprehensive transgender care appears successful, particularly in association with hormone therapy (68). Bupropion, nicotine replacement, and behavioral modification techniques are also likely to be appropriate. A comprehensive approach involves consistent smoking cessation messages from all staff, frequent supportive follow-up of cessation efforts, and direct communication of the limitations and risks that smoking imposes on hormone therapy (69).

Venous Thrombosis/Thromboembolism and Feminizing Hormones

The increased risk for venous thrombosis/pulmonary embolism is among the most serious risks in transgender women taking estrogen, although there are no prospective studies in this population (18). Retrospective studies suggest a substantial risk with the use of estrogenic compound ethinyl estradiol. One large study demonstrated a 45-fold increase in venous thrombosis/pulmonary embolism over the rate for nontrans patients, with thromboembolic episodes in 2.1% of estrogen-treated patients younger than 40 years old and in 12% of estrogen-treated patients older than age 40 (44). Later retrospective studies showed increased risk for thrombolic events with the use of oral ethinyl estradiol or conjugated equine estrogen compared with oral 17-β estradiol (38,70,71), and oral estrogen compared with transdermal estradiol (38,72). Nevertheless, the risk for venous thromboembolic events appears to remain higher with feminizing hormone therapy compared with natal women using exogenous estrogen (oral contraceptives and menopausal hormone replacement) (71). Numerous prospective studies of estrogen use in nontransgender women, in the form of oral contraceptives and postmenopausal hormone replacement, indicate that estrogen combined with progestins, smoking, body mass index, or thrombophilic disorders supports a further increased risk for venous thromboembolic events (41,73–75).

Osteoporosis

All Transgender Patients, No Hormone Use, No Surgery
No evidence shows increased or decreased risk for osteoporosis among transgender persons. Providers should follow recommended guidelines for natal females in transgender men; routine screening is not recommended for transgender women, except as indicated by additional risk factors.

Transgender Women, Past or Present Feminizing
Hormones, Pre- and Postorchiectomy
Current studies on the effects of feminizing hormone therapy on bone mineral density are mixed, with some studies finding increases, while others finding fairly dramatic decreases, especially at the lumbar spine (39,76). This variability may depend on the doses of estrogen, the type of androgen-blocking medication, and whether it is used before or simultaneously with estrogen, as well as pre-hormone therapy activity and bone density factors that may be more prevalent in transgender women (77). No long-term studies have addressed fracture risk, especially in an elderly transgender population, and routine screening is not currently recommended for preorchiectomy patients except as indicated by additional risk factors. Weight-bearing activity and calcium and vitamin D supplementation, if diet is inadequate, are recommended.

It is unclear how much estrogen is needed following gonadal removal to protect against bone loss, but studies in postmenopausal women suggest that very-low-dose estrogen (0.025 mg transdermal estradiol, for example) may be sufficient (78). Loss of bone density is most likely after orchiectomy in patients with other risk factors (e.g., white or Asian ethnicity, smoking, family history, high alcohol use, hyperthyroidism) and in those who are not fully adherent to hormone therapy. In general, estrogen therapy is advised to reduce the risk for osteoporosis. If there are contraindications to estrogen therapy, weight-bearing exercise, adequate calcium (1200 mg daily), and vitamin D (800 to 1000 units daily) are recommended to limit bone loss, as has been recommended for postmenopausal women (79). Dual x-ray absorptiometry (DEXA) screening is recommended for patients age 50 to 65 years who have been off estrogen therapy for longer than 5 years, and all patients older than age 65.

Transgender Men, Past or Present Hormone Use, Pre- or Postoophorectomy

Transgender men begin with an average of 10% to 12% less bone density than natal males, before any hormonal or surgical intervention (80). Prospective and case-control studies have found that testosterone therapy, at supraphysiologic doses, maintains or increases bone density among transgender men (54,81–83). However, most of these studies lasted between 12 and 36 months; none extended beyond 63 months. It is unclear what testosterone level is needed following gonad removal to protect against bone loss. Prospective studies of transgender patients with oophorectomy indicate that bone mineral density may decrease even with testosterone supplementation, particularly if testosterone use is interrupted or the dose is inadequate to suppress luteinizing hormone (82–84).

Progestins have been used in some transgender men patients to enhance amenorrhea before hysterectomy. This medication appears to result in bone density loss with long-term use among natal women (85) and, thus, may contribute to loss of bone density in the transgender setting. Overall, loss of bone density is most likely in patients with other risk factors (e.g., white or Asian ethnicity, smoking, family history, high alcohol use, hyperthyroidism) and those who are not fully adherent to hormone therapy, especially after oophorectomy. In general, testosterone therapy is advised to reduce the risk for osteoporosis. If there are contraindications to testosterone, weight-bearing exercise and adequate calcium (1200 mg daily) and vitamin D (800 to 1000 units daily) are recommended to limit bone loss (79). DEXA screening is recommended for patients age 50 to 65 who have been off testosterone therapy for longer than 5 years, and all patients over age 65 who are no longer receiving testosterone therapy. Patients over age 65 who continue to use testosterone probably do not benefit from DEXA.

Sexually Transmitted Infections

Transgender individuals do share many of the same concerns regarding STIs, including hepatitis B and HIV infection, found in the lesbian, gay, and bisexual communities (see Chapter 12). There are a few transgender-specific considerations, however. Transgender individuals (of any gender) who have sex with men can be considered in a population that is at increased risk for STIs (86). Sexual practices among transgender individuals vary greatly, and assumptions should not be made about the gender of a patient's sexual partner(s), sexual activities, or individual risks (87). Cofactors related to unsafe sex, such as depression, suicidal ideation, and physical or sexual abuse, are also increased among the transgender population: Studies indicate that the need to affirm one's gender identity can drive high-risk sexual behaviors (88–92). Finally, because needle-sharing with injectable hormones (or silicone) is a trans-specific potential risk factor for transmission of HIV and hepatitis B and C viruses, patients need to be educated regarding the risks as well as safe handling of needles and syringes.

STI prevention strategies should be appropriately targeted to each individual patient's anatomy and specific sexual practices. For example, nonpenetrative sexual activities with appropriate barrier protection (latex gloves, dental dams, nonmicrowaveable plastic wrap) or penetration with a dildo (covered by a condom) can be recommended for patients who are taking feminizing hormones and are unable to sustain an erection sufficiently firm for condom use. To prevent condom breakage, supplemental lubrication should be recommended for transgender women who have had vaginoplasty (as the neovagina is not self-lubricating) and transgender men patients who take testosterone (as decreased estrogen can result in vaginal atrophy and dryness). Water-based lubricants only should be used with latex barriers because oil-based products degrade latex and may therefore result in inadvertent transmission of infectious agents. For a more detailed discussion of STI and HIV prevention, please see Chapters 12, 13, and 14.

The variable anatomy of transgender persons can affect screening for STIs. A self-collected or clinician-collected vaginal swab is the recommended sample type. A first-catch urine specimen is acceptable but might detect up to 10% fewer infections when compared with vaginal and endocervical swab samples. However, this test can be used regardless of anatomy providing an acceptable alternative testing method when a vaginal, endocervical or urethral swab is not appropriate. Rectal and pharyngeal samples should be used in patients based on symptoms or on a history of high-risk oral or anal sex. Hormone therapy does not affect treatment of STIs in the transgender individual. Some HIV medications increase or decrease serum estrogen levels, but there is no evidence that cross-sex hormones interfere with the effectiveness of HIV medication or negatively affect the progression of HIV/AIDS. Little has been published regarding the risks of genital reassignment surgery among those with HIV/AIDS. HIV-infected persons have an increased risk for infection with any major surgery, with the number and severity of complications related to CD4 count. Genital surgery outcomes appear to be good with adequate patient selection and preoperative preparation (93).

Fertility Issues

Cross-sex hormones may reduce fertility, and this may be permanent even if hormones are discontinued. However, both transgender women and men have accomplished successful pregnancies with partners, sperm donors, or surrogates by discontinuing hormones. Alternative reproductive options for transgender men might include oocyte (egg) or embryo freezing. Patients should be advised that these techniques are not widely available and can be very costly. Transgender women should use sperm banking before initiation of hormone therapy for best results, as feminizing hormones can permanently affect fertility (14). Ideally, several samples should be banked. With the patient's permission, a letter of introduction should be sent to the collection center to ensure that the patient who is already cross-living will be treated in a respectful manner.

Transgender men may continue to ovulate while receiving testosterone therapy, even if menses have stopped; the risk for pregnancy is reduced but not predictably. However, it is important to recognize that testosterone can adversely affect a developing fetus (18). Depo-Provera, barrier methods, and spermicides are contraceptive options for patients at risk for pregnancy who are receiving or considering testosterone therapy. Tubal ligation, hormonal implants, and intrauterine devices are highly effective long-term alternatives for these patients.

Sexual Function

Testosterone therapy tends to increase libido among transgender men, while feminizing hormone therapy tends to reduce libido, reduce erectile function, and decrease ejaculation among transgender women (18). If a transgender woman is concerned about limiting erectile dysfunction while undergoing hormone therapy, the prescribing clinician should first consider adjusting the dose of hormones while addressing the patient's desires regarding the degree of feminization and level of erectile function. If this is unsuccessful, erection-enhancing drugs such as phosphodiesterase type 5 inhibitors (e.g., sildenafil) may be considered. Following genital surgery, sexual function (libido, arousal, pain with sex, and orgasm) varies and depends on preoperative sexual function, the type of surgery performed, and hormonal status (94).

Transgender Hormone Therapy

Transgender hormone therapy—the provision of exogenous endocrine agents to induce feminizing or masculinizing changes—is a medically necessary intervention for many transgender individuals (7,14). Some people seek maximum feminization/masculinization, while others experience relief with an androgynous presentation resulting from hormonal minimization of existing secondary sex characteristics (95). In addition to inducing physical changes, the act of using cross-gender hormones is itself an affirmation of gender identity—a powerful incentive for this population (3). Studies indicate improved psychological adjustment and quality of life with hormone therapy among transgender people before surgery (14).

Transgender patients desiring hormone therapy may ask their primary care provider to offer this treatment. Primary care providers can increase their experience and comfort in providing transgender hormone therapy through a variety of means. First, simply caring for transgender patients improves understanding of their specific health care needs. In addition, familiarity with hormone regimens and the transition/affirmation process is facilitated by co-managing care or consulting with a more experienced provider. Physicians who provide transgender hormone therapy come from many different specialties, including endocrinology, family medicine, internal medicine, obstetrics and gynecology, and psychiatry. There is no comprehensive list of experienced transgender hormone providers; physicians who publish in the medical literature and/or who are members of the World Professional Association for Transgender Health (WPATH) are most easily identified. However, physicians who provide transgender hormone therapy undergo no specific training and standard certification for this care does not exist. Thus, actual practices may vary significantly from provider to provider, making it difficult to discern which physicians are most qualified to serve as a mentor. The following section briefly explains the range of potential roles for the primary care provider in transgender hormone care.

Bridging

Patients may present for care already receiving hormones, whether obtained by prescription or through other means (e.g., purchased over the Internet). If a clinician is uncomfortable providing long-term hormone therapy, a good option is to provide a 1- to 6-month prescription for hormones while helping the patient find a clinician who can provide long-term follow-up care. Prior medical records should be requested and the history of hormone prescription documented in the current chart. The patient's current regimen should be assessed for safety and drug interactions; safer medications or doses should be substituted when indicated. Clear limits should be negotiated regarding the duration of bridging therapy.

Hormone Therapy Following Gonad Removal

Hormone replacement with estrogen or testosterone is usually continued for life after an oophorectomy or orchiectomy, unless medical contraindications arise. Estrogen and testosterone doses are often decreased after surgery, and antiandrogens for transgender women may be discontinued (4,13,18). Laboratory monitoring can be done yearly for otherwise healthy patients.

Hormone Maintenance Before Gonad Removal

Once patients have achieved maximal feminizing or masculinizing benefits from hormones (typically 2 or more years), they remain on a maintenance dose. The maintenance dose is then adjusted for change in health conditions, aging or other considerations (e.g., lifestyle changes) (96). Upon presenting for maintenance hormones, the provider should assess the patient's current regimen for safety and drug interactions and substitute safer medications or doses when indicated. The patient should be monitored by physical examinations and laboratory testing every 6 months. For patients receiving long-term therapy, the need for physical examinations may be less frequent depending on concomitant medical conditions. The dose and form of hormones should be revisited regularly with any changes in the patient's health status and available evidence on the potential long-term risk of hormones. For example, a physician prescribing maintenance hormones should feel comfortable addressing hormone adjustments related to venous thromboembolic risk and aging, hormones and cardiovascular risk factors, and hormones and fertility. It is important to discuss any reduction or interruption of hormone therapy with the patient well in advance.

Initiating Hormonal Feminization or Masculinization

Primary care providers are well suited to provide safe and effective masculinizing or feminizing hormone therapy in the setting of comprehensive health care. It is not necessary for the prescribing clinician to be an endocrine expert, but it is important to be familiar with relevant medical and psychosocial issues. This clinical situation requires commitment in terms of provider time and expertise. Hormone therapy must be individualized based on the patient's goals, the risk/benefit ratio of medications, the presence of other medical conditions, and consideration of social and economic issues. In general, the provision of hormone therapy should be consistent with the WPATH Standards of Care (SOC) 7, available online at www.wpath.org. The SOC 7 provides a flexible framework to guide the overall treatment of transsexual, transgender, and gender-nonconforming people.

Table 18-2 Commonly Used Published Transgender Hormone Protocols

	Endocrine Society, 2009*	Feldman and Safer (WPATH), 2009†	Vancouver Guidelines, 2006, Revised 2013††	Center of Excellence for Transgender Health, 2011§
Evidence-based or graded	Yes	Yes	Limited evidence base provided, but not graded or extensively reviewed	Yes, grades the evidence but does not provide extensive references or analysis
Includes puberty suppression	Yes	No	No	Limited— references Endocrine Society

*Hembree WC, Cohen-Kettenis P, Delemarre-van de Waal HA, et al; Endocrine Society. Endocrine treatment of transsexual persons: an Endocrine Society clinical practice guideline. J Clin Endocrinol Metab. 2009;94: 3132-3154.

†Feldman J, Safer J. Hormone therapy in adults: suggested revisions to the sixth version of the standards of care. Int J Transgender. 2009;11:146-82.

††Endocrine therapy for transgender adults in British Columbia: suggested guidelines. Vancouver, BC: Vancouver Coastal Health Authority, Department of Public Health; 2006, revised 2013.

A new version of the British Columbia Endocrine Guidelines are being drafted to align with the WPATH Standards of Care, Version 7. Once they are published, they will be available online at: http://transhealth. vch.ca.

§Primary Care Protocol for Transgender Patient Care. Center of Excellence for Transgender Health, University of California, San Francisco, Department of Family and Community Medicine; April 2011. www.transhealth. ucsf.edu.

There are a wide variety of published hormone regimens, but no randomized clinical trials comparing their safety and efficacy. The three most recent, widely used, and comprehensive guides to hormone therapy include "Endocrine Treatment of Transsexual Persons: An Endocrine Society Clinical Practice Guideline" (4), "Hormone Therapy in Adults: Suggested Revisions to the Sixth Version of the Standards of Care" (18), and "Physical Aspects of Transgender Endocrine Therapy" (96). The Center for Excellence in Transgender Health places their recommendations for hormone assessment, dosing, and monitoring among their larger reference material for transgender health (13). The WPATH SOC 7 guidelines are based primarily on the work of Feldman and Safer (18). It is not within the scope of this chapter to review each of these guidelines in detail, and they are fundamentally quite similar. Table 18-2 briefly summarizes these guidelines. There are nuances in each that promote varying degrees of flexibility during the steps in the process of care. Clinicians should understand the different approaches and adopt one that is both evidence based and meets the concerns of those seeking care.

The process of gender transition involves profound mental, social, emotional, economic, and legal changes in a patient's life. Hormone therapy can be both an enriching and complicating element in this transition, and "trans-competent" mental health professionals can provide a wide variety of resources to assist the transgender patient (and hormone provider) in this complex process. When a therapist is involved, and with the patient's consent, regular communication is advised to ensure that the transition process is proceeding smoothly.

Role of Behavioral Health Care in Primary Care of Transgender Patients

Transgender patients may seek mental health services for a variety reasons, including referral for medical interventions, exploration of identity, assistance in coping with stressors of dealing with stigma, mental health concerns including depression, anxiety, or other psychological concerns. Behavioral health care providers (psychologists, psychiatrists, social workers, etc.) and primary care providers can improve overall mental and physical health through collaboration to address transgender specific experiences of transition and lifetime health concerns.

Transgender people, in dealing with social stigma, can be at risk for higher levels of depressive and anxious symptoms, as well as higher rates of suicidal ideation stemming from societal, peer, or family rejection (97). A recent survey by the National Gay and Lesbian Taskforce on transgender health found that up to 41% of transgender and gender-nonconforming respondents had attempted suicide at some point in their lifetime (1). Mental health is an important area to assess and appropriately address not only as a precursor to medical intervention but at other points in transgender patients' lives.

Collaborative Relationships Between Behavioral Health and Primary Care

Transgender patients can feel at times disempowered in accessing adequate health care and may be reticent to bring up issues surrounding mental health, substance use, or higher risk behaviors. Establishing a release of information early on in treatment can be helpful to facilitate communication and encourage patients to address issues discussed in therapy that may impact their physical health with their primary care providers. Behavioral health care providers can assist clients in advocating for themselves with their primary care providers, as well as communicate areas of concern that primary care providers can then evaluate in the clinic.

On the other hand, primary care providers are often an entry point to care for transgender patients. Behavioral health providers have historically been the "gatekeepers" for medical interventions for transgender patients, and this historical context of the relationship has resulted in many transgender patients having complex feelings about the role of behavioral health providers in medical care, which may act as a barrier to care (98). Primary care providers are in a position to be able to use the rapport built with transgender patients to support accessing behavioral health care services (when needed), particularly if major surgery is not being contemplated.

Mental Health Assessment

A thorough mental health assessment will include a general mental health history, including exploration of risk for suicide as well as a history of physical, sexual, and emotional trauma; experiences in therapy; psychosocial factors; past and current symptoms; and prior treatment or medications. It is imperative that symptoms be assessed through a biopsychosocial approach, including the consideration of effect of systems of oppression on the experiences of symptoms on transgender patients' experiences. Transgender patients may be at higher risk for depression and anxiety and the use of avoidant coping strategies in dealing with social stigma or rejection (99). This must be considered not only in assessment but also in treatment. Building a social support system and developing a safe space for transgender clients to express their authentic gender expressions can be tremendously healing in remittance of mental health symptoms.

Assessment of Gender Dysphoria

Many transgender people present for mental health services with an awareness of discomfort with their birth assigned sex or secondary sex characteristics, although some become aware of dysphoric feelings during psychotherapy for other presenting concerns, such as depression. When assessing for a history of gender dysphoria, clinicians may want to explore the origin of gendered awareness feelings, asking such questions as, "When was the first time you remember being aware of transgender feelings?" Assessing the reactions of the onset of puberty can be very informative about intensity of gender dysphoric feelings as secondary sex characteristics began to develop, for example: "What were your feelings about . . . (starting menstruation, beginning to get erections, starting to grow breasts, developing pubic hair)?

Questions aimed at establishing current experiences of gender dysphoric feelings should focus on anatomic dysphoria as well as affective responses. Anatomic dysphoria can be assessed through administration of self-report measures aimed at assessing level of distress in response to different body parts, or through clinical interview exploring feelings of distress regarding secondary sex characteristics. Assessment of self-harming behaviors focused on genital or breast areas should be explored. Mental health practitioners should explore the existence of depression and anxiety in relationship to gender dysphoria in order to differentially diagnose accurately the intensity of depressive and anxious symptoms. Many times depression and anxiety symptoms can be substantially decreased through accurate diagnosis and treatment of the underlying gender dysphoria (100).

Role of Behavioral Health Care in Facilitating Transition

The WPATH SOC 7 (14) require 1 referral for hormone therapy from a professional trained to assess overall behavioral health and gender dysphoria. This can be a primary care provider who is knowledgeable and trained in behavioral health care concerns, as well as competent in assessing gender dysphoria. Providers should work to assess and diagnose gender dysphoria, work to stabilize co-occurring mental health concerns (such as substance use or depression), and assist the patient in learning about options in pursuing hormone therapy. Realistic expectations for hormone therapy, expectations about course of hormone treatment, and exploration of reproductive concerns are all areas clinicians can help patients explore before referral for hormones. Patients receiving antidepressive or psychotropic medications should work with experienced clinicians to explore the effect of hormones on their mood. Planning for initiation of hormone treatment, not only physically but also emotionally, is an important step in the transition process. Clinicians can help educate patients about the medical process, demystifying and empowering them to educate themselves about their hormone regimens, what to expect, and how to be an advocate for themselves with their providers.

The WPATH SOC 7 also requires referral from a mental health practitioner for surgical interventions for transgender patients. One referral is required for chest/breast surgery and two referrals are required for genital surgeries according to some guidelines. Some practice guidelines have introduced more flexibility for these surgeries. Letters from mental health practitioners should include information about the history of gender dysphoria and stabilization of any co-occurring mental health concerns and should address the patient's informed consent to treatment (14). Informed consent is always necessary.

Health Maintenance

Behavioral health care providers can work with primary care providers to address how any mental health symptoms may affect overall health and particularly issues such as substance use, tobacco use, depression, and anxiety symptoms. Conversely, primary care providers can assist patients in seeking out behavioral health services to help cope with issues of stigma and stress that may occur with transition and/or post-transition issues.

Surgical Interventions

Several surgical procedures exist to assist transgender persons in bringing their body into greater alignment with their gender identity. These procedures, in whole or part, are sometimes referred to as sex reassignment surgery or gender affirmation surgery. WPATH's SOC 7 includes clinical guidelines regarding surgical interventions, developed to promote optimal patient care. A detailed description of the types of surgeries and their potential complications may be found in SOC 7 and Principles of Transgender Medicine and Surgery (101).

Feminizing Procedures

Augmentation Mammoplasty
Breast augmentation, usually performed by a plastic surgeon, places saline-filled implants submuscularly via an incision under the breast (near the inframammary fold) or around the areola. Unless hormones are contraindicated, augmentation surgery is commonly delayed until after hormonal therapy has been undertaken for 12 to 18 months to allow time for hormonal breast development.

Vaginoplasty
The term *vaginoplasty* includes several procedures that transform the male external genitalia into female genitalia. Vaginoplasty includes orchiectomy, creation of a vaginal cavity and neoclitoris, labioplasty (construction of labia), and penile dissection with partial penectomy. It is usually performed by a plastic surgeon in a single operative setting, although some surgeons prefer to perform labioplasty and clitoroplasty as a second surgery following healing of the initial vaginoplasty. The penile inversion technique is most commonly used to create the neovagina (102). In this technique the majority of skin from the shaft of the penis is inverted and used to line the inner walls of the vaginal cavity. Following vaginoplasty postoperative vaginal dilatation is needed to achieve and maintain desired vaginal depth. Initially, patients are instructed to dilate three to four times per day during the first 6 weeks. Over time, the frequency decreases to daily or a few times per week, depending on the frequency of vaginal intercourse, but it is recommended that dilation be a lifelong practice.

Orchiectomy and Penectomy

Orchiectomy as a single procedure may be sought by patients who would like to reduce the risks and side effects of feminizing hormones by lowering the dosage needed to oppose endogenous testosterone (103). Patients who identify as more androgynous or "male to eunuch" in their gender identity may also pursue orchiectomy (104). Typically the testes are removed with preservation of scrotal skin in case vaginoplasty or labioplasty are sought in the future, but there is risk for shrinkage or damage of the skin. Some transgender women seek penectomy without vaginoplasty as a less invasive alternative when vaginal penetration is not desired. A shallow vaginal dimple is created that does not require dilation (as in vaginoplasty), and a new urethral opening is created to allow the patient to urinate in a sitting position. Penectomy as a separate procedure is not recommended if the patient wishes to pursue vaginoplasty at a later date.

Facial Procedures

Facial feminizing surgeries include, but are not limited to, removal of supraorbital bossing ("brow bossing"), brow elevation, rhinoplasty, ear pinning, augmentation of the lip vermilion area, cheek augmentation, chin/jaw reduction, and reduction laryngochondroplasty (also known as "tracheal shave" or "Adam's apple reduction").

Silicone Injections

Injection of free (gelatinous) silicone is extremely hazardous. Use of free silicone is not legal in many countries (including Canada and the United States), but these injections may be performed abroad or illicitly by non-medical personnel. Additionally, some laypersons may hold "pumping parties" where transwomen may be injected using even industrial-grade silicone oil with minimal or no sterile techniques. Risks associated with these procedures include local and systemic infection, embolization, painful granuloma formation, and a systemic inflammatory syndrome that can be fatal (13,105).

Masculinizing Procedures

Chest Surgery

Subcutaneous mastectomy results in a chest that has a male contour, is fully sensate, and has minimal scarring (106). The procedure consists of removal of most of the breast tissue, removal of excess skin, and removal of the inframammary fold. Reduction and repositioning of the nipple-areolar complex are often required to approximate male nipples. The choice of technique must be appropriately selected for the patient's breast size and skin quality: skin that is inelastic (often due to years of breast binding) can adversely affect the outcome and will influence (and limit) the surgeon's choice of technique. Some patients will choose a breast reduction in lieu of a subcutaneous mastectomy. Prior reduction affects options for reconstruction so should be approached cautiously for the patient who wants a full reconstruction in the future.

Hysterectomy and Oophorectomy
Patients may desire hysterectomy and oophorectomy to reduce gender dysphoria, to treat preexisting gynecologic problems, to prevent menstrual bleeding in the patient who cannot tolerate testosterone, or to eliminate the need for regular Pap testing and pelvic examinations in patients who cannot tolerate vaginal examination. Oophorectomy often allows reduction in testosterone dosage, along with associated health risks and adverse effects.

Vaginectomy and Urethral Lengthening
Some patients may request vaginectomy concurrent with a vaginal or abdominal hysterectomy. This procedure includes excision of all vaginal mucosa and approximation of the levator ani muscles in order to obliterate the previous vaginal cavity. Vaginal mucosa is then recruited to lengthen the urethra, which will then carry urine through the neo-phallus in a metoidioplasty or a phalloplasty (106). If urethral extension is sought as part of future genital reconstruction (e.g., phalloplasty) vaginectomy should not be performed, as vaginal mucosa is used to lengthen the urethra. These procedures are usually performed by the urologist and are a requisite part of a phalloplasty, but are optional in metoidioplasty.

Metoidioplasty
Metoidioplasty involves releasing the hormonally enlarged clitoris from its surrounding tissues (107). A flap of skin from the labia minora is then "wrapped around" the stalk to add bulk, resulting in a small phallus that has erogenous sensation. In addition, the fixed part of the urethra can be extended and incorporated into the microphallus by recruiting tissue from the vaginal mucosa. The procedure results in a small, sensate phallus that may allow for urination while standing. The microphallus created by metoidioplasty is typically not large enough for sexual penetration (106). Metoidioplasty is an option for patients who do not want to undergo the lengthy phalloplasty procedure with its higher rate of complications and donor-site morbidity.

Phalloplasty
Phalloplasty is a long and complex microsurgical procedure that requires free tissue transfer, usually a forearm graft, to create the neophallus (106). A small segment of the ulnar forearm is rolled into a tube to form the urethra. This is then rolled within a larger piece of the forearm

(including fat and skin) to form a "tube within a tube." The procedure results in an adult male-size phallus that transmits urine, and may later achieve rigidity by insertion of an erectile prosthesis. The native clitoris is not removed but is de-epithelialized and covered by the base of the phallus to preserve erogenous sensation. After anatomic and functional stability is ensured (approximately 1 year), an erectile prosthesis may be placed. Tattooing of the neo-glans may be performed as a later procedure to help create a visible demarcation between the penile shaft and the glans (106).

Scrotoplasty
A scrotum facilitates comfort in the male role by more closely approximating male appearance in underwear and swim trunks. Performed by the urologist or plastic surgeon, the scrotoplasty uses tissue from the labia majora to create a pouch (neo-scrotum), which is situated over the vaginal opening (108). After full healing, testicular implants may be placed. Although the skin is initially tight, over time the weight of the prosthesis stretches the redraped labial skin to create a more natural appearance (109).

Hormone Suppression Therapy for Youths

Adolescents experiencing gender dysphoria are sometimes eligible for medical intervention to suppress puberty. The goals of puberty suppression therapy are three-fold:

* To give trans youths more time to explore their gender nonconformity and other developmental issues;
* To relieve the psychological and social distress associated with development of secondary sexual characteristics and hormonal changes during puberty;
* To facilitate possible future transition by preventing the development of sex characteristics, which are difficult or impossible to reverse if adolescents continue on to pursue sex reassignment (14,110).

Hormone suppression therapy involves the use of gonadotropin-releasing hormone (GnRH) analogues to minimize estrogen or testosterone production and consequently delay the physical changes of puberty. Hormone suppression is considered fully reversible, as the patient's testicles or ovaries resume usual function once GnRH analogues are stopped. However, studies on long-term effects of puberty suppression, on bone and brain development particularly, are not yet available. Thus, before any physical interventions are considered for adolescents, extensive exploration of psychological, family, and social issues should be performed (4). Chapter 16

Table 18-3   Criteria for Puberty-Suppressing Hormones

For adolescents to receive puberty suppressing hormones, the following minimum criteria must be met:

1. The adolescent has demonstrated a long-lasting and intense pattern of gender nonconformity or gender dysphoria (whether suppressed or expressed).

2. Gender dysphoria emerged or worsened with the onset of puberty.

3. Any coexisting psychological, medical, or social problems that could interfere with treatment (e.g., that may compromise treatment adherence) have been addressed, such that the adolescent's situation and functioning are stable enough to start treatment.

4. The adolescent has given informed consent and, particularly when the adolescent has not reached the age of medical consent, the parents or other caretakers or guardians have consented to the treatment and are involved in supporting the adolescent throughout the treatment process.

Adapted with permission from: Coleman E, Bockting W, Botzer M, et al. Standards of care for the health of transsexual, transgender, and gender-nonconforming people, version 7. Int J Transgender. 2012;13: 165-232.

discusses these issues as well as the risks and benefits of pubertal suppression therapy.

It is recommended to wait until adolescents are at least Tanner stage 2 to begin puberty suppression, and studies evaluating this approach only included children who were at least 12 years of age as well (111–113). WPATH's SOC 7 (14) has established minimum criteria for initiating hormone suppression therapy (see Table 18-3).

Multiple published studies and guidelines on puberty-suppressing hormone therapy recommend the use of GnRH analogues as the backbone of therapy (4,113). The specific medications, however, vary broadly. Triptorelin has been used in the largest studies done in the Netherlands (112), but leuprolide depot is widely used in the United States (personal communication). While pregnancy, breastfeeding, and hypersensitivity are usually the only absolute contraindications to use of GnRH agonists, long-term data on bone density, final adult height, and potential resumption of sperm production in biological male trans youth are lacking (4).

Most GnRH agonists are administered by injection, although a few are available as subcutaneous implants. Measurements of gonadotropin and testosterone/estradiol guide dose adjustment. If the gonadal axis is not completely suppressed, the interval of injections is shortened or the dose increased (4). The most common clinical protocols for initiating and maintaining hormone suppression are found in the Endocrine Society guidelines (4) and the Dutch protocols, described in several publications (110,112,113). Hormone suppression therapy is generally continued until age 16 years, at which time patients may start feminizing/masculinizing hormones or discontinue suppression and resume natural puberty.

Conclusion

Many health care providers across a variety of specialties provide excellent hormonal and surgical care for transgender patients. However, comprehensive health care for transgender patients need not and cannot be delegated exclusively to "transgender specialists" or lesbian gay, bisexual, and transgender clinics. Not every primary care clinician will be able to offer all elements of comprehensive transgender care; however, with increasing availability of transgender-specific health information, every physician can become comfortable in working with transgender patients to meet their health care needs.

Summary Points

- When establishing care with a transgender patient, a thorough history of hormonal, surgical, or other gender-related interventions is essential. Risks and recommendations for preventive care often depend on the patient's hormonal and surgical status.
- Physical examinations should be structured based on the organs present rather than the perceived gender of the patient.
- Screening mammography is advisable in transgender women over age 50 with additional risk factors (e.g., estrogen and progestin use >5 years, positive family history, body mass index > 35 kg/m^2).
- Yearly chest wall and axillary examinations, along with education regarding the small but possible risk for breast cancer, are recommended for transgender men after chest reconstruction surgery.
- Pap smears should follow recommended guidelines for natal females in patients with an intact cervix and can often be as infrequent as every 3 to 5 years.
- The prostate is not removed in any of the standard feminizing genital surgeries. Routine PSA screening is not recommended. Digital rectal examinations with palpation of the prostate should be performed as per guidelines for rectal cancer screening, along with education regarding the small but possible risk of prostate cancer.
- Regardless of hormone status, the transgender population as a whole has several risk factors for cardiovascular disease; feminizing or masculinizing hormone therapy further increases cardiovascular risks such as hypertension, diabetes, and hyperlipidemia.
- Providers should screen all transgender patients for past and present tobacco use and provide appropriate cessation interventions.
- Transgender women receiving any form of estrogen are at increased risk for venous thromboembolic events. Avoidance of ethinyl estradiol in all patients and oral estrogens in at-risk patients may reduce this risk.

- STI prevention strategies should be appropriately targeted to each individual patient's anatomic needs and specific sexual practices.

References

1. **Grant JM, Mottet LA, Tanis J, et al.** Injustice at every turn: A report of the National Transgender Discrimination Survey. Washington DC: National Center for Transgender Equality and National Gay and Lesbian Task Force; 2011.
2. **Institute of Medicine.** The Health of Lesbian, Gay, Bisexual, and Transgender People: Building a Foundation for Better Understanding. Washington DC: National Academies Press; 2011.
3. **Kammerer N, Mason T, Connors M.** Transgender health and social service needs in the context of HIV risk. Int J Transgender. 1999;3.
4. **Hembree WC, Cohen-Kettenis P, Delemarre-van de Waal HA, et al.** Endocrine treatment of transsexual persons: an Endocrine Society Clinical practice guideline. J Clin Endocrinol Metab. 2009;94:3132-54.
5. **Feldman J.** Preventive care of the transgendered patient. In: Ettner R, Monstrey S, Eyler AE, eds. Principles of Transgender Surgery and Medicine. New York: Haworth Press; 2007: 33-72.
6. **Smith YLS, Van Goozen SHM, Kuiper AJ, Cohen-Kettenis PT.** Sex reassignment: outcomes and predictors of treatment for adolescent and adult transsexuals. Psychol Med. 2005;35: 89-99.
7. **Newfield E, Hart S, Dibble S, Kohler L.** Female-to-male transgender quality of life. Qual Life Res. 2006;15:1447-57.
8. **Feldman JL, Goldberg JM.** Transgender primary medical care. Int J Transgender. 2006;9: 3-34.
9. **Baba T, Endo T, Honnma H, et al.** Association between polycystic ovary syndrome and female-to-male transsexuality. Hum Reprod. 2007;22:1011-6.
10. **Mueller A, Gooren LJ, Naton-Schötz S, et al.** Prevalence of polycystic ovary syndrome and hyperandrogenemia in female-to-male transsexuals. J Clin Endocrinol Metab. 2008;93: 1408-11.
11. **Lombardi EL, Wilchins RA, Priesing D, Malouf D.** Gender violence. J Homosex. 2002;42: 89-101.
12. **Sperber J, Landers S, Lawrence S.** Access to health care for transgendered persons: results of a needs assessment in Boston. Int J Transgender. 2005;8:75-91.
13. **Center of Excellence for Transgender Health.** Primary Care Protocol for Transgender Patient Care. San Francisco, CA: University of California; 2011.
14. **Coleman E, Bockting W, Botzer M, et al.** Standards of care for the health of transsexual, transgender, and gender-nonconforming people, version 7. Int J Transgend. 2012;13: 165-232.
15. **Schlatterer K, Yassouridis A, Werder KV, et al.** A follow-up study for estimating the effectiveness of a cross-gender hormone substitution therapy on transsexual patients. Arch Sex Behav. 1998;27:475-92.
16. **Institute of Medicine.** Collecting Sexual Orientation and Gender Identity Data in Electronic Health Records: Workshop Summary. Washington, DC: National Academies Press; 2013.
17. **Asscheman H, Giltay EJ, Megens JA, et al.** A long-term follow-up study of mortality in transsexuals receiving treatment with cross-sex hormones. Eur J Endocrinol. 2011;164:635-42.
18. **Feldman J, Safer J.** Hormone therapy in adults: suggested revisions to the sixth version of the standards of care. Int J Transgender. 2009;11:146-82.
19. **Calonge N, Petitti D, DeWitt T, et al.** Screening for breast cancer: U.S. Preventive Services Task Force recommendation statement. Ann Intern Med. 2009;151:716-26.

20. **Deapen D, Hamilton A, Bernstein L, Brody GS.** Breast cancer stage at diagnosis and survival among patients with prior breast implants. Plast Reconstr Surg. 2000;105:535-40.

21. **Eyler AE, Whittle S.** FTM breast cancer: community awareness and illustrative cases. Paper presented at 17th Biennial Symposium of the Harry Benjamin International Gender Dysphoria Association, Galveston, TX, November 2001.

22. **Brinton LA, Persson I, Boice JD Jr, et al.** Breast cancer risk in relation to amount of tissue removed during breast reduction operations in Sweden. Cancer. 2001;91:478-83.

23. **Lawrence A.** Vaginal neoplasia in a male-to-female transsexual: case report, review of the literature, and recommendations for cytological screening. Int J Transgender. 2001;5.

24. **van Trotsenburg MA.** Gynecological aspects of transgender healthcare. Int J Transgender. 2009;11:238-46.

25. **Moyer VA.** Screening for cervical cancer: U.S. Preventive Services Task Force recommendation statement. Ann Intern Med. 2012;156:880-91.

26. **Fiumara N, Di Mattia A.** Gonorrhoea and condyloma acuminata in a male transsexual. Br J Vener Dis. 1973;49:478-9.

27. **van Engeland AA, Hage JJ, van Diest PJ, Karim RB.** Colpectomy after vaginoplasty in transsexuals. Obstet Gynecol. 2000;95:1006-8.

28. **Miller N, Bedard YC, Cooter NB, Shaul DL.** Histological changes in the genital tract in transsexual women following androgen therapy. Histopathology. 1986;10:661-9.

29. **Melnikow J, Nuovo J, Willan AR, et al.** Natural history of cervical squamous intraepithelial lesions: a meta-analysis. Obstet Gynecol. 1998;92:727-35.

30. **Sherman ME, Lorincz AT, Scott DR, et al.** Baseline cytology, human papillomavirus testing, and risk for cervical neoplasia: a 10-year cohort analysis. J Natl Cancer Inst. 2003;95: 46-52.

31. **Bosinski HA, Peter M, Bonatz G, et al.** A higher rate of hyperandrogenic disorders in female-to-male transsexuals. Psychoneuroendocrinology. 1997;22:361-80.

32. **Cibula D, Cifkova R, Fanta M, et al.** Increased risk of non-insulin dependent diabetes mellitus, arterial hypertension and coronary artery disease in perimenopausal women with a history of the polycystic ovary syndrome. Hum Reprod. 2000;15:785-9.

33. **Moyer VA.** Screening for prostate cancer: U.S. Preventive Services Task Force recommendation statement. Ann Intern Med. 2012;157:120-34.

34. **Morgentaler A, Bruning CO, DeWolf WC.** Occult prostate cancer in men with low serum testosterone levels. JAMA. 1996;276:1904-6.

35. **Blanchard R.** A structural equation model for age at clinical presentation in nonhomosexual male gender dysphorics. Arch Sex Behav. 1994;23:311-20.

36. **Nieder TO, Herff M, Cerwenka S, et al.** Age of onset and sexual orientation in transsexual males and females. J Sex Med. 2011;8:783-91.

37. **Feldman JL.** Initiating feminizing hormone therapy over age 50: results and challenges. Paper presented at World Professional Association for Transgender Health Biennial Symposium; September 27, 2011; Atlanta, GA.

38. **van Kesteren PJ, Asscheman H, Megens JA, Gooren LJ.** Mortality and morbidity in transsexual subjects treated with cross-sex hormones. Clin Endocrinol. 1997;47:337-42.

39. **Wierckx K, Mueller S, Weyers S, et al.** Long–term evaluation of cross–sex hormone treatment in transsexual persons. J Sex Med. 2012;9:2641-51.

40. **Gooren LJ, Giltay EJ, Bunck MC.** Long-term treatment of transsexuals with cross-sex hormones: extensive personal experience. J Clin Endocrinol Metab. 2008;93:19.

41. **Rossouw JE, Anderson GL, Prentice RL, et al.** Risks and benefits of estrogen plus progestin in healthy postmenopausal women: principal results From the Women's Health Initiative randomized controlled trial. JAMA. 2002;288:321-33.

42. **Grady D, Herrington D, Bittner V, et al.** Cardiovascular disease outcomes during 6.8 years of hormone therapy: Heart and Estrogen/progestin Replacement Study follow-up (HERS II). JAMA. 2002;288:49-57.

43. **Scarabin PY, Oger E, Plu-Bureau G.** Differential association of oral and transdermal oestrogen-replacement therapy with venous thromboembolism risk. Lancet. 2003;362:428-32.

44. **Asscheman H, Gooren LJ.** Hormone treatment in transsexuals. J Psychol Hum Sex. 1992; 5:39-54.
45. **Inoue H, Nishida N, Ikeda N, et al.** The sudden and unexpected death of a female-to-male transsexual patient. J Forensic Leg Med. 2007;14:382-6.
46. **Parssinen M, Seppala T.** Steroid use and long-term health risks in former athletes. Sports Med. 2002;32:83-94.
47. **James PA, Oparil S, Carter BL, et al.** 2014 evidence-based guideline for the management of high blood pressure in adults: report from the panel members appointed to the Eighth Joint National Committee (JNC 8). JAMA. 2014;311: 507-20.
48. **Rhoden EL, Morgentaler A.** Risks of testosterone-replacement therapy and recommendations for monitoring. N Engl J Med. 2004;350:482-92.
49. **Steinbeck A.** Hormonal medication for transsexuals. Venereology. 1997;10:175-7.
50. **Tangredi JF, Buxton IL.** Hypertension as a complication of topical testosterone therapy. Ann Pharmacother. 2001;35:1205-7.
51. **Giorgi A, Weatherby RP, Murphy PW.** Muscular strength, body composition and health responses to the use of testosterone enanthate: a double blind study. J Sci Med Sport. 199912; 2:341-55.
52. **Elbers JMH, Giltay EJ, Teerlink T, et al.** Effects of sex steroids on components of the insulin resistance syndrome in transsexual subjects. Clin Endocrinol. 2003;58:562-71.
53. **Giltay EJ, Lambert J, Gooren LJ, et al.** Sex steroids, insulin, and arterial stiffness in women and men. Hypertension. 1999;34:590-7.
54. **Mueller A, Kiesewetter F, Binder H, et al.** Long-term administration of testosterone undecanoate every 3 months for testosterone supplementation in female-to-male transsexuals. J Clin Endocrinol Metab. 2007;92:3470-5.
55. **Feldman J.** New onset of type 2 diabetes mellitus with feminizing hormone therapy: case series. Int J Transgender. 2002;6.
56. **Elbers JM, Asscheman H, Seidell JC, Gooren LJ.** Effects of sex steroid hormones on regional fat depots as assessed by magnetic resonance imaging in transsexuals. Am J Physiol. 1999; 276:E317-25.
57. **Koh-Banerjee P, Wang Y, Hu FB, et al.** Changes in body weight and body fat distribution as risk factors for clinical diabetes in U.S. men. Am J Epidemiol. 2004;159:1150-9.
58. **Resnick HE, Valsania P, Halter JB, Lin X.** Relation of weight gain and weight loss on subsequent diabetes risk in overweight adults. J Epidemiol Commun Health. 2000;54: 596-602.
59. **Elbers JM, Asscheman H, Seidell JC, et al.** Long-term testosterone administration increases visceral fat in female to male transsexuals. J Clin Endocrinol Metab. 1997;82:2044-7.
60. **Glueck CJ, Lang J, Hamer T, Tracy T.** Severe hypertriglyceridemia and pancreatitis when estrogen replacement therapy is given to hypertriglyceridemic women. J Lab Clin Med. 1994; 123:59-64.
61. **Goldenberg NM, Wang P, Glueck CJ.** An observational study of severe hypertriglyceridemia, hypertriglyceridemic acute pancreatitis, and failure of triglyceride-lowering therapy when estrogens are given to women with and without familial hypertriglyceridemia. Clin Chim Acta. 2003;332:11-9.
62. **Erenus M, Karakoc B, Gurler A.** Comparison of effects of continuous combined transdermal with oral estrogen and oral progestogen replacement therapies on serum lipoproteins and compliance. Climacteric 2001;4:228-34.
63. **Sanada M, Tsuda M, Kodama I, et al.** Substitution of transdermal estradiol during oral estrogen-progestin therapy in postmenopausal women: effects on hypertriglyceridemia. Menopause 2004;11:331-6.
64. **Stone NJ, Robinson JG, Lichtenstein AH, et al.** 2013 ACC/AHA guideline on the treatment of blood cholesterol to reduce atherosclerotic cardiovascular risk in adults. Circulation. 2014; 129(25 Suppl 2):S1-45.
65. **Expert Panel on Detection, Evaluation, and Treatment of High Blood Cholesterol in Adults.** Executive summary of the Third Report of the National Cholesterol Education Program

(NCEP) Expert Panel on Detection, Evaluation, and Treatment of High Blood Cholesterol in Adults (Adult Treatment Panel III). JAMA. 2001;285:2486-97.

66. **Ott J, Aust S, Promberger R, et al**. Crosssex hormone therapy alters the serum lipid profile: a retrospective cohort study in 169 transsexuals. J Sex Med. 2011;8:2361-9.

67. **Whitsel EA, Boyko EJ, Matsumoto AM, et al**. Intramuscular testosterone esters and plasma lipids in hypogonadal men: a meta-analysis. Am J Med. 2001;111:261-9.

68. **Feldman J, Bockting W, Allen S, Brintell D**. Smoking cessation among persons receiving transgender hormone therapy. Paper presented at the Harry Benjamin International Symposium on Gender Dysphoria; September 10-13, 2003; Gent, Belgium.

69. **Feldman J, Bockting WO**. Transgender health. Minn Med. 2003;86:25-32.

70. **Toorians AW, Gooren LJ, Asscheman H**. Venous thromboembolism and (oral) estrogen use. Int J Transgender. 2001;5.

71. **Asscheman H, T'Sjoen G, Lemaire A, et al**. Risk of venous thromboembolism (VTE) in estrogen-treated male-to-female transsexuals: a review of literature and observations from 9 European centers for gender dysphoria. J Sex Med. 2011;8:118.

72. **Toorians A, Thomassen M, Zweegman S, et al**. Venous thrombosis and changes of hemostatic variables during cross-sex hormone treatment in transsexual people. J Clin Endocrinol Metab. 2003;88:5723-9.

73. **Gomes MP, Deitcher SR**. Risk of venous thromboembolic disease associated with hormonal contraceptives and hormone replacement therapy: a clinical review. Arch Intern Med. 2004; 164:1965-76.

74. **Jick H**. Incidence of venous thromboembolism in users of combined oral contraceptives. Methods for identifying cases and estimating person time at risk must be detailed. BMJ. 2000;320:57-8.

75. **Peverill RE**. Hormone therapy and venous thromboembolism. Best Pract Res Clin Endocrinol Metab. 2003;17:149-64.

76. **Jones R, Schultz C, Chatterton B**. A longitudinal study of bone density in reassigned transsexuals. Bone. 2009;44:S126.

77. **Van Caenegem E, Taes Y, Wierckx K, et al**. Low bone mass is prevalent in male-to-female transsexual persons before the start of cross-sex hormonal therapy and gonadectomy. Bone. 2013;54:92-7.

78. **Dören M, Samsioe G**. Prevention of postmenopausal osteoporosis with oestrogen replacement therapy and associated compounds: update on clinical trials since 1995. Hum Reprod Update. 2000;6:419-26.

79. **National Osteoporosis Foundation**. Clinician's Guide to Prevention and Treatment of Osteoporosis. Washington DC: National Osteoporosis Foundation; 2010.

80. **Campion JM, Maricic MJ**. Osteoporosis in men. Am Fam Physician. 2003;67:1521-6.

81. **Haraldsen I, Haug E, Falch J, et al**. Cross-sex pattern of bone mineral density in early onset gender identity disorder. Horm Behav. 2007;52:334-43.

82. **Turner A, Chen TC, Barber TW, et al**. Testosterone increases bone mineral density in female-to-male transsexuals: a case series of 15 subjects. Clin Endocrinol (Oxf). 2004;61: 560-6.

83. **van Kesteren P, Lips P, Gooren LJ, et al**. Long-term follow-up of bone mineral density and bone metabolism in transsexuals treated with cross-sex hormones. Clin Endocrinol. 1998; 48:347-54.

84. **Goh HH, Ratnam SS**. Effects of hormone deficiency, androgen therapy and calcium supplementation on bone mineral density in female transsexuals. Maturitas. 1997;26: 45-52.

85. **Scholes D, LaCroix AZ, Ichikawa LE, et al**. Change in bone mineral density among adolescent women using and discontinuing depot medroxyprogesterone acetate contraception. Arch Pediatr Adolesc Med. 2005;159:139-44.

86. **Feldman JL, Robinson B, Grey J, Bockting W**. HIV risk among transgender persons: a national internet-based study. Paper presented at XXI Symposium of World Professional Association for Transgender Health; June 28, 2009; Oslo, Norway.

87. **Bauer GR, Travers R, Scanlon K, Coleman TA.** High heterogeneity of HIV-related sexual risk among transgender people in Ontario, Canada: a province-wide respondent-driven sampling survey. BMC Public Health. 2012;12:292.

88. **Bockting W, Robinson B, Rosser B.** Transgender HIV prevention: a qualitative needs assessment. AIDS Care. 1998;10:505-25.

89. **Crosby RA, Pitts NL.** Caught between different worlds: how transgendered women may be "forced" into risky sex. J Sex Res. 2007;44:43-8.

90. **Melendez RM, Pinto R.** "It's really a hard life": love, gender, and HIV risk among male-to-female transgender persons. Cult Health Sex. 2007;9:233-45.

91. **Nemoto T, Operario D, Keatley J, et al.** HIV risk behaviors among male-to-female transgender persons of color in San Francisco. Am J Public Health. 2004;94:1193-9.

92. **Sausa LA, Keatley JA, Operario D.** Peceived risks and benefits of sex work among transgender women of color in San Francisco. Arch Sex Behav. 2007;36:768-77.

93. **Kirk S.** Guidelines for selecting HIV positive patients for genital reconstructive surgery. Int J Transgender. 1999;3.

94. **Klein C, Gorzalka BB.** Continuing medical education: sexual functioning in transsexuals following hormone therapy and genital surgery: a review. J Sex Med. 2009;6:2922-39.

95. **Factor RJ, Rothblum E.** Exploring gender identity and community among three groups of transgender individuals in the United States: MTFs, FTMs, and genderqueers. Health Sociol Rev. 2008;17:235-53.

96. **Dahl M, Feldman J, Goldberg J, Jaberi A.** Physical aspects of transgender endocrine therapy. Int J Transgender. 2006;9:111-34.

97. **Nuttbrock L, Rosenblum A, Blumenstein R.** Transgender identity affirmation and mental health. Int J Transgender. 2002;6:1-11.

98. **Corneil TA, Eisfeld JH, Botzer M.** Proposed changes to diagnoses related to gender identity in the DSM: a World Professional Association for Transgender Health consensus paper regarding the potential impact on access to health care for transgender persons. Int J Transgender. 2010;12:107-14.

99. **Budge SL, Adelson JL, Howard KA.** Anxiety and depression in transgender individuals: the roles of transition status, loss, social support, and coping. J Consult Clin Psychol. 2013;81: 545-57.

100. **Gómez-Gil E, Zubiaurre-Elorza L, Esteva I, et al.** Hormone-treated transsexuals report less social distress, anxiety and depression. Psychoneuroendocrinology. 2012;37:662-70.

101. **Ettner R, Monstrey S, Eyler AE.** Principles of Transgender Medicine and Surgery. Binghamton, NY: Haworth Press; 2007.

102. **Takata L, Meltzer T.** Procedures, postoperative care, and potential complications of gender reassignment surgery for the primary care physician. Prim Psychiatry. 2000;7:74-8.

103. **Reid RW.** Orchiectomy as a first stage towards gender reassignment: a positive option. Paper presented at Gendys '96: The Fourth International Gender Dysphoria Conference; 1996; Manchester, United Kingdom.

104. **Johnson TW, Wassersug RJ.** Gender identity disorder outside the binary: when gender identity disorder-not otherwise specified is not good enough. Arch Sex Behav. 2010;39:597-8.

105. **Gaber Y.** Secondary lymphoedema of the lower leg as an unusual side-effect of a liquid silicone injection in the hips and buttocks. Dermatology. 2004;208:342-4.

106. **Monstrey SJ, Ceulemans P, Hoebeke P.** Sex reassignment surgery in the female-to-male transsexual. Semin Plast Surg. 2011;25:229-44.

107. **Perovic S, Djordjevic M.** Metoidioplasty: a variant of phalloplasty in female transsexuals. BJU Int. 2003;92:981-5.

108. **Sengezer M, Sadove RC.** Scrotal construction by expansion of labia majora in biological female transsexuals. Ann Plast Surg. 1993;31:372-6.

109. **Hage JJ, Bouman FG, Bloem J.** Constructing a scrotum in female-to-male transsexuals. Plast Reconstr Surg. 1993;91:914-21.

110. **de Vries AL, Cohen-Kettenis PT, Delemarre-van de Waal H.** Clinical management of gender dysphoria in adolescents. Int J Transgender. 2006;9:83-94.

111. **Cohen-Kettenis PT, Schagen SEE, Steensma TD, et al.** Puberty suppression in a gender-dysphoric adolescent: a 22-year follow-up. Arch Sex Behav. 2011;40:843-7.

112. **de Vries ALC, Steensma TD, Doreleijers TAH, Cohen-Kettenis PT.** Puberty suppression in adolescents with gender identity disorder: a prospective follow-up study. J Sex Med. 2011;8: 2276-83.

113. **Delemarre-van de Waal HA, Cohen-Kettenis PT.** Clinical management of gender identity disorder in adolescents: a protocol on psychological and paediatric endocrinology aspects. Eur J Endocrinol. 2006;155:S131-7.

Policy Issues and Global LGBT Health

Chapter 19

Policy and Legal Issues Affecting LGBT Health

SEAN CAHILL, PhD
HECTOR L. VARGAS JR., JD

Introduction

Primary care providers are critical to better understanding, reducing, and, one day, eliminating health disparities affecting lesbian, gay, bisexual, and transgender (LGBT) patients. However, many important structural barriers continue to impede LGBT people's access to better care and better health outcomes. These include a reluctance of LGBT patients to disclose their sexual and gender identity, often due to fear that they will experience discriminatory treatment (1–3); a lack of providers trained to address the specific health care needs of LGBT people (4,5); lack of access to health insurance, such as the outlawing of domestic partner health benefits for public sector employees in Michigan, Ohio, Georgia, and other states (6); much lower rates of health insurance coverage for same-sex couples (7); and a lack of culturally appropriate prevention services (8).

Since the publication of the first edition of the *Fenway Guide*, there have been significant strides in the legal and policy arenas to overcome these barriers and address health disparities facing LGBT people. At the federal level, for example, the U.S. government committed to eliminate health disparities in LGBT people by including LGBT health as a new topic area in Healthy People 2020 (9). In addition, the Patient Protection and Affordable Care Act (hereafter referred to as the Affordable Care Act or ACA) has been a hub for activity to address LGBT health. The Obama administration has also taken substantial executive branch actions to promote LGBT health, and private, nongovernmental organizational initiatives have been developed to improve the health and well-being of LGBT people. This chapter will review these and other recent legal and policy changes, which have the potential to bring the United States several steps closer to eliminating health disparities among LGBT people.

The Affordable Care Act and Expanded Health Care Access for LGBT People

Lack of access to health care is likely a major factor contributing to LGBT disparities. Studies have shown that lesbians and transgender people are less likely to access preventive care (10,11); they are also less likely to have health insurance (12). Insurance companies have historically denied coverage for pre-existing conditions such as HIV infection, thus affecting coverage for many gay and bisexual men as well as transgender women. In 2012, only 13% of the estimated 1.2 million Americans living with HIV had private insurance, and 25% had no insurance (13). Moreover, same-sex couples are insured at much lower rates than heterosexual couples (7). Many LGBT people have been denied coverage under their same-sex partners' employee benefits programs. In fact, more than 3 dozen states passed laws or constitutional amendments that outlawed spousal and domestic partner benefits for public sector workers; it was not until 2014 that many of these laws and amendments were struck down (14).

The ACA is benefitting LGBT people because it counters these barriers to affordable insurance by requiring insurance companies to cover all who apply and to offer the same rates without regard to pre-existing health conditions (15). The ACA also provides support for preventive care and HIV testing, treatment, and prevention services. The pre-existing condition provision means that thousands of people living with HIV will be able to access health coverage, which should help improve treatment outcomes, a key goal of the National HIV/AIDS Strategy.

Nondiscrimination Protections under the Affordable Care Act

The ACA and regulations adopted as part of its implementation also include new health care protections for LGBT people. ACA section 1557 prohibits discrimination on the basis of existing civil rights law by any entity taking money from the U.S. government. This would include any hospital receiving Medicaid or Medicare funding, for example. Section 1557 explicitly refers to Title IX of the Education Amendments of 1972. Title IX, often used to protect girls and women from sex discrimination in school sports, has been interpreted by the courts and the U.S. Department of Health and Human Services (HHS) to also cover gender identity and, therefore, transgender people (16).

In addition, a 2012 federal regulation outlaws sexual orientation and gender identity discrimination by qualified health plans (QHPs) traded on state health insurance marketplaces (HIMs). This regulation also bans "marketing practices or benefit designs that will have the effect of discouraging the enrollment of individuals with significant health needs in QHPs," which could potentially help protect people living with HIV/AIDS (17). However, note that this 2012 regulation protects against insurance discrimination, not against discrimination in health care. Most Americans—about 55%—have insurance that is large group coverage offered by their employer (18). This insurance is regulated by the Employee Retirement Income Security Act, which does not prohibit sexual orientation and gender identity discrimination.

Nondiscrimination protections in health care and insurance coverage are important given that in much of the country it is still legal to deny a person a job, promotion, housing, or access to a public accommodation, such as a health care facility, because of real or perceived sexual orientation and gender identity. As of October 2014, 21 states and the District of Columbia have outlawed discrimination on the basis of sexual orientation, as have hundreds of municipalities, and 17 of these states also have outlawed discrimination on the basis of gender identity (19). While most of these laws cover public accommodations, including health care access, not all do. For example, New York City's gender identity nondiscrimination law protects against discrimination in health care access and access to homeless shelters. Massachusetts' gender identity nondiscrimination law does not.

Medicaid and Medicare

Medicare and Medicaid provide critical support to many thousands of LGBT people, including many living with HIV. Most LGBT elders qualify for Medicare if they have paid into the system sufficiently during their working lives. Some people living with HIV in the United States are also Medicare beneficiaries, while others receive Medicaid (20). However, until the ACA, childless adults could not qualify for Medicaid unless they were disabled. This meant that they had to have an AIDS diagnosis. The Medicaid expansion to individuals who earn up to 138% of the poverty level, a key component of the ACA, is changing this and allowing many childless low-income LGBT individuals to access Medicaid. However, those in states without Medicaid expansion will not receive this coverage (21,22). Further expansion would benefit many low-income LGBT people and people living with HIV, as well as millions of other low-income Americans.

Health Insurance Marketplaces

State HIMs are the mechanism whereby low- and moderate-income individuals and families eligible for federal subsidies and employees of small businesses are able to purchase affordable health insurance (23). The marketplaces became active in January 2014. As mentioned previously, rules promulgated by HHS in 2012 require nondiscrimination on the basis of sexual orientation and gender identity by insurers whose products are offered on HIMs. In addition, efforts are underway to ensure HIMs reach out to LGBT consumers, collect confidential patient data on sexual orientation and gender identity, ensure that subsidies and enrollment systems include same-sex couples and children of same-sex couples, and prohibit exclusions of transgender people's health care needs. For example, in Massachusetts, the Division of Insurance issued a directive in June 2014 requiring private insurers to cover medically necessary gender reassignment surgery and cross-sex hormones (24).

It is also critical that people with HIV/AIDS and other vulnerable populations have access to essential care and treatment through the QHPs traded on the HIMs. People with HIV/AIDS must take at least three antiretroviral drugs to effectively suppress HIV. However, the HHS Informational Bulletin of December 2011 proposed that plans are allowed to cover only 1 drug in each category covered by the benchmark (25). This could mean that people with HIV are not able to access the life-saving medications. Utilization controls, such as requiring prior authorization to access antiretrovirals, could also hinder access to treatment. In May 2014 the National Health Law Program and the AIDS Institute sued 4 Florida insurance companies for allegedly pricing medications in such a way that discourages people with HIV/AIDS from selecting their policies (26).

The Ryan White Care Act

With full implementation of the ACA, thousands of people currently receiving health care through Ryan White Program–funded providers are now eligible for Medicaid coverage or subsidized insurance offered through state exchanges (the Ryan White Program is the country's grant program for uninsured and underinsured people living with HIV/AIDS). The protection against insurance discrimination based on pre-existing condition is a welcome development that is increasing access to coverage and health care for the 1.2 million Americans living with HIV, but it does not mean that the Ryan White Program is no longer needed. Key essential enabling services funded by Ryan White are not funded by any other source. These include case management, treatment adherence, prevention and outreach in nontraditional settings, legal services and benefits advocacy, and dental care. The number of patients receiving health care from Ryan White providers increased 56% from 2001 to 2009, even as funding remained flat in real dollar terms (27). Given these substantial unmet needs, continued funding for Ryan White is critical. The Ryan White reauthorization expired September 30, 2013. There is no sunset provision, and funding continues through continuing resolutions into 2015 and beyond. The consensus among policy makers, providers, and advocates is that the Ryan White Program is still needed even as many low-income people living with HIV access medical care because of the expanded access brought about by the ACA.

The Prevention and Public Health Fund

Another potential benefit for LGBT people through the ACA is the Prevention and Public Health Fund, which supports community prevention through community transformation grants and other mechanisms as well as clinical prevention, infrastructure, and research. Priority issues include reducing the structural causes of chronic illness, such as tobacco use and obesity. Because tobacco use rates are higher among LGBT people and obesity is higher among lesbians (11), there may be opportunities for community transformation grant–funded work that targets LGBT people.

Access to Substance Use and Mental Health Services

Access to mental health and substance use treatment is particularly important for LGBT people, as the research literature shows higher rates of mental health issues and substance use among LGBT populations than among heterosexuals (28–31) (see also Chapters 10 and 11). Despite the need for mental health and addiction services, several studies show that LGBT people experience discrimination or lack of provider cultural competency when accessing care (1,32). The ACA could dramatically expand access to behavioral health services for LGBT people because it mandates that an insurer's essential health benefits package cover 10 categories of benefits—including mental health and substance abuse services. However, it is vital that mental health and substance use service providers receive training to be clinically competent with LGBT patients.

New Models of Service Delivery and Payment

Two new models of service delivery and payment are being taken up across the U.S. health care system: patient-centered medical homes (PCMHs), or health homes, and accountable care organizations (ACOs). As an essential element of the ACA, PCMHs offer comprehensive, coordinated, accessible care and are committed to quality and safety. Central to the PCMH model is the need to "know your patient." Given the level of health disparities among LGBT people, collection of data on sexual orientation and gender identity and patient–provider conversations about LGBT identity and sexual behavior are critical to the PCMH model because they offer an opportunity to increase provider knowledge of LGBT patients and their health needs.

Ryan White Part C clinics, which provide comprehensive primary health care in an outpatient setting for people living with HIV disease, are a "strong example" of a "medical home" model (33). In these clinics, "access to primary and specialty care is coordinated and monitored by the HIV primary care team, as are psychosocial and social services for patients based on their needs" (34).

In November 2012, HHS Secretary Kathleen Sebelius announced that HIV infection would be added to a list of chronic health conditions that could be addressed through the health home model. The health home model is a variation on the PCMH model, in which "person-centered" or "whole-person" care is provided to an individual with a chronic condition. This is significant in that it provides an opportunity to adapt the success of the Ryan

White Program to an insurance model, which has traditionally been focused on a fee-for-service system (35).

While the health home model is a service delivery model, the ACO model aims to rein in growth in health care costs while concurrently improving health outcomes. The ACO model was introduced in the context of the ACA as part of Medicare; it has since been "rapidly adopted by commercial payers around the country as a tool for improving patient outcomes and controlling runaway health care spending" (36). ACOs are "an evolving model of care in which physicians and hospitals accept joint responsibility for the quality and cost of care delivered to a population of patients . . . [leading to] better coordination of care among physicians and across settings of care, leading to better quality and greater safety, more appropriate and efficient care services" (37).

ACOs are expected to ensure cost savings "not from stinting on needed care, but rather through improving the quality of care" (38). Yet there are significant concerns that "vulnerable populations," including "those with complex medical problems or social needs," face potential risks as well as benefits from ACOs (38). Most analyses, however, do not examine the particular risks that LGBT people and people living with HIV face. LGBT people have experienced obstacles to getting health coverage, and lesbians and transgender people are less likely than others to access preventive care (39,40).

Providers will have a critical role to play to ensure that the complex and expensive needs of people living with HIV and LGBT people are met by ACOs, even as growth in health care costs is reduced. Among the most costly health issues facing LGBT people are HIV care, behavioral health, and transgender care. For ACOs to ensure clinically competent care for LGBT people and improved treatment outcomes for people with HIV—improving the quality of care, while at the same time reducing the cost curve—it is also essential that LGBT-competent providers be included in the provider networks that make up ACOs.

Other Federal Actions and Initiatives That Support LGBT Health

In addition to the implementation of the ACA, the federal government has taken several other actions in recent years with the goal of further promoting the health and health care access of LGBT individuals, couples, and families. These are highlighted below.

Healthy People 2020

As previously referenced at the outset of this chapter, after years of advocacy efforts (41), the federal government included a new Healthy People 2020 topic area for "Lesbian, Gay, Bisexual and Transgender Health." This topic area, accessible online, provides a brief overview of health disparities facing LGBT populations, including an emphasis on social determinants, such as "oppression and discrimination," that affect the health of LGBT people (9). The LGBT-specific objectives in Healthy People 2020 currently relate to increasing the number of "population-based data systems" and surveys that specifically ask questions that identify LGBT populations. Under section 4302 of the ACA, the HHS Secretary can require the collection of data to document health disparities. In June 2011, HHS Secretary Sebelius indicated that these disparities include LGBT disparities (42). As part of these efforts, a sexual orientation question is now being asked on the National Health Interview Survey (NHIS). HHS is also cognitively testing a gender identity question to be added to NHIS in the future (43).

Domestic Partner Benefits for Public Sector Employees

Although many private-sector employers offer health insurance coverage to same-sex spouses and/or partners of their employees, not all do. In addition, many municipal and state government employers offer partner health benefits, although, as mentioned above, many states outlaw domestic partner benefits for public sector workers (14). It is in this context that in 2010, President Obama issued an executive order extending domestic partner health insurance to federal civilian employees in same-sex relationships (44), allowing thousands of federal employees to provide coverage for their same-sex partners or spouses.

Centers for Medicare & Medicaid Services Hospital and Nursing Home Visitation Policies

Inspired by the story of Janice Langbehn who, along with her children, was denied access to her dying partner at a Miami hospital, President Obama issued a presidential memorandum in April 2010 ordering HHS to develop regulations ensuring the right of every patient to designate visitors regardless of sexual orientation or gender identity (45). The rules, issued as "Conditions of Participation" in Medicare and Medicaid and effective in 2011, require nearly every hospital in the country to establish written policies allowing patients to choose visitors who may "enjoy 'full and equal visitation privileges . . . regardless of whether the visitor is a family member, a spouse, a domestic partner (including a same-sex domestic partner), or other type of visitor'" (46). The rules, and accompanying guidance issued by the Centers for Medicare & Medicaid Services (CMS), also require hospitals to inform patients of their right to choose a representative who can make decisions on behalf of the patient. The guidance instructs hospitals to give "deference to patients' wishes . . . whether expressed in writing, orally, or through other evidence" and "is intended to make it easier for family members, including a same-sex domestic partner, to make informed care decisions for loved ones who have become incapacitated" (47).

In 2013, the CMS clarified that the 2010 presidential memorandum covering hospital visitation rights for same-sex spouses and partners also applies to nursing homes and long-term care facilities. "Residents must be notified of their rights to have visitors on a 24-hour basis, who could include, but are not limited to, spouses (including same-sex spouses), domestic partners (including same-sex domestic partners), other family members, or friends," the guidance states (48).

CLAS Standards Incorporation of LGBT Cultural Competency

In 2013, the HHS Office of Minority Health issued newly revised National Standards for Culturally and Linguistically Appropriate Services in Health and Health Care (also known as the CLAS Standards) along with its Blueprint for implementing the CLAS Standards (49). Through its broad definition of "culture," the Blueprint "fully incorporates" LGBT cultural competency into the CLAS Standards (50). The standards are an important tool in ensuring that providers address LGBT health issues and will have a large effect on the implementation of the ACA (50).

Designation of LGBT People as a Medically Underserved Population and Designation of Providers Trained in LGBT Health as a Health Professional Shortage Area

In fall 2011, the Negotiated Rulemaking Committee considered revising the definitions of Medically Underserved Populations and Health Professional Shortage Areas (HPSA). The Fenway Institute submitted written and oral testimony to the Committee in support of designating LGBT people as a Medically Underserved Population and as a HPSA population group. In October 2011, the Negotiated Rulemaking Committee recommended, by an overwhelming vote of 23-2, to HHS that LGBT people be designated a medically underserved population, and as an HPSA population group (51). If HHS adopts these recommendations, these designations could mean significant resources to health centers that serve large numbers of LGBT patients, as well as to providers who develop a specialization in LGBT health care (52). As of October 2014, HHS had not yet taken action on these recommendations.

Gathering Sexual Orientation and Gender Identity Data in Electronic Health Records as Part of Meaningful Use Guidelines

A provider's knowledge of a patient's sexual orientation and gender identity is essential to providing appropriate prevention screening and care (53).

Patients who disclose their sexual orientation identity to health care providers may feel safer discussing their health and risk behaviors as well (54). A sample of New York City men who have sex with men (MSM) from the 2004–2005 National HIV Behavioral Surveillance system found that 61% had not disclosed their same-sex orientation or behavior to their medical providers. White MSM and native-born MSM were more likely to have disclosed than black, Latino, Asian, and immigrant MSM. Disclosure correlated with having tested for HIV (55).

The Institute of Medicine (IOM) Committee on Lesbian, Gay, Bisexual, and Transgender Health Issues and Research Gaps and Opportunities recommended in 2011 that sexual orientation and gender identity questions be asked in clinical settings and be standardized to allow for the comparison and pooling of data to analyze the unique needs of LGBT people (11). In 2012, the IOM hosted a follow-up workshop to discuss best practices in collecting sexual orientation and gender identity data in electronic health record (EHR) systems (56). Healthy People 2020 also calls for gathering sexual orientation data by clinicians, suggesting that health care providers "appropriately inquire about and be . . . supportive of a patient's sexual orientation to enhance the patient-provider interaction and regular use of care" (9). Gathering LGBT data in clinical settings is also consistent with HHS efforts to gather health data on LGBT populations as authorized under section 4302 of the ACA (42).

As this book went to press, the Office of the National Coordinator of Health Information Technology (ONCHIT) was considering whether to include sexual orientation and gender identity questions in the core demographic section of stage 3 meaningful use guidelines. At a February 6, 2013, public meeting, an ONCHIT staff person noted that there was "overwhelming support" in public comment submitted for requiring that providers ask these questions. In March 2014, the Health Information Technology Policy Committee submitted recommendations to ONCHIT, including the recommendation that "CEHRT [certified EHR technology] provides the functionality to capture . . . sexual orientation, gender identity" (57). In late February 2014, ONCHIT issued proposed 2015 EHR Certification Criteria and 2017 Certified EHR Technology (CEHRT) proposals, which suggest SNOMED code sets for sexual orientation and gender identity (58). Many health care organizations are already moving forward with efforts to gather such data in EHRs, including the Mayo Clinic in Minnesota and Beth Israel Hospital in New York City.

The Veterans Affairs Health Care System and LGBT Veterans

With more than 8 million individuals enrolled in the VA health care system, many LGBT people receive health care there. The VA is also the largest single provider of medical care to people with HIV in the United States (59). It has served 64,000 HIV-infected veterans since 1981 and currently serves 23,000

HIV-infected veterans. Little is known about the experiences and needs of LGBT veterans. A few state Behavioral Risk Factor Surveillance Surveys ask about sexual orientation; all ask about veteran status. An analysis of Massachusetts Behavioral Risk Factor Surveillance System data from 2005 through 2010 found that lesbian, gay, and bisexual veterans reported higher rates of suicidal ideation compared with heterosexual veterans (29). Other issues that may disproportionately affect gay veterans are "trauma from childhood adversity interacting with military trauma" (60). Because so many gay veterans associate their military service with hiding their sexual orientation, and because some were dishonorably discharged under the prior policies banning homosexuals from serving, the VA has begun to undertake affirmative outreach to LGBT veterans to ensure that they access the health care services and benefits to which they are entitled. In 2013 the VA issued a directive regarding "the respectful delivery of health care to transgender and intersex Veterans" (61). The directive clarifies that veterans are eligible for mental health services and hormone treatments, but not sex reassignment surgery. A year later the VA issued a similar directive regarding gay, lesbian, and bisexual veterans (62). Training of VA staff in LGBT issues so they can provide clinically competent care is occurring in New York, Massachusetts, and elsewhere. There are also two LGBT program officers who act as ombudspersons for LGBT veterans seeking services and point persons for VA staff looking to increase their competency in caring for LGBT veterans. In September 2013, U.S. Attorney General Eric Holder announced that, in the wake of the *Windsor v. U.S.* ruling striking down federal nonrecognition of same-sex marriages, the VA would provide spousal benefits to same-sex spouses (63). These benefits include health care and survivor benefits.

Insurance Coverage of Transgender Health Care

Transgender people have health needs that require access to nondiscriminatory health care. The widespread failure of most insurance plans to cover transgender health needs, including surgery and cross-sex hormones, is based on the commonly held misconception that treatment of transgender people is merely "cosmetic" or "elective" in nature. There is a consensus in the mainstream medical community that gender dysphoria is a recognized medical condition requiring medical and mental health care. Gender dysphoria is a persistently and deeply felt cross-gender identification, including an enduring sense that a person's body is of the wrong sex. Gender reassignment surgery and cross-sex hormone treatment are considered medically necessary by many physicians for their transgender patients. The American Medical Association adopted a resolution in 2008 supporting public and private health insurance coverage for treatment of gender identity disorder as recommended by the patient's physician. These treatments also significantly improve transgender patients' long-term health out-comes—including significantly improving quality of life, general health, social functioning, and mental health. Many transgender people report that they are happier and more productive following their transition to express their current gender identity. Better health outcomes for transgender indi-viduals could, in the long run, actually decrease costs for care. As noted earlier, the Massachusetts Division of Insurance mandated that private insurance plans cover transgender health needs in 2014. At the direction of Governor Deval Patrick, the Massachusetts Medicaid Department was also considering covering gender reassignment surgery and cross-sex hormones as this book went to press. California's and Vermont's Medicaid plans cover transgender health needs, and Connecticut was also considering such coverage as of late 2014 (64).

Health Care Private Sector Policies That Support LGBT People

Health Professional Associations

Many health professional associations have begun to address matters of LGBT health, including adopting policies that ensure members of these associations do not discriminate against patients on the basis of sexual ori-entation or gender identity. In addition, many of these associations have adopted policies that not only address specific health disparities affecting LGBT people but also have taken positions in support of laws and public policies that ensure equal treatment for LGBT people as a means to improve the health and well-being of LGBT people and their families. These policies address a wide range of topics—from eliminating health disparities for LGBT people, to supporting health care for transgender populations, to endorsing nondiscrimination laws and marriage equality. "Compendium of Health Profession Association LGBT Policy & Position Statements" is available on the glma.org website (65).

The Joint Commission

Another important development in recent years was the implementation of the Joint Commission's new patient-centered communication standards, including 2 new standards designed to improve LGBT health (66). The Joint Commission, the nation's largest and oldest health care accrediting body, began requiring hospitals it accredits to establish nondiscrimination poli-cies that are inclusive of sexual orientation and gender identity and expres-sion and to implement equal visitation policies. A nondiscrimination policy that covers sexual orientation and gender identity is an important baseline step for hospitals, clinics, and other health care organizations to take: Not only does it show a commitment that discrimination will not be tolerated, but it also helps to create a welcoming environment for LGBT patients. In connection with these new standards, the Joint Commission published a field guide for hospitals and health care organizations "for creating processes, policies, and programs that are sensitive and inclusive of LGBT patients and families" (67).

Legal Protections for LGBT People and Families

Because discrimination and stigma directed against the LGBT community contribute to health disparities among LGBT populations (11,68), it is important to recognize the larger legal landscape for LGBT people. LGBT individuals continue to suffer from discrimination in employment, housing, and basic civil rights. As discussed earlier, no federal law consistently protects LGBT individuals from employment and other forms of discrimination (with the exception of hate crimes); in 29 states the statewide nondiscrimination laws are not inclusive of sexual orientation, and in 32 states gender identity or expression is not specifically included in those laws (19). This section addresses this broader legal landscape.

Marriage, Civil Unions, and Domestic Partnerships

Legal recognition of same-sex relationships and marriages of same-sex couples directly affects the health and wellness of LGBT people (69). As of October 2014, 32 states and the District of Columbia recognized marriage for same-sex couples. Three other states had court rulings that cleared the way for marriage equality. In 8 additional states, rulings await further action, and in the other 7 states lawsuits are pending (14).

Several important federal policies that until 2013 treated same-sex spouses and partners differently from heterosexual spouses have changed in the wake of the 2013 *U.S. v. Windsor* Supreme Court ruling striking down as unconstitutional the federal nonrecognition part of the Defense of Marriage Act (DOMA). Before *Windsor*, DOMA prevented the federal government from recognizing marriages of same-sex couples for the purposes of federal benefits and programs. According to a 2004 report of the General Accounting Office, there are 1138 federal statutory provisions in which marital status is a factor in determining or receiving benefits, rights, and privileges, and all of these benefits, rights, and privileges were denied to legally married same-sex couples (70). One example was the inequitable federal tax treatment of health insurance benefits provided to a same-sex spouse or domestic partner through an employee's workplace. These health insurance benefits were treated as taxable income under federal law. Some employers recognized this inequity and tried to ameliorate these negative consequences by "grossing up" income to the employee, a practice that involved the employer reporting a higher value of the benefit to ensure that the employee receives the true value of the benefit after taxes (71).

The 2013 *U.S. v. Windsor* ruling opened up federal benefits to same-sex couples who are legally married, and even possibly for couples who have consecrated a civil union or domestic partnership but have not been married. Same-sex couples in states with same-sex marriage recognition are now being treated equally under the Family and Medical Leave Act, Social Security spousal and survivor benefits, immigration policy, veteran's spousal benefits, and other important policy areas. While some federal agencies, such as the U.S. Immigration and Customs Enforcement Agency, recognize same-sex marriages based on where they were performed regardless of where the couple currently lives (known as the "state of celebration" standard), other agencies, such the Social Security Administration and the Department of Veterans Affairs, are statutorily required to use the "state of residence" standard. This means that same-sex couples who live in a state that does not recognize their marriage cannot access federal spousal protections or benefits. The U.S. Congress would need to change this statutory language for same-sex couples in all 50 states to be treated equally under these federal policies.

In addition to these concrete protections and benefits, policies that protect spousal relationships potentially have important mental and physical health benefits for same-sex couples (72). As GLMA noted in a 2008 research brief titled "Same-Sex Marriage and Health": "Married individuals report more emotional support and are more likely to have a close confidant than the unmarried. Emotional support is directly associated with health and wellbeing and provides protection against the negative health consequences of stress" (69).

Family and Adoption Laws

According to a report by the Williams Institute, nearly 6 million children and adults have an LGBT parent, and more than 125,000 same-sex couple households include 220,000 children under 18 (73). The report also shows that LGBT individuals and same-sex couples raising children face some economic disadvantages. These disadvantages point to how marriage, adoption, and other legal institutions that recognize LGBT families can provide "crucial protections for children from a financial, legal and psychosocial stability perspective, along with increased degrees of social acceptance and support" (69).

As noted in the Williams Institute report:

> Second-parent and joint adoptions protect children in same-sex parent families by giving the child the legal security of having two legal parents, entitling them to crucial financial benefits, including inheritance rights, wrongful death and other tort damages, Social Security benefits, and child support. In many situations, second-parent adoptions are

important to ensure health insurance coverage for the child and to allow both parents to make medical decisions for the child (73).

A second-parent adoption is a process in which one partner adopts the child of the second partner who is already recognized as a legal parent (through birth or adoption) without severing the second partner's parental relationship to the child. A joint adoption, as the phrase implies, is when a couple jointly adopts a child. Second-parent adoptions are available in a growing number of states and local county jurisdictions. Appellate courts in 4 states have held that second-parent adoptions are not available (Nebraska, Ohio, Wisconsin, and North Carolina). Until recently, Florida was the only state that prohibited an individual homosexual from adopting. Now, only Mississippi has a specifically antigay adoption policy, prohibiting adoption by "couples of the same-gender." Utah also prohibits adoption by couples that are "cohabitating" outside of marriage (73). The Human Rights Campaign website keeps updated maps of state parenting and marriage laws (www.hrc.org/resources/entry/maps-of-state-laws-policies).

Health Care Decision-Making

The question of who can make health care decisions if a person is incapacitated is of particular concern for LGBT people and same-sex couples. There are many stories like that of Bill Flanigan, who was refused access to his dying partner and therefore unable to tell doctors that his partner did not want life-prolonging measures. This was despite the fact that Flanigan and his partner were registered domestic partners and that Flanigan had been made his partner's medical power of attorney (74). In states where same-sex couples can marry, a legal spouse can make health care decisions on behalf of an incapacitated partner. But the outcome may change if the couple is traveling in a state where marriage is not recognized. When there are no legal directives or documents, state laws often designate relatives to make those decisions even though the LGBT individual may have been estranged from his family.

It is highly advisable for all LGBT people, regardless of the relationship recognition laws in the state where they reside, to secure a medical power of attorney (or health care proxy) that designates a partner or friend to make health care decisions on their behalf. It is also recommended that LGBT people complete a living will that specifies the type of life-saving or life-prolonging measures a person wants if they are unable to communicate their wishes. The previously mentioned CMS regulations on medical decision-making and the Joint Commission standards and field guide provide some assurances that these documents should be respected and followed by hospitals and providers. As the guidance to the CMS rules indicate, a patient's wishes, whether communicated in writing, verbally or through some other means, should be given considerable weight and deference.

Family and Medical Leave

Family and medical leave is designed to help employees balance their family obligations, enabling them to schedule unpaid leave to recuperate from a serious illness or care for a sick family member. The federal Family and Medical Leave Act (FMLA), which was adopted in 1993, allows an employee working for an employer with 50 or more employees to take "12 weeks of unpaid job-protected leave to recover from a serious illness, care for a seriously ill family member, or stay at home following the birth or adoption of a child" (75). For transgender people, the law's definition of "serious medical condition" may not cover treatment needed to address "gender dysphoria" (formerly called *gender identity disorder*), the distress that individuals may experience when their gender identity does not match their physical anatomy (75). Until 2013, because of DOMA (as discussed above), a worker in a same-sex marriage could not take leave to care for her spouse, although the Obama administration in 2010 adopted guidance clarifying that an individual who is parenting may take leave to care for the child, regardless of the legal relationship between parent and child (75). Where the federal law was lacking until the 2013 *U.S. v. Windsor* ruling, states and local jurisdictions, as well as employers, had stepped in to allow family and medical leave for same-sex spouses and partners. At least 13 states, plus the District of Columbia, had LGBT-inclusive family and medical leave laws as of early 2014 (76). In response to the *Windsor* ruling, in 2014 the U.S. Department of Labor published a Notice of Proposed Rulemaking that would change from a "state of residence" standard to a "state of celebration" standard for the definition of spouse (77). This would allow same-sex couples married in states that recognize same-sex marriage to access the protections of the FMLA to care for their spouse in any of the 50 states, regardless of whether their current state of residence recognizes same-sex marriage.

Conclusion

In conclusion, a wide array of social practices and public policies affect LGBT people's ability to access health care for themselves and their families. LGBT people, who have lower rates of health insurance coverage and experience other barriers to care, stand to benefit from the changes brought about by the Affordable Care Act. Changes in key government agencies—such as the VA health system, which serves 8 million Americans—will improve culturally competent care for LGBT people. Moves by nongovernmental organizations such as the Joint Commission will increase access to quality care. Finally, recognition of same-sex spouses as a result of the 2013 *U.S. v. Windsor* ruling is already providing important protections for same-sex couples, especially older LGBT people.

Summary Points

- Social discrimination and stigma related to homosexuality, bisexuality, gender variance, and HIV remain strong in U.S. society.
- Lower rates of health insurance coverage, lack of culturally competent care, and discrimination in health care limit access to care and contribute to significant health disparities.
- In recent years, the federal government has taken many steps to address LGBT health and reduce disparities in insurance coverage, access to health care, and health outcomes, including inclusion of LGBT health in Healthy People 2020, visitation protections for same-sex spouses in nursing homes, greater attention to LGBT veterans by the VA, and non-discrimination protections for LGBT people in relation to the state health insurance marketplaces.
- Many provisions of the ACA will benefit LGBT people and people living with HIV.
- Private organizations have also taken steps to improve LGBT people's experiences in the health care system, including the Joint Commission and many health professional associations, which have adopted non-discrimination standards.
- The federal government has taken steps to increase data collection on sexual orientation and gender identity in health surveys. Data collection in clinical settings, and in EHRs, is also critical to understand and address LGBT disparities.
- The landmark *U.S. v. Windsor* Supreme Court decision in 2013 striking down federal nonrecognition of same-sex marriages is having a ripple effect across federal family protection policies; same-sex spouses living in states with same-sex marriage recognition are now treated equally under the Family and Medical Leave Act, Social Security benefits, immigration policy, and other important areas.

References

1. **Lambda Legal.** When Health Care Isn't Caring: Lambda Legal's Survey of Discrimination Against LGBT People and People with HIV. New York: Lambda Legal; 2010.
2. **D'Emilio J.** Sexual Politics, Sexual Communities: The Making of a Homosexual Minority in the United States, 1940-1970. Chicago: University of Chicago Press; 1998.
3. **Badgett L, Lau H, Sears B, Ho D.** Bias in the workplace: consistent evidence of sexual orientation and gender identity discrimination. Williams Institute. 2007. Available at: http://escholarship.org/uc/item/5h3731xr.
4. **Obedin-Maliver J, Goldsmith ES, Stewart L, et al.** Lesbian, gay, bisexual and transgender-related content in undergraduate medical education. JAMA. 2011;306:971-7.
5. **HIV Medicine Association.** The looming crisis in HIV care: who will provide the care? June 2010. Available at: www.hivma.org/uploadedFiles/HIVMA/Policy_and_Advocacy/Policy_Priorities/HIV_Medical_Workforce/Briefs/The%20Looming%20Crisis%20in%20HIV%20Care.pdf.

6. Cahill S. The role of antigay family amendments in the 2004 election. In: Strasser M, ed. Defending Same-Sex Marriage, Volume 1."Separate But Equal" No More: A Guide to the Legal Status of Same-Sex Marriage, Civil Unions, and Other Partnerships. Westport, CT: Praeger; 2007:119-40.

7. Ponce N, Cochran S, Pizer J, Mays V. The effects of unequal access to health insurance for same-sex couples in California. Health Aff. 2010;29:1539-48.

8. Mayer K, Bradford J, Makadon H, et al. Sexual and gender minority health: what we know and what needs to be done. Am J Public Health. 2008;98:989-95.

9. U.S. Department of Health and Human Services. Office of Disease Prevention and Health Promotion. Healthy People 2020. Lesbian, gay, bisexual, and transgender health. Available at: www.healthypeople.gov/2020/topicsobjectives2020/overview.aspx?topicid=25.

10. Valanis BG, Bowen DJ, Bassford T, et al. Sexual orientation and health: comparisons in the women's health initiative sample. Arch Fam Med. 2000;9:843-53.

11. Institute of Medicine. The Health of Lesbian, Gay, Bisexual, and Transgender People: Building a Foundation for Better Understanding. Washington, DC: The National Academies Press; 2011.

12. Ranji U, Beamesderfer A, Kates J, Salganicoff A. Health and access to care and coverage for lesbian, gay, bisexual, and transgender individuals in the U.S. The Henry J. Kaiser Family Foundation. 2014. Available at: http://kff.org/report-section/health-and-access-to-care-and-coverage-for-lgbt-individuals-in-the-u-s-health-challenges/.

13. HIV Health Reform. Implications of the Supreme Court's Affordable Care Act decision for people with HIV. June 2012. Available at: www.hivhealthreform.org/wp-content/uploads/2012/06/ACA-SCOTUS-Final-HHR.pdf.

14. National Conference of State Legislatures. Same-sex marriage laws. Available at: www.ncsl.org/research/human-services/same-sex-marriage-laws.aspx.

15. U.S. Department of Health and Human Services. Health coverage rights and protections. Available at: www.hhs.gov/healthcare/rights/index.html.

16. Cianciotto J, Cahill S. LGBT Youth in America's Schools. Ann Arbor: University of Michigan Press; 2012:63-5.

17. Rosenbaum S. Essential health benefits update: proposed regulations implementing the ACA; and application of the proposed EHB regulations to Medicaid benchmark plans. Health Reform GPS. George Washington University's Hirsh Health Law and Policy Program and the Robert Wood Johnson Foundation. November 29, 2012. Available at: http://healthreformgps.org/resources/essential-health-benefits-update-proposed-regulations-implementing-the-aca-and-application-of-the-proposed-ehb-regulations-to-medicaid-benchmark-plans/

18. Janiki H. Employment-based health insurance: 2010. Household Economic Studies. US Census Bureau. 2013. Available at: www.census.gov/prod/2013pubs/p70-134.pdf.

19. National Gay and Lesbian Task Force. State nondiscrimination laws in the U.S. Last updated May 21, 2014. Available at: www.thetaskforce.org. www.thetaskforce.org/nondiscrimination-laws-map

20. Henry J. Kaiser Family Foundation. HIV/AIDS policy fact sheet: Medicare and HIV/AIDS. 2009. Available at: www.kff.org/hivaids/7171.cfm.

21. Supreme Court of the United States. National Federation of Independent Business et al. v. Sebelius, Secretary of Health and Human Services, et al. June 28, 2012.

22. Washington Post Staff. Landmark: The Inside Story of America's New Health-Care Law and What It Means for Us All. New York: Public Affairs (Perseus); 2010.

23. Weil A, Shafir A, Zemel S. Health insurance exchange basics. Briefing. National Academy for State Health Policy. 2011. Available at: www.nashp.org/sites/default/files/health.insurance.exchange.basics.pdf.

24. Murphy J, Commissioner of Insurance. Guidance regarding prohibited discrimination on the basis of gender identity or gender dysphoria including medically necessary transgender surgery and related health care services. Bulletin 2014-3. June 20, 2014. Available at: www.mass.gov/ocabr/docs/doi/legal-hearings/bulletin-201403.pdf.

25. **U.S. Department of Health and Human Services.** Essential health benefits: HHS informational bulletin fact sheet. Available at: www.ncsl.org/documents/health/EHBhhsInfFactSheet.pdf.

26. **PR Newswire/Reuters.** NHeLP and The AIDS institute file HIV/AIDS discrimination complaint against Florida health insurers; advocates seek enforcement of ACA anti-discrimination provisions. May 29, 2014. Available at: www.prnewswire.com/news-releases/nhelp-and-the-aids-institute-file-hivaids-discrimination-complaint-against-florida-health-insurers-261103901.html.

27. **Weddle A, Hauschild B.** HIV medical provider experiences: results of a survey of Ryan White Part C programs. Presentation to the Institute of Medicine, Committee on HIV Screening and Access to Care. September 29, 2010. HIV Medical Association and Forum for Collaborative HIV Research. Available at: www.hivma.org/uploadedFiles/HIVMA/Policy_and_Advocacy/Policy_Priorities/HIV_Medical_Workforce/Resources/Ryan%20White%20Part%20C%20Survey%20IOM%209%2026%2010.pdf.

28. **Gilman SE, Cochran SD, Mays VM, et al.** Risk of psychiatric disorders among individuals reporting same-sex sexual partners in the National Comorbidity Survey. Am J Public Health. 2001;91:933-9.

29. **Blosnich J.** Suicidal ideation among sexual minority veterans: results from the 2005-2010 Massachusetts Behavioral Risk Factor Surveillance Survey. Am J Public Health. 2012;102:44-7.

30. **Centers for Disease Control and Prevention.** HIV risk, prevention, and testing behaviors among men who have sex with men—National HIV Behavioral Surveillance System, 21 U.S. cities, 2008. MMWR Morb Mortal Wkly Rep. 2011;60:1-34.

31. **King M, Semlyen J, Tai SS, et al.** A systematic review of mental disorder, suicide, and deliberate self harm in lesbian, gay and bisexual people. BMC Psychiatry. 2008;8:70.

32. **Cochran SD, Mays VM.** Physical health complaints among lesbians, gay men, and bisexual and homosexually experienced heterosexual individuals: results from the California Quality of Life Survey. Am J Public Health. 2007;97:2048-55.

33. **Patient-Centered Primary Care Collaborative.** Defining the medical home. Available at: www.pcpcc.org/about/medical-home.

34. **Gallant J, Adimora A, Carmichael J, et al.** Essential components of effective HIV care: a policy paper of the HIV Medicine Association of the Infectious Diseases Society of America and the Ryan White Medical Providers Coalition. Clin Infect Dis. 2011;53:1043-50.

35. **Kaiser Family Foundation.** Quick take: an update on the ACA & HIV: Medicaid health homes. December 2012. Available at: www.kff.org/hivaids/quicktake_mhh_hiv.cfm.

36. **Kuntz M.** Meeting the ACO challenge head on. Health Management Technology. July 2012. Available at: www.healthmgttech.com/articles/201207/meeting-the-aco-challenge-head-on.php.

37. **Crosson FJ.** The Accountable Care Organization: whatever its growing pains, the concept is too vitally important to fail. Health Affairs. 2011;30:1250-5.

38. **Lewis VA, Larson BK, McClurg AB, Boswell RG, Fisher ES.** The promise and peril of accountable care for vulnerable populations: a framework for overcoming obstacles. Health Aff. 2012; 31:1777-85.

39. **Cochran SD, Mays VM, Bowen D, et al.** Cancer-related risk indicators and preventive screening behaviors among lesbians and bisexual women. Am J Public Health. 2001;91:591.

40. **Diamant AL, Schuster MA, Lever J.** Receipt of preventive health care services by lesbians. Am J Prev Med. 2000;19:141.

41. **Gay and Lesbian Medical Association (GMLA) and LGBT Health Experts.** Healthy People 2010: a companion document for lesbian, gay, bisexual, and transgender (LGBT) health. 2001. www.glma.org/_data/n_0001/resources/live/HealthyCompanionDoc3.pdf.

42. **U.S. Department of Health and Human Services.** Affordable Care Act to improve data collection, reduce health disparities. News release. June 29, 2011. Available at: http://miamiherald.typepad.com/gaysouthflorida/2011/06/us-affordable-care-act-to-improve-lgbt-data-collection-reduce-health-disparities.html.

43. **Cahill S.** The public policy significance of data collection on sexual orientation and gender identity. August 24, 2013. Society for the Scientific Study of Sexuality Annual Symposium, San Francisco, California.

44. **The White House.** Presidential Memorandum: extension of benefits to same-sex domestic partners of federal employees. June 2, 2010. Available at: www.whitehouse.gov/the-press-office/presidential-memorandum-extension-benefits-same-sex-domestic-partners-federal-emplo.

45. **The White House.** Presidential Memorandum: Hospital visitation. April 15, 2010. Available at: www.whitehouse.gov/the-press-office/presidential-memorandum-hospital-visitation.

46. **U.S. Department of Health and Human Services.** Medicare finalizes new rules to require equal visitation rights for all hospital patients. Press Release. November 17, 2010. Available at: www.businesswire.com/news/home/20101117006577/en/Medicare-Finalizes-Rules-Require-Equal-Visitation-Rights#.U_vixPldX-E.

47. **Centers for Medicare & Medicaid Services.** Medicare steps up enforcement of equal visitation and representation rights in hospitals. Press Release. September 8, 2011. Available at: www.cms.gov/Newsroom/MediaReleaseDatabase/Press-Releases/2011-Press-Releases-Items/2011-09-08.html.

48. **Centers for Medicare & Medicaid Services.** Reminder: access and visitation rights in long term care (LTC) facilities. Ref: S&C: 13-42-NH. June 28, 2013. Available at: www.cms.gov/Medicare/Provider-Enrollment-and-Certification/SurveyCertificationGenInfo/Downloads/Survey-and-Cert-Letter-13-42.pdf.

49. **U.S. Department of Health and Human Services.** Office of Minority Health. Think cultural health. Available at: https://www.thinkculturalhealth.hhs.gov/Content/clas.asp.

50. **Baker K.** New health services standards ensure respect for LGBT patients. ThinkProgress. April 24, 2013. Available at: http://thinkprogress.org/lgbt/2013/04/24/1916631/new-health-services-standards-ensure-respect-for-lgbt-patients/?mobile=nc.

51. **Negotiated Rulemaking Committee on the Designation of Medically Underserved Populations and Health Professional Shortage Areas.** Final Report to the Secretary. October 31, 2011.

52. The case for designating LGBT people as a medically underserved population and as a health professional shortage area population group. Boston: The Fenway Institute, the Center for American Progress, Human Rights Campaign, GLMA. August 2014. Available at: http://thefenwayinstitute.org/wp-content/uploads/MUP_HPSA-Brief_v11-FINAL-081914.pdf.

53. **Makadon HJ.** Ending LGBT invisibility in health care: the first step in ensuring equitable care. Cleve Clin J Med. 2011;78:220-4.

54. **Klitzman RL, Greenberg JD.** Patterns of communication between gay and lesbian patients and their health care providers. J Homosex. 2002;42:65-75.

55. **Berstein KT, Liu KL, Begier EM, et al.** Same-sex attraction disclosure to health care providers among New York City men who have sex with men. Arch Intern Med. 2008;168: 1458-64.

56. **Institute of Medicine.** Collecting Sexual Orientation and Gender Identity Data in Electronic Health Records: Workshop Summary. Washington, DC: The National Academies Press; 2013.

57. **Cahill S, Makadon H.** Sexual orientation and gender identity data collection update: U.S. government takes steps to promote sexual orientation and gender identity data collection through meaningful use guidelines. LGBT Health. 2014:1-4.

58. **U.S. Federal Register.** Notice of Proposed Rule Making, RIN 0991-AB92. The Voluntary 2015 Edition Electronic Health Record Certification Criteria; Interoperability Updates and Regulatory Improvements. March 19, 2014. Available at: https://www.federalregister.gov/articles/2014/03/19/2014-06041/voluntary-2015-edition-electronic-health-record-ehr-certification-criteria-interoperability-updates.

59. **U.S. Department of Veterans Affairs.** The state of care for veterans with HIV/AIDS. 2009. Available at: www.hiv.va.gov/provider/policy/state-of-care/veterans.asp.

60. **Blosnich JR, Bossarte RM, Silenzio VM.** Improved health care for sexual minority and transgender veterans; Blosnich et al. respond. Am J Public Health. 2012;102:E10-E11.

61. **U.S. Department of Veterans Affairs.** Providing health care for transgender and intersex veterans. February 8, 2013. Available at: www.va.gov/vhapublications/ViewPublication.asp?pub_ID=2863.

62. **U.S. Department of Veterans Affairs.** Guidance regarding the provision of health care for lesbian, gay and bisexual veterans. July 1, 2014. Available at: http://www1.va.gov/VHAPUBLICAtIONs/ViewPublication.asp?pub_ID=3013

63. **U.S. Department of Justice.** Attorney General Holder announces move to extend veterans benefits to same-sex married couples. Press Release. September 4, 2013. Available at: www.justice.gov/opa/pr/2013/September/13-ag-991.html.

64. **The Fenway Institute.** Public comment re: Proposed amendments to regulations found at 130 CMR 415.000, 130 CMR 410.000, 130 CMR 405.000, 130 CMR 423.000, 130 CMR 406.000, 130 CMR 433.000, and 130 CMR 424.000 to allow coverage for treatment of gender dysphoria, including gender reassignment surgeries and hormone therapies. October 28, 2014. Available at: http://thefenwayinstitute.org/wp-content/uploads/Fenway-Health-MA-Medicaid-Gender-Dysphoria-Comment-Oct-28-2014.pdf.

65. **GLMA.** Compendium of Health Profession Association LGBT Policy & Position Statements. Updated 2013. Available at: http://glma.org/index.cfm?fuseaction=Page.viewPage&pageId=1037&parentID=568&nodeID=1.

66. **The Joint Commission.** Advancing effective communication, cultural competence, and patient- and family-centered care: a roadmap for hospitals. Joint Commission Resources. 2011. Available at: www.jointcommission.org/assets/1/6/ARoadmapforHospitalsfinalversion727.pdf.

67. **The Joint Commission.** Advancing effective communication, cultural competence, and patient- and family-centered care for the lesbian, gay, bisexual, and transgender (LGBT) community: a field guide. Joint Commission Resources. 2011. Available at: www.jointcommission.org/assets/1/18/LGBTFieldGuide.pdf.

68. **Meyer IH.** Prejudice, social stress, and mental health in lesbian, gay, and bisexual populations: conceptual issues and research evidence. Psychol Bull. 2003;129:674-97.

69. **Gay and Lesbian Medical Association Marriage Equality Initiative.** Same-Sex Marriage and Health. GLMA, September 2008. Available at: www.lgbthealthinitiative.com/pdf/Same-Sex_Marriage_and_Health.GLMA.08%5B1%5D.pdf.

70. **U.S. General Accounting Office.** GAO-04-353R. Defense of Marriage Act: Update to Prior Report. 2004. Available at: www.gao.gov/products/GAO-04-353R.

71. **Human Rights Campaign.** Domestic partner benefits: grossing up to offset imputed income tax. Available at: www.hrc.org/resources/entry/domestic-partner-benefits-grossing-up-to-offset-imputed-income-tax.

72. **Buffie WC.** Public health implications of same-sex marriage. Am J Public Health. 2011;101:986-90.

73. **Gates GJ.** Research. LGBT parenting in the United States. The Williams Institute. February 2013. Available at: http://williamsinstitute.law.ucla.edu/wp-content/uploads/LGBT-Parenting.pdf.

74. **Lambda Legal.** Cases. *Flanigan v. University of Maryland Hospital System.* Available at: www.lambdalegal.org/in-court/cases/flanigan-v-university-of-maryland.

75. **Burns C, Baker K.** Despite 20 years of progress, Family and Medical Leave Act fails to protect gay and transgender families. Center for American Progress. 2013. Available at: www.americanprogress.org/issues/labor/news/2013/02/05/51781/despite-20-years-of-progress-family-and-medical-leave-act-fails-to-protect-gay-and-transgender-families/.

76. **Family Equality Council.** Equality Maps. State medical leave laws. Available at: www.familyequality.org/get_informed/equality_maps/state_medical_leave_laws/.

77. **U.S. Department of Labor.** Family and Medical Leave Act. Notice of Proposed Rulemaking to revise the definition of "spouse" under the FMLA. Available at: www.dol.gov/whd/fmla/nprm-spouse/.

Chapter 20

LGBT Health: Global Perspectives and Experiences

STEFAN BARAL, Msc, MD, MPH, MBA
ERIN PAPWORTH, MPH
CARMEN LOGIE, MSW, PhD
CHRIS BEYRER, MD, MPH

Introduction

Diverse sexual and gender minorities live in every human society and country. They are welcomed in some settings and forcibly penalized in others. All over the world they are finding their voices and are organizing–sometimes in the face of intense and brutal repression–for the rights and benefits to full participation in their societies. This includes, at a minimum, acknowledgment of their basic human rights, as well as inclusion in education, health care, and other government services, to participation in political life. A striking feature of this global movement is that it has emerged in the context of the HIV and AIDS pandemic and has been shaped and supported by HIV activism and engagement. Nevertheless, the needs of lesbian, gay, bisexual, and transgender (LGBT) populations are much broader than HIV or other aspects of sexual health, and they embrace the full range of human health needs.

Conceptualizations of sexuality and gender are continually evolving and differ greatly across cultures and countries, thus making it difficult to develop both standardized portraits of reality and visions for change. These issues are particularly relevant when exploring the needs of transgender people. Transgender people exist on every continent and are increasingly organizing for rights and recognition (1). Nevertheless, gender presentations and local cultural understandings vary around the world, and many different terms are used to describe individuals who live between or outside a male–female gender binary (2–4). Transgender identity in the developed world, notably the United States, is only starting to become a topic for mainstream dialogue (5). Globally, certain countries around the world have historical narratives and figures that represent diverse gender identities, such as in Thailand (6). However, the general knowledge of transgender people and their health needs is negligible worldwide.

Detailed knowledge regarding the health status and needs of all LGBT communities globally is just starting to emerge. The United States and other high-income countries, such as Canada, Sweden, and Norway, have set a precedent for research and health programming for LGBT communities over the past few decades; however, health disparities continue to be found among these populations, and few countries have systematically incorporated LGBT health into national programming, research, and policy (7,8).

In low- and middle-income countries, LGBT persons have been described as neglected and under-represented within health research, policy, and program development (9). The best data are arguably from the literature on HIV and sexually transmitted infections (STIs), a function of the tremendous research activity in this domain of global health; however, such data provide only a snapshot of the overall health status of LGBT people worldwide. The data that do exist consistently demonstrate limited access to essential services for LGBT populations, caused by entrenched societal and systemic discrimination in these settings. Around the world, 76 countries criminalize same-sex practices. The penalties range from $300 (USD) fines and incarceration to death. Aside from violating international human rights norms of universality and nondiscrimination, these laws and institutionalized policies adversely affect the health of marginalized sexual minorities (10–13). In most contexts, such penal codes were inherited; nevertheless, over time, countries have embraced these laws or complacently allowed them to exist, and government policies have evolved to accommodate integrated cultural and political intolerance of same-sex practices in the organizational structure of health care services. Even in recent years, some sub-Saharan African countries have seen new laws introduced to enact the death penalty for some same-sex practices and lengthy prison terms for others.

Lack of funding for sexual and gender minority issues also contributes to the shortage of research conducted among LGBT populations in low- and middle-income countries (14). Yet it is critical to examine LGBT health in these countries: "The combination of social marginality and large-scale structural inequality often leads to particularly acute manifestations of structural violence among marginalized genders and sexualities in the developing world, and the disadvantaged position of LGBTQs is a crucial factor—perhaps the most crucial factor—in shaping LGBT health outcomes" (15).

Research shows that large-scale structural inequality in developing countries has devastating effects on the lives of those most vulnerable, such as sexual and gender minorities (16,17). Structural factors refer to social, economic, organizational, and political issues that contribute to inequality, such as criminalization of homosexuality, sex work, and substance use (18). Exacerbated by conditions of poverty and underdevelopment, structural inequality in low- and middle-income countries often leads to further constraints—such as dependence on family/kin networks, lack of housing, low access to education, and high unemployment—and heightened marginalization of sexual and gender minorities (19). Understanding the root causes of health disparities can guide the development of health promotion initiatives (20). A reduction of stigma, better access to health service and provision of appropriate health services around the world for LGBT will occur only with a commitment to do the research and educate professionals on how to implement change in both public health and clinical practice.

Stigma, Discrimination, and Health Outcomes Among LGBT People Globally

When discussing health outcomes for LGBT people, particularly in low- and middle-income countries, perceived and experienced stigma and discrimination must be discussed as contributing factors to the overall health of these communities. Sexual stigma refers to devaluing sexual minorities and the negative attitudes and lower status afforded to same-sex behaviors, identities, relationships, and communities (21). Sexual stigma is embedded within power relations and may result in multiple levels of social and institutional discrimination towards sexual minorities (16). The complexity of defining, understanding, and measuring stigma in part stems from its interaction with cross-cultural differences, structural inequalities, discrimination by health care professionals, and social processes that are not always integrated into stigma research focusing on the individual (11,22–24). Stigma may be particularly detrimental to the well-being of LGBT persons in low- and middle-income countries, affecting both the ability to attend school (as reported by Wade and colleagues [25]) and to obtain employment: "The structures of gender inequality are typically replicated through the stigmatization of particularly effeminate homosexual men and transgendered persons, who often have few employment options outside of sex work and who frequently are subjected to socially sanctioned physical violence" (26).

Relationships with family members may significantly contribute to health outcomes in cross-cultural contexts; experiencing rejection or abuse from family members due to sexual orientation may be therefore detrimental to health outcomes (25). Social inequities contribute to increased morbidity and mortality among LGBT persons (25,27). As discussed in other chapters of this book, a range of clinical health issues disproportionately affect LGBT persons in the United States and other high-income countries, including increased risk for STIs, HIV infection, depression, substance use (including tobacco use), human papillomavirus infection, suicidal ideation, anxiety, and body image concerns (28–33). However, much less is known about increased morbidity among LGBT persons in low- and middle-income countries.

Chronic stress resulting from stigma and discrimination contributes to these health disparities (30,34,35). Understanding risk factors for depression and other behavioral health disorders is key to decreasing global behavioral health morbidity (36,37). A recent articulation of grand challenges in global mental health highlighted the identification of modifiable social risk factors as a chief priority (20).

Meyer's minority stress model (30,38) outlines multiple stressors in the lives of sexual minorities: internalized homophobia, in which negative social attitudes contribute to shame and reduced self-worth; perceived stigma, referring to fear and expectations of rejection; and discrimination, including violence. Internalized homophobia has been associated with increased relationship problems (39) and depression (40) among sexual minorities. The minority stress model was tested for applicability with men who have sex with men (MSM) in South India, where stigma and discrimination significantly predicted higher rates of depression (35). Information on stigma and mental health outcomes among LGBT populations in developing countries remains scarce (41). Thus, our knowledge of LGBT health psychology "does not reflect the plurality and complexity of sexual cultures outside the developed world" (42).

Sexual and physical violence targeting sexual and gender minorities is a global phenomenon (35,43–46). Higher risk for onset of post-traumatic stress disorder among LGB people compared to heterosexuals in a national United States study ($n = 34,653$) was in part attributed to LGB people's greater exposure to interpersonal violence (47). LGBT persons in low- and middle-income countries experience multiple types of violence (e.g., physical, sexual), at times systematically perpetrated by government (25), family, and community. Intimate partner violence among same-sex partners has been explored in North America, but there are gaps in low- and middle-income countries (25). A study in Brazil reported intimate partner violence between women in same-sex relationships (48). Discrimination by authorities may contribute to underreporting of intimate partner violence among sexual and gender minorities in low- and middle-income countries (15,49,50).

Stigma and Discrimination in Health Care Settings in Low- and Middle-Income Countries

Discrimination by health care providers toward LGBT persons has been reported across low- and middle-income countries. This discrimination appears to be associated with sexual orientation, gender identity, and perceived HIV serostatus. Researchers have highlighted sexual stigma, as well as misconceptions and biases, among health professionals in India (51–53), leading mental health practitioners to call for further research to enhance understanding of the mental health needs of sexual minorities in India (51,52) in order to adequately meet their needs. In a survey in 2004, out of 627 Chinese medical students, one quarter believed homosexuality was a psychiatric disorder that required therapy (54). Forty percent of these respondents thought homosexual residents would negatively affect the reputation of their medical school (54). If attitudes such as these exist in middle-income countries, it is easy to extrapolate that in lower-income countries, where the majority of penal laws inhibiting sex-same practices exist, these sentiments not only occur but are significantly more prominent in the medical profession.

Reseachers have found an association with perceived or enacted stigma and decreased attendance at health clinics, return for follow-up treatment if needed, and an overall avoidance of medical services by LGBT (55,56). While a breach in confidentiality is often a concern cited by LGBT people, intense stigma reported when accessing services cannot be ignored. LGBT people throughout low- and middle-income countries recount negative experiences in health settings that include hearing clinic personnel discussing their sexual orientation, receiving insults and aggressive behaviors from health providers, and being subjected to attempts to convert them into religious activity with the assumption this would change their sexual behaviors (55).

In China, homophobia within community and social norms, and HIV-related stigma within MSM communities, act as barriers to MSM participating in HIV prevention programs (57). Discrimination by health care providers was highlighted as a key barrier to accessing health/HIV care among MSM in several countries, including Brazil, India, and Peru (58–67). In South Africa, internalized homophobia has been associated with reduced HIV knowledge among MSM (68). A survey from the Joint United Nations (U.N.) Programme on HIV/AIDS (UNAIDS) survey of HIV-related stigma among people living with HIV in 9 countries and Asia and the Pacific, including gay/bisexual men, revealed widespread stigma, discrimination, and human rights violations and low rates of post-test counseling (69). Another study with MSM in India revealed that HIV-related stigma among MSM outreach workers was so high many refused to get an HIV test because they would rather die than know they were HIV positive (70). HIV-related stigma research in the Caribbean region has also highlighted the connections between HIV-related stigma and homophobia (67,71–73). Paxton and colleagues' review of HIV-related stigma in several countries (India, Indonesia, Thailand, and the Philippines) underscored the salience of addressing HIV-related stigma among health care providers across these diverse contexts (74).

In sub-Saharan Africa, fear of discrimination, stigma, and blackmail impede access to HIV prevention, treatment, and care among MSM (11,56,75), and stigma and discrimination associated with sexuality and HIV are exacerbated among HIV-positive MSM (56,76). In a study with MSM communities conducted in Malawi, Bostwana, and Zambia, a strong association was found between ever experiencing discrimination, including denial of health care services and blackmail based on sexuality, and fear of health care in general (56). In another study from South Africa, community members reported that verbal abuse from health care workers negatively influenced appropriate use of health care services, including adherence to visits and follow-up (77). Concurrently, Fay and colleagues found that previous diagnosis and treatment of STIs in a clinic setting for MSM were associated with a greater odds of reporting fear of seeking health care and being denied health services on the basis of sexuality (56). In Kenya, stigma surrounding HIV, homosexuality, and gender nonconformity contributed to reduced HIV knowledge and HIV testing and limited access to medical and HIV services (78–80). In Senegal, MSM reported sexual stigma, discrimination, and homophobia in larger society (13,81,82); discriminatory and incompetent care by health care providers has also been reported there (83,84). Poteat and colleagues reported that criminalization reduces access to HIV prevention and exacerbates stigma among MSM in Senegal (13). Similar results have been observed in North Africa and the Middle East, where HIV-related stigma, combined with sexual stigma and homophobia, reduce access to HIV prevention services among sexual minorities (85–87). Sadly, these trends have also been observed throughout Central and South America as well (58,59,88).

Through the HIV Lens: LGBT in Low- and Middle-Income Countries Within the Context of the Epidemic

The global response to HIV provides a framework for understanding the relationship between the limited epidemiologic data and health resources available to LGBT people in low- and middle-income countries. Epidemiologic surveillance of HIV among LGBT people in low- and middle-income countries suffers in response to conditions of criminalization, repression, and social stigma often found in these countries. In low- and middle-income countries, most data on HIV are collected through demographic and health surveys. These surveys are household-based studies designed to collect nationally representative data focused on 4 core areas: reproductive health, communicable diseases, nutrition, and HIV/AIDS. The results of these surveys provide the foundation for health policy and particularly the national strategic response to the HIV epidemic in the country. Since 1984, over 250 surveys including HIV testing have been conducted in more than 30 countries (www.measureDHS.com). Demographic and health surveys measure several risk factors for HIV but generally have not assessed same-sex practices, and they have rarely been used to conduct meaningful assessments of sex work or substance use outside of alcohol use. Because same-sex practices, sex work, and drug use are the primary risk factors for the acquisition and transmission of HIV in much of the world, the omission of these practices has probably resulted in risk misclassification and, more generally, a limited understanding of the actual drivers of the HIV epidemic across many low- and middle-income countries. This brings into question the common characterization of HIV in certain regions, such as sub-Saharan Africa, as being predominately in heterosexual populations.

As a result, the HIV prevalence among LGBT people is often unavailable. The few studies that do target LGBT people are often small samples of urban populations. Therefore, comparing the HIV prevalence among LGBT persons with that in the general population leads to inherently conservative estimates of disease burden. HIV prevalence provided for the general population is typically age-standardized to model the average prevalence of HIV among those age 15 to 49 years. However, most LGBT people typically sampled are younger than age 30. When HIV prevalence is assessed among those age 30 and older, it tends to be significantly higher among LGBT people than among all reproductive-age adults, even in very widespread HIV epidemics (55). Moreover, highly stigmatized settings, found in a large percentage of low- and middle-income countries, limit the collection of high-quality data as well as participation in these studies, biasing sampling in ways that increase uncertainty. The inability to secure significant research support and the fear of personal adverse events in response to mainstream entities supporting LGBT studies have been major additional barriers to understanding the burden of HIV in these populations. When studies have been launched, many LGBT people avoid participating in fear of their sexual practices or orientation being exposed. This is especially true among LGBT people older than age 30, thus limiting our understanding of the actual burden of disease across the life course.

Taken together, it appears that epidemiologic data in low- and middle-income countries gravely misrepresent the health realities of LGBT people, particularly in the context of HIV risk. Available evidence from these countries suggests that structural factors—social, economic, political, or legal factors—in addition to individual-level risk factors are likely to play important roles in shaping infectious disease risks, as well as treatment and care options for LGBT populations (18).

Although data are sparse, some important information has begun to emerge regarding barriers to health care for gay men and other MSM within the context of HIV prevention globally; however, there continues to be an immense deficiency of data on lesbians, other women who have sex with women (WSW), and transgender persons in low- and middle-income countries. Where possible, this chapter draws from known studies and examples in low- and middle-income countries as to the health status of these populations. While couched in the global response to HIV, these studies provide a baseline understanding of the social reality of LGBT in low- and middle-income countries. Where there is a lack of epidemiologic examples, data from high-income countries are used and extrapolated to assume reality in low- and middle-income countries.

Burden of HIV and Other Sexually Transmitted Infections among LGBT

Men Who Have Sex With Men

In the public health construct, *MSM* has become the term used to define sexual behaviors in which male-to-male sex occurs; this approach moves away from identity-based categorization of persons (e.g., gay, bisexual) toward a focus on sexual practices to account for the complexity of sexuality as well as cross-cultural differences in conceptualizing sexuality. As explained in the USAID Measure Evaluation guideline, perhaps the most important nuance of this public health definition is the inclusion of men who self-identify as heterosexuals but who engage in sex with other men for various reasons (e.g., sexual attraction, isolation, economic compensation, gender scripts, incarceration), along with men who share a nonheterosexual identity (i.e., gay, homosexual, bisexual, or other culture-specific concepts that equate with attraction to other men) (89). This inclusion is important at the individual risk level because recognizing the biological and behavioral practices that facilitate increased risk for disease is an essential step in creating effective prevention programs to reduce risk.

In low- and middle-income country settings, the limited data available suggest that MSM have nearly 20 times higher odds of living with HIV than other reproductive-age adults (90). In high-income settings, this ratio is far higher given the limited background epidemics seen in many high-income settings. Results from a systematic review indicated that MSM in countries with very low HIV prevalence have 58.4 times higher odds for HIV infection compared with the general population (90). The odds were 14.4 in countries with low HIV prevalence and 9.6 in medium-high prevalence settings (10).

A systematic review in 2012 showed aggregated HIV prevalence estimates per regions of the world, with pooled HIV prevalence among MSM ranging from 3.0% (95% CI, 2.4% to 3.6%) in the Middle East and North Africa region (where general population rates are reported as roughly 0.09%) (91), to 25.4% (95% CI, 21.4% to 29.5%) in the Caribbean region (compared with roughly 1.5% in the adult population) (91). Specific studies in sub-Saharan Africa have reiterated this disproportionate burden of HIV in MSM. For example, in 2 studies in Senegal in 2004 and 2007 conducted in 4 urban settings, prevalence in MSM was 21.5% (95% CI, 18% to 25%) and 21.8% (95% CI, 18% to 25%), respectively, compared with the UNAIDS estimates of 0.7% prevalence in the adult male population (>15 years of age) in 2007 (25). In 2008 in the 2 main cities of Malawi, Blantyre and Lilongwe, a research team found a 21.4% (95% CI, 16% to 28%) HIV prevalence in MSM in contrast to UNAIDS 2007 adult male estimates of 9.6% (55).

The disproportionate burden of HIV in MSM populations displays the inadequacy of public policies worldwide to actively promote care, treatment, and prevention for MSM (91,92). Less than 10% of MSM globally have access to services for HIV prevention, treatment, and care (93). The Foundation for AIDS Research (14) special report "MSM, HIV, and the Road to Universal Access—How Far Have We Come?" described the lack of leadership in the response to HIV among MSM globally as "an epidemic of denial, indifference and inaction."

Transgender Women

Transgender women have elevated risks for HIV and STIs (94). A 2012 meta-analysis of data from 15 mostly middle- or high-income countries found the pooled global HIV prevalence for transgender women was 19.1% (95% CI, 17.4% to 20.7%) and the odds ratio for HIV infection in transgender women compared with all adults of reproductive age was 48.8 (95% CI, 21.2 to 76.3) (95) (Table 20-1). The authors subsequently deconstructed these data to show rates of 17.7% (95% CI, 15.6% to 19.8%) in low- and middle-income countries and 21.6% (95% CI, 18.8% to 24.3%) in high-income countries (95). The authors noted that constraints in this review included a dearth of data throughout the world; in addition, studies available were mainly from countries where the HIV epidemic was concentrated in the male population, while the pooled results masked the wide geographic variations within diverse countries such as India or Brazil (95). Nevertheless, the results indicate that transgender women have a substantially high risk for HIV infection compared with other adults of reproductive age in both high- and low-income countries for which data were available. The authors also noted that there are effectively no data from countries with generalized epidemics and that the reality of the burden of disease for this population in those contexts is completely unknown. Another systematic review indicated that transgender women who were sex workers had significantly higher HIV infection risks in comparison with transgender women not involved in sex work, male sex workers, and nontransgender sex workers (96).

The risk factors associated with transgender people remain understudied; however, there is evidence that biological risk factors are closely associated with the birth sex (rather than gender identity) of the person (95). Transgender women, for instance, share some biological risk factors with MSM, and the rare data that do exist for transgender people mainly include transgender women studied as a subpopulation of MSM.

Transgender women's exacerbated vulnerability to HIV has been attributed to social and systemic factors, such as widespread violence; discrimination; and inadequate access to housing, employment, education, and health care (97–99). These factors, combined with low social support, are associated with transgender women's involvement in survival sex work in the United States. Clearly, inclusion of transgender women is needed in both medical training and epidemiologic research worldwide (100). Few health care providers receive education and training on the health needs of transgender people. While medical provider attitudes and knowledge have improved over time, bias and lack of knowledge persist (101). Provider attitudes toward transgender people are barriers to care and limit access to early testing and treatment for HIV (102–104). Lack of access to legitimate medical sources for transition-related care leads many transgender women to use and share syringes for illicit hormone and silicone injections, which may increase risk for HIV (104).

Women Who Have Sex With Women

The epidemiology of HIV offers further examples of insufficient and/or inequitable public policies globally for WSW (105). The term *WSW* attempts to

Table 20-1   Meta-Analyses of Aggregate Country Data Comparing HIV Prevalence Among Transgender Women and All Reproductive-Age Adults in Countries With Data on HIV Prevalence in Transgender Women, 2000–2011

Country	Sample Size	HIV Prevalence Among Transgender Women (95% CI), %	Odds Ratio (95% CI)	HIV Prevalence Among Reproductive-Age Adults, %	HIV Prevalence Among Reproductive-Age Males, %	Percentage of Total HIV Infections That Are Among Men, %	Income Level	References
Argentina	931	33.5 (28.3–38.8)	92.4 (80.6–105.8)	0.54	0.73	67.3	M	164–167
Brazil	638	33.1 (26.7–39.4)	85.3 (72.3–100.6)	0.58	0.68	59.2	M	168–170
El Salvador	67	19.4 (0.0–40.9)	23.2 (12.7–42.5)	1.03	1.42	65.6	M	171
Peru	450	28.9 (21.1–36.7)	84.7 (69.1–103.9)	0.48	0.73	75.3	M	172
Uruguay	260	18.8 (7.9–29.8)	38.3 (28.1–52.3)	0.60	0.82	67.7	M	173,174
Australia	133	4.5 (0.0–21.1)	24.9 (11.0–56.5)	0.19	0.26	69.0	H	175
India	135	43.7 (31.0–56.4)	208.0 (148.0–292.3)	0.37	0.44	61.7	M	176,177
Indonesia	1384	26.1 (21.6–30.6)	180.3 (159.9–203.3)	0.20	0.32	70.7	M	178–180
Pakistan	2643	2.2 (0.0–6.0)	21.9 (16.9–28.4)	0.10	0.14	70.5	M	85,181–183
Thailand	614	12.5 (5.1–19.9)	9.9 (7.8–12.6)	1.43	1.71	59.6	M	184,185
Vietnam	75	6.7 (0.0–28.5)	15.6 (6.3–38.8)	0.45	0.73	70.0	M	186
Italy	826	24.5 (18.5–30.4)	65.8 (56.1–77.1)	0.49	0.65	65.7	H	187,188
Netherlands	69	18.8 (0.0–40.1)	81.8 (44.7–149.5)	0.28	0.39	68.6	H	189
Spain	136	18.4 (3.2–33.6)	40.9 (26.5–63.1)	0.55	0.81	75.4	H	190,191
United States	2705	21.7 (18.4–25.1)	34.2 (31.2–37.5)	0.81	1.18	74.2	H	97,192–199
Pooled estimate*	11066	19.1 (17.4–20.7)	48.8 (31.2–76.3)	0.44	0.58	—	—	—

H = high income; M = middle income. Table reprinted from *Lancet Infectious Diseases*, 13(3), Baral SD, Poteat T, Stromdahl S, Wirtz AL, Guadamuz TE, Beyrer C, Worldwide burden of HIV in transgender women: a systematic review and meta-analysis, pp. 214–22, Copyright 2013 with permission from Elsevier.

*Degrees of freedom = 14, heterogeneity chi-square = 914.7, I^2 = 98.5%, test of odds ratio = 1, z = 16.21, P = 0.0001.

include women who do not self-identify as lesbians, homosexual, bisexual, or other culture-specific concepts that equate with attraction to other women. In Africa, WSW in some settings have been targets of sexual violence, which have led to considerable HIV risks for these women (106,107). The litany of examples of reported rights violations of WSW in South Africa includes the death of Zoliswa Nkonyana after being stoned, beaten, and stabbed in February 2006 for being a lesbian. Before this, a 22-year-old WSW was raped in Soweto in 2004, the same month as another teenage lesbian was raped in Mohlakeng (108). An ActionAID report highlighted that there are currently as many as 10 new cases of "corrective rape" (the criminal practice of raping a lesbian in order to "cure" her of her sexual orientation) per week and that the rate is rising in South Africa (109). Women most vulnerable to sexual assault in South Africa often live in poor, black communities with a burden of high HIV infection (76,110). In a country where general HIV prevalence is reported to be 17.30% (95% CI, 16.60% to 18.10%) for the adult population, sexual violence exacerbates the risk of HIV transmission for WSW in this context (111).

In a study in Lesotho conducted in 2010, Johns Hopkins University researchers found that rights violations among WSW were common, with the majority of women reporting at least 1 abuse (11). While study participants reported that care was denied less often among MSM in other southern African countries, fear of seeking health care services and gossiping among health care workers were commonly reported. Blackmail was a very common threat to these women and notably was highly associated with having disclosed their sexual orientation to a health care worker. Less than 1 in 10 women reported having been raped, and most knew their rapist; only 1 of these rapists had used a condom during forced intercourse. Approximately a third of women who reported being raped felt that they were targeted because they were lesbian. Given the high risk for HIV acquisition associated with rape, this is both a significant human rights violation and public health issue. While same-sex practices are legal in South Africa, the passivity of police and justice systems in the persecution and arrest of sexual violence cases, for both WSW and women in general, shows inept public policy and political will to protect these vulnerable populations.

WSW have been described as neglected and understudied in HIV/STI research (112-114)—overshadowed by the focus on MSM (115). Reports in the medical literature have noted that because of the lack of penetrating sexual practices among WSW, this subgroup was less at risk for exposure to HIV and other STIs. However, research conducted primarily in the United States has shown a complex array of various risks among WSW, including sex with men (most self-identified lesbian women reported 1 or more lifetime male sex partners) (116), sex work, injection drug use, and/or experience of sexual violence (117-119). For instance, studies report higher HIV incidence among WSW injection drug users in comparison with other female injection drug users, in part due to social isolation, poverty, higher-risk injection practices, and sexual risk behavior (120–122). In addition, research suggests sexual minority women may not engage in routine gynecologic appointments (123,124) or HIV/STI testing (117).

Ample evidence indicates sexual transmission of STI between women, including trichomoniasis, human papillomavirus, bacterial vaginosis, herpes, and hepatitis B (117,118,120,121,123,125). Researchers have in fact described similar STI prevalence among sexual minority and heterosexual women (114,121). In a study in Brazil ($n = 145$), almost half of WSW did not use condoms when sharing sex toys. While the risk for STI transmission cannot equate to the risk seen in male-to-male or male-to-female sex, further research is needed to understand the risk associated with same-sex female practices (123). Work with WSW in Toronto, Canada, revealed associations between sexual stigma and HIV/STI risk (17). This implies that a lack of training for clinicians on the health needs of WSW may create barriers to appropriate health service access.

LGBT Health in Low- and Middle-Income Countries: The Modified Social Ecological Model Framework

As discussed thus far, structural drivers of negative health outcomes among LGBT people include social, political, and economic factors that contribute to social inequities, such as stigma (126–130). These structural drivers do not directly cause disease; rather, they contextualize individual behavioral risks. For example, as stated in Beyrer (91) and Baral (131) and colleagues, emerging data suggest that sexual behavior cannot fully elucidate high-transmission dynamics within MSM HIV outbreaks, particularly in the era of highly active antiretroviral therapy distribution and accessibility. Other factors, including biological, couple, network-level, community, and policy-level drivers, are essential to understanding how HIV transmission rates remain high in this subpopulation (91).

To better understand individual risks that emerge from structural factors, researchers have developed a Modified Social Ecological Model (MSEM). This model (Figure 20-1) attempts to depict the complex nature of HIV risk among LGBT people through a multidimensional framework that includes policy, community, network, and individual levels of influence on health (129). Although specific to HIV, this model could potentially be applied to other LGBT health outcomes. In addition, the model is not specific to any setting, but the higher levels of discrimination found in low- and middle-income countries on the policy and community levels potentially exacerbate individual risk.

At the public policy level, which includes national laws and state health strategies, the MSEM asserts that policies regulating the health sector have a direct effect on access to appropriate health services for all citizens. At the community level, norms and values that stigmatize same-sex behavior and

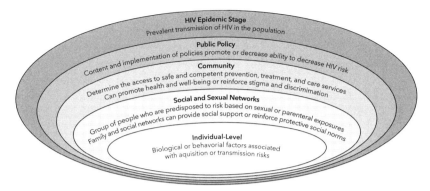

Figure 20-1 Modified social ecological model for HIV risk in vulnerable populations.

gender nonconformity can affect LGBT knowledge of, and delivery and access to, appropriate treatments for HIV and other STIs (7,13,23,35,90, 130–133). For example, fear of discrimination within HIV services can limit knowledge of unprotected anal intercourse risks and access to prevention methods. Large sexual networks have also been shown to be an important risk factor for HIV among MSM, especially in the context of rapid transmission related to acute HIV infections affecting even single members of those sexual networks. Similarly, limited engagement in the continuum of HIV care among LGBT people secondary to lack of targeted programs and stigma results in likely high mean and total community viral load and, in turn, higher risk for HIV acquisition and transmission among members of the network. Social networks are also important, often through enhanced social capital linked to increased health literacy and safer sexual practices among LGBT people (10,25). At the core of the MSEM, individual factors are fundamental to HIV/STI acquisition and transmission, including condom use, number of sexual partners, and genital ulcerative diseases (13,129). HIV, while a bloodborne virus, is more closely linked to social and structural contexts than other infectious diseases given the longstanding ability to prevent the acquisition and transmission of the virus. The different levels of risk factors are significantly interlinked, highlighting the importance of assessing contexts of individual-level risk factors if there is a plan to address those risk factors. Information on individual- and network-level risk for HIV are covered in detail in Chapters 13 and 14. Furthermore, the following sections detail the macro-level structural factors that facilitate individual risk for LGBT persons in low- and middle-income countries.

Public Policy and LGBT Health in Low- and Middle-Income Countries

Public health policies provide the framework for health delivery in any given country (134). These policies dictate what type of health services are subsidized at the national level, what health priorities receive concentrated funding and, in principle, ensure that quality of service delivery meets standards set out by the state. From the perspective of sexual and gender minorities, these policies also either promote or decrease society's ability to provide appropriate services, such as preventive or harm reduction programs (e.g., relevant messaging and condom and lubricant provision) by passing laws that make such activity legal or illegal, or by providing or disrupting funding mechanisms supporting these programs (135–137).

Inadequate legal policies have historically inhibited the delivery of best health practices for groups around the world (138). There are numerous examples of laws—including criminalization of sex work and substance use, or criminalization of prevention practices, such as needle exchange—founded in morals, cultural relativism, and politics rather than in the results of public health science. In such contexts, marginalized populations such as sex workers, people who inject drugs, and LGBT persons have a higher baseline risk for acquiring infectious diseases because of the lack of scientifically proven targeted prevention and harm reduction strategies (138).

The limitations in health policy for LGBT persons around the world materialize in intricate ways and are not restricted to criminalized settings. Countries where same-sex practices are not illegal but lack coherent and evidenced-based policies to promote LGBT health and human rights also limit the health sector's ability to provide necessary focused prevention and treatment services for LGBT people (137). National policies dictate national medical curricula for health care providers, including clinicians and clinical support staff. Often, curricula do not address sexual or gender minorities, as these populations are automatically excluded by virtue of the illegal or ignored status of their sexual practices. Even when access to health care is present, health care providers are not trained in the health needs of sexual and gender minorities populations, which facilitates inadequacy in clinical services and ultimately reluctance to seeking health care by those in need (56,139). This is true in all countries but is especially difficult in low-income countries, where clinical care is often provided by perimedical practitioners (e.g., nurses and midwives) because of a lack of trained physicians and clinical providers (140).

In some contexts, public policies go so far as to actively obstruct health professionals in providing services to sexual minorities and to prosecute providers who are found or accused of doing so. In December 2008 in Senegal, 9 community health workers providing HIV prevention information and condoms were detained and charged with engaging in homosexual conduct as prohibited by the state (13). Throughout Senegal as a result, MSM-specific service providers suspended their HIV prevention work out of fear for their programs' and their staff's personal safety; those who continued their services reported an immediate decline in MSM participation (13). Further studies showed that this detention led to increased stigma and fear of violence in health settings for MSM and reduced uptake of services (13).

State-sponsored crackdowns against homosexuality in countries such as Senegal, Malawi, Cameroon, Kenya, Thailand, Cambodia, Uganda, and Zimbabwe have received widespread international press and have had serious implications in the provision of health services to LGBT (13,141,142). In some countries, policies even mandate reporting of same-sex practices if disclosed in health care settings, which leaves health care providers the extremely conflicting choice of fulfilling their professional obligation to care and treat or be legally prosecuted for such provision (141). For example, on October 13, 2009, Ugandan legislator David Bahati introduced the Anti-Homosexuality Bill No. 18 in the Ugandan Parliament (143). The aim was to enhance existing antihomosexuality laws. It included heavier punishments and criminalization for direct and indirect support for same-sex practices, including a requirement to report perceived homosexuals and deny shelter to and punish those who do not comply. In February 2014, Uganda's president signed the bill into law. The law was subsequently declared null and void by the Ugandan Supreme Court in August 2014, based on a technicality (142). Nonetheless, the bill had already had tangible effects on the health and well-being of MSM and other sexual and gender minorities in Uganda. There is a clause in the bill that could apply to health care consultations when sexual practices and/or orientation are disclosed, voluntarily or not; it reads: "To 'impose a burden on the community to report homosexuals', all 'persons in authority', defined as one with 'power or control over other people because of your knowledge and official position . . . including . . . social authority' are by law required to report them within 24 hours to authorities. Failure to report leaves one liable to a fine or imprisonment" (141).

Standard of care in health care settings implies that confidentiality is maintained unless there is imminent risk to self or others posed by nondisclosure. Such violation of the Hippocratic Oath, and of professional ethics across many fields, would decrease the likelihood that clients would disclose their sexuality to receive appropriate care or services, and increase the likelihood that a health care provider would be unwilling to provide services to LGBT persons.

The law specifically defined and criminalized "promotion of homosexuality," targeting the "funding," "sponsoring," "offering premises for . . . homosexuality or promotion of homosexuality." A service provider of HIV risk-reduction counselling, peer education, condom and condom-compatible lubricant distribution, irrespective of the source of funds, risked fines and/or imprisonment. This portion of the law potentially prohibited all HIV prevention, treatment, and care services for acknowledged MSM and even sexual health education programs mentioning homosexuality. The Ministry of Health in Uganda has a program for most at-risk populations in Kampala focused on HIV prevention, which includes MSM. In the context of the law, this program would have been likely considered illegal. In April 2009, a UNICEF teenage peer education handbook, focused on providing sexual health education, was vilified as promoting homosexuality because it included a passage on same-sex attraction (141).

Further penalties for LGBT people living with HIV include life imprisonment for "attempted aggravated homosexuality" compared with 7 years for those who are HIV negative. Moreover, measures by the person living with HIV to limit transmission, including use of condoms, disclosure of HIV status to sexual partners, and undetectable viral load through treatment with antiretroviral therapy, are not mitigating. Thus, disclosing HIV serostatus and same-sex practices to anybody, including health care workers, would result in those workers being forced to report the patient within 24 hours, potentially resulting in life imprisonment. This clause would very likely have reduced disclosure of sexual practices and HIV status to health care workers, as well as to sexual partners and could therefore likely have resulted in increased stigma and HIV infection rates.

In addition, potentially any charge of homosexuality is to be followed by legally mandated HIV testing of the accused. HIV status would then be disclosable in a court of law, a public space, whether the person is guilty or not guilty of homosexuality. In effect, the law wrote state-sponsored homophobia into law, which has now been established as a significant risk factor for HIV among LGBT, and specifically MSM, in Uganda (141).

Health and Human Rights in Public Policy

The policies developed or adopted within any one country or state often have roots within international legal frameworks, which often include explicit human rights language. The modern human rights movement had its origins in the same atrocities as modern medical ethics: the crimes against humanity perpetrated by the Nazis in Germany and their allies during World War II. In response to the Holocaust and the crimes of Nazi doctors, the United Nations General Assembly adopted a visionary set of principles articulating those fundamental rights of human beings that no state could take away. These were articulated in the 1948 Universal Declaration of Human Rights (UDHR) and supported by all of the existing United Nations member states (144). The UDHR was developed as a founding document of human rights law and policy; it is an aspirational declaration, however, not an enforceable treaty. The UDHR was intended to set the stage for the development of binding treaties that would support the core tenets of a treaty included in the UDHR. The UDHR says little specifically in regard to health but does articulate in Article 25 that all persons have a right to a minimum standard of living, which includes access to health care (144): "Everyone has the right to a standard of living adequate for the health and well-being of himself and of his family, including food, clothing, housing and medical care and necessary social services, and the right to security in the event of unemployment, sickness, widowhood, old age or other lack of livelihood in circumstances beyond his control."

The human rights document that does speak most specifically to the right to health is the 1976 International Covenant on Economic, Social and Cultural Rights (ICESCR), again of the United Nations (145). Article 12 of the ICESCR refines the right to health with new precision:

1. The States Parties to the present Covenant recognize the right of everyone to the enjoyment of the *highest attainable standard* of physical and mental health.

The steps to be taken to achieve the full realization of this right shall include:

a) The provision for the reduction of the still-birth rate and of infant mortality and for the healthy development of the child

b) The improvement of all aspects of environmental and industrial hygiene

c) The prevention, treatment and control of epidemic, endemic, occupational and other diseases

d) The creation of conditions which would assure to all medical service and medical attention in the event of sickness.

General Comment 14 of article 12 of the Covenant was made in 2000, in part to address the special issues raised by the AIDS pandemic and reproductive health more broadly (146). Article 8 of the General Comment 14 speaks both to a more precise explanation of the right to health, and of the right to sexual and reproductive freedom: "The right to health is not to be understood as a right to be *healthy*. The right to health contains both freedoms and entitlements. The freedoms include the right to control one's health and body, *including sexual and reproductive freedom*, and the right to be free from interference, such as the right to be free from torture, nonconsensual medical treatment and experimentation."

While General Comment 14 of the ICESCR is traditionally assumed to be focused on sexual and reproductive health rights of women, it is also useful for advocacy for freedoms related to sexual rights for lesbian, gay, and bisexual people. Moreover, it is relevant for advocating for freedoms of gender identities for transgender people as the document explicitly highlights the right to control one's body. While General Comment 14 contains useful language to support advocacy efforts, these comments are not binding and not developed through a United Nations member state process.

The International Covenant on Civil and Political Rights (ICCPR) generally deals with political rights, including such basic rights as freedom from slavery, torture, persecution, and discrimination. It includes nondiscrimination on the basis of sex as a basic right but did not originally directly address sexual orientation or gender identities. In 1994, the U.N. Human Rights Committee offered an opinion on *Toonen v. Australia*, a case in which the

Australian state of Tasmania overturned legislation allowing discrimination against gay and lesbian citizens (147). The Committee's conclusion was that discrimination based on sex included sexual orientation, and so the law was in violation of the Convention. The opinion suggested that U.N. member states expand the right to freedom from discrimination to sexual and gender minority populations within international human rights law. Moreover, Article 26 of the ICCPR asserts prohibition of "discrimination . . . on any ground such as race, colour, sex, language, religion, political or other opinion, national or social origin, property, birth or other status" (148). The ICCPR has been signed by 174 U.N. member states, including many of the same where state-sponsored discrimination targeting transgender women is significant. Because the ICCPR does not specifically mention sexual orientation and gender identity, state-sponsored discrimination targeting transgender women does not imply violation of the letter of the covenant, even if it does violate the spirit of it.

The Yogyakarta Principles

The Yogyakarta Principles, formally known as the "Yogyakarta Principles on the Application of International Human Rights Law in relation to Sexual Orientation and Gender Identity," were released in 2007 and have been widely cited since. The principles detail and affirm those fundamental rights and dignities inherent to all human beings, which should never be abrogated on the basis of real or perceived sexual orientation or gender identity and which have status in existing conventions. The Yogyakarta Principles draw on existing human rights law to lay out a series of fundamental rights already extant in international human rights conventions and treaties. They were invoked in both the Indian and Nepali decisions to strike down antihomosexual/antisodomy laws. In the Indian case it was stated that:

> The [Yogyakarta] principles are intended as a coherent and comprehensive identification of the obligation of States to respect, protect and fulfill the human rights of all persons regardless of their sexual orientation or gender identity . . . . The Constitution of India recognizes, protects and celebrates diversity. To stigmatize or to criminalize homosexuals only on account of their sexual orientation would be against the constitutional morality.

—The Delhi High Court, July 2, 2009.

The Yogyakarta Principles have had significant traction within the U.N. family, having been cited by UNAIDS, United Nations Office on Drugs and Crime, and the Office of the High Commissioner for Human Rights (149). In Latin America, legal briefs invoking the Yogyakarta Principles have been filed in Argentina and Colombia, and national legislatures have invoked them in several countries, including Argentina, Brazil, Mexico, and Uruguay (149).

In June 2011, the U.N. Human Rights Council narrowly passed a nonbinding resolution to support equal rights for all people irrespective of sexual orientation or gender identity. While these resolutions are focused more on addressing the immediate needs of gay and lesbian people, their passing sets the stage to support laws and policies that would fulfill the rights of transgender people as well to live with nondiscrimination.

There are some recent examples of protective and enabling laws, most notably in Asia and the Pacific (150). Recent court judgments have improved the legal environment in Nepal, India, Pakistan, the Philippines, Fiji, South Korea, and Hong Kong Special Administrative Region of China (150). More specifically, the government of Nepal is considering proposals to introduce comprehensive legal protections from discrimination relating to sexuality and gender identity in the context of the drafting of a new constitution (151). The core thesis presented here is that transgender women experience discrimination based on the difference between their birth sex and their gender identity. This discrimination violates their basic rights of nondiscrimination and manifests in disproportionate HIV risk and consequent disease burden. Even in settings where the discrimination is not specifically state-sponsored, the lack of recognition of and protections for transgender peoples interferes with access to comprehensive preventive HIV-related services.

Community-Level Determinants of Risk Among LGBT in Low- and Middle-Income Countries

Community environments can promote or diminish health and well-being (131). The definition of who or what constitutes a "community" is contested but tends to include network ties, relationships between organizations and groups, and geographic/political regions (131,152). Cultural, economic, religious, geographic lines, prison walls, or any combination of the above may bind communities. Sociocultural norms and values, social cohesion, and network structures are shaped by larger social-structural forces and influence interpersonal processes and individual behaviors (135,153). In the realm of public health infectious disease prevention programs, community-level concepts have been used in various ways to prevent disease transmission. The gold standard of large-scale immunization campaigns using community resistance or herd immunity as key outcome indicators plays an important role in reducing the spread of infectious diseases (131). For example, interventions focused on establishing condom use norms or hand washing have demonstrated efficacy in increasing condom use and reducing communicable diseases, respectively (135,154). Within the framework of the MSEM presented in Figure 20-1, community-level factors associated with infectious disease risk revolve around safe provision of services, the confidentiality of services, and access to appropriate services in a given context.

However, antigay community norms can impede the provision of safe, high-quality services (155). As Beyrer notes, deep roots of homophobia may be entrenched in the tensions of changing gender norms, changes in socio-economic status of a country, or the residual misogyny of many societies (155). Societal emotions at the community level can also be manipulated by political and other leaders, often politically motivated and for self-interest. In recent years in Malawi, the late President Bingu wa Mutharika used anti-homosexual rhetoric whenever his administration was accused of corruption and mismanagement, resulting in aggressive community-level backlash against LGBT persons (155,156). In Uganda, evangelical Christian leaders from the United States have clearly influenced the national debate on discriminatory legislation by promoting antigay legislators and their own political agendas (155,157). The use of anti-LGBT rhetoric as a political wedge has a long history in the United States and was shown to be a political topic used repeatedly by political strategists to assist in elections (155). As political systems in low- and middle-income countries grow, and voters gain in education and tolerance, one hopes that continued attempts to manipulate hatred and fear of vulnerable sexual minorities eventually will become a part of the political past (155). Unfortunately, for now they remain galvanizing tools in political systems and debates, and consequently have added to the exclusion of LGBT populations from normal societal structures, including health services (13,56,155,158).

In health care settings, stigmatizing community norms affect 2 important issues that cause inadequate health service provision for LGBT people: 1) health knowledge and norms of LGBT people at the provider level and 2) assumptions and knowledge of health risk for the populations within their own communities. The availability and type of services for LGBT persons at the community level propagate stigma and discrimination toward LGBT persons if negative health care experiences occur, and thus reduce efficacy of prevention programs and messages within society (139,159).

The invisibility of WSW in health services around the world is exemplified at the community level by the lack of knowledge of WSW individual health risks, both by health providers and by the community itself (116). In the United States, medical curricula are not mandated to include education on MSM, WSW, or transgender specific care and treatment. Even if full sexual histories are obtained (which is also not always the case), providers may incorrectly assume WSW have little risk for STI transmission and neglect to provide risk reduction information to the patient. Concurrently, lesbians and other WSW might perceive themselves to be at low risk for STI compared with their heterosexual counterparts as a result of complex social messages of typical transmission, perceptions of sex partners and fidelity, and perceive or enacted stigma (116). Qualitative data has anecdotally shown misconceptions by lesbians include the belief that STI prevention or risk reduction behavior is mainly a heterosexual female issue (116,160). If these misconceptions are prevalent within WSW communities, their ability to proactively protect themselves, their networks, and their communities is limited. The final contributing factor noted by King and colleagues that directly affects the individual health and well-being of WSW is the reality that at the community level, women living in single-female or two-female households have lower socioeconomic status compared with households with one male. In high-income countries this compounds community health risks by reducing accessibility to health insurance or the ability to pay for health services. If this is the case in high-income countries, the reality for women in low- and middle-income countries is significantly worse, as exemplified by the international communities priority approach to empowering and economically enhancing the status of women, in hopes of equalizing the economic earning power between men and women globally (161). Thus, the compilation of the invisibility of LGBT in epidemiologic and medical practice, and actualized stigma and discrimination at the community-level, facilitates an increased risk for individual risk for the LGBT community worldwide (137,162).

Service Delivery for LGBT People in Low- and Middle-Income Countries

Given that current health services are currently not meeting the needs of LGBT people throughout the world, what other types of service delivery models at the community level would be more appropriate? Researchers have proposed different models for provision of health services to LGBT people that could mitigate community level stigma and discrimination in low- and middle-income countries, including fully integrated, stand-alone, and hybrid models of services. Beyrer and colleagues assert that because LGBT groups are key populations at risk in the HIV epidemic, health services for LGBT people that are *fully integrated* into general HIV or primary care programs are optimal in certain settings throughout the world (139). In other settings, *stand-alone models* that provide tailored, nondiscriminatory services only to LGBT populations within a community may work well. Some find stand-alone models to be easier to implement, while others argue against these models, believing they can lead to involuntary and coercive services; others stress that in highly homophobic environments, stand-alone services could be potential targets for anti-homosexual campaigns, political agendas, and community-level discrimination (139). The *hybrid model* links LGBT community-based educational outreach and prevention programs to clinical services that serve the entire population but have providers that are well trained in LGBT health issues. Hybrid models have seen success in certain regions, such as Malawi, Senegal, and Lesotho (139). It is likely that a mix of these 3 models will be needed to meet the specific contexts of different low- or middle-income countries. No matter which model is used, it is essential that all levels of staff receive training in providing sensitive, nondiscriminatory care to LGBT people (139). In addition, it is necessary for low- and middle-income countries to create policies that address and protect LGBT rights, as it is public policies that determine allocation of economic resources to health care (135).

Moving Forward

It is now clear that LGBT communities worldwide face an array of challenges to their well-being. Their health and their struggle for human rights, full citizenship, and full participation in society are inextricably linked. For many, the struggle for equality and dignity is just beginning and is fraught with risks at the partner, family, community, and national levels. Nevertheless, LGBT people are taking those risks. Their communities are organizing, and their invisibility in much of the world is coming to an end. The interconnectedness of our world has allowed for LGBT people to communicate and engage in ways that were literally unimaginable just a few short years ago—rapidly eroding isolation and expanding access to information, global solidarity, and support for their advocacy in health and rights. But with demands for health rights, and for inclusion and acceptance, have come perhaps inevitable setbacks, backlash from civil and religious authorities, and the many tensions that emerge for any social change movement among stigmatized minorities. But in 2013, LGBT rights are firmly on the world's agenda as a civil and political rights issue. There is no clearer indication of this level of attention than the fact that the 2012 International Human Rights Event, Chaired by U.N. Secretary General Ban Ki-moon, was dedicated to LGBT human rights. With the U.S. pop star Ricky Martin and the South African Singer Cha at his side, Ban gave a ringing endorsement of global solidarity with LGBT people saying:

> The very first article of the UDHR proclaims that "All human beings are born free and equal in dignity and rights." All human beings—not some, not most, but all. No one gets to decide who is entitled to human rights and who is not. Let me say this loud and clear: lesbian, gay, bisexual, and transgender people are entitled to the same rights as everyone else. They, too, are born free and equal (163).

It will be a long time before LGBT people worldwide enjoy their full freedom, "the same rights as everyone else," including the right to culturally competent health care in settings that are safe, inclusive, and fully supportive of human dignity. But the movement toward acceptance is surely unstoppable, and the emerging global solidarity among our communities is a source of critical strength for the fights ahead. Access to health care, along with the right to an education, are among the most critical rights for the enjoyment of all other rights, and so play fundamental roles in the realization of well-being for LGBT people worldwide. As LGBT people emerge from the shadows in country after country, the health movement that has been developed by LGBT people and their allies in the global north will provide critical models, training and capacity building, technical support and research collaboration that will benefit all partners and begin to realize the right to health for those most in need. This is truly one of the signature human and civil rights efforts of our time—but is a struggle we can, and must, begin to win.

Summary Points

- LGBT people in low and middle-income countries possess complex, multidimensional health outcomes that must be defined within an integrated structural-level, community-level, and individual-level framework.
- The burden of STIs, and particularly HIV infection, among LGBT people in low- and middle-income countries is significantly higher than among other reproductive-age adults.
- The needs of transgender women and men have largely been ignored in terms of characterizing HIV risks as well as health service needs in low- and middle-income countries.
- Given the focus on funding HIV-related programming, the health and human rights needs of lesbian women and other WSW have been understudied and underserved in most low- and middle-income countries.
- Understanding HIV-related risks among LGBT people in low- and middle-income countries necessitates characterizing multiple levels of risk transcending just individual practices and including community-level stigma and discrimination, limited clinical provider competency, and stigmatizing and even criminalizing public policies.
- Optimal health service delivery for LGBT people will differ by socio-economic and cultural contexts and may include fully integrated, stand-alone, and hybrid models of health services.
- Health services tailored to mitigate stigma, facilitate health care access, ensure appropriate care delivery, and promote the health and human rights of LGBT people globally are essential for long-term service delivery for LGBT people in low- and middle-income countries.
- Preservice and in-service training to increase both clinical and cultural competency of health care workers to better address the health needs of LGBT people is an urgent priority across the world.

References

1. **International Gay & Lesbian Human Rights Commission**. Available at: http://iglhrc.org/.
2. **Blackwood E, Wieringa S**. Female Desires: Same-Sex Relations and Transgender Practices Across Cultures. New York: Columbia University Press; 1999.
3. **Herdt GH**. Same Sex, Different Cultures: Gays and Lesbians Across Cultures. Boulder, CO: Westview Press; 1997.

4. **Nanda S.** Gender Diversity: Crosscultural Variations. Long Grove, IL: Waveland Press; 2000.
5. **Talbot M.** About a boy. The New Yorker. March 18, 2013. Available at: www.newyorker.com/ magazine/2013/03/18/about-a-boy-2.
6. **Beyrer C.** War in the blood. In: Sex, Politics and HIV/AIDS in SouthEast Asia. London: Zed Books; 1998.
7. **Bränström R, van der Star A.** All inclusive public health—what about LGBT populations? Eur J Public Health. 2013;23:353-4.
8. **European Union Agency for Fundamental Rights.** EU LGBT survey - European Union lesbian, gay, bisexual and transgender survey - results at a glance. May 2013. Available at: http://fra.europa.eu/en/publication/2013/eu-lgbt-survey-european-union-lesbian-gay-bisexual-and-transgender-survey-results.
9. **Beyrer C, Wirtz A, Walker D, et al.** The Global HIV Epidemics Among Men Who Have Sex With Men: Epidemiology, Prevention, Access to Care and Human Rights. Washington, DC: World Bank Publications; 2011.
10. **Baral S, Sifakis F, Cleghorn F, Beyrer C.** Elevated risk for HIV infection among men who have sex with men in low- and middle-income countries 2000-2006: a systematic review. PLoS Med. 2007;4:e339.
11. **Baral S, Adams D, Lebona J, et al.** A cross-sectional assessment of population demographics, HIV risks and human rights contexts among men who have sex with men in Lesotho. J Int AIDS Soc. 2011;14:36.
12. **Beyrer C.** Global prevention of HIV infection for neglected populations: men who have sex with men. Clin Infect Dis. 2010;50 Suppl 3:S108-13.
13. **Poteat T, Diouf D, Drame FM, et al.** HIV risk among MSM in Senegal: a qualitative rapid assessment of the impact of enforcing laws that criminalize same sex practices. PLoS One. 2011;6:e28760.
14. **amfAR AIDS Research.** MSM, HIV, and the Road to Universal Access—How Far Have We Come? 2008. Available at: www.amfar.org/uploadedFiles/In_the_Community/Publications/ MSM%20HIV%20and%20the%20Road%20to%20Universal%20Access.pdf.
15. **Padilla M.** Carribean Pleasure Industry: Tourism, Sexuality, and AIDS in the Dominican Republic. Chicago: University of Chicago Press; 2007.
16. **Chakrapani V, Newman PA, Shunmugam M, McLuckie A, Melwin F.** Structural violence against Kothi-identified men who have sex with men in Chennai, India: a qualitative investigation. AIDS Educ Prev. 2007;19:346-64.
17. **Logie C.** The case for the World Health Organization's Commission on the Social Determinants of Health to Address Sexual Orientation. Am J Public Health. 2012.
18. **Baral S, Logie CH, Grosso A, Wirtz AL, Beyrer C.** Modified social ecological model: a tool to guide the assessment of the risks and risk contexts of HIV epidemics. BMC Public Health. 2013;13:482.
19. **Padilla M, Aguila AD, Parker R.** Globalization, structural violence, and LGBT health: a cross-cultural perspective. In: Meyer I, Northridge M, eds. The Health of Sexual Minorities. New York: Springer:209-41.
20. **Collins P, Patel V, Joestl S, et al.** Grand challenges in global mental health. Nature. 2011;475:27-30.
21. **Herek GM.** Science, public policy, and legal recognition of same-sex relationships. Am Psychol. 2007;62:713-5.
22. **Campbell C, Deacon H.** Unraveling the contexts of stigma: from iternalisation to resistance to change. J Commun Appl Soc Psychol. 2006;16:411-7.
23. **Mahajan A, Sayles JN, Patel V, Remien R, Sawires S.** Stigma in the HIV/AIDS epidemic: a review of the literature and recommendations for the way forward. AIDS. 2008;22(Suppl 2): S67-9.
24. **Van Brakel WH.** Measuring health-related stigma—a literature review. Psychol Health Med. 2006;11:307-34.
25. **Wade AS, Larmarange J, Diop AK, et al.** Reduction in risk-taking behaviors among MSM in Senegal between 2004 and 2007 and prevalence of HIV and other STIs. ELIHoS Project, ANRS 12139. AIDS Care. 2010;22:409-14.

26. **Parker RG, Easton D, Klein CH.** Structural barriers and facilitators in HIV prevention: a review of international research. AIDS. 2000;14 Suppl 1:S22-32.

27. **Farmer P, Connors M, Simmons J, eds.** Women, Poverty, and AIDS: Sex, Drugs, and Structural Violence. Monroe, ME: Common Courage Press; 1996.

28. **King M, Semlyen J, Tai S, et al.** A systematic review of mental disorder, suicide, and deliberate self harm in lesbian, gay and bisexual people. BMC Psychiatry. 2008;8:70.

29. **Cochran SD, Mays VM.** Burden of psychiatric morbidity among lesbian, gay, and bisexual individuals in the California Quality of Life Survey. J Abnorm Psychol. 2009;118:647-58.

30. **Meyer IH.** Prejudice, social stress, and mental health in lesbian, gay, and bisexual populations: conceptual issues and research evidence. Psychol Bull. 2003;129:674-97.

31. **Frisell T, Lichtenstein P, Rahman Q, Langstrom N.** Psychiatric morbidity associated with same-sex sexual behaviour: influence of minority stress and familial factors. Psychol Med. 2010;40:315-24.

32. **Lewis NM.** Mental health in sexual minorities: recent indicators, trends, and their relationships to place in North America and Europe. Health Place. 2009;15:1029-45.

33. **Plöderl M, Kralovec K, Fartacek R.** The relation between sexual orientation and suicide attempts in Austria. Arch Sex Behav. 2010;39:1403-14.

34. **Diaz RM, Ayala G, Bein E, Henne J, Marin BV.** The impact of homophobia, poverty, and racism on the mental health of gay and bisexual Latino men: findings from 3 US cities. Am J Public Health. 2001;91:927-32.

35. **Logie C, Newman P, Chakrapani V, Shunmugam M.** Adapting the minority stress model: associations between gender non-conformity stigma, HIV-related stigma and depression among men who have sex with men in South India. Soc Sci Med. 2012;74:1261-8.

36. **Lee PT, Henderson M, Patel V.** A UN summit on global mental health. Lancet. 2010;376:516.

37. **World Health Organization.** Depression. 2010. Available at: www.who.int/topics/depression/en/.

38. **Meyer IH.** Minority stress and mental health in gay men. J Health Soc Behav. 1995;36:38-56.

39. **Frost DM, Meyer IH.** Internalized homophobia and relationship quality among lesbians, gay men, and bisexuals. J Counsel Psychol. 2009;56:97-109.

40. **Hatzenbuehler M, Nolen-Hoeksema S, Erickson S.** Minority stress predictors of HIV risk behavior, substance use, and depressive symptoms: results from a prospective study of bereaved gay men. Health Psychol. 2008;27:455-62.

41. **amfAR.** Global Consultation on MSM and HIV/AIDS Research. 2008. Available at: www.amfar.org/content.aspx?id=7157.

42. **Flowers P.** How does an emergent LGBTQ health psychology reconstruct its subject? Feminism Psychol. 2009;19:555-60.

43. **Rothman EF, Exner D, Baughman AL.** The prevalence of sexual assault against people who identify as gay, lesbian, or bisexual in the United States: a systematic review. Trauma Viol Abuse. 2011;12:55-66.

44. **Logie C, James L, Tharao W, Loutfy M.** "We don't exist": a qualitative study of marginalization experienced by HIV-positive lesbian, bisexual, queer, and transgender women in Toronto, Canada. J Int AIDS Soc. 2012;15:17392.

45. **Newman PA, Chakrapani V, Cook C, Shunmugam M, Kakinami L.** Determinants of sexual risk behavior among men who have sex with men accessing public sex environments in Chennai, India. J LGBT Health Res. 2008;4:81-7.

46. **Baral S, Burrell E, Scheibe A, et al.** HIV risk and associations of HIV infection among men who have sex with men in peri-urban Cape Town, South Africa. BMC Public Health. 2011; 11:766.

47. **Roberts AL, Austin SB, Corliss HL, Vandermorris AK, Koenen KC.** Pervasive trauma exposure among US sexual orientation minority adults and risk of posttraumatic stress disorder. Am J Public Health. 2010;100:2433-41.

48. **Eiven L.** Lesbians, health and human rights: a Latin American perspective: a contribution for discussion and reflection. Women's Health Collection. 2003;7:44-54.

49. **Kulick D.** The gender of Brazilian transgendered prostitutes. Am Anthropol. 1997;99:574-85.

50. **Prieur A.** Mema's house, Mexico City: On Transvestites, Queens, and Machos. Chicago: University of Chicago Press; 1998.

51. **Chandra PS, Ravi V, Desai A, Subbakrishna DK.** Anxiety and depression among HIV-infected heterosexuals—a report from india. J Psychosom Res. 1998;45:401-9.

52. **Chandran V.** From judgment to practice: section 377 and the medical sector. Indian J Med Ethics. 2009;1:198-9.

53. **Parekh S.** Researching LGB youths in India: still a distant dream. J Gay Lesbian Issues Educ. 2006;3:147-50.

54. **Hon KL, Leung TF, Yau AP, et al.** A survey of attitudes toward homosexuality in Hong Kong Chinese medical students. Teach Learn Med. 2005;17:344-8.

55. **Baral S, Trapence G, Motimedi F, et al.** HIV prevalence, risks for HIV infection, and human rights among men who have sex with men (MSM) in Malawi, Namibia, and Botswana. PLoS One. 2009;4:e4997.

56. **Fay H, Baral SD, Trapence G, et al.** Stigma, health care access, and HIV knowledge among men who have sex with men in Malawi, Namibia, and Botswana. AIDS Behav. 2011;15:1088-97.

57. **Feng Y, Wu Z, Detels R.** Evolution of men who have sex with men community and experienced stigma among men who have sex with men in Chengdu, China. J Acquir Immune Defic Syndr. 2010;53:S98-S103.

58. **Araujo M, Montagner MA, da Silva R, Lopes F, de Freitas M.** Symbolic violence experienced by men who have sex with men in the primary health service in Fortalez, Ceara, Brazil: negotiation identity under stigma. AIDS Patient Care STDs. 2009;23:663-8.

59. **Berkman A, Garcia J, Muñoz-Laboy M, Paiva V, Parker R.** A critical analysis of the Brazilian response to HIV/AIDS: lessons learned for controlling and mitigating the epidemic in developing countries. Am J Public Health. 2005;95:1162-72.

60. **Konkle-Parker DJ, Erlen JA, Dubbert PM.** Barriers and facilitators to medication adherence in a southern minority population with HIV disease. J Assoc Nurses AIDS Care. 2008;19:98-104.

61. **Rao D, Kekwaletswe TC, Hosek S, Martinez J, Rodriguez F.** Stigma and social barriers to medication adherence with urban youth living with HIV. AIDS Care. 2007;19:28-33.

62. **Rintamaki LS, Davis TC, Skripkauskas S, Bennett CL, Wolf MS.** Social stigma concerns and HIV medication adherence. AIDS Patient Care STDS. 2006;20:359-68.

63. **Ware NC, Wyatt MA, Tugenberg T.** Social relationships, stigma and adherence to antiretroviral therapy for HIV/AIDS. AIDS Care. 2006;18:904-10.

64. **Malta M, Beyrer C.** The HIV epidemic and human rights violations in Brazil. J Int AIDS Soc. 2013;16:18817.

65. **Bradford JB, Coleman S, Cunningham W.** HIV system navigation: an emerging model to improve HIV care access. AIDS Patient Care STDS. 2007;21 Suppl 1:S49-58.

66. **Naar-King S, Bradford J, Coleman S, et al.** Retention in care of persons newly diagnosed with HIV: outcomes of the Outreach Initiative. AIDS Patient Care STDS. 2007;21 Suppl 1:S40-8.

67. **White RC, Carr R.** Homosexuality and HIV/AIDS stigma in Jamaica. Cult Health Sex. 2005; 7:347-59.

68. **Vu L, Tun W, Sheehy M, Nel D.** Levels and correlates of internalized homophobia among men who have sex with men in Pretoria, South Africa. AIDS Behav. 2012;16:717-23.

69. **UNAIDS.** People Living with HIV Stigma Index: Asia Pacific regional analysis 2011. Available at: www.unaids.org/en/media/unaids/contentassets/documents/unaidspublication/2011/20110829_PLHIVStigmaIndex_en.pdf.

70. **Safren S, Martin C, Menon S, et al.** A survey of MSM HIV prevention outreach workers in Chennai, India. AIDS Educ Prev. 2006;18:323-32.

71. **Abell N, Rutledge S, McCann T, Padmore J.** Examining HIV/AIDS provider stigma: assessing regional concerns in the islands of the Eastern Caribbean. AIDS Care. 2007;19:242-7.

72. **Carr R.** Stigmas, gender, and coping: a study of HIV+ Jamaicans. Race Gender Class. 2002; 9:122-44.

73. **Norman LR, Carr R, Jimenez J.** Sexual stigma and sympathy: attitudes toward persons living with HIV in Jamaica. Cult Health Sex. 2006;8:423-33.

74. **Paxton S, Gonzales G, Uppakaew K, et al.** AIDS-related discrimination in Asia. AIDS Care. 2005;17:413-24.

75. **Sandfort TG, Nel J, Rich E, Reddy V, Yi H.** HIV testing and self-reported HIV status in South African men who have sex with men: results from a community-based survey. Sex Transm Infect. 2008;84:425-9.

76. **Cloete A, Simbayi LC, Kalichman SC, Strebel A, Henda N.** Stigma and discrimination experiences of HIV-positive men who have sex with men in Cape Town, South Africa. AIDS Care. 2008;20:1105-10.

77. **Lane T, Shade SB, McIntyre J, Morin SF.** Alcohol and sexual risk behavior among men who have sex with men in South african township communities. AIDS Behav. 2008; 12(4 Suppl):S78-S85.

78. **Okal J, Luchters S, Geibel S, Chersich MF, Lango D, Temmerman M.** Social context, sexual risk perceptions and stigma: HIV vulnerability among male sex workers in Mombasa, Kenya. Cult Health Sex. 2009:1.

79. **Onyango-Ouma W, Birungi H, Geibel S.** Understanding the HIV/STI risks and prevention needs of men who have sex with men in Nairobi, Kenya. Nairobi: Population Council; 2005.

80. **Sharma A, Bukusi E, Gorbach P, Cohen CR, Muga C, Kwena Z, et al.** Sexual identity and risk of HIV/STI among men who have sex with men in Nairobi. Sex Transm Dis. 2008;35:352-4.

81. **Niang CI, Tapsoba P, Weiss E, et al.** "It's raining stones": stigma, violence and HIV vulnerability among men who have sex with men in Dakar, Senegal. Culture Health Sexual. 2003; 5:499-512.

82. **Teunis N.** Same-sex sexuality in Africa: a case study from Senegal. AIDS Behav. 2001;5(2):173.

83. **Moreau A, Tapsoba P, Niang C, Diop AK.** Implementing STI/HIV prevention and care interventions for men who have sex with men in Dakar, Senegal. Washington, DC: Population Council; 2007.

84. **Niang C, Moreau A, Kostermans K, et al., eds.** Men who have sex with men in Burkina Faso, Senegal, and The Gambia: the multi-country HIV/AIDS program approach [Abstract]. The XV International AIDS Conference, 2004; Bangkok.

85. **Hawkes S, Collumbien M, Platt L, et al.** HIV and other sexually transmitted infections among men, transgenders and women selling sex in two cities in Pakistan: a cross-sectional prevalence survey. Sex Transm Infect. 2009;85 Suppl 2:ii8-16.

86. **Rajabali A, Khan S, Warraich HJ, Khanani MR, Ali SH.** HIV and homosexuality in Pakistan. Lancet Infect Dis. 2008;8:511-5.

87. **Shawky S, Soliman C, Kassak KM, et al.** HIV surveillance and epidemic profile in the Middle East and North Africa. J Acquir Immune Defic Syndr. 2009;51 Suppl 3:S83-95.

88. **Caceres CF, Stall R.** Commentary: The human immunodeficiency virus/AIDS epidemic among men who have sex with men in Latin America and the Caribbean: it is time to bridge the gap. Int J Epidemiol. 2003;32:740-3.

89. **Betron M, Gonzalez-Figueroa E.** Gender Identity, Violence, and HIV among MSM and TG: A Literature Review and a Call for Screening. Washington, DC: Futures Group International; 2009.

90. **Baral S, Sifakis F, Cleghorn F, Beyrer C.** Elevated risk for HIV infection among men who have sex with men in low- and middle-income countries 2000-2006: a systematic review. PLoS Med. 2007;4:e339.

91. **Beyrer C, Baral SD, van Griensven F, et al.** Global epidemiology of HIV infection in men who have sex with men. Lancet. 2012;380:367-77.

92. **Baral SS, Diouf D, Trapence G, et al.** Criminalization of same sex practices as a structural driver of HIV risk among men who have sex with men (MSM): the cases of Senegal, Malawi, and Uganda (MOPE0951). International AIDS Conference 2010; Vienna, Austria.

93. **UNAIDS. Report on the Global AIDS Epidemic.** 2006. Available at: www.unaids.org/en/media/ unaids/contentassets/documents/unaidspublication/2010/20101123_globalreport_en.pdf.

94. **Herbst JH, Jacobs ED, Finlayson TJ, et al.** Estimating HIV prevalence and risk behaviors of transgender persons in the United States: a systematic review. AIDS Behav. 2008;12:1-17.

95. **Baral SD, Poteat T, Stromdahl S, et al.** Worldwide burden of HIV in transgender women: a systematic review and meta-analysis. Lancet Infect Dis. 2013;13:214-22.

96. **Operario D, Soma T, Underhill K.** Sex work and HIV status among transgender women: systematic review and meta-analysis. J Acquir Immune Defic Syndr. 2008;48:97-103.

97. **Clements-Nolle K, Marx R, Guzman R, Katz M.** HIV prevalence, risk behaviors, health care use, and mental health status of transgender persons: implications for public health intervention. Am J Public Health. 2001;91:915-21.

98. **Nemoto T, Operario D, Keatley J, Han L, Soma T.** HIV risk behaviors among male-to-female transgender persons of color in San Francisco. Am J Public Health. 2004;94:1193-9.

99. **Price MA, Rida W, Mwangome M, et al.** Identifying at-risk populations in Kenya and South Africa: HIV incidence in cohorts of men who report sex with men, sex workers, and youth. J Acquir Immune Defic Syndr. 2012;59:185-93.

100. **Wilson PA, Moore TE.** Public health responses to the HIV epidemic among black men who have sex with men: a qualitative study of US Health Departments and Communities. Am J Public Health. 2009;99:1013-22.

101. **Lurie S.** Identifying training needs of health-care providers related to treatment and care of transgendered patients: a qualitative needs assessment conducted in New England. Int J Transgender. 2005;8:93-112.

102. **Rachlin K, Green J, Lombardi E.** Utilization of health care among female-to-male transgender individuals in the United States. J Homosex. 2008;54:243-58.

103. **Sanchez NF, Sanchez JP, Danoff A.** Health care utilization, barriers to care, and hormone usage among male-to-female transgender persons in New York City. Am J Public Health. 2009;99:713-9.

104. **Wallace PM.** Finding self: a qualitative study of transgender, transitioning, and adulterated silicone. Health Educ J. 2010;69:439-46.

105. **Ward H.** Prevention strategies for sexually transmitted infections: importance of sexual network structure and epidemic phase. Sex Transm Infect. 2007;83 Suppl 1:i43-9.

106. **Gontek I.** Sexual violence against lesbian women in South Africa [Thesis]. 2007. Available at: http://asiphephe.org/modules/MDCatalogue/resources/98_40_sexual_violence_against_lesbian_women_in_sa_ines_gontek.pdf

107. **Beyrer C.** Lesbian, gay, bisexual, and transgender populations in Africa: a social justice movement emerges in the era of HIV. SAHARA J. 2012;9:177-9.

108. **Kelly A.** Raped and killed for being a lesbian: South Africa ignores 'corrective' attacks. The Guardian. March 12, 2009. Available at: www.theguardian.com/world/2009/mar/12/eudy-simelane-corrective-rape-south-africa.

109. **Action Aid.** Hate Crimes: The Rise of 'Corrective Rape' in South Africa. London: Action Aid, 2009.

110. **Lenke K, Piehl M.** Women who have sex with women in the global HIV pandemic. Development. 2009;52:91-4.

111. **UNAIDS. UNAIDS strategy 2011–2015.** 2010. Available at: www.unaids.org/en/aboutunaids/unaidsstrategygoalsby2015/.

112. **Vandepitte J, Bukenya J, Weiss HA, et al.** HIV and other sexually transmitted infections in a cohort of women involved in high-risk sexual behavior in Kampala, Uganda. Sex Transm Dis. 2011;38:316-23.

113. **Arend ED.** The politics of invisibility: homophobia and low-income HIV-positive women who have sex with women. J Homosex. 2005;49:97-122.

114. **Marrazzo J.** Dangerous assumptions: lesbians and sexual death. Sex Transm Dis. 2005;32:570-1.

115. **Altman D, Aggleton P, Williams M, et al.** Men who have sex with men: stigma and discrimination. Lancet. 2012;12:91-7.

116. **Holmes K, Sparling F, Stamm W, et al.** Sexually Transmitted Diseases. 4th ed. New York: McGraw-Hill; 2008.

117. **Bauer GR, Welles SL.** Beyond assumptions of negligible risk: sexually transmitted diseases and women who have sex with women. Am J Public Health. 2001;91:1282-6.

118. **Marrazzo J.** Sexually transmitted infections in women who have sex with women: who cares? Sex Transm Infect. 2000;76:330-2.

119. **Morrow K, Allsworth J.** Sexual risk in lesbians and bisexual women. J Gay Lesbian Med Assoc. 2002;6:159-65.

120. **Bailey JV, Farquhar C, Owen C, Mangtani P.** Sexually transmitted infections in women who have sex with women. Sex Transm Infect. 2004;80:244-6.

121. **Fethers K, Marks C, Mindel A, Estcourt E.** Sexually transmitted infections and risk behaviours in women who have sex with women. Sex Transm Infect. 2000;76:345-9.

122. **Friedman SR, Ompad DC, Maslow C, et al.** HIV prevalence, risk behaviors, and high-risk sexual and injection networks among young women injectors who have sex with women. Am J Public Health. 2003;93:902-6.

123. **Pinto AP, Baggio HC, Guedes GB.** Sexually-transmitted viral diseases in women: clinical and epidemiological aspects and advances in laboratory diagnosis. Braz J Infect Dis. 2005;9: 241-50.

124. **Diamant AL, Schuster MA, Lever J.** Receipt of preventive health care services by lesbians. Am J Prev Med. 2000;19:141-8.

125. **Lindley LL, Barnett CL, Brandt HM, Hardin JW, Burcin M.** STDs among sexually active female college students: does sexual orientation make a difference? Perspect Sex Reprod Health. 2008;40:212-7.

126. **Auerbach JD, Parkhurst JO, Cáceres CF.** Addressing social drivers of HIV/AIDS for the long-term response: conceptual and methodological considerations. Global Public Health. 2011;6(suppl 3):S293-309.

127. **Kippax S, Holt M, Friedman S.** Bridging the social and the biomedical: engaging the social and political sciences in HIV research. J Int AIDS Soc. 2011;14:S1.

128. **Parker R, Aggleton P.** HIV and AIDS-related stigma and discrimination: a conceptual framework and implications for action. Soc Sci Med. 2003; 57:13e24.

129. **Beyrer C, Villar JC, Suwanvanichkij V, Singh S, Baral SD, Mills EJ.** Neglected diseases, civil conflicts, and the right to health. Lancet. 2007;370:619-27.

130. **Beyrer C.** HIV epidemiology update and transmission factors: risks and risk contexts. Clin Infect Dis. 2007;44:981-7.

131. **Baral S, Logie C, Grosso A, Wirtz A, Beyrer C.** Modified social ecological model: a tool to guide the assessment of the risks and risk contexts of HIV epidemics. BMC Public Health. 201317;13:482.

132. **Beyrer C, Baral SD, Walker D, et al.** The expanding epidemics of HIV type 1 among men who have sex with men in low- and middle-income countries: diversity and consistency. Epidemiol Rev. 2010;32:137-51.

133. **Smith AD, Tapsoba P, Peshu N, Sanders EJ, Jaffe HW.** Men who have sex with men and HIV/AIDS in sub-Saharan Africa. Lancet. 2009;374:416-22.

134. **Berkman LF, Glass T, Brissette I, Seeman TE.** From social integration to health: Durkheim in the new millennium. Soc Sci Med. 2000;51:843-57.

135. **Wellings K, Collumbien M, Slaymaker E, et al.** Sexual behaviour in context: a global perspective. Lancet. 2006;368:1706-28.

136. **Beyrer C, Wirtz AL, Baral S, Peryskina A, Sifakis F.** Epidemiologic links between drug use and HIV epidemics: an international perspective. J Acquir Immune Defic Syndr. 2010; 55 Suppl 1:S10-6.

137. **Degenhardt L, Mathers B, Vickerman P, et al.** Prevention of HIV infection for people who inject drugs: why individual, structural, and combination approaches are needed. Lancet. 2010;376:285-301.

138. **Baral S, Beyrer C, Muessig K, et al.** Burden of HIV among female sex workers in low-income and middle-income countries: a systematic review and meta-analysis. Lancet Infect Dis. 2012;12:538-49.

139. **Beyrer C, Baral S, Kerrigan D, et al.** Expanding the space: inclusion of most-at-risk populations in HIV prevention, treatment, and care services. J Acquir Immune Defic Syndr. 2011; 57 Suppl 2:S96-9.

140. **Beyrer C, Sullivan PS, Sanchez J, et al.** A call to action for comprehensive HIV services for men who have sex with men. Lancet. 2012;380:424-38.

141. **Semugoma P, Beyrer C, Baral S.** Assessing the effects of anti-homosexuality legislation in Uganda on HIV prevention, treatment, and care services. SAHARA J. 2012;9:173-6.

142. **Smith D.** Uganda anti-gay law declared 'null and void' by constitutional court. The Guardian. August 1, 2014. Available at: www.theguardian.com/world/2014/aug/01/uganda-anti-gay-law-null-and-void.

143. **Olukya G.** David Bahati, Uganda lawmaker, refuses to withdraw anti-gay bill. Huffington Post. March 18, 2010. Available at: www.huffingtonpost.com/2010/01/08/david-bahati-uganda-lawma_n_416084.html.

144. **U.N. General Assembly.** Universal Declaration of Human Rights. December 10, 1948, 217A (III).

145. **U.N. General Assembly.** International Covenant on Economic, Social and Cultural Rights. December 16, 1966. United Nations Treaty Series 1966;993:3.

146. **U.N. Committee on Economic, Social and Cultural Rights.** General comment no. 14: The right to the highest attainable standard of health. 2000. Available at: www.nesri.org/resources/general-comment-no-14-the-right-to-the-highest-attainable-standard-of-health.

147. **Kirby M.** Respecting the basic human rights. Integration. 1997:30-3.

148. **United Nations.** International Covenant on Civil and Political Rights. New York: OHCHR; 2008.

149. **Dittrich BO.** Yogyakarta principles: applying existing human rights norms to sexual orientation and gender identity. HIV AIDS Policy Law Rev. 2008;13:92-3.

150. **Godwin J.** Legal environments, human rights and HIV responses among men who have sex with men and transgender people in Asia and the Pacific: an agenda for action. United Nations Development Programme. 2010. Available at: www.undp.org/content/undp/en/home/librarypage/hiv-aids/legal-environments-human-rights-and-hiv-responses-among-men-who/.

151. **U.N. General Assembly.** Constitutional Process in Nepal Considers Inclusion of Anti-Discrimination Measures, Minority Protections in Draft, Women's Committee Assured. July 20, 2011. Available at: www.un.org/News/Press/docs/2011/wom1873.doc.htm.

152. **McLeroy KR, Bibeau D, Steckler A, Glanz K.** An ecological perspective on health promotion programs. Health Educ Q. 1988;15:351-77.

153. **Auerbach JD, Parkhurst JO, Caceres CF.** Addressing social drivers of HIV/AIDS for the long-term response: conceptual and methodological considerations. Global Public Health. 2011; 6 Suppl 3:S293-309.

154. **Wang K, Brown K, Shen SY, Tucker J.** Social network-based interventions to promote condom use: a systematic review. AIDS Behav. 2011;15:1298-308.

155. **Beyrer C.** LGBT Africa: a social justice movement emerges in the era of HIV. SAHARA-J 2012;9:177-9.

156. **Kasunda A.** OPC blesses US-funded survey to determine Malawi's gay population. The Nation. February 24, 2012.

157. **Gettleman J.** Americans' role seen in Uganda anti-gay push. New York Times. January 3, 2010. Available at: www.nytimes.com/2010/01/04/world/africa/04uganda.html?_r=0.

158. **Trapence G, Collins C, Avrett S, et al.** From personal survival to public health: community leadership by men who have sex with men in the response to HIV. Lancet. 2012;380:400-10.

159. **Wolfe D, Carrieri MP, Shepard D.** Treatment and care for injecting drug users with HIV infection: a review of barriers and ways forward. Lancet. 2010;376:355-66.

160. **Marrazzo JM, Coffey P, Bingham A.** Sexual practices, risk perception and knowledge of sexually transmitted disease risk among lesbian and bisexual women. Perspect Sex Reprod Health. 2005;37:6-12.

161. **Kabeer N.** Gender Mainstreaming in Poverty Eradication and the Millennium Development Goals. London: Marlborough House; 2003.

162. **Strathdee SA, Hallett TB, Bobrova N, et al.** HIV and risk environment for injecting drug users: the past, present, and future. Lancet. 2010;376:268-85.

163. **Ki-moon B.** Governments have duty to fight prejudice, not fuel it. United Nations. December 11, 2012. Available at: www.un.org/News/Press/docs/2012/sgsm14717.doc.htm.

164. **Toibaro JJ, Ebensrtejin JF, Parlante A, et al.** Sexually transmitted infections among transgender individuals and other sexual identities. Medicina. 2009;69:327-30.

165. **Dos Ramos Farias MS, Garcia MN, Reynaga E, et al.** First report on sexually transmitted infections among trans (male to female transvestites, transsexuals, or transgender) and male sex workers in Argentina: high HIV, HPV, HBV, and syphilis prevalence. Int J Infect Dis 2011;15:e635-40.

166. **Pando MA, Gomez-Carrillo M, Vignoles M, et al.** Incidence of HIV type 1 infection, —anti-retroviral drug resistance, and molecular characterization in newly diagnosed individuals in Argentina: a global fund project. AIDS Res Human Retrovir. 2011;27:17-23.

167. **Sotelo J, Claudia B.** P2-287 seroprevalence and incidence study of HIV in transgender in Argentina—2009. J Epidemiol Commun Health. 2011;65(Suppl 1):A301.

168. **Grandi JL, Goihman S, Ueda M, Rutherford GW.** HIV infection, syphilis, and behavioral risks in Brazilian male sex workers. AIDS Behav. 2000;4:129-35.

169. **Lobato MI, Koff WJ, Schestatsky SS, et al.** Clinical characteristics, psychiatric comorbidities and sociodemographic profile of transsexual patients from an outpatient clinic in Brazil. Int J Transgender. 2008;10:69-77.

170. **Carballo-Dieuez A, Balan I, Dolezal C, Mello MB.** Recalled sexual experiences in childhood with older partners: a study of Brazilian men who have sex with men and male-to-female transgender persons. Arch Sex Behav. 2012;41:363-76.

171. **Barrington C, Wejnert C, Guardado ME, Nieto AI, Bailey GP.** Social network characteristics and HIV vulnerability among transgender persons in San Salvador: identifying opportunities for HIV prevention strategies. AIDS Behav. 2012;16:214-24.

172. **Silva-Santisteban A, Raymond HF, Salazar X, et al.** Understanding the HIV/AIDS epidemic in transgender women of Lima, Peru: results from a sero-epidemiologic study using respondent driven sampling. AIDS Behav. 2012;16:872-81.

173. **Russi JC, Serra M, Vinoles J, et al.** Sexual transmission of hepatitis B virus, hepatitis C virus, and human immunodeficiency virus type 1 infections among male transvestite comercial sex workers in Montevideo, Uruguay. Am J Trop Med Hyg. 2003;68:716-20.

174. **Vinoles J, Serra M, Russi JC, et al.** Seroincidence and phylogeny of human immunodeficiency virus infections in a cohort of commercial sex workers in Montevideo, Uruguay. Am J Trop Med Hyg. 2005;72:495-500.

175. **Pell C, Prone I, Vlahakis E.** A clinical audit of male to female (MTF) transgender patients attending taylor square private clinic in Sydney, Australia, aiming to improve quality of care. J Sex Med. 2011;8:179.

176. **Shinde S, Setia M, Row-Kavi A, Anand V, Jerajani H.** Male sex workers: are we ignoring a risk group in Mumbai, India? Indian J Dermatol Venereol Leprol. 2009;75:41-6.

177. **Sahastrabuddhe S, Gupta A, Stuart E, et al.** Sexually transmitted infections and risk behaviors among transgender persons (Hijras) of Pune, India. J Acquir Immune Defic Syndr. 2011; 59:72-8.

178. **Pisani E, Girault P, Gultom M, et al.** HIV, syphilis infection, and sexual practices among transgenders, male sex workers, and other men who have sex with men in Jakarta, Indonesia. Sex Transm Infect. 2004;80:536-40.

179. **Guy R, Mustikawati DE, Wijaksono DB, et al.** Voluntary counselling and testing sites as a source of sentinel information on HIV prevalence in a concentrated epidemic: a pilot project from Indonesia. Int J STD AIDS. 2011;22:505-11.

180. **Prabawanti C, Bollen L, Palupy R, et al.** HIV, sexually transmitted infections, and sexual risk behavior among transgenders in Indonesia. AIDS Behav. 2011;15:663-73.

181. **Altaf A.** Explosive expansion of HIV and associated risk factors among male and hijra sex workers in Sindh, Pakistan. J Acquir Immune Defic Syndr. 2009;51:158.

182. **Bokhari A, Nizamani NM, Jackson DJ, et al.** HIV risk in Karachi and Lahore, Pakistan: an emerging epidemic in injecting and commercial sex networks. Int J STD AIDS. 2007;18: 486-92.

183. **Shaw SY, Emmanuel F, Adrien A, et al.** The descriptive epidemiology of male sex workers in Pakistan: a biological and behavioural examination. Sex Transm Infect. 2011;87:73-80.

184. HIV prevalence among populations of men who have sex with men—Thailand, 2003 and 2005. MMWR Morb Mortal Wkly Rep. 2006;55:844-8.

185. **Chariyalertsak S, Kosachunhanan N, Saokhieo P, et al.** HIV incidence, risk factors, and motivation for biomedical intervention among gay, bisexual men, and transgender persons in Northern Thailand. PLoS One. 2011;6:e24295.

186. **Nguyen TA, Nguyen HT, Le GT, Detels R.** Prevalence and risk factors associated with HIV infection among men having sex with men in Ho Chi Minh City, Vietnam. AIDS Behav. 2008;12:476-82.

187. **Spizzichino L, Zaccarelli M, Rezza G, et al.** HIV infection among foreign transsexual sex workers in Rome—prevalence, behavior patterns, and seroconversion rates. Sex Transm Dis. 2001;28:405-11.

188. **Zaccarelli M, Spizzichino L, Venezia S, Antinori A, Gattari P.** Changes in regular condom use among immigrant transsexuals attending a counselling and testing reference site in central Rome: a 12 year study. Sex Transm Infect. 2004;80:541-5.

189. **van Veen MG, Gotz HM, van Leeuwen PA, Prins M, van de Laar MJW.** HIV and sexual risk behavior among commercial sex workers in the Netherlands. Arch Sex Behav. 2010;39:714-23.

190. **Belza MJ, Grp EVS.** Risk of HIV infection among male sex workers in Spain. Sex Transm Infect. 2005;81:85-8.

191. **Gutierrez M, Tajada P, Alvarez A, et al.** Prevalence of HIV-1 non-B subtypes, syphilis, HTLV, and hepatitis B and C viruses among immigrant sex workers in Madrid, Spain. J Med Virol. 2004;74:521-7.

192. **Kellogg TA, Clements-Nolle K, Dilley J, Katz MH, McFarland W.** Incidence of human immunodeficiency virus among male-to-female transgendered persons in San Francisco. J Acquir Immune Defic Syndr. 2001;28:380-4.

193. **Murrill CS, Liu KL, Guilin V, et al.** HIV prevalence and associated risk behaviors in New York City's house ball community. Am J Public Health. 2008;98:1074-80.

194. **Nuttbrock L, Hwahng S, Bockting W, et al.** Lifetime risk factors for HIV/sexually transmitted infections among male-to-female transgender persons. J Acquir Immune Defic Syndr. 2009; 52:417-21.

195. **Reback CJ, Lombardi EL, Simon PA, Frye DM.** HIV seroprevalence and risk behaviors among transgendered women who exchange sex in comparison with those who do not. J Psychol Human Sexual. 2005;17:5-22.

196. **Schulden JD, Song BW, Barros A, et al.** Rapid HIV testing in transgender communities by community-based organizations in three cities. Public Health Rep. 2008;123:101-14.

197. **Shrestha RK, Sansom SL, Schulden JD, et al.** Costs and effectiveness of finding new HIV diagnoses by using rapid testing in transgender communities. AIDS Educ Prev. 2011:49-57.

198. **Simon PA, Reback CJ, Bemis CC.** HIV prevalence and incidence among male-to-female transsexuals receiving HIV prevention services in Los Angeles County. AIDS. 2000;14:2953-5.

199. **Stephens SC, Bernstein KT, Philip SS.** Male to female and female to male transgender persons have different sexual risk behaviors yet similar rates of STDs and HIV. AIDS Behav. 2011;15:683-6.

Appendix A

Suggestions for Creating an Inclusive and Welcoming Environment for LGBT Patients and Staff

Nondiscrimination Policies

- Include sexual orientation and gender identity/expression in nondiscrimination policies; publicly display and/or distribute these policies
- Have a clear and specific mechanism for reporting and addressing discrimination if it occurs

Care and Services

- Offer specific services and programs to meet the needs of LGBT patients (e.g., support groups; HIV and sexually transmitted infection screening, prevention, and treatment; transgender health care programs)
- Create and maintain a list of LGBT-welcoming referrals for services you do not provide
- Ensure that registration and medical history forms are inclusive of LGBT relationships, identities, and families
- Collect patient demographic data on sexual orientation and gender identity and enter it in the electronic health record
- Ask patients to indicate on registration forms what names and pronouns they prefer to use

Physical Space

- Have brochures, posters, and/or periodicals on LGBT topics available in waiting rooms
- Offer single-stall gender-neutral (unisex) bathrooms, or develop policies that allow transgender people to use bathrooms that match their gender identity

Community Engagement

- Include LGBT imagery (e.g., rainbow flag; pictures of same-sex couples) in marketing and educational materials, websites, brochures, etc.
- Recognize LGBT days of observance (e.g., Pride, World AIDS Day) and cohost events with community groups
- Include LGBT needs in patient surveys and community assessments
- Market your organization in LGBT periodicals and local service directories

Sustainability

- Ensure that senior management and the governing board are actively engaged in change efforts
- Train all staff, including clinical staff, front-line staff, and administrative staff, in LGBT-affirmative care and cultural competency
- Incorporate LGBT issues into other mandated trainings
- Identify an LGBT "champion" (a staff member knowledgeable about serving LGBT patients who can help patients feel represented and comfortable and can keep the organization moving forward on improving LGBT health)

LGBT Employee Benefits and Recruitment

- Extend benefits to unmarried same-sex partners of employees
- Offer transgender health care coverage
- Have an affirmative action policy that includes equal hire for LGBT people
- Include LGBT issues in employee satisfaction surveys
- Advertise open positions in LGBT periodicals and at LGBT events

See also *Advancing Effective Communication, Cultural Competence, and Patient- and Family-Centered Care for the Lesbian, Gay, Bisexual, and Transgender (LGBT) Community* (www.jointcommission.org/lgbt).

Sample Sexual Orientation and Gender Identity Questions for Patient Registration and Intake Forms

---

Sexual Orientation Question*[†]

Do you think of yourself as:
- ☐ Lesbian, gay, or homosexual
- ☐ Straight or heterosexual
- ☐ Bisexual
- ☐ Something else
- ☐ Don't know

Two-Step Gender Identity and Birth Sex Question*[‡]

What is your current gender identity? (Check and/or circle all that apply)
- ☐ Male
- ☐ Female
- ☐ Transgender male/Trans man/FTM
- ☐ Transgender female/Trans woman/MTF
- ☐ Genderqueer
- ☐ Additional category (please specify): _____
- ☐ Decline to answer

What sex were you assigned at birth? (Check one)
- ☐ Male
- ☐ Female
- ☐ Decline to answer

Additional Transgender-Sensitive Questions

Do you have a name or nickname that you prefer to be called that is different from what is listed in your patient registration information?

_____

What gender pronoun(s) do you prefer? (e.g., she, he, they, zie)

_____

---

*A 2013 survey tested similar sexual orientation and gender identity questions with patients at 4 health centers. Study respondents found the questions to be acceptable and important to ask. (Cahill S, Singal R, Grasso C, et al. Do ask, do tell: high levels of acceptability by patients of routine collection of sexual orientation and gender identity data in four diverse American community health centers. PLoS ONE. 2014;9:e107104).

†The sexual orientation question was adapted from the National Health Interview Survey and is used on Fenway Health's registration form.

‡The two-step gender identity and birth sex question is recommended by leading transgender medical and research experts, including the University of California San Francisco's Center of Excellence for Transgender Health and the World Professional Association for Transgender Health. The use of 2 questions instead of 1 both validates a person's present gender identity and aids in understanding their history. It is important to understand that some transgender people do not currently identify their gender identity as transgender for a variety of reasons: Some believe it is part of their past and not a present identification; others may not identify with the word *transgender* because of cultural beliefs, social networks, and linguistic norms in geographic locations.

Appendix C

Selected Resources on LGBT Health

National Organizations

These organizations offer information, tools, and/or training on lesbian, gay, bisexual, and transgender (LGBT) people and their health care needs. For more resources, visit: www.lgbthealtheducation.org/publications/lgbt-health-resources

General LGBT
- National LGBT Health Education Center: www.lgbthealtheducation.org
- The Fenway Institute: www.thefenwayinstitute.org
- Human Rights Campaign: www.hrc.org
- National Gay and Lesbian Task Force: www.thetaskforce.org
- GLMA: Health Professionals Advancing LGBT Equality: www.glma.org
- CDC: Lesbian, Gay, Bisexual, and Transgender Health: www.cdc.gov/lgbthealth
- The Williams Institute: williamsinstitute.law.ucla.edu
- SAMHSA: LGBT Resources: www.samhsa.gov/behavioral-health-equity/lgbt

Transgender
- Center of Excellence for Transgender Health: www.transhealth.ucsf.edu
- National Center for Transgender Equality: www.transequality.org
- World Professional Association for Transgender Health: www.wpath.org

Youth and Their Families
- Gay, Lesbian, & Straight Education Network (GLSEN): www.glsen.org
- The Trevor Project: www.thetrevorproject.org
- Parents, Families, and Friends of LGBT People (PFLAG): www.pflag.org
- Family Acceptance Project: familyproject.sfsu.edu
- American Institutes for Research – LGBT Youth: www.air.org/page/lgbtq-youth

LGBT Parents
- Family Equality Council: www.familyequality.org
- Children of Lesbians and Gays Everywhere: www.colage.org
- American Fertility Association: www.theafa.org/family-building/lgbt-family-building

Aging
- Services & Advocacy for Gay, Lesbian, Bisexual & Transgender Elders (SAGE): www.sageusa.org
- National Resource Center on LGBT Aging: www.lgbtagingcenter.org
- LGBT Aging Project: www.lgbtagingproject.org

Bisexuality
- Bisexual Resource Center: www.biresource.net

LBT Women
- Mautner Project of Whitman-Walker Health: http://whitman-walker.thankyou4caring.org/mautnerproject

HIV and Sexually Transmitted Infections
- National Network of STD Clinical Prevention Training Centers (NNPTC): www.nnptc.org
- CDC: HIV/AIDS Prevention: www.cdc.gov/hiv
- CDC: Sexually Transmitted Diseases: www.cdc.gov/std
- AIDS Education and Training Centers: www.aids-ed.org
- National Minority AIDS Council: www.nmac.org
- The Global Forum on MSM & HIV – Provider Curriculum: www.msmgf.org/index.cfm/id/369/training-for-healthcare-providers/
- Joint United Nations Programme on HIV and AIDS: www.UNAIDS.org

Violence Prevention
- GLBTQ Domestic Violence Project: www.glbtqdvp.org
- The Network La Red: www.tnlr.org

LGBT Community Centers
- CenterLink LGBT Community Center Directory: www.lgbtcenters.org

Medical Professional Associations and Committees

- GLMA: Health Professionals Advancing LGBT Equality www.glma.org
- World Professional Association for Transgender Health www.wpath.org
- American Medical Student Association – Gender and Sexuality Committee www.amsa.org/AMSA/Homepage/About/Committees/Genderand Sexuality.aspx
- American Medical Association – LGBT Advisory Committee www.ama-assn.org/ama/pub/about-ama/our-people/member-groups-sections/glbt-advisory-committee.page
- Association of Gay and Lesbian Psychiatrists (AGLP) www.aglp.org

- Lesbian and Gay Child and Adolescent Psychiatric Association (LAGCAPA)
  www.lagcapa.org
- American Psychological Association (APA) – LGBT Concerns
  www.apa.org/pi/lgbt/
- LGBT Caucus of Public Health Professionals
  www.aphalgbt.org
- LGBT PA Caucus
  www.lbgpa.org
- National Association of Social Workers – National Committee on Lesbian, Gay, Bisexual, and Transgender Issues (NCLGBTI)
  www.socialworkers.org/governance/cmtes/nclgbi.asp
- The Association of Lesbian, Gay, Bisexual, Transgender Addiction Professionals and their Allies (NALGAP)
  www.nalgap.org

Selected Publications

- Institute of Medicine (IOM). The Health of Lesbian, Gay, Bisexual, and Transgender People: Building a Foundation for Better Understanding
  www.iom.edu/Reports/2011/The-Health-of-Lesbian-Gay-Bisexual-and-Transgender-People.aspx
- The Joint Commission. Advancing Effective Communication, Cultural Competence, and Patient- and Family-Centered Care for the Lesbian, Gay, Bisexual, and Transgender (LGBT) Community: A Field Guide
  www.jointcommission.org/lgbt
- American Academy of Child and Adolescent Psychiatry (AACAP). Practice Parameter on Gay, Lesbian, or Bisexual Sexual Orientation, Gender Nonconformity, and Gender Discordance in Children and Adolescents
  download.journals.elsevierhealth.com/pdfs/journals/0890-8567/PIIS089085671200500X.pdf
- World Professional Association for Transgender Health. Standards of Care for the Health of Transsexual, Transgender, and Gender Nonconforming People
  www.wpath.org/site_page.cfm?pk_association_webpage_menu=1351
- Association of American Medical Colleges. Implementing Curricular and Institutional Climate Changes to Improve Health Care for Individuals Who Are LGBT, Gender Nonconforming, or Born with DSD: A Resource for Medical Educators
  http://offers.aamc.org/lgbt-dsd-health
- LGBT Health (peer-reviewed journal)
  www.liebertpub.com/overview/lgbt-health/618/

Hotlines

- GLBT National Help Center
  www.glbtnationalhelpcenter.org (online peer support)
  888-843-4564 (all ages)
  800-246-7743 (youth up to 25)

- Lesbian, Gay, Bisexual and Transgender Helpline
  888-340-4528 (all ages)

- Peer Listening Line
  800-399-PEER (youth)

- Trevor Lifeline for LGBTQ Youth
  www.thetrevorproject.org (text and chat support)
  866-488-7386 (youth)

- GLBTQ Domestic Violence Project Hotline
  800-832-1901

Patient Registration and Medical History Forms

1. REGISTRATION FORM

Please provide information in this section so that providers and staff may address you correctly and bill for services correctly.

Name on Insurance or Legal Government Records: _____
Preferred Name/Nickname (if different): _____
Date of Birth: _____
Current Address: _____
Mailing Address (if different from above):_____
Phone Number: _____ (home) _____ (mobile) _____ (other)
Email: _____
Preferred method of contact: ☐ Phone (home/mobile/other)   ☐ Email   ☐ US Mail
Emergency Contact: Name_____ Phone: _____ Relationship: _____

What is your current gender identity? (Check and/or circle all that apply)
☐ Male   ☐ Female   ☐ Transgender Male/Trans Man/FTM
☐ Transgender Female/Trans Woman/MTF
☐ Genderqueer   ☐ Additional Category, please specify: _____
☐ Decline to Answer

What sex were you assigned at birth on your original birth certificate? (Check one)
☐ Male   ☐ Female   ☐ Decline to Answer

What sex is listed on your health insurance or government records?   ☐ Male   ☐ Female

What gender pronoun(s) do you prefer? (he, she, they, zie, etc.): _____

What best describes your race?
           ☐ African American or Black   ☐ Asian   ☐ Caucasian or White
           ☐ Multiracial ☐ Native American or Alaskan Native or Inuit ☐ Pacific Islander
           ☐ Other: _____

What best describes your ethnicity?
           ☐ Hispanic/Latino/Latina
           ☐ Not Hispanic/Latino/Latina

What is your country of birth? _____

What is your primary language?
   ☐ English   ☐ Spanish   ☐ French   ☐ Portuguese
   ☐ Russian   ☐ Other: _____

Do you think of yourself as:
   ☐ Lesbian, gay, or homosexual   ☐ Straight or heterosexual
   ☐ Bisexual   ☐ Something else   ☐ Don't know

What is the highest level of education you have completed?
   ☐ Some high school   ☐ High school or equivalent
   ☐ Some college or technical/professional school
   ☐ Bachelor's degree   ☐ At least some graduate school

What is your current employment status?
   ☐ Working full-time   ☐ Working part-time   ☐ Student full-time
   ☐ Student part-time   ☐ Retired   ☐ Disabled/unable to work
   ☐ Searching for work

Are you a U.S. veteran? ☐ Yes   ☐ No

Which of the following categories best describes your current annual income?
   ☐ Less than $10,000   ☐ $10,000-15,000   ☐ $15,001-20,000
   ☐ $20,001-30,000   ☐ $30,001-50,000   ☐ $50,001-80,000
   ☐ More than $80,000

Please tell us about any special needs for your health care appointment.

Do you require a foreign language translator with you during your health care appointment?
   ☐ Yes   ☐ No
   If Yes, what language? _____

Would you like to request/have a chaperone or companion be with you during your
health care appointment?
   ☐ Yes   ☐ No
   If Yes, would you prefer: ☐ Male   ☐ Female or Name: _____

Do you require any other special services or assistance during your health care appointment?
   ☐ Yes   ☐ No
   If Yes, describe your need: _____

2. MEDICAL HISTORY FORM

Please take a few moments to complete the questions below. This form will become part of your medical record. Your answers on this form will help your health care provider better understand your medical concerns and conditions. If you are uncomfortable with any question, do not answer it. If you cannot remember specific details, please approximate. Add any notes you think are important. All the information that you provide on this form will be considered protected health information and will be treated in accordance with our policies on patient confidentiality.

BIOGRAPHICAL INFORMATION

Name on Insurance or Legal Government Records: _____

Preferred Name/Nickname (if different): _____

Date of Birth: _____

What is your current gender identity? (Check and/or circle all that apply)
- ☐ Male   ☐ Female   ☐ Transgender Male/Trans Man/FTM
- ☐ Transgender Female/Trans Woman/MTF
- ☐ Genderqueer   ☐ Additional Category, please specify: _____
- ☐ Decline to Answer

What sex were you assigned at birth on your original birth certificate? (Check one)
- ☐ Male   ☐ Female   ☐ Decline to Answer

What gender pronoun(s) do you prefer? (he, she, they, zie, etc.): _____

What best describes your race?
- ☐ African American or Black   ☐ Asian   ☐ Caucasian or White
- ☐ Multiracial   ☐ Native American or Alaskan Native or Inuit
- ☐ Pacific Islander   ☐ Other: _____

What best describes your ethnicity?
- ☐ Hispanic/Latino/Latina
- ☐ Not Hispanic/Latino/Latina

What is your country of birth? _____

What is your primary language?
- ☐ English   ☐ Spanish   ☐ French   ☐ Portuguese
- ☐ Russian   ☐ Other: _____

Do you think of yourself as...
    ☐ Lesbian, gay, or homosexual ☐ Straight or heterosexual
    ☐ Bisexual   ☐ Something else: _____   ☐ Don't know

Do you have a health condition or disability that limits your activity or requires that you have some additional assistance with daily activities?
    ☐ Yes   ☐ No
    If Yes, describe: _____

CURRENT HEALTH

What brings you in today? _____
Have you seen another provider in the past for this concern? .... ☐ Yes ☐ No
    If Yes: Where?_____ When? _____ Outcome: _____
Do you have any specific goals for your health? .... ☐ Yes ☐ No
    Please describe: _____
Has there been any change in your general health in the past year? .... ☐ Yes ☐ No
    If Yes, describe:_____
Are you now under a provider's care for a particular problem? .... ☐ Yes ☐ No
    If Yes, describe: _____
Have you **ever** had any serious illnesses or surgery?.. ☐ Yes ☐ No
    If Yes, describe _____
    _____

Please list your current medications: prescription, over-the-counter, vitamins, supplements and herbal products you take regularly

Medication/Supplement Name	Dose	How Often	Reason for Medication/Supplement

Do you have any allergies?... ☐ Yes ☐ No

    List with reaction: _____

PERSONAL AND FAMILY MEDICAL HISTORY

Health History – Please check if appropriate and indicate your age when diagnosed.

Condition	Age of Diagnosis	Is This Ongoing?	
___Arthritis	_____	☐ Yes	☐ No
___Asthma	_____	☐ Yes	☐ No
___Cancer (type):	_____	☐ Yes	☐ No
___Diabetes	_____	☐ Yes	☐ No
___Emphysema/COPD	_____	☐ Yes	☐ No
___Gastrointestinal problems	_____	☐ Yes	☐ No
___Heart problems (type):	_____	☐ Yes	☐ No
___Kidney problems	_____	☐ Yes	☐ No
___Liver problems or hepatitis	_____	☐ Yes	☐ No
___Mental health problems	_____	☐ Yes	☐ No
___Migraines	_____	☐ Yes	☐ No
___Osteoporosis	_____	☐ Yes	☐ No
___Thyroid problems	_____	☐ Yes	☐ No
___Other (list):	_____	☐ Yes	☐ No

HOSPITALIZATIONS   ☐ None

Operation or Illness	Year	Hospital/Outcome

FAMILY HISTORY OF ILLNESS (please list relative and age of diagnosis or death if known. Please consider parents, siblings, children, grandparents, aunts and uncles)

Asthma: _____

Cancer: _____

Diabetes: _____

Heart disease: _____

High blood pressure: _____

Genetic disorder: _____

Blood disease: _____

Mental health: _____

Other: _____

Family deaths at an early age (under 60): _____

PREVENTION (please answer the questions to the best of your ability):

When was your last physical exam: _____

Date of last flu shot: _____   Date of shingles shot: (over 60) _____

Date of last pneumonia shot: _____   Dates of HPV shots: (9-26+) _____

Date of last tetanus shot: _____   Dates of Hepatitis B shots: _____

Have you ever had chickenpox or the chickenpox vaccine? ☐ Yes ☐ No ☐ Unsure

Date of last cholesterol check: _____ Results: ☐ Normal ☐ Borderline ☐ High ☐ Unknown

Date of last colon cancer screening (age 50+): _____ Type of screening: _____

Date of last mammogram (age 40+): _____ Results: ☐ Normal ☐ Other: _____

Date of last Pap test: _____   Results: ☐ Normal ☐ Other: _____

Date of last vision exam: _____   Date of last dental exam: _____

Do you have a living will? .... ☐ Yes ☐ No ☐ Unsure

Do you have a power of attorney or health care proxy? .... ☐ Yes ☐ No ☐ Unsure

    If Yes, list name and describe relationship to you _____

Would you like information on living wills or power of attorney/health care proxy?

    ☐ Yes ☐ No

LIFESTYLE AND WELLNESS

Are you happy/satisfied with your current weight? .... ☐ Yes ☐ No ☐ Unsure

    If No, please describe: _____

Do you currently follow a special diet? ...:............................ ☐ Yes ☐ No

    If Yes, what type? _____ (ex: vegetarian, vegan, low calorie, diabetic, Weight Watchers)

Do you worry that you have lost control over how much you eat?

    ☐ Yes ☐ No ☐ Unsure

    If Yes or Unsure, explain:_____

Does your weight affect the way you feel about yourself?   ☐ Yes ☐ No ☐ Unsure

Do you ever feel guilt, shame or anxiety about your weight or food you eat?

    ☐ Yes ☐ No ☐ Unsure

How many meals do you eat out during an average week? ☐ None ☐ 1-3 ☐ 4-6 ☐ 7-10 ☐ >10

With whom do you take most of your meals?

    ☐ Alone   ☐ Family/partner   ☐ Friends   ☐ Community setting

How much time do you spend exercising or doing physical activity which markedly increases your breathing such as vigorous walking, cycling, running, swimming:

Daily _____	Weekly _____
☐ More than 7 hours	☐ More than 7 hours
☐ 3-7 hours	☐ 3-7 hours
☐ 1-3 hours	☐ 1-3 hours
☐ About 1 hour	☐ About 1 hour
☐ Less than 1 hour	☐ Less than 1 hour
☐ Not at all	☐ Not at all

What kinds of exercise or physical activity do you participate in?

      Type: _____

Do you think you exercise: ☐ Too much   ☐ Just the right amount   ☐ Not enough
                          ☐ I don't think about it

With whom do you exercise?   ☐ Alone   ☐ Friend/family   ☐ Coworker
                        ☐ Gym acquaintance ☐ Group sports ☐ Trainer

If you do not exercise, can you describe why you don't? _____

Would you like to increase physical activity in your life?
                        ☐ Yes   ☐ No   ☐ Unsure   ☐ No need

Hour many hours of uninterrupted sleep do you get each night?   _____ hours

How many hours of uninterrupted sleep would you like each night? _____ hours

What part of the day do you get most of your sleep? ☐ Daytime ☐ Nighttime

Do you normally wake up feeling rested? ☐ Most of the time ☐ Sometimes ☐ Never

Are you concerned about your sleep? ☐ Yes ☐ No ☐ Unsure

    Do you have problems: ☐ Falling asleep ☐ Staying asleep
                    ☐ Waking up too early   ☐ Other   ☐ No problem

    Does your sleep interfere with your daily functioning? ☐ Often ☐ Sometimes ☐ Never

Is there anything in your life that <u>keeps you</u> from getting enough sleep, engaging in physical activity, or making changes to your diet?   ☐ Yes   ☐ No

    If Yes, please describe: _____

Is there anything that <u>helps you</u> get enough sleep, stay physically active, or eat healthfully?   ☐ Yes   ☐ No

    If Yes, please describe: _____

Do you work or go to school? .... ☐ Yes   ☐ No

If Yes:

    Do you enjoy your work/school on most days? .... ☐ Yes   ☐ No

    Do you feel you have a healthy work/school and life balance? .... ☐ Yes   ☐ No

Do you make time for relaxation in your day? .... ☐ Yes   ☐ No

    If Yes, what do you do to relax? _____

    If No, what would you like to do to relax? _____

BODY IMAGE

Are you happy with the way you look/appear?

    ☐ Often   ☐ Sometimes   ☐ Never/infrequently

If you could, what would you change about your body or appearance? (please list): _____

_____

Are you others' opinions about your appearance important to you?

    ☐ Often   ☐ Sometimes   ☐ Never/infrequently

Do you feel that what/who you see in the mirror is how others see you? ...... ☐ Yes   ☐ No

    If No, can you describe? _____

_____

Do concerns about your body get in the way of your participating in physical activity, employment, dating, being intimate, or other things?

☐ Often   ☐ Sometimes   ☐ Never/infrequently

Have you ever done anything to change your body appearance or shape?   ☐ Yes   ☐ No
If Yes:
What things have you already done to change your body's appearance or shape?
☐ Diet ☐ Exercise   ☐ Plastic surgery   ☐ Hormones   ☐ Medications/supplements
☐ Silicone   ☐ Supplements   ☐ Steroids   ☐ Other: _____

Would you or have you considered changing your body appearance or shape?   ☐ Yes   ☐ No
If Yes:
What things have you or might you consider doing to change your body's appearance or shape?
☐ Diet ☐ Exercise   ☐ Plastic surgery   ☐ Hormones   ☐ Medications/supplements
☐ Silicone   ☐ Supplements   ☐ Steroids   ☐ Other: _____

FAMILY AND RELATIONSHIPS

What is your relationship/marital status?
☐ Single   ☐ Married/Monogamous   ☐ Married/Open
☐ Partnered/Monogamous   ☐ Partnered/Open   ☐ Divorced   ☐ Separated

Who are the major support persons in your life (please list)? _____

_____

Are you satisfied with the quality and quantity of support you get from these persons?
☐ Yes   ☐ No   ☐ Unsure

Do you plan and enjoy time with these and other family and friends?
☐ Always   ☐ Sometimes
☐ Rarely   ☐ Never

With whom do you live? (Check all that apply)
☐ Alone   ☐ Partner/spouse   ☐ Parent/sibling
☐ Roommate(s)   ☐ Children   ☐ Other:_____
Do you have any pets?   ☐ Yes   ☐ No
If Yes, what kind?_____
Are you happy/comfortable in your current living situation? .... ☐ Yes   ☐ No   ☐ Unsure
If No, please explain: _____
Do you have any children? .... ☐ Yes   ☐ No
(if Yes, check below)
☐ I have children under the age of 18 who live with me
☐ I have children under the age of 18 who do not live with me
☐ I have adult children over 18
Do you want to add children to your family in the
next 5 years? .... ☐ Yes   ☐ No   ☐ Unsure

Are you a primary care taker to any children or adults in your life? ☐ Yes ☐ No

  If Yes, describe: _____

Are you in a committed/serious relationship with an intimate partner? ☐ Yes ☐ No

  If No: Are you satisfied with this?

    ☐ Very satisfied   ☐ Somewhat satisfied   ☐ Dissatisfied

  If Yes: Is your partner... ☐ Male   ☐ Female   ☐ Transgender

    What is the length of time of this relationship?: _____

    Are you satisfied with your relationship?

    ☐ Very satisfied   ☐ Somewhat satisfied   ☐ Dissatisfied

Are you coping with the loss of a partner, family member or the ending of a relationship? ☐ Yes ☐ No

  Please describe: _____

MENTAL HEALTH

Do you have a history of depression, anxiety, or other mental health problems?... ☐ Yes ☐ No

Have you ever taken medication for anxiety, depression, or other mental health problems?.. ☐ Yes ☐ No

Are you interested in speaking to a mental health provider?...................... ☐ Yes ☐ No

Over the past 2 weeks, have you experienced little interest or pleasure in doing things during several or more days?................................. ☐ Yes ☐ No

Over the past 2 weeks, have you experienced feeling down, depressed, or hopeless during several or more days?.............................. ☐ Yes ☐ No

Over the past 2 weeks, have you felt nervous, anxious, or on edge on several or more days?.. ☐ Yes ☐ No

Over the past 2 weeks, have you not been able to stop or control worrying or worried too much about different things on several or more days? ..... ☐ Yes ☐ No

Over the past 2 weeks, have you had trouble relaxing or been so restless it's hard to sit still on several or more days? .... ☐ Yes ☐ No

In your life, have you ever had any experience that was so frightening, horrible, or upsetting that you had nightmares, thought about it when you did not want to, were constantly on guard, or felt numb/detached? .... ☐ Yes ☐ No

When you are feeling stressed, anxious, overwhelmed or depressed, what do you do to take care of yourself?

  Describe:_____

  How well do these strategies work for you? _____

SUBTANCE USE

How many cigarettes do you smoke per day? _____
   If none, have you ever smoked?   ☐ No   ☐ Yes — When did you quit? _____
Do you use any other forms of tobacco?   ☐ Yes ☐ No
   If Yes: please describe:_____
Do you ever hide your smoking or tobacco use?   ☐ Yes ☐ No ☐ N/A
Do you want to cut down or quit smoking or tobacco use?   ☐ Yes ☐ No ☐ N/A
Do others want you to cut down or quit smoking or using tobacco? ☐ Yes ☐ No ☐ N/A
Are there any activities or times that trigger your smoking
   or using tobacco?   ☐ Yes ☐ No ☐ N/A
   If Yes, describe:_____

How many alcoholic drinks do you have in an average week? _____
How many alcoholic drinks do you have on an average day? _____
Have you ever been concerned about your drinking?   ☐ Yes ☐ No
Do you use recreational drugs?   ☐ Yes ☐ No
   If Yes, what recreational drugs do you use?
      ☐ Marijuana ☐ Ecstasy (X) ☐ Crystal methamphetamine/amphetamines
      ☐ Cocaine ☐ GHB ☐ Poppers ☐ Opiates/Heroin Hallucinogens
      ☐ Other: _____
How often do you use? _____
What is your preferred method of delivery ?   ☐ Smoking ☐ Oral ☐ Injection
                                              ☐ Snorting/bumping ☐ Booty bumping
                                              ☐ Other: _____
Do you use alcohol or drugs when you have sex?............................ ☐ Yes ☐ No
Do you ever take prescription drugs to feel high?............................ ☐ Yes ☐ No

Has anyone, including a family member, friend, or health care
   worker been concerned about your drinking or drug use? .... ☐ Yes ☐ No
Have you or someone else been injured as a result of your
   drinking or drug use?.. ☐ Yes ☐ No
Has drinking or drug use caused problems between you and
   your family or friends? .... ☐ Yes ☐ No
Has drinking or drug use caused problems at work or at school?....... ☐ Yes ☐ No
Has drinking or drug use ever led to criminal/legal action? .... ☐ Yes ☐ No
Do you ever feel guilt or remorse because of your drinking or
   drug use?.. ☐ Yes ☐ No
Have you ever engaged in any substance use treatment?................. ☐ Yes ☐ No
   When and where? _____
Are you interested in cutting down or quitting your
   drinking or drug use? .... ☐ Yes ☐ No

SAFETY & SOCIAL STRESS

Do you feel safe at home?... ☐ Always   ☐ Sometimes   ☐ Never

Do you avoid people, places, or situations because you think you
something unpleasant might happen?.. ☐ Yes   ☐ No

Have you ever been hit, kicked, or otherwise physically hurt by someone? ...... ☐ Yes   ☐ No

   If yes, did this happen in the past 12 months?...................................... ☐ Yes   ☐ No

Has your partner or anyone else ever isolated you from friends and family?..... ☐ Yes   ☐ No

   If yes, did this happen in the past 12 months?...................................... ☐ Yes   ☐ No

Have you ever felt forced into having any type of sexual activity, even if it
wasn't penetration? .... ☐ Yes   ☐ No

   If yes, did this happen in the past 12 months?...................................... ☐ Yes   ☐ No

Has a partner ever forced you to have unsafe sex, to use drugs
during sex, or to do something you didn't want to do during sex? .... ☐ Yes   ☐ No

   If yes, did this happen in the past 12 months?...................................... ☐ Yes   ☐ No

Have you ever been treated with less courtesy/respect or discriminated
against because of your gender, physical appearance, sexual
orientation, race/ethnicity, or other attribute?.. ☐ Yes   ☐ No

   If yes, did this happen in the past year?   ☐ Often   ☐ Sometimes   ☐ Rarely or never

Do you expect that you will be treated with less courtesy/respect or
discriminated against because of your gender, physical
appearance, sexual orientation, race/ethnicity, or other attribute?

                       ☐ Often   ☐ Sometimes   ☐ Rarely or never

SEXUAL HISTORY

Have you been sexually active in the past year?   ☐ Yes   ☐ No

Are you currently sexually active with (check all that apply):

    ☐ Men   ☐ Women   ☐ Transgender persons

In the past have you been sexually active with (check all that apply):

    ☐ Men   ☐ Women   ☐ Transgender persons

Are you currently sexually active with:

    ☐ One person   ☐ More than one person   ☐ Not applicable

How many sexual partners have you had in the past 6 months? _____

How many sexual partners have you had in the past year? _____

Please note below the specific type of sex you are having and if you use a condom or other barrier:

    If you prefer not to answer this question, please mark here: ☐

Sexual Activity	Yes	No	Not Applicable	Barrier Use (condoms/dental dams/other)		
Oral Sex (Perform)				☐ Always	☐ Sometimes	☐ Never
Oral Sex (Receive)				☐ Always	☐ Sometimes	☐ Never
Vaginal Sex Penetrate				☐ Always	☐ Sometimes	☐ Never
Vaginal Sex Receive Penetration				☐ Always	☐ Sometimes	☐ Never
Anal Receptive Sex (bottom)				☐ Always	☐ Sometimes	☐ Never
Anal Insertive Sex (top)				☐ Always	☐ Sometimes	☐ Never
Use Dildos/Toys/etc.....				☐ Always	☐ Sometimes	☐ Never

What other sexual activities do you participate in?_____

_____

Do you have questions or concerns about any sexual activities?   ☐ Yes   ☐ No

    If Yes, describe: _____

Do you ever have a need for a contraceptive method to help you or your partner avoid pregnancy?

    ☐ Yes   ☐ No   ☐ Not applicable

    If so, what do you usually use? _____

Do you ever have sex with someone you don't know or just met?   ☐ Yes   ☐ No

    If Yes, where do you find these partners: ☐ Internet   ☐ Mobile app   ☐ Bar/club/out

                    ☐ Public sex venue

                    ☐ Other:_____

Do you or have you given/received sex for money or drugs in the past 3 months?   ☐ Yes   ☐ No

Do you use drugs or alcohol when having sex?   ☐ Yes   ☐ No

Have you ever been tested for a sexually transmitted infection?   ☐ Yes   ☐ No

Have you ever been diagnosed with a sexually transmitted infection?   ☐ Yes   ☐ No

What sexually transmitted infections were you diagnosed with:

Sexually Transmitted Infection	Location	Diagnosed in Past Year
Gonorrhea	☐ Oral ☐ Genital ☐ Anal	☐ Yes ☐ No
Chlamydia	☐ Oral ☐ Genital ☐ Anal	☐ Yes ☐ No
Nonspecific urethritis		☐ Yes ☐ No
Herpes	☐ Oral ☐ Genital ☐ Anal	☐ Yes ☐ No
Syphilis		☐ Yes ☐ No
Human papillomavirus/warts	☐ Oral ☐ Genital ☐ Anal	☐ Yes ☐ No
Trichomonas		☐ Yes ☐ No
Other:_____	☐ Oral ☐ Genital ☐ Anal	☐ Yes ☐ No

Have you ever been tested for HIV?   ☐ Yes   ☐ No

    If yes, when was your last test: _____

    What were the results: ☐ Negative   ☐ Positive   ☐ Indeterminate   ☐ Don't know

What do you do to protect yourself from HIV and sexually transmitted infections?

    Please describe: _____

Are you satisfied with your sex life?   ☐ Often   ☐ Sometimes   ☐ Rarely or never

Are there any things about your sex life you would like to change? _____
_____

Is there anything you would like to talk about regarding your sex life or sexual functioning with a health care provider?   ☐ Yes   ☐ No

    If Yes, describe: _____

Thank you for taking the time to complete this health and wellness questionnaire. Your responses will help your medical provider address your specific need, questions, and concerns. Your feedback about the questions asked is very important to us so that we may continually address your needs. Please let your provider know if you have any thoughts or concerns about the questions asked or not asked.

Index

Note: Page numbers followed by *t* indicate table, those followed by *f* indicate figure.